AF361024

Advances in Forensic Genetics

Advances in Forensic Genetics

Editor

Niels Morling

MDPI • Basel • Beijing • Wuhan • Barcelona • Belgrade • Manchester • Tokyo • Cluj • Tianjin

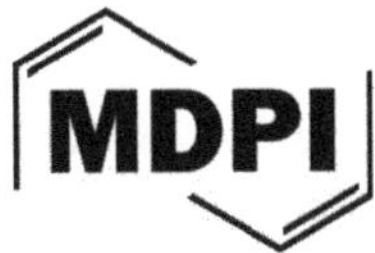

Editor
Niels Morling
University of Copenhagen
Denmark

Editorial Office
MDPI
St. Alban-Anlage 66
4052 Basel, Switzerland

This is a reprint of articles from the Special Issue published online in the open access journal *Genes* (ISSN 2073-4425) (available at: https://www.mdpi.com/journal/genes/special_issues/Advances_Forensic_Genetics).

For citation purposes, cite each article independently as indicated on the article page online and as indicated below:

LastName, A.A.; LastName, B.B.; LastName, C.C. Article Title. *Journal Name* **Year**, *Volume Number*, Page Range.

ISBN 978-3-0365-4697-1 (Hbk)
ISBN 978-3-0365-4698-8 (PDF)

Contents

About the Editor

Niels Morling

Niels Morling is a professor of forensic genetics at the Section of Forensic Genetics, Department of Forensic Medicine, University of Copenhagen, and an Adjunct Professor at the Department of Mathematical Sciences, Aalborg University, Denmark. He has been a part-time professor of forensic genetics at the University of Tromsø, Norway. He is an MD, a general practitioner, and a specialist in clinical immunology.

In 1989, Niels Morling was appointed chief of the Institute of Forensic Genetics, University of Copenhagen, Denmark. He introduced DNA investigations in forensic genetics in Denmark. Later, he was chief of the Department of Forensic Medicine, University of Copenhagen, Denmark, for many years.

Niels Morling has been a member of Danish law commissions concerning the use of forensic genetic DNA investigations, establishing the Danish crime DNA database, and the Danish Children's Act. He has served on international human rights panels.

Niels Morling has been chairman of several Danish and international scientific organizations, including the International Society for Forensic Genetics. Presently, he is Chairman of the European DNA Profiling Group.

Niels Morling is a doctor of medical sciences from the University of Copenhagen. He has published over 500 scientific articles, book chapters, etc., in forensic and medical genetics, forensic genetic statistics, and immunology. He has supervised more than 100 postdocs, PhD, and masterstudents and lectured in more than 30 countries. He is a member of the editorial board of several scientific journals.

Niels Morling's current research focuses on forensic genetics, forensic genetic statistics, the genetics and epigenetics of sudden cardiac death, melanoma, and other malignant skin diseases.

Preface to "Advances in Forensic Genetics"

Since the first publications of DNA typing with restriction fragment length polymorphisms detected with radioactive multilocus DNA probes in forensic genetics in the mid-1980s, forensic genetics has undergone impressive development leading to exciting possibilities in work in criminal cases, relationship testing, identification of human remains, animal and plant forensics, etc. The scientific progress in forensic genetics has been characterised by the constant development of new methods that have improved the efficiency of forensic genetic examinations to a degree that was unthinkable 40 years ago.

The new methods are being introduced with a speed that makes it complicated for newcomers and professionals in the field to get an overview of the many aspects within it. Thus, high-quality reviews of the status of forensic genetic methods, as well as new ones, are welcome.

This book includes 25 reviews and original research articles concerning forensic genetics published in the Special Issue "Advances in Forensic Genetics" of Genes (ISSN 2073-4425), a Special Issue belonging to the section "Molecular Genetics and Genomics". The book is dedicated to presenting the current status of some forensic genetic areas by invited review articles and original research articles. I sincerely thank the authors of the invited reviews and original research articles for their contributions.

Niels Morling
Editor

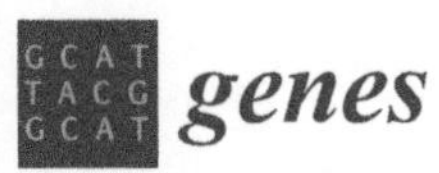

Review

Assessing the Forensic Value of DNA Evidence from Y Chromosomes and Mitogenomes

Mikkel M. Andersen [1,2,*] and **David J. Balding** [3,4]

[1] Department of Mathematical Sciences, Aalborg University, 9220 Aalborg, Denmark
[2] Section of Forensic Genetics, Department of Forensic Medicine, University of Copenhagen, 1165 Copenhagen, Denmark
[3] Melbourne Integrative Genomics, University of Melbourne, Melbourne 3010, Australia; dbalding@unimelb.edu.au
[4] Genetics Institute, University College London, London WC1E 6BT, UK
[*] Correspondence: mikl@math.aau.dk

Abstract: Y chromosome and mitochondrial DNA profiles have been used as evidence in courts for decades, yet the problem of evaluating the weight of evidence has not been adequately resolved. Both are lineage markers (inherited from just one parent), which presents different interpretation challenges compared with standard autosomal DNA profiles (inherited from both parents). We review approaches to the evaluation of lineage marker profiles for forensic identification, focussing on the key roles of profile mutation rate and relatedness (extending beyond known relatives). Higher mutation rates imply fewer individuals matching the profile of an alleged contributor, but they will be more closely related. This makes it challenging to evaluate the possibility that one of these matching individuals could be the true source, because relatives may be plausible alternative contributors, and may not be well mixed in the population. These issues reduce the usefulness of profile databases drawn from a broad population: larger populations can have a lower profile relative frequency because of lower relatedness with the alleged contributor. Many evaluation methods do not adequately take account of distant relatedness, but its effects have become more pronounced with the latest generation of high-mutation-rate Y profiles.

Keywords: evidence; Y-STR; mtDNA; mitochondria

Citation: Andersen, M.M.; Balding, D.J. Assessing the Forensic Value of DNA Evidence from Y Chromosomes and Mitogenomes. *Genes* **2021**, *12*, 1209. https://doi.org/10.3390/genes12081209

Academic Editor: David Caramelli

Received: 7 July 2021
Accepted: 2 August 2021
Published: 5 August 2021

Publisher's Note: MDPI stays neutral with regard to jurisdictional claims in published maps and institutional affiliations.

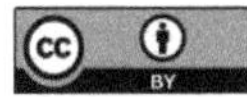

1. Weight of Evidence for Lineage Marker Profiles

Standard DNA profiles use autosomal DNA, inherited from both parents. We focus here on DNA profiles obtained from the Y chromosome and the mitochondrial genome (mitogenome/mtDNA), which are inherited only from the father and from the mother, respectively. Because of this uniparental inheritance over generations, these DNA profiles are called lineage markers. We outline the forensic value of lineage markers in general, give a brief, historical review and critique of evaluation methods and make recommendations for improved practice. A key message is that the high mutation rates of the latest generation of Y chromosome short tandem repeat (STR) profiles have effects that exaggerate the deficiencies of previous methods of analysis, but understanding these effects highlights ways forward. The mutation rate of even the whole mitogenome is lower, but insights from the high-mutation-rate setting are also informative for evaluating and communicating the weight of evidence.

We focus on the simplest scenario in which there is a good-quality, single-contributor DNA profile (either Y or mitogenome) obtained from an evidence sample, and a matching reference profile from a known individual Q who is alleged to be the source of the evidence sample (sometimes Q is called the person of interest, PoI). Hypotheses of interest are:

$$H_Q : \text{the evidence profile came from } Q,$$
$$H_X : \text{the evidence profile came from } X,$$

where X is an alternative to Q as the source of the DNA whose profile is not available. The likelihood ratio (LR) comparing the strength of the DNA profile evidence for H_Q relative to H_X is then

$$\text{LR}(X, Q) = \frac{\text{P(profile evidence} \mid H_Q)}{\text{P(profile evidence} \mid H_X)} = \frac{1}{\text{P}(X \text{ has profile } q)}, \tag{1}$$

where q is the profile of Q. We omit background information and other evidence from the notation; see [1] for a discussion. The denominator of (1) is a probability for the unknown profile of X, given the observed q and possibly a database of profiles.

1.1. The Effect of Relatedness and Mutation Rate on the LR

For lineage markers, the relatedness of two individuals is fully captured by a single number, G, of generations (or germline transfers, or meioses) that separate X and Q, following either female-only or male-only ancestors. Degree-1 ($G = 1$) relative pairs are parent/offspring, $G = 2$ for siblings and grandparent/grandchild, while $G = 3$ for avuncular relationships such as aunt/niece as well as great-grandparent/great-grandchild. As G increases, the relatedness becomes less likely to be known, but there is a female-lineage G and a male-lineage G for all pairs of individuals, "unrelated" only means that G is large and/or unknown.

Given $G = g$ for X and Q, we can approximate (1) by

$$\text{LR}(X, Q) = \frac{1}{(1-\mu)^g} \approx e^{g\mu} \tag{2}$$

where μ is the profile mutation rate, which is the probability that parent and child have non-matching profiles. For Y-STR loci with mutation rates $\mu_l, l = 1, \ldots, L$, and assuming independence of mutation events across loci, we have

$$\mu = 1 - \prod_{l=1}^{L}(1-\mu_l) < \sum_{l=1}^{L} \mu_l. \tag{3}$$

For the mitogenome, the lower mutation rate, larger number of sites, and possible germline selection events as part of the mitochondrial bottleneck [2] make it impractical to use (3) at individual sites, but it can be employed over genome regions [3,4].

The LR Formula (2) is not exact for at least two reasons. Firstly, it assumes that μ is constant over generations and independent of the current profile state. In fact, accurate estimates are hard to obtain but the STR mutation rate is likely to depend on the allele sequence (including its length and presence of a partial repeat) [5]. However, these effects are relatively unimportant for the total mutation rate over many loci. Secondly, it is based on assuming no mutations in the lineage path connecting X and Q, whereas a match can also arise following an even number of mutations between X with Q such that the effect of each mutation is reversed by another mutation. However, profiles consisting of many loci and with multiple possible mutation events at each locus are very unlikely to match if there is any mutation between X and Q [6,7].

For G unknown, in place of (2), we have (see also [8]):

$$\text{LR}(X, Q) = \frac{1}{\sum_{g=1}^{\infty}(1-\mu)^g \text{P}(G = g)} \qquad \text{where} \quad \sum_{g=1}^{\infty} \text{P}(G = g) = 1. \tag{4}$$

Equation (4) requires a probability distribution for G, which can be informed by population genetic models and by the available information about alternative possible sources of the DNA profile. We introduced X as a specific alternative individual but, in practice, there are usually many alternative sources of the DNA. In either case, $P(G = g)$ can be interpreted as the probability that the unknown alternative source of the DNA is a degree-g relative of Q. If, for example, it is known that all of the degree-g relatives of Q are excluded as possible sources, then $P(G = g) = 0$ in (4), and the other values must be assigned to maintain $\sum_{g=1}^{\infty} P(G = g) = 1$.

Although we can rarely compute it accurately, (4) tells us how to evaluate a lineage marker profile match: we need to assess, given the known circumstances, the probability that an alternative source of the DNA has relatedness g with the alleged source Q, and weight this probability by $(1-\mu)^g$, which means that individuals with $g \gg 1/\mu$ contribute little to the LR.

Most presentations of lineage marker DNA profile evidence mention something like "maternally-related individuals will share the same mitochondrial DNA profile" and then proceed to assess weight of evidence assuming that X and Q are unrelated. This practice is potentially misleading, because we are all maternally related and we are also all paternally related, what is important is the degree g of the relatedness (or that $g \gg 1/\mu$).

1.2. The Role of Databases in Evidence Evaluation

Most methods reviewed below make some use of a database of profiles to provide information about population profile frequencies. When multiple databases are available, the one with ancestry closest to that of Q should usually be chosen [9,10], unless the database size is very small and there is an alternative database of larger size drawn from a population with similar ancestry.

Databases are usually not random samples [7,11], and not drawn from the population relevant to a specific case. For lineage markers, the important role of relatedness implies that the way the database is sampled can have a big impact on inferences. On the one hand, databases sampling may be biased towards including more sets of related individuals, for example because relatives of a suspected contributor may also be suspects. On the other hand, some databases implement a policy of excluding close relatives.

For Y and the mitogenome, the most important international databases, both highly respected for their data quality [12], are available online at www.YHRD.org (accessed on 1 August 2021) [13] and www.EMPOP.online (accessed on 1 August 2021) [14,15]. In July 2021, EMPOP had 48,572 mtDNA sequences (of which 4289 cover the entire mitogenome, the rest span some or all of the control region, which is the most variable part of the mitogenome [15]). YHRD had 337,449 minimal (8 STR loci) profiles, of which 97,087 were 27-locus Yfiler Plus profiles. Both databases contain samples from multiple worldwide populations—in some cases, including several subpopulations.

1.3. The Probability of Matching Profiles

Equation (4) has profound implications for the role of databases in computing the LR. For any of the lineage markers in Table 1, the space of possible profiles is so vast that it is extremely unlikely that two distinct lineages will generate the same (complete) profile by neutral mutations. Although matching Y-STR profiles have been reported between males with different single-nucleotide polymorphism (SNP) subhaplotypes, the matching males were in the same geographic region and relatedness is the most likely explanation [16,17], noting that the Y chromosome accumulates several single-nucleotide mutations per generation [18]. Unless μ is very low, the possibility of a match between distantly-related individuals is negligible relative to the much more likely event of a match between pairs of individuals who are related closely enough to generate the match, but distantly enough that the relatedness is not recognised. Relatedness also affects match probabilities for autosomal profiles, but recombination weakens its effects, except in the case of monozygotic twins [19].

Table 1. Estimates of μ for lineage marker profiles. The per-year mitogenome mutation rates in [3,4] have been multiplied by a generation time of 25 years.

Type	Markers	Profile Mutation Rate μ [% Per Generation]	Reference
Ychr	PowerPlex Y (12 loci)	2.5%	[7,20]
Ychr	Yfiler (17 loci)	4.4%	[7,20]
Ychr	PowerPlex Y23 (23 loci)	8.3%	[7,20]
Ychr	Yfiler Plus (27 loci)	13.5%	[7,20]
Mitogenome	16,070 sites	0.3–1.9%	[3,21]
Mitogenome	16,494 sites	0.4–2.3%	[4,21]

For the mitogenome, μ is estimated to be approximately 1 per 70 generations (Table 1). Thus, alternative sources X will almost certainly be female-line relatives of Q with G up to a few hundred [21]. This is greatly beyond the known relatives of Q, but is still closer than a random pair of individuals in a large population, who are typically separated by thousands of generations [21]. For older Y profile kits, μ is a small multiple of the mitogenome value; but for more recent Y profile kits, μ can be an order of magnitude higher, approximately 1 per 7.5 generations for Yfiler Plus profiles (Table 1). In that case, profile matches occur between pairs of individuals separated by at most a few tens of generations [7].

Therefore, the majority of profiles in broadly-defined databases such as YHRD or EMPOP are drawn from individuals that are too distantly related to Q to be relevant to a particular case. The frequency of q can depend sensitively on the choice of population, according to its average relatedness with Q. Alternative sources of the DNA may be concentrated in the same subpopulation as Q, defined by geographical origin and/or social factors such as ethnicity and religion. A relevant consideration is that if Q is in fact not the source of the DNA, the false allegation may in part be due to Q resembling the true source in some characteristics such as appearance, place of residence, or social background, which tends to increase $P(G = g)$ for small values of g.

2. Review of Evaluation Methods

Most methods have not addressed the fundamental effects of relatedness, mutation rate and database sampling frame discussed above. We will review methods assuming, as most authors have done, that the available database is appropriate, and return to these issues in the Discussion.

2.1. Adjusted Database Counts

The denominator of the LR (1), is often assumed to equal the *match probability*, π_q, the relative frequency of q in a population of alternative sources of the DNA. Many approaches aim to estimate π_q based on the count k_q of q in a database of size n. The database relative frequency k_q/n has long been recognised as an unsatisfactory estimator of π_q, because we often have $k_q = 0$ and yet Q has the profile and so $\pi_q > 0$.

Further, the requirement to avoid overstatement of evidence converts here to preferring a "conservative" over-estimate of π_q rather than an under-estimate. Excessive conservativeness wastes information, and our goal should be to evaluate the evidence as accurately as possible, while taking care to guard against being anti-conservative. However, the latter requirement is difficult to satisfy, and there is no agreement about to what extent we should seek to eliminate any risk of being anti-conservative.

Various adjustments to k_q and n have been proposed to avoid zero estimates and introduce an upward bias. We will discuss them in order of increasing conservativeness as measured by $\hat{\pi}_q$ when $k_q = 0$.

2.1.1. Adjustment Based on the Database Frequency Spectrum

Brenner's κ (kappa) estimate [22] (based on [23]) is $\hat{\pi}_q = (1-\kappa)/n$ when $k_q = 0$, where κ is the fraction of singleton profiles (observed only once in the database). Intuitively, a large κ corresponds to high profile diversity, which justifies a low estimate for π_q. The estimator can be very small if the database consists mainly of singletons, which is the case for high-mutation-rate Y profiles. In particular, if the database consists only of singletons, then $\kappa = 1$ and $\hat{\pi}_q = 0$. Cereda's estimators [24,25] are based on the numbers of both singletons and doubletons (profiles observed exactly twice). All of these approaches take no account of individuals that share profile q due to relatedness with Q, and the estimates can be strongly influenced by the way the database is sampled, as discussed above.

2.1.2. Augmenting the Database

If we compute the database relative frequency after adding q, then both k_q and n are augmented by one to obtain $\hat{\pi}_q = (k_q+1)/(n+1)$. If we add two copies of q to the database, corresponding to the profiles of both Q and X under H_X, we obtain [26]

$$\hat{\pi}_q = \frac{k_q + 2}{n + 2}. \tag{5}$$

Other methods can be modified similarly by augmenting the database with one or two copies of q.

Use of (5) is conservative in the sense that we do not know whether we have observed one or two individuals with q (that is, we do not know whether H_X is true). Both the above estimators can alternatively be derived as Bayesian posterior probabilities given a uniform prior for π_q, the first using the original database, while (5) uses the database augmented with one copy of q. A uniform prior is conservative in that it assigns weight to unrealistically high values of π_q.

2.1.3. Upper Confidence Limit (UCL)

An alternative to (5) is an upper confidence limit (usually 95%) for π_q [27,28]. This is the smallest binomial "success" probability π such that the probability of observing up to k_q successes in n trials is ≤ 0.05. That is, the UCL is the largest π such that

$$\sum_{x=0}^{k_q} \binom{n}{x} \pi^x (1-\pi)^{n-x} \leq 0.05 \tag{6}$$

which is sometimes called the Clopper–Pearson formula [29]. The UCL represents a standard scientific approach to controlling the risk of overstating the evidence: it provides an answer to the question of how big the unknown π_q could reasonably be, given observations k_q and n. The 95% UCL is larger (more conservative) than (5). For example, when $k_q = 0$, from (6) and $\ln(0.05) \approx -3$, the UCL is just under $3/n$, whereas (5) is just under $2/n$.

2.2. The Discrete Laplace Method

The Discrete Laplace method [30,31] models π_q for all possible q, making it also useful for model-based clustering and mixture analyses [32,33]. Intuitively, based on the database profiles, clusters are identified corresponding to the descendants of a recent common ancestor, and probabilities are computed for the observed profiles to belong to each cluster. The ancestors are treated as unrelated and so their profiles are independent. Profile probabilities are then computed by assuming that profiles descend independently from each ancestor according to a Discrete Laplace (double geometric) distribution.

2.3. Coancestry Adjustment for Population Substructure

The population genetic parameter F_{ST}, often referred to as θ in forensic DNA profiling, has been widely used to correct match probabilities for autosomal DNA profiles [34]. An analogous adjustment for lineage marker profiles [1,35] is

$$\text{LR} = \frac{1}{\theta + (1-\theta)\pi_q} \tag{7}$$

There are several interpretations of θ—one is that it represents the average level of relatedness of individuals within a subpopulation, relative to a larger population. In forensic settings, the larger population can be interpreted as the population from which the available profile database was drawn, while the subpopulation is not usually well defined but it is assumed to include Q and some or all of the alternative possible sources of the evidence sample. The denominator of (7) can be loosely interpreted as follows. Under H_X, there is probability θ that X is a relative of Q, sufficiently close that a match is very likely, while with probability $1-\theta$, X comes from the broader population which includes more distant relatives of Q such that the match probability is well estimated by the database relative frequency.

Equation (7) can be used in conjunction with the Discrete Laplace or adjusted database count methods to estimate π_q. However, θ cannot be directly estimated because the value will depend on the available case-specific background information as well as the population that the reference database was drawn from. For example, if the database is drawn from a broad population that extends greatly beyond the population relevant to the case, then a larger θ would be needed than if the database came from a smaller more homogeneous region that includes most alternative donors of the DNA in a particular case.

Population-genetic estimates of θ have been reported for many human subpopulation-population pairs [36,37] and from simulation scenarios [9]. Most available estimates of θ are for autosomal loci. For lineage markers, the smaller effective population size (there are 4 copies of each autosome for every Y chromosome) tends to increase the value of θ, but the higher mutation rate of the Y tends to act in the opposite direction. Many population genetic studies do not estimate θ relative to a forensic database, but instead use a hypothetical ancestral reference population which leads to smaller estimates. Further, few studies are available at the fine geographical scale relevant for many cases.

In general, every alternative X can have a different value of θ reflecting their level of ancestry shared with Q relative to the database population. However, rather than try to choose a distribution of θ values appropriate for the alternative contributors in a case, usual practice is to take a single value from the upper tail of that distribution. Ref. [36] argued for $\theta = 0.03$ as a conservative, default value for autosomal profiles, finding through simulations based on real data that it remains appropriate even if X in fact comes from a different continent than the database population.

2.4. Estimating the Number of Matches in the Population

If we knew that K_q individuals have a profile matching Q, and these are well-mixed in a population of alternative sources of the DNA of size N, then the LR would equal the inverse of the match probability, which is

$$\text{LR} = \frac{N}{K_q}. \tag{8}$$

We have noted above that this is not directly useful in practice, in contrast with the central role of the LR in the interpretation of autosomal profiles, because the choice of population and hence the value of N is problematic for lineage marker profiles. As we consider larger suspect populations, K_q tends to increase at a slower rate than N, because the matching individuals are relatives of Q and they are expected to form a smaller proportion of the population when it is more broadly defined.

An alternative to reporting the LR is to report estimates of K_q. A precise estimate is not usually possible, but probability distributions for K_q can be obtained using simulation under different population genetic models [7,21,38], which can include various mutation rates and mechanisms, and demographic factors such as population growth and structure, as well as variance in offspring number. The simulations can also take into account database frequencies, provided the database sampling scheme is known, which is only feasible in practice if the database can be assumed to be a random sample from the population. Often conditioning on k_q and n from a database does not greatly alter the distribution of K_q, since it merely confirms that the profile is rare, as expected from the mutation rate [7].

A further advantage of the simulation approach is that it can easily incorporate available information about the numbers of close relatives of Q, and about their profiles if available [38].

Using the malan (MAle Lineage ANalysis) software [20], the distribution of K_q was found in high-mutation-rate settings to be insensitive to the modelling assumptions [7,38]. In the case of Yfiler Plus, the number of matching males is typically <10 and rarely more than a few tens. This approach has been extended to mitogenomes [21], but due to their lower mutation rate, the distribution of K_q was spread over a wider range, and was more sensitive to the population genetic model. While there remains merit in reporting to jurors an estimate of K_q, the arguments for this are less compelling than in high-mutation-rate settings, and conversely problems with the match probability and LR are lessened.

Given the estimates of K_q, a juror can assess how likely it is that one of these matching individuals was the source of the evidence profile, rather than Q. The population size N may play some role in these considerations, but is relatively unimportant. Since K_q is a count, it is likely to be more interpretable to a juror than an LR or a match probability [39]: it can be presented using phrases such as "the number of individuals with profile q is unlikely to be more than...".

2.5. Methods Not Widely Used

2.5.1. Population Genetic Modelling Using the Coalescent

The first method for computing match probabilities using an explicit genetic model was based on a genealogical tree with $n + 2$ leaves, representing the database augmented with one copy of q plus a leaf node representing an unobserved profile [40]. Given a mutation model and a demographic model describing the population size, growth rates and structure, a Markov chain Monte Carlo algorithm updates the tree structure and branch lengths, as well as the profiles at the internal nodes of the tree and the unobserved leaf node. The distribution of profiles in the population is estimated from equilibrium frequencies at the unobserved leaf. The method was found to perform well in comparison to methods available at the time [41], but it is computationally demanding, particularly for large databases. This is because the whole profile space is explored, whereas only the probability of q is needed for forensic identification.

2.5.2. Frequency Surveying

The frequency surveying method [42–44] is based on pairwise distances, measured in mutational steps, between the Y profiles from individual i and j. An exponential regression is then based on these distances and used to establish a Beta prior distribution in a Bayesian model with a binomial likelihood. One disadvantage of this approach is that the differences in mutation rates across Y-STR loci are ignored, and only counting the number of mutational steps discards information. This method is still available at www.YHRD.org (accessed on 1 August 2021) [13], but is no longer recommended [11].

2.5.3. Graphical Statistical Models

These Y profile models [45,46] are computationally fast and allow intermediate alleles, which the population-genetic models above cannot accommodate. However, they do not exploit much genetic information and alleles are merely assumed to be different categories.

3. Recommendations from Forensic Authorities

For Y profiles, the Discrete Laplace method (Section 2.2) is currently recommended in the Philippines [47] and in Germany [48], where it was first used in court in a case from 2015 [49]. In that case, profiles were available for some male-line relatives of the suspected contributor, which can be taken into account in assessing the strength of the evidence by the malan simulation approach [38] (Section 2.4). The Polish Speaking Working Group of the International Society for Forensic Genetics (ISFG) [50] currently recommends using the κ method (Section 2.1.1). The UK Forensic Regulator has recently commended use of (5), the adjusted database frequency [10].

Below we briefly summarise and comment on recommendations from two other forensic authorities.

3.1. Scientific Working Group on DNA Analysis Methods (USA, Canada)
3.1.1. Y Profiles

The SWGDAM 2014 guidelines [51] note that "the profile probability is not the same as the match probability", but they do not distinguish between low- and high-mutation-rate profiles. They recommend that the profile probability is estimated by the unadjusted database relative frequency k_q/n, or with a UCL (Section 2.1.3), and that this value be used within (7) to adjust for population structure (Section 2.3).

The guidelines also discuss the importance of identifying the relevant population(s) and the difficulty in choosing an appropriate θ value, and they suggest default values for three kits. For PowerPlex Y23, the most discriminatory (highest profile mutation rate) of the three, they suggest $\theta = 2 \times 10^{-5}$ for African Americans, Asians, Caucasians and Hispanics; and $\theta = 3 \times 10^{-4}$ when Native Americans are considered.

3.1.2. mtDNA

The SWGDAM 2019 guidelines for mtDNA [52] are similar to those for Y profiles [51], except for the θ adjustment. They write: *"It is recognized that population substructure exists for mtDNA haplotypes. However, determination of an appropriate theta (θ) value is complicated by the variety of primer sets, covering different portions of HV1 and/or HV2, which may be applied to forensic casework. SWGDAM has not yet reached consensus on the appropriate statistical approach to estimating θ for mtDNA comparisons"*.

3.2. International Society for Forensic Genetics (ISFG)
3.2.1. Y Profiles

The ISFG 2020 guidelines [11] state that "Information on the degree of paternal relatedness in the suspect population as well as on the familial network is, however, needed to interpret Y chromosome results in the best possible way" but did not delineate how to achieve this. The guidelines focus on estimating a profile relative frequency from a database, for which they recommend the Discrete Laplace method (Section 2.2), which we support in low-mutation-rate settings, but the guidelines do not distinguish low- and high-mutation-rate settings. They note arguments for avoiding estimates of the match probability π_q, referencing [7], but they write "the appropriate wording for statements not relying on population databases need to be validated in the context of the national guidelines".

3.2.2. mtDNA

The ISFG 2014 guidelines on mtDNA [15] focus on estimates of π_q. They do not recommend a particular estimator, but they mention (5) (Section 2.1.2) and the UCL (Section 2.1.3).

4. Some Further Issues
4.1. Combination with Autosomal Evidence

In many respects, lineage marker profiles resemble a single locus of an autosomal profile, with a higher mutation rate and hence greater allelic diversity than for typical autosomal loci but only one allele rather than two. The problem of the strong role for relatedness that we have highlighted in this review also arises at a single autosomal locus, although, due to diploidy, there are four lineages connecting Q and X at an autosomal locus, one for each pairing of an allele from Q with one from X.

It is possible to compute a combined LR for autosomal and lineage marker profiles that both match Q. This is rarely done in practice, perhaps because an autosomal profile match is typically so informative that the relatively small additional evidential strength of the lineage marker match is outweighed by the additional interpretation issues. One possible approach would be to multiply a conservative estimate of K_q by the autosomal match probability, to obtain an estimate of the expected number of individuals matching Q at both lineage marker and autosomal profiles. Alternatively, if the lineage marker profile mutation rate is low, it may be acceptable to multiply autosomal and lineage marker LRs, each obtained using a suitable value of θ.

4.2. Locus Order for Duplicated Y Loci

The STR loci that form a Y profile have known locations on the Y chromosome, except for the ordering of some pairs of duplicated loci including DYS385a and DYS385b. Two males with the same pair of alleles DYS385a/b may or may not match because of the unknown order. When the two alleles from Q are the same as those from the evidence profile, the evaluation problem can be overcome by omitting the duplicated loci, which tends to underestimate evidential strength, or by assuming a match at both loci, which tends to overstate evidential strength, by at most a factor of two and arguably much less.

4.3. Consistency

A consistency principle has been proposed requiring that the strength of evidence for a Y profile cannot be less than that for any of the subprofiles obtained by omitting one or more loci [53]. This reasonable requirement is not enforced by most of the methods discussed here, because a Y profile is treated as a single allele and subprofiles are not considered. The problem can be important when there is a good sample size for a particular DNA profiling kit, but a reduced sample size for a more detailed profile that includes additional loci [10,51]. The method of Section 2.4 based on the distribution of the number K_q of matching individuals does respect the principle, because adding additional loci to a profile increases the mutation rate, and hence stochastically reduces K_q.

4.4. Partial Profiles

Often the DNA from a contributor of interest is at a very low level and/or degraded, so that a partial profile can arise if no allele is observed at some Y-STR loci, due to allele drop-out and/or masking by the alleles of a known contributor. The principles of interpretation are unchanged, using only the loci at which an allele is observed. The fewer the loci observed, the lower the profile mutation rate, which increases the number of matching individuals and decreases their average relatedness with Q. These quantities can be assessed using simulation including only the observed loci [20,54].

4.5. Mixtures

Many evidence profiles come from multiple unknown contributors. When there is a large discrepancy in the amounts of DNA, it may be possible to deconvolve the mixture (assign alleles to distinct, unknown contributors) based on peak heights. Mixture examples with peak height information are included in [55].

Surprisingly, for high-mutation-rate Y profiles, a two-male mixture profile in which q is fully represented is almost as powerful as observing q as a single-source evidence profile [38]. Although many pairs of possible Y profiles could give rise to the observed mixture, the great majority of these possible profiles do not exist in the worldwide human population, which is minuscule compared with the vast number of possible profiles. Since we know that q does exist in the population, the pair of profiles that includes q can be much more likely than all the other profile pairs combined, unless one or more of the other profiles has been observed in a database [38].

For low-mutation-rate Y profiles, the Discrete Laplace method (Section 2.2) can be used to deconvolve mixtures using estimated population frequencies [33].

A "profile-centred" (HC) method [55] is based on (4) and focusses on the number of generations G in the lineage linking Q with alternative contributor X. Beyond some threshold on G, the method assumes that the match probability is low and uses a population frequency estimator similar to the Discrete Laplace method. The HC method assumes a constant-size, random mating population of size N to assign weights for the mixture donors (using formulas for the probability that two random persons are g generations apart). The HC method uses the κ method (Section 2.1.1) for calibration, so that these methods are the same in the special case of good-quality single-source profiles.

5. Discussion

Our review of methods for assessing the forensic value of DNA evidence from lineage markers, namely Y profiles and mitogenomes, has emphasised the key roles of the profile mutation rate and the (male-line or female-line) relatedness G, which are not adequately addressed by many methods. In particular, it is unsatisfactory to inform courts that, for example, a Y profile match is likely for male-line relatives and then to proceed as if the alleged contributor Q is unrelated to the alternative contributors, because (4) highlights that the evidential weight depends on the relatedness of Q with each alternative source of the evidence sample DNA profile.

Values of G are typically unknown in actual populations except when G is very small, but the distribution of G can be investigated via simulation in population genetic models (Section 2.4). There are also some well documented actual human populations that can be studied in more detail. To date these are relatively isolated and not typical of many cosmopolitan urban populations. A national-scale project is underway in Denmark aimed at tracing lineages over a century for almost the whole population [56]. At this time-depth, lineage paths up to about $G = 8$ for two contemporary young adults can be traced, provided that there are no migrants in the lineage.

When the profile mutation rate is low (say below 0.05 per generation, which holds for the mitogenome and older Y-STR profiling kits), most of the individuals with profiles matching Q are separated by at least several tens of generations. There are typically hundreds of matching individuals—in some cases, thousands of them [21]. That is enough individuals and at sufficient genetic distance that many of them will differ from Q in many characteristics, thus lessening the problems discussed above. In these cases, methods based on estimating the population match probability π_q, such as the Discrete Laplace method recommended by the ISFG (Section 2.2) may be acceptable, provided that the role of relatedness is also adequately explained possibly through a θ adjustment. As discussed in Section 2.3, appropriate values for θ can depend on case-specific details and the reference database.

For high-mutation-rate profiles (say above 0.1 per generation), most males matching Q are related to him within a few generations, and there seems no satisfactory alternative to summarising to a court the distribution of the number of close relatives of Q expected to match, as well as their degree of relatedness (Section 2.4). The UCL, for example, will be conservative if the alternative sources of the DNA include few close relatives of Q, but without addressing that question directly we cannot be sure. Methods that rely on a database may be affected by a non-conservative bias, because a broad database population may have lower average relatedness with Q than the alternative sources of the DNA in a particular case, and they may be adversely affected by the role of relatives in the database sampling frame.

Better models and rate estimates for mutation will improve the simulation-based approach to approximating the number of matching individuals. Some data are available but details such as the dependence of mutation rate on current profile state have been little studied, particularly for mitogenomes. Mutation models allowing for allele-specific mutation rates have been investigated [5], but the available data were insufficient to estimate the model parameters accurately.

We believe that the relatedness, mutation and database issues that we have highlighted here can be adequately addressed, and that fair and comprehensible evaluation of lineage marker profile evidence is now within reach.

Author Contributions: Conceptualization, M.M.A. and D.J.B.; methodology, M.M.A. and D.J.B.; formal analysis, M.M.A. and D.J.B.; investigation, M.M.A. and D.J.B.; resources, M.M.A. and D.J.B.; data curation, M.M.A. and D.J.B.; writing—original draft preparation, M.M.A. and D.J.B.; writing—review and editing, M.M.A. and D.J.B.; visualization, M.M.A. and D.J.B.; supervision, M.M.A. and D.J.B. All authors have read and agreed to the published version of the manuscript.

Funding: This research received no external funding.

Institutional Review Board Statement: Not applicable.

Informed Consent Statement: Not applicable.

Data Availability Statement: Not applicable.

Conflicts of Interest: The authors declare no conflict of interest.

References

1. Balding, D.J.; Steele, C.D. *Weight-of-Evidence for Forensic DNA Profiles*, 2nd ed.; Wiley: Chichester, UK, 2015.
2. Johnston, I.; Burgstaller, J.; Havlicek, V.; Kolbe, T.; Rülicke, T.; Brem, G.; Poulton, J.; Jones, N. Stochastic modelling, Bayesian inference, and new in vivo measurements elucidate the debated mtDNA bottleneck mechanism. *Elife* **2015**, *4*, e07464. [CrossRef] [PubMed]
3. Rieux, A.; Eriksson, A.; Li, M.; Sobkowiak, B.; Weinert, L.A.; Warmuth, V.; Ruiz-Linares, A.; Manica, A.; Balloux, F. Improved Calibration of the Human Mitochondrial Clock Using Ancient Genomes. *Mol. Biol. Evol.* **2014**, *31*, 2780–2792. [CrossRef] [PubMed]
4. Översti, S.; Onkamo, P.; Stoljarova, M.; Budowle, B.; Sajantila, A.; Palo, J.U. Identification and analysis of mtDNA genomes attributed to Finns reveal long-stagnant demographic trends obscured in the total diversity. *Sci. Rep.* **2017**, *7*, 6193. [CrossRef]
5. Jochens, A.; Caliebe, A.; Rösler, U.; Krawczak, M. Empirical Evaluation Reveals Best Fit of a Logistic Mutation Model for Human Y-chromosomal Microsatellites. *Genetics* **2011**, *189*, 1403–1411. [CrossRef] [PubMed]
6. Brenner, C.H. Understanding Y haplotype matching probability. *Forensic Sci. Int. Genet.* **2014**, *8*, 233–243. [CrossRef]
7. Andersen, M.M.; Balding, D.J. How convincing is a matching Y-chromosome profile? *PLoS Genet.* **2017**, *13*, e1007028. [CrossRef]
8. Caliebe, A.; Krawczak, M. Match probabilities for Y-chromosomal profiles: A paradigm shift. *Forensic Sci. Int. Genet.* **2018**, *37*, 200–203. [CrossRef]
9. Steele, C.D.; Balding, D.J. Choice of population database for forensic DNA profile analysis. *Sci. Justice* **2014**, *54*, 487–493. [CrossRef]
10. Forensic Science Regulator. Guidance for Y-STR Analysis Delivered into the Criminal Justice System in England and Wales: Forensic Science Regulator Guidance Y-STR Profiling (FSR-G-227). 2021. Available online: https://www.gov.uk/government/publications/y-str-profiling (accessed on 1 August 2021).
11. Roewer, L.; Andersen, M.M.; Ballantyne, J.; Butler, J.M.; Caliebe, A.; Corach, D.; D'Amato, M.E.; Gusmão, L.; Hou, Y.; de Knijff, P.; et al. DNA commission of the International Society of Forensic Genetics (ISFG): Recommendations on the interpretation of Y-STR results in forensic analysis. *Forensic Sci. Int. Genet.* **2020**, *48*, 102308. [CrossRef] [PubMed]
12. Zimmermann, B.; Röck, A.; Huber, G.; Krämer, T.; Schneider, P.M.; Parson, W. Application of a west Eurasian-specific filter for quasi-median network analysis: Sharpening the blade for mtDNA error detection. *Forensic Sci. Int. Genet.* **2011**, *5*, 133–137. [CrossRef] [PubMed]
13. Willuweit, S.; Roewer, L. The New Y Chromosome Haplotype Reference Database. *Forensic Sci. Int. Genet.* **2015**, *15*, 43–48. [CrossRef]
14. Parson, W.; Dür, A. EMPOP—A forensic mtDNA database. *Forensic Sci. Int. Genet.* **2007**, *1*, 88–92. [CrossRef]
15. Parson, W.; Gusmão, L.; Hares, D.; Irwin, J.; Mayr, W.; Morling, N.; Pokorak, E.; Prinz, M.; Salas, A.; Schneider, P.; et al. DNA Commission of the International Society for Forensic Genetics: Revised and extended guidelines for mitochondrial DNA typing. *Forensic Sci. Int. Genet.* **2014**, *13*, 134–142. [CrossRef]
16. Larmuseau, M.; Vanderheyden, N.; Van Geystelen, A.; van Oven, M.; de Knijff, P.; Decorte, R. Recent Radiation within Y-chromosomal Haplogroup R-M269 Resulted in High Y-STR Haplotype Resemblance. *Ann. Hum. Genet.* **2014**, *78*, 92–103. [CrossRef] [PubMed]
17. Solé-Morata, N.; Bertranpetit, J.; Comas, D.; Calafell, F. Recent Radiation of R-M269 and High Y-STR Haplotype Resemblance Confirmed. *Ann. Hum. Genet.* **2014**, *78*, 253–254. [CrossRef] [PubMed]

18. Balanovsky, O. Toward a consensus on SNP and STR mutation rates on the human Y-chromosome. *Hum. Genet.* **2017**, *136*, 575–590. [CrossRef] [PubMed]

19. Tvedebrink, T.; Morling, N. Identical twins in forensic genetics—Epidemiology and risk based estimation of weight of evidence. *Sci. Justice* **2015**, *55*, 408–414. [CrossRef] [PubMed]

20. Andersen, M.M. malan: MAle Lineage ANalysis. *J. Open Source Softw.* **2018**, *3*. [CrossRef]

21. Andersen, M.M.; Balding, D.J. How many individuals share a mitochondrial genome? *PLoS Genet.* **2018**, *14*, e1007774. [CrossRef]

22. Brenner, C.H. Fundamental problem of forensic mathematics—The evidential value of a rare haplotype. *Forensic Sci. Int. Genet.* **2010**, *4*, 281–291. [CrossRef]

23. Robbins, H.E. Estimating the Total Probability of the Unobserved Outcomes of an Experiment. *Ann. Math. Stat.* **1968**, *39*, 256–257. [CrossRef]

24. Cereda, G. Impact of model choice on LR assessment in case of rare haplotype match (frequentist approach). *Scand. J. Stat.* **2017**, *44*, 230–248. [CrossRef]

25. Cereda, G. Bayesian approach to LR assessment in case of rare type match. *Stat. Neerl.* **2017**, *71*, 141–164. [CrossRef]

26. Balding, D.J. *Weight-of-Evidence for Forensic DNA Profiles*, 1st ed.; Wiley: Chichester, UK, 2005.

27. Holland, M.; Parsons, T. Mitochondrial DNA Sequence Analysis—Validation and Use for Forensic Casework. *Forensic Sci. Rev.* **1999**, *11*, 21–50. [PubMed]

28. Budowle, B.; Ge, J.; Chakraborty, R. Basic Principles for Estimating the Rarity of Y-STR Haplotypes Derived from Forensic Evidence. In *18th International Symposium on Human Identification*; Promega: Madison, WI, USA, 2007; Available online: https://www.promega.com/products/pm/genetic-identity/ishi-conference-proceedings/18th-ishi-oral-presentations-mvc/ (accessed on 1 August 2021).

29. Clopper, C.; Pearson, E. The use of confidence or fiducial intervals illustrated in the case of the binomial. *Biometrika* **1934**, *26*, 404–413. [CrossRef]

30. Andersen, M.M.; Eriksen, P.S.; Morling, N. The discrete Laplace exponential family and estimation of Y-STR haplotype frequencies. *J. Theor. Biol.* **2013**, *329*, 39–51. [CrossRef]

31. Andersen, M.M. Discrete Laplace mixture model with applications in forensic genetics. *J. Open Source Softw.* **2018**, *3*. [CrossRef]

32. Andersen, M.M.; Eriksen, P.S.; Morling, N. Cluster analysis of European Y-chromosomal STR haplotypes using the discrete Laplace method. *Forensic Sci. Int. Genet.* **2014**, *11*, 182–194. [CrossRef] [PubMed]

33. Andersen, M.M.; Eriksen, P.S.; Mogensen, H.S.; Morling, N. Identifying the most likely contributors to a Y-STR mixture using the discrete Laplace method. *Forensic Sci. Int. Genet.* **2015**, *15*, 76–83. [CrossRef]

34. Balding, D.J.; Nichols, R.A. DNA profile match probability calculation: How to allow for population stratification, relatedness, database selection and single bands. *Forensic Sci. Int.* **1994**, *64*, 125–140. [CrossRef]

35. Buckleton, J.; Krawczak, M.; Weir, B. The interpretation of lineage markers in forensic DNA testing. *Forensic Sci. Int. Genet.* **2011**, *5*, 78–83. [CrossRef]

36. Steele, C.D.; Syndercombe Court, D.; Balding, D.J. Worldwide Estimates Relative to Five Continental-Scale Populations. *Ann. Hum. Genet.* **2014**, *78*, 468–477. [CrossRef]

37. Buckleton, J.; Curran, J.; Goudet, J.; Taylor, D.; Thiery, A.; Weir, B. Population-specific FST values for forensic STR markers: A worldwide survey. *Forensic Sci. Int. Genet.* **2016**, *23*, 91–100. [CrossRef]

38. Andersen, M.M.; Balding, D.J. Y-profile evidence: Close paternal relatives and mixtures. *Forensic Sci. Int. Genet.* **2019**, *38*, 48–53. [CrossRef] [PubMed]

39. Hoffrage, U.; Lindsey, S.; Hertwig, R.; Gigerenzer, G. Communicating Statistical Information. *Science* **2000**, *290*, 2261–2262. [CrossRef] [PubMed]

40. Wilson, I.J.; Weale, M.E.; Balding, D.J. Inferences from DNA Data: Population Histories, Evolutionary Processes and Forensic Match Probabilities. *J. R. Stat. Soc. Ser. A* **2003**, *166*, 155–201. [CrossRef]

41. Andersen, M.M.; Caliebe, A.; Jochens, A.; Willuweit, S.; Krawczak, M. Estimating trace-suspect match probabilities for singleton Y-STR haplotypes using coalescent theory. *Forensic Sci. Int. Genet.* **2013**, *7*, 264–271. [CrossRef]

42. Roewer, L.; Kayser, M.; de Knijff, P.; Anslinger, K.; Betz, A.; Caglia, A.; Corach, D.; Füredi, S.; Henke, L.; Hidding, M.; et al. A new method for the evaluation of matches in non-recombining genomes: Application to Y-chromosomal short tandem repeat (STR) haplotypes in European males. *Forensic Sci. Int.* **2000**, *114*, 31–43. [CrossRef]

43. Krawczak, M. Forensic evaluation of Y-STR haplotype matches: A comment. *Forensic Sci. Int.* **2001**, *118*, 114–115. [CrossRef]

44. Willuweit, S.; Caliebe, A.; Andersen, M.; Roewer, L. Y-STR frequency surveying method: A critical reappraisal. *Forensic Sci. Int. Genet.* **2011**, *5*, 84–90. [CrossRef]

45. Andersen, M.M.; Curran, J.; de Zoete, J.; Taylor, D.; Buckleton, J. Modelling the dependence structure of Y-STR haplotypes using graphical models. *Forensic Sci. Int. Genet.* **2018**, *37*, 29–36. [CrossRef]

46. Andersen, M.M.; Caliebe, A.; Kirkeby, K.; Knudsen, M.; Vihrs, N.; Curran, J.M. Estimation of Y haplotype frequencies with lower order dependencies. *Forensic Sci. Int. Genet.* **2020**, *46*, 102214. [CrossRef]

47. Rodriguez, J.; Laude, R.; De Ungriaa, M. An integrated system for forensic DNA testing of sexual assault cases in the Philippines. *Forensic Sci. Int. Synerg.* **2021**, *3*, 100133. [CrossRef] [PubMed]

48. Willuweit, S.; Anslinger, K.; Bäßler, G.; Eckert, M.; Fimmers, R.; Hohoff, C.; Kraft, M.; Leuker, C.; Molsberger, G.; Pich, U.; et al. Joint recommendations of the project group "Statistical analysis of DNA" and the German Stain Commission on the statistical analysis of Y-chromosomal DNA typing results. *Rechtsmedizin* **2018**, *28*, 138–142. [CrossRef]

49. Roewer, L. Y-chromosome short tandem repeats in forensics—Sexing, profiling, and matching male DNA. *WIREs Forensic Sci.* **2019**, *1*, e1336. [CrossRef]

50. Rębała, K.; Branicki, W.; Pawłowski, R.; Spólnicka, M.; Kupiec, T.; Parys-Proszek, A.; Woźniak, M.; Grzybowski, T.; Boroń, M.; Wróbel, M.; et al. Recommendations of the Polish Speaking Working Group of the International Society for Forensic Genetics on forensic Y chromosome typing. *Arch. Forensic Med. Criminol.* **2020**, *70*, 1–18. [CrossRef]

51. SWGDAM. SWGDAM Interpretation Guidelines for Y-Chromosome STR Testing. 2014. Available online: https://www.swgdam.org/publications (accessed on 1 August 2021).

52. SWGDAM. SWGDAM MtDNA Interpretation Guidelines. 2019. Available online: https://www.swgdam.org/publications (accessed on 1 August 2021).

53. Cowell, R.G. Consistent estimation of Y STR haplotype probabilities. *Forensic Sci. Int. Genet.* **2020**, *49*, 102365. [CrossRef]

54. Andersen, M.M. mitolina: MITOchondrial LINeage Analysis. *J. Open Source Softw.* **2019**, *4*, 1266. [CrossRef]

55. Taylor, D.; Curran, J.M.; Buckleton, J. Likelihood ratio development for mixed Y-STR profiles. *Forensic Sci. Int. Genet.* **2018**, *35*, 82–96. [CrossRef]

56. Using Artificial Intelligence for Mapping the Danish Genealogy and Strengthening Research. Available online: https://novonordiskfonden.dk/en/news/kunstig-intelligens-skal-kortlaegge-danskernes-stam-trae-og-styrke-forskning/ (accessed on 17 June 2021).

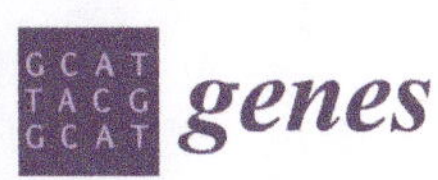 *genes*

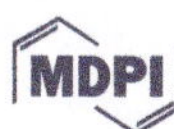

Article

Towards Forensic DNA Phenotyping for Predicting Visible Traits in Dogs

Cordula Berger [1,*,†], Josephin Heinrich [1,†], Burkhard Berger [1], Werner Hecht [2], Walther Parson [1,3] and on behalf of CaDNAP [‡]

[1] Institute of Legal Medicine, Medical University of Innsbruck, 6020 Innsbruck, Austria; josephin.heinrich@live.com (J.H.); burkhard.berger@i-med.ac.at (B.B.); walther.parson@i-med.ac.at (W.P.)
[2] Institute of Veterinary Pathology, Justus-Liebig-University Giessen, 35390 Giessen, Germany; wernerhecht@web.de
[3] Forensic Science Program, The Pennsylvania State University, University Park, PA 16801, USA
* Correspondence: cordula.berger@i-med.ac.at; Tel.: +43-512-9003-70640
† These authors contributed equally to this work.
‡ Collaborators of CaDNAP are listed in Appendix A.

Abstract: The popularity of dogs as human companions explains why these pets regularly come into focus in forensic cases such as bite attacks or accidents. Canine evidence, e.g., dog hairs, can also act as a link between the victim and suspect in a crime case due to the close contact between dogs and their owners. In line with human DNA identification, dog individualization from crime scene evidence is mainly based on the analysis of short tandem repeat (STR) markers. However, when the DNA profile does not match a reference, additional information regarding the appearance of the dog may provide substantial intelligence value. Key features of the dog's appearance, such as the body size and coat colour are well-recognizable and easy to describe even to non-dog experts, including most investigating officers and eyewitnesses. Therefore, it is reasonable to complement eyewitnesses' testimonies with externally visible traits predicted from associated canine DNA samples. Here, the feasibility and suitability of canine DNA phenotyping is explored from scratch in the form of a proof of concept study. To predict the overall appearance of an unknown dog from its DNA as accurately as possible, the following six traits were chosen: (1) coat colour, (2) coat pattern, (3) coat structure, (4) body size, (5) ear shape, and (6) tail length. A total of 21 genetic markers known for high predicting values for these traits were selected from previously published datasets, comprising 15 SNPs and six INDELS. Three of them belonged to SINE insertions. The experiments were designed in three phases. In the first two stages, the performance of the markers was tested on DNA samples from dogs with well-documented physical characteristics from different breeds. The final blind test, including dogs with initially withheld appearance information, showed that the majority of the selected markers allowed to develop composite sketches, providing a realistic impression of the tested dogs. We regard this study as the first attempt to evaluate the possibilities and limitations of forensic canine DNA phenotyping.

Keywords: domestic dog (*Canis familiaris*); canine DNA phenotyping; forensic; proof of concept study

Citation: Berger, C.; Heinrich, J.; Berger, B.; Hecht, W.; Parson, W.; on behalf of CaDNAP. Towards Forensic DNA Phenotyping for Predicting Visible Traits in Dogs. *Genes* **2021**, *12*, 908. https://doi.org/10.3390/genes12060908

Academic Editor: Emiliano Giardina
Received: 25 May 2021
Accepted: 8 June 2021
Published: 11 June 2021

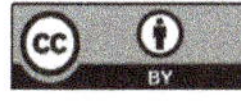

1. Introduction

DNA phenotyping in a forensic context was developed as meaningful enhancement to standard human DNA profiling, where STRs are mainly used to identify individuals [1,2]. In cases where DNA profiles do not match a suspect's profile or a criminal DNA database record, forensic DNA phenotyping (FDP) aims to predict externally visible characteristics of a person by analyzing suitable DNA markers. It provides new investigative leads irrespective of the presence of any other information such as eyewitness testimonies [1]. DNA-based appearance prediction within forensics started in the early 2000s [3] and so far, tests on human iris, hair, and skin pigmentation were successfully validated for routine casework investigations [1,4–8]. Their implementation within legislative frameworks of different countries is now discussed intensively [9].

In this study, we aim at outlining an approach for Canine DNA phenotyping in forensic settings as it is an appealing idea to test if the concept of FDP can be transferred to non-human DNA. As a first step, we generated proof of concept data to explore ways and possibilities for developing a molecular genetic tool to predict externally visible traits of dogs from DNA customized to the special needs of forensic issues. The choice fell on the domestic dog because of its extreme morphological diversity and its forensic significance.

The diverse appearance of dogs is the result of a long-standing and intensive domestication process. Although still being discussed with controversial arguments, it is broadly accepted that all contemporary dogs were domesticated from the Eurasian grey wolf (*Canis lupus*) and that they accompanied humans over millennia [10–21]. Dogs have performed a variety of roles starting from ancestral dogs that were primarily valued for their hunting or protective skills [22,23]. The desire to develop dogs with particular physical traits was the driving force behind selective breeding practices. During the last 200 years, the focus of breeding changed from working ability to outward appearance and resulted in the formation of modern dog breeds [24–26]. At present, more than 400 breeds exist, and this diversity is even leveraged by inter-breeds and mongrels. Dogs exhibit a vast array of phenotypic traits, with varying body sizes, skull shapes, hair structure, coat colours, etc. [27–56]. As a result, even an untrained eye can easily identify and describe some significant characteristics of a dog. This leads one to expect that the output of a canine DNA phenotyping test could provide practical information about the appearance of a dog of interest, which is comparable to an eye-witness testimony.

Today, there is an estimated number of almost 700 million to 1 billion dogs worldwide [57,58]. The dog density varies considerably among countries, with much higher numbers across the United States or Europe [57]. In these countries, dogs are kept almost exclusively within the home, underlining the dog's major role as a companion. This explains why canine-source material is relevant to diverse forensic cases. Dogs can cause accidents or attack humans, wildlife and domestic animals. For a recent overview concerning dog-related fatalities, see [59]. Probably forensically more relevant, and more challenging to analyse, are cases in which the transfer of canine DNA evidence occurs. Such instances can identify links between victims, suspects, and/or crime scenes and thus contribute to generating evidence in human forensic cases. Due to the close contact with humans, canine transfer samples can be plentiful. This may include, for example, saliva on trousers or hair left on the back seat of a vehicle. As dogs shed more hairs than humans, the probability of finding dog hairs can be higher than finding hairs of the dog owner.

DNA fingerprinting methods provide strong evidence for individual identification of the involved dog(s). Accordingly, a number of approaches have been published using canine STR loci for dog individualization from crime scene evidence [60–68] and guidelines have been established for forensic validation requirement [69,70]. STR profiling allows to answer questions such as: "was this dog the perpetrator of the attack?" or "does the hair found on the victim originate from the suspect's dog?". However, cases where crime scene DNA does not match a suspected dog or where reference material is not available occur frequently. Consequently, statements such as "the attack was perpetrated by a large dog with black coat colour" or "the hair comes from a black/white spotted dog with long fur" would be typical examples for helpful leads. Traditionally, such statements come from eyewitness reports. However, eyewitness testimony is not always available and can be subjective or unreliable [71–74]. DNA analysis, particularly when tailored toward canine DNA phenotyping, could counteract these limitations by answering questions similar to the above-mentioned examples based on an objective and quantifiable methodology.

2. Materials and Methods

2.1. Sampling, Documentation and DNA Extraction

Our sample collection was established based on direct inquiries to private dog owners, by visiting dog shows, dog schools and dog breeders. Buccal swabs were taken by the dog owner to minimize disturbing effects to the animals. Alphanumeric unique sample IDs were used for unambiguous sample assignment. Metadata, including all relevant externally visible characteristics, were recorded as displayed exemplarily in Table S1. In addition, tissues from dead dogs were collected at the Institute for Veterinary Pathology, Justus-Liebig-University Gießen, Germany, as described in [61]. In total, 84 dog samples were included in the study.

DNA was extracted from buccal swabs according to routine procedures on a Qiagen EZ1 Advanced XL Nucleic Acid Automated Purification System (Qiagen, Hilden, Germany) using the DNeasy Blood & Tissue Kit (Qiagen) or using Gentra Puregene reagents and protocols (Qiagen), according to the manufacturers' recommendations. The DNA of the tissue samples was extracted in a class 2 biological safety cabinet using the Gentra Puregene Tissue Kit (Qiagen, Hilden, Germany) [61,75]. Nuclear DNA quantities were determined with a spectral photometer (Nanodrop 2000; Peqlab GmbH, Erlangen, Germany) or by applying a quantitative real-time PCR assay according to [76]. The assay was performed in a total volume of 10 µL on an AB 7500 Fast Real-Time PCR System (Thermo Fisher Scientific [TFS], Waltham, MA, USA).

2.2. Marker Selection and Study Design

A total of 21 markers were selected, comprising 15 SNPs and six INDELS. The latter two were microINDELS (each with a length of 3 bp), one was of intermediate-size (167 bp) and three belong to SINE insertions. The complete marker set is listed in Table 1, which contains relevant molecular genetic information as well as metadata regarding the related phenotypes. The primer sequences and positions according to CanFam3.1 are provided in Table S2a.

The implementation of the proof of concept study was divided into three phases or experimental tests that built on one another: the pilot test, the marker test, and the blind test. Within each test, Sanger sequencing of all markers was carried out on a set of canine DNA samples in order to create molecular data for downstream phenotype interpretations.

2.3. PCR Amplification and Sanger Sequencing

Where possible, primer sequences were directly adopted from published data or were redesigned to reduce amplicon lengths. Detailed information on the primers is provided in Table S2a. Primer design was performed with the OligoAnalyzer Tool (Integrated DNA Technologies, Coralville, IA, USA) based on the CanFam3.1 (EMBL-EBI, Hinxton, Cambridgeshire, UK) reference sequences and was checked for secondary structure formation using Mfold (University at Albany, NY, USA).

PCR amplifications were carried out in 20 µL assays, containing 0.4 µL 50X Advantage 2 Polymerase Mix, 2 µL 10X Advantage 2 PCR Buffer (both Takara, Kyoto, Japan), 0.25 mg/mL BSA (Serva, Heidelberg, Germany), 200 µM each dNTP (TFS), 0.6 µL of each 10 µM primer (Microsynth, Balgach, Switzerland, Table S2a). Two to 30 ng of DNA extract were used for amplification. Thermal cycling was performed on a DNA Engine Dyad thermal cycler (Bio-Rad, Hercules, CA, USA) or a Gene Amp PCR System 9700 (TFS), comprising initial denaturation at 95 °C for 2 min, followed by 37 cycles of 95 °C for 15 s, 58 to 67 °C for 30 s (see Table S2a) and 72 °C for 45 s. PCR products were purified using ExoSAP-IT (Amersham, Bucks, UK) according to the manufacturer's recommendations.

Sanger sequencing was accomplished by combining 2 µL of BigDye Terminator v1.1 Ready Reaction Mix, 2 µL 5X Sequencing Buffer (both TFS), 1 µL 5 µM amplification primer and 5 µL amplification product to a total volume of 10 µL. Cycling conditions were 95 °C for 2 min, and 30 cycles of 96 °C for 1 min, 50 °C for 5 s and 60 °C for 4 min. Products were purified using the Performa DTR Ultra 96-Well Plate Kit (EdgeBio, San Jose, CA,

USA) according to the manufacturer's recommendations. Capillary electrophoresis was performed on an AB 3500xl Genetic Analyzer using POP6, 50 cm capillary arrays and default instrument settings (all TFS). Sequencing data were analysed using Sequencing Analysis Version 5.4 (TFS) and Sequencher Version 5.1 (GeneCodes, Ann Arbor, MI, USA). SNP data were formatted in Excel 2016 (Microsoft Corporation, Redmond, WA, USA).

The genotypes relevant for predicting visible traits comprised single nucleotide polymorphisms (SNPs) and insertion/deletion markers (INDELS) including short interspersed nuclear elements (SINEs; sequences are provided in Table S2b). The polymorphic sites were addressed by sequence analysis of the amplified DNA fragments. The interpretation of the allelic states at homo- and heterozygous SNP sites proved unambiguous. The same held true for short INDELS (up to three base pairs). However, long INDEL markers, ASIP SINE, MITF SINE, PMEL SINE, and the RSPO2 insertion caused difficult-to-interpret raw data when heterozygous. In these cases, short and long amplicon sequences (derived from both, the allele without insertion and with insertion) overlapped and caused out of phase sequence data. For interpretation of the heterozygous state, the overlapping nucleotides within the chromatogram—reflecting both sequence variants—were considered separately (see Figure S1a–d).

3. Results

For a phenotypic description of individual dogs, genetic markers for the following six traits were selected: (1) coat colour, (2) coat pattern, (3) coat structure, (4) body size, (5) ear shape, and (6) tail length. In total, a set of 21 markers was applied (Table 1). Figure 1 provides a schematic representation of the possible phenotypic manifestations that could, in principle, be deduced from this marker set. This information is based on the published explanatory power of the markers (Table 1). In general, our results confirmed the published effects of alleles at the tested loci on the phenotypic appearance of dogs.

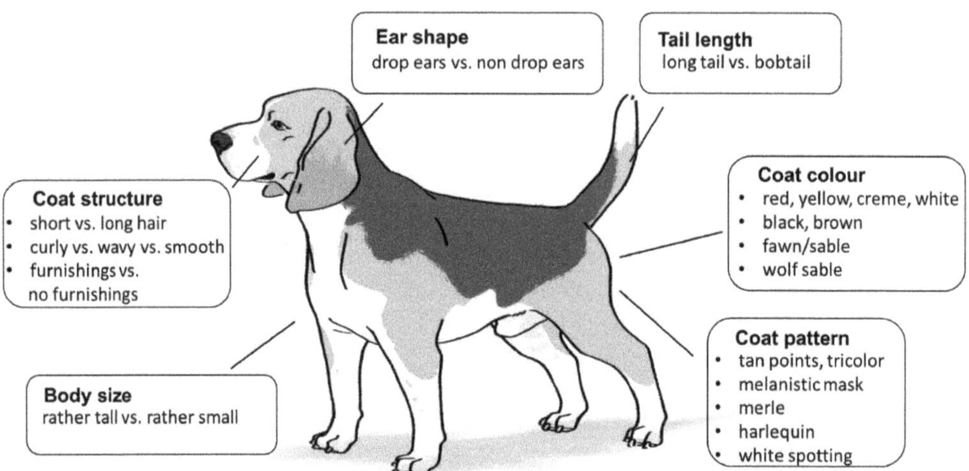

Figure 1. Schematic illustration of the trait categories selected to deduce a dog's appearance by applying canine DNA phenotyping. The six trait categories include the most obvious characteristics of a dog that can easily be recognized and described even by an untrained eyewitness. Each box refers to one trait category and contains clearly distinguishable externally visible characteristics predictable from a particular genotype. The listings should provide an overview of the standardized terminology used here to characterize the appearance. vs.—versus (picture copyright: Larissa Hasenheit).

3.1. Pilot Test

The pilot test included DNA samples from twelve dogs selected from a sample collection comprising approximately 1200 dogs [75]. Each of the 12 samples were analysed in 21 markers, resulting in 252 genotypes. This test was performed to verify the SNP and INDEL positions provided in the literature and to optimize the laboratory workflow, including PCR and sequencing conditions as well as primer redesign, if necessary (see Table S2a). All 21 markers were successfully sequenced and all SNPs/INDELS could be unambiguously assigned. In all but three markers (PMEL, PSMB7, and T-box), all previously described allelic states were found within the pilot test sample set (Table S3a).

3.2. Marker Test

In the marker test, the reliability of predicting the phenotype for each of the 21 markers representing the six trait categories was determined. Therefore, the test samples were selected from the full sample collection (n = 1200) with respect to the phenotypical appearance of the dogs to include the different phenotypic manifestations of a particular trait. A detailed list of possible genotypes at all markers and the resulting genetic-based phenotype prediction is given in Tables S4a–k.

The following presentation of the marker test outcomes is accompanied by an overview of the genetic basis and nomenclature commonly used for each trait. The simplified chart given in Figure S2 summarizes the dominance hierarchy of loci and alleles involved in the manifestation of coat colour and pattern.

3.2.1. Coat Colour and Coat Pattern

The nomenclature for the genetics of coat colours and coat patterns in dogs is based on the system established by [77] and with later adaptations (e.g., [38,55,78,79]). The term "Locus" is preceded by an alphabetical character which refers to the main characteristic realized by the particular locus (e.g., A-Locus: "A" stands for "Agouti"). Since the introduction of this naming convention by Little (1957) [77], all loci were assigned to genes, as described below.

As in most mammals, the synthesis of eumelanin (black, brown) or phaeomelanin (yellow, red) is regulated by the two genes *MC1R* (E-Locus) and *ASIP* (A-Locus). In addition to these two genes, *CBD103* (K-Locus) is of particular importance for black fur [28,80,81]. The genes *MITF* (S-Locus), *MLPH* (D-Locus), *PMEL* (M-Locus), and *PSMB7* (H-Locus) modify the coat colour and pattern that is provided by the three main loci described above and are therefore called "modifiers" [82].

For testing the coat colour markers, one set of sixteen dog samples was used. It consisted of five solid brown, two solid black, two fawn/sable with white spotting, and two brown dogs with white spotting, as well as one wild type agouti, one brown sable, one black with white spotting, one black merle, and one blue (grey) dog.

E-Locus ("Extension"); see Table S4a: The *MC1R* (Melanocortin 1 receptor) gene is epistatic to the K- and A-loci and responsible for a red, yellow, creme, and sometimes white coat colour in dogs (genotype: e/e) [31–34,83]. Alleles of the E-Locus are the dominant E (establishing a brown or black coat colour), and the recessive e. The allele for the coat pattern "melanistic mask" E^m is dominant over the E allele. Therefore, a melanistic mask is present in all E^m dogs, even if phenotypically not so well recognizable as in solid black dogs [79].

K-Locus ("dominant black"); see Table S4b: The *CBD103* (β-defensin) gene is responsible for black coat colour [28]. The effect of the K-Locus is dependent on the E-Locus and is only expressed when at least one E allele is present in a genotype. The dominant K^B allele inhibits the expression of the A-Locus. That results in solid coloured phenotype when no modifier gene (e.g., *MLPH*) is expressed [40,79]. The coat pattern "brindle" (K^{br}), in which stripes of red-yellow hair alternate with black-brown hair, was not included in this study.

A-Locus ("Agouti"); see (Table S4c): The Agouti signaling protein gene has four alleles identified so far, hierarchically ordered according to their dominance: A^y (fawn/sable)

> a^w (agouti/wild type- wild type, black banded hairs) > a^t (tan points) >a (recessive black) [27,29]. The A-Locus is expressed when the K-Locus is homozygous for the recessive k^y allele. The coat pattern "sable" arises from hairs with tips darker in colour than the light-coloured base. Three main sable patterns are common in dog breeds: (1) clear sable—completely fawn dogs with just a few eumelanin (black/brown) hairs; (2) tipped sable—fawn dogs with eumelanin (black/brown) hairs usually on the back, head, ears and tail; (3) shaded sable—fawn dogs with eumelanin (black/brown) hairs covering the top of the head, ears and back; shading can be very light or very dark and distinct [http://www.doggenetics.co.uk/tan.html#sable] (accessed on 10 June 2021).

Agouti (a^w—"w" stands for "wild type") is characterized by hairs showing alternating colours along the hair shaft ("banding"; Fawn/black or brown).

B-Locus ("<u>B</u>rown"); see Table S4d: The gene *TYRP1* (Tyrosinase-related protein 1) affects only eumelanin, causing all black areas to turn to a brownish colour [33,55]. Brown is expressed by recessive alleles. It can be expressed when two of the three brown alleles are present in a genotype (b^s/b^s, b^s/b^d, b^s/b^c, b^d/b^d, b^d/b^c, b^c/b^c) [55]. The gene also affects the colour of the nose and eyes, making them brownish (liver).

D-Locus ("<u>D</u>ilution"); see Table S4e: The *MLPH* (Melanophilin) gene affects both eumelanin and phaeomelanin [30,56,84]. As the allele causing dilution is recessive, a dilution is only expressed when a dog is homozygous for this allele. In this case, a black dog will become dark grey (also called "blue"), and a brown dog will become pale cream-brown ("Isabella").

S-Locus ("<u>S</u>potting"); see Table S4f: The *MITF* gene (microphthalmia associated transcription factor) is associated with one or more spotting patterns in dogs [47,55,85]. The range of spotting patterns is large, starting from no spotting and minimal white spotting, known as wild type (S/S), pseudo irish spotting (S/S^p), to piebald spotting and extremely white spotting (S^p/S^p). This is mainly caused by a SINE insertion on the *MITF* gene [85].

M-Locus ("<u>M</u>erle"); see Table S4g: The premelanosome protein (*PMEL*) gene is responsible for merle coats described by the following features: (1) a light, diluted base colour and (2) random patches of fully pigmented fur of various size and location [39–41]. As the variant is semi-dominant, heterozygous individuals have at least a mild dilution of eumelanin areas, whereas m/m animals are normally pigmented and M/M individuals are mainly white (the latter occasionally exhibit deafness and ocular problems) [79]. A variety of merle phenotypes is known among dog breeds, such the classic, double, hidden, harlequin, cryptic and dilute forms. The hidden form possesses the M allele but the phenotypic merle pattern is invisible due to the epistatic impact of the e allele at the *MC1R* gene, when homozygous [39,41,86].

H-Locus ("<u>H</u>arlequin"); Table S4g: The *PSMB7* (Proteasome 20S Subunit β7) gene is a dominant modifier gene of the merle *SILV* gene (M-Locus) that removes the dilute pigment and increases the size of the fully pigmented regions (dark spots on a white background) [37]. Harlequin is only expressed on a Merle background and is a well-known and easily recognizable coat pattern almost exclusively found in Great Danes.

Applying the just-described genetic foundations of coat colour traits to the results of the marker test, in 12 out of 16 analysed dogs, the genotypes predicted the expected phenotypes correctly (Tables S3b and S5).

For six of the 16 dogs, the phenotypic interpretation of the genotypic data obtained was straightforward, and for the other six dogs, heterozygous alleles in Q331 (b^s) were detected. Three of the latter group had a brown coat colour, one had a black coat colour and one showed a grey coat that is in accordance with the recessive inheritance of the coat colour modifier gene *MLPH*. One dog had an "e/e" *MC1R* genotype and a "B/b^s" *TYPR1* genotype and showed brown eye rims and brown nose leather, which is in accordance with the description given in [55].

For three dog samples, the sequence analyses failed in the ASIP SINE markers. However, due to the hierarchical gene expression of the coat colour genes, it was deducible that the *ASIP* gene was of no account in these cases. Dog DE02_20 showed an e/e genotype at the E-locus and both dogs DE01_006 and DE01_052 had a K^B/K^B genotype at the K-locus (Figure S2, Table S3b).

The only discrepancy within the group of 16 dogs refers to the genotype interpretation of markers TYRP1_Q331ter and TYRP1_345delP, which refer to a black coat colour instead of actually brown (dog individuals AT0282, DE01_006, DE01_052, and DE02_017).

For the coat pattern trait, consistent results for all tested samples between the genotypic data and the physical visible traits of the dogs were achieved. Only individual AT0134 showed no results in both MITF markers. (Tables S3b and S5).

It should be noted that three dogs (AT0062, AT0183, AT0257) were heterozygous at the K-Locus (K^B/k^y), indicating that their coat pattern could be brindled [80], but this pattern was not observed in these individuals. AT0062 showed a black with white spotting phenotype and AT0183 and AT0257 had a solid black phenotypic appearance.

The markers of the remaining trait categories were tested with 10 dog samples each. For each category, the dogs were selected by their appearance, in order to include both manifestations of the particular phenotypic characteristics in question, e.g., smooth vs. curly dogs, small vs. tall dogs.

3.2.2. Coat Structure

Three genes, *RSPO2*, *FGF5*, and *KRT71* (encoding for R-spondin–2, fibroblast growth factor–5, and keratin-71, respectively), together account for most coat structure phenotypes (Table S4h): The *RSPO2* gene is strongly associated with wired hair as well as the "furnishings", phenotypically characterized by a moustache and pronounced eyebrows as well as increased hair growth on the face and legs [36,87]. Variations in the *FGF5* gene control the hair length in many dog breeds, the short hair mutation being of dominant inheritance [40]. The *KRT71* gene is found to be associated with a curly hair phenotype. As the mutation is semi-dominant, animals heterozygous for this gene have an at least so-called "wavy" coat [40].

The analyses for the three above-mentioned **coat structure trait** markers were straight forward and the genotype data were in accordance with the phenotypical appearance of all 10 dogs (Tables S3b and S5).

3.2.3. Tail Length

The C189G mutation in exon 1 of the *T-Box* transcription factor T gene was found to be strongly correlated with a short-tail phenotype for dogs belonging to specific breeds if heterozygous for this mutation. The T gene mutation can cause both anury (absence of tail) and brachyury (very short tail) [48,54]. Homozygosity for the mutation causes either embryonic or early postnatal lethality [48,88] (Table S4i).

For the prediction of the tail length, the success-rate amounted to 70%. Three of 10 dogs showed no correct genotype–phenotype correlation for the bobtail phenotype (Tables S3b and S5). These samples came from an English Bulldog (AT0056), a Boston Terrier (AT0062) and a French Bulldog (AT0210).

3.2.4. Ear Shape

Wild canines have upright ears, whereas hanging ears are a characteristic of dog domestication. The marker IGF2BP2_BICFPJ1062878 used for ear shape determination was described in [89] (Table S4j).

The interpretation of this single ear shape marker included in the marker set proved to be unreliable (Tables S3b and S5). Only two dogs reflected the genotype in their phenotypical appearance. One dog did not show drop ears as genotypically indicated. No clear interpretation was possible for the six heterozygote dogs, as three of them had drop ears, and the other three exhibited non-drop ears. For one sample, no sequence data were obtained (AT0274).

Table 1. Detailed information on the selected 21 phenotype-specific markers allocated to the respective trait category. For the coat colour and coat pattern markers, the commonly used locus (Locus) and allele names (Allele) are listed (see, for example, reviews [38,40]). Upper case letters of an allele refer to dominant inheritance, lower case letters to recessive inheritance. For a detailed description of external visible traits (phenotype), see Sections 3.2.1–3.2.3. Additionally, the phenotypic manifestation is given as well as the corresponding references. Sequence information for the marker types INDEL and SINE are given in Table S2b. n.a. not applicable.

Trait Category	Marker ID	Locus	Allele	Marker Type	Nucleotide	Dominance (x)	Phenotype	Reference
	MC1R_306ter	E (extension)	e	SNP	T		red, yellow, cream, white	[33–55]
			E		C	x	black, brown	
	MC1R_M264V	**E (exten-sion)**	E	**SNP**	A		**no melanistic mask (black, brown)**	[32,34]
			E^m		G	x	**melanistic mask (black, brown)**	
	CBD103_S54	K (from 'dominant black')	k^y	INDEL	GGG		yellow—expression of agouti alleles	[28,80]
			K^B		DelGGG	x	black, brown, blue	
	CBD103_S53	**K (from 'dominant black')**	k^y	**SNP**	G		**yellow—expression of agouti alleles**	[28,80]
			K^B		C	x	**black, brown, blue**	
Coat colour, coat pattern	ASIP S82	A (agouti)	A^y	SNP	T	x	fawn/sable	[27]
			a^w		G		wild type/agouti (black, brown)	
	ASIP H83	**A (agouti)**	A^y	**SNP**	A	x	**fawn/sable**	[27]
			a^w		G		**wild type/agouti (black, brown)**	
	ASIP_SINE	A (agouti)	a^t	SINE	SINE		tan points (black, brown), tricolour	[29]
			a^w		no SINE		wild type/agouti (black, brown)	
	ASIP_R96	**A (agouti)**	a^t	**SNP**	C		**tan points (black, brown), tricolour**	[27]
			a		T		recessive black	
	TYRP1_Q331ter	B (brown)	B	SNP	C	x	black	[33,55]
			b^s		T		brown	

Table 1. *Cont.*

Trait Category	Marker ID	Locus	Allele	Marker Type	Nucleotide	Dominance (x)	Phenotype	Reference
	TYRP1_345delP B (brown)		**B**	**INDEL**	**CCT**	x	**black**	[33,55]
			b^d		**DelCCT**		**brown**	
	MLPH_157471_c.-22G>A	D (dilutes eumelanin)	D	SNP	G	x	not diluted pigmentation	[30,56,84]
			d		A		diluted pigmentation	
	MITF_SNP	**S (spotting)**	**S**	**SNP**	**A**	**not clarified**	**solid colorred, minimal white spotting**	[47]
			S		**G**		**white spotting**	
	MITF_INS	S (spotting)	S	SINE	no SINE		solid coloured, minimal white spotting	[85]
			S^P		SINE		white spotting (S^P—piebald)	
			S/S^P				pseudo irish spotting	
	PMEL	**M (merle)**	**M**	**SINE**	**SINE**	**semi dominant**	**merle**	[39–41,46]
			m		**no SINE**		**no merle**	
			M/m		SINE/no SINE		mild merle	
	PSMB7	H (harlequin)	H	SNP	G	x	harlequin	[35,37]
			h		T		no harlequin	
Coatcoat structure	**FGF5**	**n.a.**	**n.a.**	**SNP**	**G**	x	**short hair**	[36]
					T		**long hair**	
	RSPO2	n.a.	n.a.	INDEL	no Ins		no furnishings	[36]
					Ins	x	furnishings	
	KRT71	**n.a.**	**n.a.**	**SNP**	**A**	**semi dominant**	**smooth coat**	[36,40]
					G		**curly coat**	
					A/G		wavy coat	
Tail length	T-Box_C295G	n.a.	n.a.	SNP	G	x	bobtail	[48,54]
					C		long tail	
Ear shape	**BICFPJ1062878**	**n.a.**	**n.a.**	**SNP**	**G**	**not clarified**	**non drop ears**	[89]
					A		**drop ears**	
Body size	IGF1R	n.a.	n.a.	SNP	G		rather tall	[49]
					A	x	rather small	

3.2.5. Body Size

The insulin-like growth factor 1 receptor (*IGF1R*) has a strong effect on the size of a dog. The allele "A" of the nonsynonymous SNP at 41,849,479 (CanFam 3.1) is a causal mutation for small body size in dogs (Table S4k) and is present in many tiny breeds [49].

IGF1R could be successfully genotyped for all dogs in the marker study. Even though only this single body size marker was included in the marker set, an accurate prediction of the body size in seven out of 10 dogs was possible (Tables S3b and S5).

3.3. Blind Test

In the course of the blind test, nine samples from dogs of blinded phenotypes were analysed with the 21-marker set, resulting in 189 genotypes. For this test, nine canine DNA extracts (D4925–D4931, D4933–D4934) were collected and prepared in a second lab—which also recorded the associated metadata including a photographic documentation—and were sent to the laboratory performing the tests. All samples were successfully genotyped in all markers (Table S3c). Subsequently, sketches of the nine dogs were drawn based on the genetic information obtained and compared to the dogs' phenotypes as displayed on photos, which were disclosed after the completion of the genetic analyses and the drawing of the sketches. Figure 2 shows a comparison between the photographical documentation and the images drawn based solely on the genetic data. Additionally, the outcome of the test is summarized as a heatmap (Table S5).

Three dogs had an identical genotype for all markers (D4926, D4928 and D4931) except for the ear shape marker, which showed a heterozygous state in D4931. Indeed, their phenotypical appearance was very similar, as all three individuals had black and tan points and minimal white spotting (S/S and a^t/a^t) fur, long smooth hair, a long tail, and a rather tall body size. In all three cases, the ear shape could not be traced by the provided photo documentation.

Dog D4927 showed a very similar genotype as the three dogs described above except the two E-locus markers, both being heterozygous, resulting in a correctly predicted "black tan points" fur including a melanistic mask (Figure 2).

For dog D4925, a high genotype–phenotype concordance was observed, except for the tail length. The genotype indicates a long tail, which is in contrast to the tail on the reference photo. However, the tail seemed to be artificially cropped.

For the light-coloured dog, D4929, with obvious upright ears, a high correspondence between genotypic prediction and phenotypic appearance could be achieved.

D4930 showed, in all but two markers, a high concordance between the genotypic predication and phenotypic appearance. The state of the body size marker suggested a tall body size that obviously did not match the dog's appearance. The heterozygous state at the ear shape marker led to inconclusive phenotypic interpretation.

Five of the six physical visible traits of D4933 were successfully predicted by the genetic data. Only the ear shape—non-drop ears—could not be unambiguously identified based on the reference photo. The K-Locus showed a heterozygous allelic state (K^B/k^y), which in some cases would indicate a brindle coat pattern, but the coat pattern of this individual was black with white spotting.

D4934 had a high correspondence between genotypic predication and phenotypic appearance for coat colour, coat pattern and coat structure, but for the body size, tail length, and ear shape, the assignments were discrepant or inconclusive, respectively.

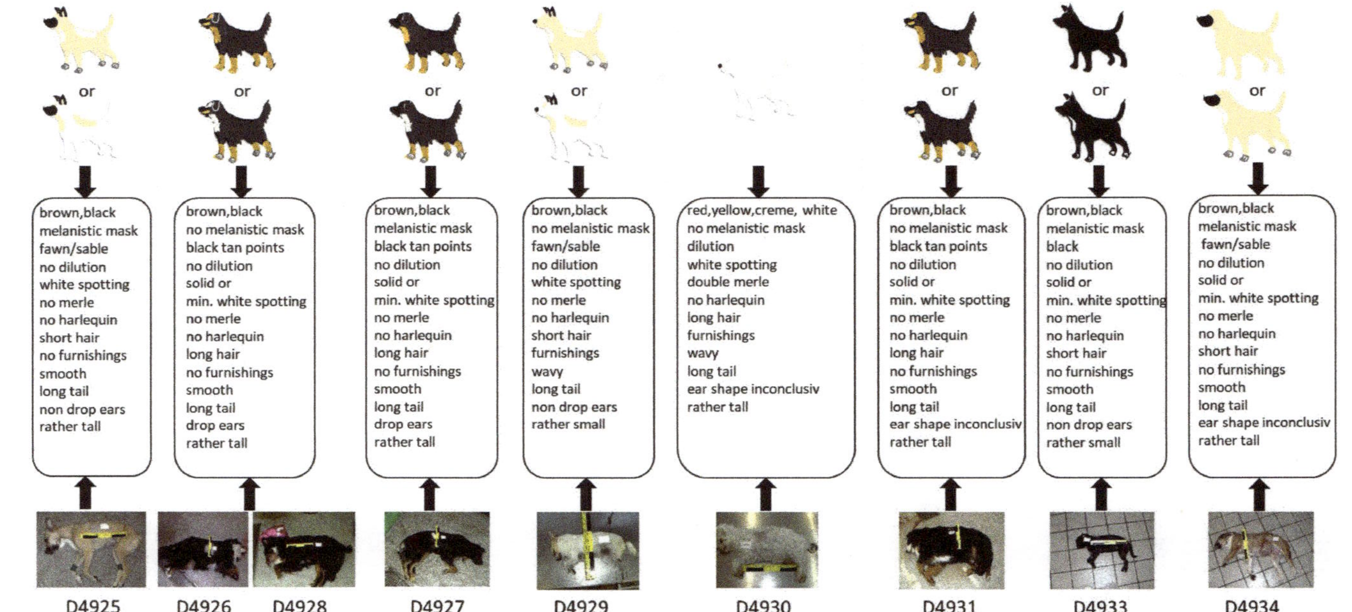

Figure 2. Results of the blind test: Identikit pictures (sketches) were drawn based on the genotypes and subsequently compared with photos of the nine tested dogs. Uncertainties in the manifestation of some visible characteristics required up to two versions of the identikit pictures. For all but one dog (D4930), two versions were necessary in order to reflect the possible phenotypes obtained from the genotype data. Dogs D4926 and D4928 showed the same genotype and therefore identical sketches. In general, identikit pictures and photos showed high levels of similarity. min. = minimal.

4. Discussion

The canine DNA phenotyping approach introduced here builds on established knowledge mainly gained in genome-wide association studies [49,50,90–94] and further advances in canine genetics, in particular, the sequencing of the dog genome [24,95–97]. Hence, there was no requirement to search for new candidate markers possibly associated with morphological traits; rather, a panel of published markers was selected, as summarized in Table 1. Genotyping of various visible traits in dogs has already been established in the context of medical research [98] or to support breeding efforts within particular breeds [82,99]. Existing applications of genomic prediction, some of which are commercially available, are mainly intended to verify pedigrees or breeds, to select specific phenotypes according to market demands or studbook policies, and to avoid associated inherited diseases. Obviously, the objectives of these approaches differ from forensic needs. One fundamental issue relates to sample quality. DNA evidence from crime scenes can be notoriously difficult to assess due to the low quantity and/or quality of DNA and the possibility of contamination with other DNA sources or substances (e.g., PCR inhibitors). Therefore, the aims of the pilot test included the optimization of the laboratory workflow and the verification of the published SNP or INDEL positions. This optimization step comprised the redesign of several published PCR primers, resulting in shortened amplicons (Table S2a), which are known to be more successful when analysing degraded DNA [100–102]. The successful completion of the pilot test was the methodological basis for the subsequent experiments.

Based on the idea of a proof of concept study, a relatively small selection of 21 genetic markers described in the literature as causative or highly correlated to externally visible traits was used. The reliability of predicting the phenotype was determined in the marker test. Given the relatively small number of markers addressed herein, the ability to differentiate visible traits turned out to be promising. However, the performance of the individual markers to correctly predict particular trait categories varied considerably. The choice of 15 markers selected for the categories coat colour and coat structure proved to be adequate, as shown by the high predictive accuracy for most of the dogs in this study. The coat colour and structure of nearly all dogs was predicted precisely as shown in Table S5. However, the results of the test also suggest that a targeted expansion of the number of markers could improve the predictions. An example for this assertion can be given for the *TYRP1* gene. Schmutz et al. [55] described the three *TYRP1* alleles—Q331ter, 345delP and S41C—that express a brown coat colour when a combination of any two of the recessive *TYRP1* alleles occurs. Our marker set included only the two markers TYRP1_Q331ter and TYRP1_345delP, which might explain the low performance of colour prediction under some allele combinations (Table S3). Therefore, the inclusion of at least a third *TYRP1* marker (allele "b^c"), a base substitution in exon 2 that causes a serine to cysteine exchange (S41C; c.121T>A), would probably increase the accuracy of coat colour prediction. Furthermore, it is possible that there are additional rare alleles of TYRP1 causing brown that were not detected in our original survey of dogs, but such alleles would likely be quite rare [55]. On the other hand, the category coat structure seems to be nearly perfectly covered by the three markers included in our marker set. In this category, all samples of the marker test and the blind test were correctly assigned. This is promising, as the category coat structure comprised eye-catching traits such as long hairs and curled coats, which were predicted accurately by only three markers.

For testing body size, only the IGF1R marker was applied. The body size from seven out of 10 dogs was predicted correctly based on simple classification "rather small" versus "rather tall". Hoopes et al. [49] hypothesized that the IGF1R nonsynonymous SNP is a causal mutation for tiny size in dogs. In their study, Allele A was present in many, but not all, of the tiny breeds. This indicates that the inclusion of more body size-associated markers may help to prevent a possible breed-specific bias. Breed-specific genotypes might also be the reason for false predicted tail length in three of 10 tested dogs. Some breeds including English bulldogs and Boston Terriers have bobtails without the mutation at the *T-Box* gene [48]. This could explain the observed discrepancy in samples AT0056 and AT0062, which belong to both breeds, respectively.

The marker with the lowest explanatory power proved to be IGF2BP2_BICFPJ1062878 which was selected to differentiate between drop ears and non-drop ears. Particularly, the heterozygous state, which was established in 60% of the tested dogs, did not allow for firm conclusions.

In a final step, the practical forensic applicability of our approach was evaluated in the blind test, comprising samples from nine dogs. To illustrate the global outcome of the 21-marker set, a sketch of each dog was prepared on bases of the genotypes observed, which included all characteristics deduced from the genetic data. The real phenotypical appearance was disclosed after the completion of the sketches by providing reference photos. A direct comparison between the sketches and the photos showed a high recognition effect, as laid out in Figure 2. The results of the blind test reflected those obtained in the marker test with a very high accuracy for coat colour, coat pattern and coat structure prediction. The discrepancies observed in the remaining traits may be related to the small number of genetic markers used for these traits, particularly for ear shape, body size and tail length. Additionally, the effect of (cosmetic) manipulation was observed as evident in the incorrect tail length prediction (long tail) of dog D4925, which was caused by cropping. Although prohibited in some countries, tail docking cannot be excluded. The same applies to ear cropping, which is also commonly observed. Such artificially altered body parts cannot be predicted but should be taken into consideration when translating the genetic information into a phenotypic sketch.

5. Conclusions

This proof of concept study for the first time presents an experimental approach to predict externally visible traits in dogs from DNA for forensic purposes. We used six trait categories that were selected on the bases of an untrained person´s ability to recognize them, as an eyewitness would probably be. The experiments were successful for the majority of the selected markers and predicted traits allowed for a realistic impression of the general appearance of the tested dogs. These promising results stimulate future research that requires an increased set of markers and individuals. We note that an extensive phenotypical documentation of the studied individuals is crucial for the interpretation of the predicted traits. Finally, we suggest the development of molecular genetic tools that allow for a stream-lined laboratory workflow compatible with forensic quality sample types.

Supplementary Materials: Supporting materials are available online at https://www.mdpi.com/2073-4425/12/6/908/s1, Figure S1a–d: sanger sequencing chromatograms of dog samples with heterozygous genotypes in length variant markers. The base circled indicates from where it is possible to distinguish alleles with (+) and without (−) the insertion. The arrow indicates the interpretation reading direction. The sequences of all SINEs and the insertion are provided in Table S2b. Table S1a: ASIP SINE, heterozygous state: SINE (−) and SINE (+), Table S1b: MITF SINE, heterozygous state: heterozygote SINE (−) and SINE (+), Table S1c: RSPO2 INS, heterozygous state: Insertion (−) and Insertion (+), Table S1d: PMEL SINE, heterozygous state: SINE (−) and SINE (+). Figure S2: Simplified chart of coat colour loci and alleles in the dog (modified according to Embark Veterinary https://embarkvet.com/breeders/resources/canine-genetics-for-dog-breeders/coat-color/genetics-101/) (accessed on 10 June 2021). It summarizes the dominance hierarchy of loci and alleles involved in the manifestation of coat colour and pattern. The colouring of the boxes ("Loci") and the coloured circles below the allele designations indicate the deducible coat colours. For simplicity, coat colour modifiers "S-locus" (white spotting), "D-locus" (dilution), "M-locus" (merle), and "H-locus" (harlequin) were not included.

Author Contributions: Conceptualization: C.B., B.B., W.H. and W.P.; Laboratory work: C.B. and J.H.; Data analysis: C.B. and J.H.; Provided Samples: CaDNAP and J.H.; Writing—original draft preparation: C.B., B.B. and J.H.; Writing—review and editing: W.H. and W.P.; Supervision: W.P. All authors have read and agreed to the published version of the manuscript.

Funding: This research received no external funding.

Institutional Review Board Statement: Not applicable.

Acknowledgments: Harald Niederstätter (Medical University of Innsbruck) is greatly acknowledged for his helpful assistance and discussion. Larissa Hasenheit is greatly acknowledged for her design of the dog drawing in Figure 1.

Conflicts of Interest: The authors declare no conflict of interest.

Appendix A

Collaborators (in alphabetic order) of CaDNAP (Canine DNA Profiling Group): Andreas Hellmann (Bundeskriminalamt, Kriminaltechnisches Institut, Wiesbaden, Germany), Nadja Morf (Institute of Forensic Medicine, University of Zurich, Switzerland), Udo Rohleder (Bundeskriminalamt, Kriminaltechnisches Institut, Wiesbaden, Germany); Uwe Schleenbecker (Bundeskriminalamt, Kriminaltechnisches Institut, Wiesbaden, Germany).

References

1. Kayser, M. Forensic DNA Phenotyping: Predicting human appearance from crime scene material for investigative purposes. *Forensic Sci. Int. Genet.* **2015**, *18*, 33–48. [CrossRef] [PubMed]
2. Kayser, M.; de Knijff, P. Improving human forensics through advances in genetics, genomics and molecular biology. *Nat. Rev. Genet.* **2011**, *12*, 179–192. [CrossRef]
3. Grimes, E.A.; Noake, P.J.; Dixon, L.; Urquhart, A. Sequence polymorphism in the human melanocortin 1 receptor gene as an indicator of the red hair phenotype. *Forensic Sci. Int.* **2001**, *122*, 124–129. [CrossRef]
4. Chaitanya, L.; Breslin, K.; Zuniga, S.; Wirken, L.; Pospiech, E.; Kukla-Bartoszek, M.; Sijen, T.; Knijff, P.; Liu, F.; Branicki, W.; et al. The HIrisPlex-S system for eye, hair and skin colour prediction from DNA: Introduction and forensic developmental validation. *Forensic Sci. Int. Genet.* **2018**, *35*, 123–135. [CrossRef] [PubMed]
5. Walsh, S.; Chaitanya, L.; Clarisse, L.; Wirken, L.; Draus-Barini, J.; Kovatsi, L.; Maeda, H.; Ishikawa, T.; Sijen, T.; de Knijff, P.; et al. Developmental validation of the HIrisPlex system: DNA-based eye and hair colour prediction for forensic and anthropological usage. *Forensic Sci. Int. Genet.* **2014**, *9*, 150–161. [CrossRef] [PubMed]
6. Walsh, S.; Kayser, M. A Practical Guide to the HIrisPlex System: Simultaneous Prediction of Eye and Hair Color from DNA. In Forensic DNA Typing Protocols. *Methods Mol Biol.* **2016**, *1420*, 213–231. [CrossRef]
7. Walsh, S.; Lindenbergh, A.; Zuniga, S.B.; Sijen, T.; de Knijff, P.; Kayser, M.; Ballantyne, K.N. Developmental validation of the IrisPlex system: Determination of blue and brown iris colour for forensic intelligence. *Forensic Sci. Int. Genet.* **2011**, *5*, 464–471. [CrossRef]
8. Walsh, S.; Liu, F.; Ballantyne, K.N.; van Oven, M.; Lao, O.; Kayser, M. IrisPlex: A sensitive DNA tool for accurate prediction of blue and brown eye colour in the absence of ancestry information. *Forensic Sci. Int. Genet.* **2011**, *5*, 170–180. [CrossRef]
9. Schneider, P.M.; Prainsack, B.; Kayser, M. The Use of Forensic DNA Phenotyping in Predicting Appearance and Biogeographic Ancestry. *Dtsch. Ärzteblatt Int.* **2019**, *116*, 873–880. [CrossRef]
10. Ostrander, E.A.; Wayne, R.K.; Freedman, A.H.; Davis, B.W. Demographic history, selection and functional diversity of the canine genome. *Nat. Rev. Genet.* **2017**, *18*, 705–720. [CrossRef]
11. Freedman, A.H.; Gronau, I.; Schweizer, R.M.; Ortega-Del Vecchyo, D.; Han, E.; Silva, P.M.; Galaverni, M.; Fan, Z.; Marx, P.; Lorente-Galdos, B.; et al. Genome sequencing highlights the dynamic early history of dogs. *PLoS Genet.* **2014**, *10*, e1004016. [CrossRef]
12. Freedman, A.H.; Wayne, R.K. Deciphering the Origin of Dogs: From Fossils to Genomes. *Annu. Rev. Anim. Biosci.* **2017**, *5*, 281–307. [CrossRef]
13. Thalmann, O.; Shapiro, B.; Cui, P.; Schuenemann, V.J.; Sawyer, S.K.; Greenfield, D.L.; Germonpre, M.B.; Sablin, M.V.; Lopez-Giraldez, F.; Domingo-Roura, X.; et al. Complete mitochondrial genomes of ancient canids suggest a European origin of domestic dogs. *Science* **2013**, *342*, 871–874. [CrossRef] [PubMed]
14. Frantz, L.A.; Mullin, V.E.; Pionnier-Capitan, M.; Lebrasseur, O.; Ollivier, M.; Perri, A.; Linderholm, A.; Mattiangeli, V.; Teasdale, M.D.; Dimopoulos, E.A.; et al. Genomic and archaeological evidence suggest a dual origin of domestic dogs. *Science* **2016**, *352*, 1228–1231. [CrossRef] [PubMed]
15. Perri, A.R.; Feuerborn, T.R.; Frantz, L.A.F.; Larson, G.; Malhi, R.S.; Meltzer, D.J.; Witt, K.E. Dog domestication and the dual dispersal of people and dogs into the Americas. *Proc. Natl. Acad. Sci. USA* **2021**, *118*, 6. [CrossRef] [PubMed]
16. Vilà, C.; Leonard, J.A. Canid Phylogeny and Origin of the Domestic Dog. In *The Genetics of the Dog*; Ostrander, E.A., Ruvinsky, A., Eds.; CABI: Wallingford, UK, 2012.
17. Perri, A. A wolf in dog's clothing: Initial dog domestication and Pleistocene wolf variation. *J. Archaeol. Sci.* **2016**, *68*, 1–4. [CrossRef]

18. Baumann, C.; Pfrengle, S.; Munzel, S.C.; Molak, M.; Feuerborn, T.R.; Breidenstein, A.; Reiter, E.; Albrecht, G.; Kind, C.J.; Verjux, C.; et al. A refined proposal for the origin of dogs: The case study of Gnirshohle, a Magdalenian cave site. *Sci. Rep.* **2021**, *11*, 5137. [CrossRef]

19. Botigue, L.R.; Song, S.; Scheu, A.; Gopalan, S.; Pendleton, A.L.; Oetjens, M.; Taravella, A.M.; Seregely, T.; Zeeb-Lanz, A.; Arbogast, R.M.; et al. Ancient European dog genomes reveal continuity since the Early Neolithic. *Nat. Commun.* **2017**, *8*, 16082. [CrossRef]

20. Bergstrom, A.; Frantz, L.; Schmidt, R.; Ersmark, E.; Lebrasseur, O.; Girdland-Flink, L.; Lin, A.T.; Stora, J.; Sjogren, K.G.; Anthony, D.; et al. Origins and genetic legacy of prehistoric dogs. *Science* **2020**, *370*, 557–564. [CrossRef]

21. Skoglund, P.; Ersmark, E.; Palkopoulou, E.; Dalen, L. Ancient wolf genome reveals an early divergence of domestic dog ancestors and admixture into high-latitude breeds. *Curr. Biol.* **2015**, *25*, 1515–1519. [CrossRef]

22. Parker, H.G.; Gilbert, S.F. From caveman companion to medical innovator: Genomic insights into the origin and evolution of domestic dogs. *Adv. Genom. Genet.* **2015**, *5*, 239–255. [CrossRef]

23. Moody, J.A.; Clark, L.A.; Murphy, K.E. Working Dogs: History and Applications. In *The Dog and Its Genome*; Ostrander, E., Giger, U., Lindblad-Toh, E., Eds.; Cold Springer Harbor Laboratory Press: New York, NY, USA, 2006; pp. 1–18.

24. Lindblad-Toh, K.; Wade, C.M.; Mikkelsen, T.S.; Karlsson, E.K.; Jaffe, D.B.; Kamal, M.; Clamp, M.; Chang, J.L.; Kulbokas, E.J., 3rd; Zody, M.C.; et al. Genome sequence, comparative analysis and haplotype structure of the domestic dog. *Nature* **2005**, *438*, 803–819. [CrossRef]

25. Parker, H.G. Genomic analyses of modern dog breeds. *Mamm. Genome* **2012**, *23*, 19–27. [CrossRef]

26. Parker, H.G.; Dreger, D.L.; Rimbault, M.; Davis, B.W.; Mullen, A.B.; Carpintero-Ramirez, G.; Ostrander, E.A. Genomic Analyses Reveal the Influence of Geographic Origin, Migration, and Hybridization on Modern Dog Breed Development. *Cell Rep.* **2017**, *19*, 697–708. [CrossRef]

27. Berryere, T.G.; Kerns, J.A.; Barsh, G.S.; Schmutz, S.M. Association of an Agouti allele with fawn or sable coat color in domestic dogs. *Mamm. Genome* **2005**, *16*, 262–272. [CrossRef]

28. Candille, S.I.; Kaelin, C.B.; Cattanach, B.M.; Yu, B.; Thompson, D.A.; Nix, M.A.; Kerns, J.A.; Schmutz, S.M.; Millhauser, G.L.; Barsh, G.S. A β-defensin mutation causes black coat color in domestic dogs. *Science* **2007**, *318*, 1418–1423. [CrossRef]

29. Dreger, D.L.; Schmutz, S.M. A SINE insertion causes the black-and-tan and saddle tan phenotypes in domestic dogs. *J. Hered.* **2011**, *102*, S11–S18. [CrossRef] [PubMed]

30. Philipp, U.; Hamann, H.; Mecklenburg, L.; Nishino, S.; Mignot, E.; Gunzel-Apel, A.R.; Schmutz, S.M.; Leeb, T. Polymorphisms within the canine MLPH gene are associated with dilute coat color in dogs. *BMC Genet.* **2005**, *6*, 34. [CrossRef] [PubMed]

31. Schmutz, S.M.; Berryere, T.G. The genetics of cream coat color in dogs. *J. Hered.* **2007**, *98*, 544–548. [CrossRef]

32. Schmutz, S.M.; Berryere, T.G.; Ellinwood, N.M.; Kerns, J.A.; Barsh, G.S. MC1R studies in dogs with melanistic mask or brindle patterns. *J. Hered.* **2003**, *94*, 69–73. [CrossRef] [PubMed]

33. Schmutz, S.M.; Berryere, T.G.; Goldfinch, A.D. TYRP1 and MC1R genotypes and their effects on coat color in dogs. *Mamm. Genome* **2002**, *13*, 380–387. [CrossRef]

34. Newton, J.M.; Wilkie, A.L.; He, L.; Jordan, S.A.; Metallinos, D.L.; Holmes, N.G.; Jackson, I.J.; Barsh, G.S. Melanocortin 1 receptor variation in the domestic dog. *Mamm. Genome* **2000**, *11*, 24–30. [CrossRef]

35. Clark, L.A.; Starr, A.N.; Tsai, K.L.; Murphy, K.E. Genome-wide linkage scan localizes the harlequin locus in the Great Dane to chromosome 9. *Gene* **2008**, *418*, 49–52. [CrossRef] [PubMed]

36. Cadieu, E.; Neff, M.W.; Quignon, P.; Walsh, K.; Chase, K.; Parker, H.G.; Vonholdt, B.M.; Rhue, A.; Boyko, A.; Byers, A.; et al. coat variation in the domestic dog is governed by variants in three genes. *Science* **2009**, *326*, 150–153. [CrossRef]

37. Clark, L.A.; Tsai, K.L.; Starr, A.N.; Nowend, K.L.; Murphy, K.E. A missense mutation in the 20S proteasome beta2 subunit of Great Danes having harlequin coat patterning. *Genomics* **2011**, *97*, 244–248. [CrossRef]

38. Kaelin, C.B.; Barsh, G.S. Genetics of pigmentation in dogs and cats. *Annu. Rev. Anim. Biosci.* **2013**, *1*, 125–156. [CrossRef] [PubMed]

39. Murphy, S.C.; Evans, J.M.; Tsai, K.L.; Clarke, L.A. Length variations within the Merle retrotransposon of canine PMEL: Correlating genotype with phenotype. *Mob. DNA* **2018**, *9*, 1. [CrossRef] [PubMed]

40. Saif, R.; Iftekhar, A.; Asif, F.; Alghanem, M.S. Dog Coat Colour Genetics: A Review. *Adv. Life Sci.* **2020**, *7*, 215–224.

41. Varga, L.; Lenart, X.; Zenke, P.; Orban, L.; Hudak, P.; Ninausz, N.; Pelles, Z.; Szoke, A. Being Merle: The Molecular Genetic Background of the Canine Merle Mutation. *Genes* **2020**, *11*, 660. [CrossRef] [PubMed]

42. Vaysse, A.; Ratnakumar, A.; Derrien, T.; Axelsson, E.; Rosengren Pielberg, G.; Sigurdsson, S.; Fall, T.; Seppala, E.H.; Hansen, M.S.; Lawley, C.T.; et al. Identification of genomic regions associated with phenotypic variation between dog breeds using selection mapping. *PLoS Genet.* **2011**, *7*, e1002316. [CrossRef]

43. Boyko, A.R. The domestic dog: Man's best friend in the genomic era. *Genome Biol.* **2011**, *12*, 216. [CrossRef]

44. Boyko, A.R.; Quignon, P.; Li, L.; Schoenebeck, J.J.; Degenhardt, J.D.; Lohmueller, K.E.; Zhao, K.; Brisbin, A.; Parker, H.G.; vonHoldt, B.M.; et al. A simple genetic architecture underlies morphological variation in dogs. *PLoS Biol.* **2010**, *8*, e1000451. [CrossRef]

45. Shearin, A.L.; Ostrander, E.A. Canine morphology: Hunting for genes and tracking mutations. *PLoS Biol.* **2010**, *8*, e1000310. [CrossRef] [PubMed]

46. Clark, L.A.; Wahl, J.M.; Rees, C.A.; Murphy, K.E. Retrotransposon insertion in SILV is responsible for merle patterning of the domestic dog. *Proc. Natl. Acad. Sci. USA* **2006**, *103*, 1376–1381. [CrossRef]

47. Leegwater, P.A.; van Hagen, M.A.; van Oost, B.A. Localization of white spotting locus in boxer dogs on CFA20 by genome-wide linkage analysis with 1500 SNPs. *J. Hered.* **2007**, *98*, 549–552. [CrossRef] [PubMed]

48. Hytonen, M.K.; Grall, A.; Hedan, B.; Dreano, S.; Seguin, S.J.; Delattre, D.; Thomas, A.; Galibert, F.; Paulin, L.; Lohi, H.; et al. Ancestral T-Box Mutation Is Present in Many, but Not All, Short-Tailed Dog Breeds. *J. Hered.* **2009**, *100*, 236–240. [CrossRef]

49. Hoopes, B.C.; Rimbault, M.; Liebers, D.; Ostrander, E.A.; Sutter, N.B. The insulin-like growth factor 1 receptor (IGF1R) contributes to reduced size in dogs. *Mamm. Genome* **2012**, *23*, 780–790. [CrossRef] [PubMed]

50. Karlsson, E.K.; Baranowska, I.; Wade, C.M.; Salmon Hillbertz, N.H.C.; Zody, M.C.; Anderson, N.; Biagi, T.M.; Patterson, N.; Pielberg, G.R.; Kulbokas, E.J.; et al. Efficient mapping of mendelian traits in dogs through genome-wide association. *Nat. Genet.* **2007**, *39*, 1321–1328. [CrossRef]

51. Thomas, R.; Duke, S.E.; Karlsson, E.K.; Evans, A.; Ellis, P.; Lindblad-Toh, K.; Langford, C.F.; Breen, M. A genome assembly-integrated dog 1 Mb BAC microarray: A cytogenetic resource for canine cancer studies and comparative genomic analysis. *Cytogenet. Genome Res.* **2008**, *122*, 110–121. [CrossRef]

52. Sutter, N.B.; Bustamante, C.D.; Chase, K.; Gray, M.M.; Zhao, K.Y.; Zhu, L.; Padhukasahasram, B.; Karlins, E.; Davis, S.; Jones, P.G.; et al. A single IGF1 allele is a major determinant of small size in dogs. *Science* **2007**, *316*, 112–115. [CrossRef]

53. Parker, H.G.; VonHoldt, B.M.; Quignon, P.; Margulies, E.H.; Shao, S.; Mosher, D.S.; Spady, T.C.; Elkahloun, A.; Cargill, M.; Jones, P.G.; et al. An Expressed Fgf4 Retrogene Is Associated with Breed-Defining Chondrodysplasia in Domestic Dogs. *Science* **2009**, *325*, 995–998. [CrossRef]

54. Haworth, K.; Putt, W.; Cattanach, B.; Breen, M.; Binns, M.; Lingaas, F.; Edwards, Y.H. Canine homolog of the T-box transcription factor T; failure of the protein to bind to its DNA target leads to a short-tail phenotype. *Mamm. Genome* **2001**, *12*, 212–218. [CrossRef] [PubMed]

55. Schmutz, S.M.; Berryere, T.G. Genes affecting coat colour and pattern in domestic dogs: A review. *Anim. Genet.* **2007**, *38*, 539–549. [CrossRef]

56. Welle, M.; Philipp, U.; Rufenacht, S.; Roosje, P.; Scharfenstein, M.; Schutz, E.; Brenig, B.; Linek, M.; Mecklenburg, L.; Grest, P.; et al. MLPH Genotype-Melanin Phenotype Correlation in Dilute Dogs. *J. Hered.* **2009**, *100*, S75–S79. [CrossRef]

57. Sykes, N.; Beirne, P.; Horowitz, A.; Jones, I.; Kalof, L.; Karlsson, E.; King, T.; Litwak, H.; McDonald, R.A.; Murphy, L.J.; et al. Humanity's Best Friend: A Dog-Centric Approach to Addressing Global Challenges. *Animals* **2020**, *10*, 502. [CrossRef] [PubMed]

58. Hughes, J.; Macdonald, D.W. A review of the interactions between free-roaming domestic dogs and wildlife. *Biol. Conserv.* **2013**, *157*, 341–351. [CrossRef]

59. Sarenbo, S.; Svensson, P.A. Bitten or struck by dog: A rising number of fatalities in Europe, 1995–2016. *Forensic Sci. Int.* **2021**, *318*, 110592. [CrossRef]

60. Berger, B.; Berger, C.; Hecht, W.; Hellmann, A.; Rohleder, U.; Schleenbecker, U.; Parson, W. Validation of two canine STR multiplex-assays following the ISFG recommendations for non-human DNA analysis. *Forensic Sci. Int. Genet.* **2014**, *8*, 90–100. [CrossRef]

61. Berger, B.; Berger, C.; Heinrich, J.; Niederstätter, H.; Hecht, W.; Hellmann, A.; Rohleder, U.; Schleenbecker, U.; Morf, N.; Freire-Aradas, A.; et al. Dog breed affiliation with a forensically validated canine STR set. *Forensic Sci. Int. Genet.* **2018**, *37*, 126–134. [CrossRef]

62. Eichmann, C.; Berger, B.; Parson, W. A proposed nomenclature for 15 canine-specific polymorphic STR loci for forensic purposes. *Int. J. Leg. Med.* **2004**, *118*, 249–266. [CrossRef]

63. Wictum, E.; Kun, T.; Lindquist, C.; Malvick, J.; Vankan, D.; Sacks, B. Developmental validation of DogFiler, a novel multiplex for canine DNA profiling in forensic casework. *Forensic Sci. Int. Genet.* **2013**, *7*, 82–91. [CrossRef] [PubMed]

64. Van Asch, B.; Pereira, F. State-of-the-Art and Future Prospects of Canine STR-Based Genotyping. *Open Forensic Sci. J.* **2010**, *3*, 45–52. [CrossRef]

65. Kanthaswamy, S.; Oldt, R.F.; Montes, M.; Falak, A. Comparing two commercial domestic dog (Canis familiaris) STR genotyping kits for forensic identity calculations in a mixed-breed dog population sample. *Anim. Genet.* **2019**, *50*, 105–111. [CrossRef]

66. Kanthaswamy, S.; Tom, B.K.; Mattila, A.-M.; Johnston, E.; Dayton, M.; Kinaga, J.; Erickson, B.J.-A.; Halverson, J.; Fantin, D.; DeNise, S.; et al. Canine population data generated from a multiplex STR kit for use in forensic casework. *J. Forensic Sci.* **2009**, *54*, 829–840. [CrossRef]

67. Hellmann, A.P.; Rohleder, U.; Eichmann, C.; Pfeiffer, I.; Parson, W.; Schleenbecker, U. A Proposal for Standardization in Forensic Canine DNA Typing: Allele Nomenclature of Six Canine-Specific STR Loci. *J. Forensic Sci.* **2006**, *51*, 274–281. [CrossRef]

68. Van Asch, B.; Alves, C.; Gusmao, L.; Pereira, V.; Pereira, F.; Amorim, A. A new autosomal STR nineplex for canine identification and parentage testing. *Electrophoresis* **2009**, *30*, 417–423. [CrossRef]

69. Budowle, B.; Garofano, P.; Hellman, A.; Ketchum, M.; Kanthaswamy, S.; Parson, W.; van Haeringen, W.; Fain, S.; Broad, T. Recommendations for animal DNA forensic and identity testing. *Int. J. Leg. Med.* **2005**, *119*, 295–302. [CrossRef]

70. Linacre, A.; Gusmao, L.; Hecht, W.; Hellmann, A.P.; Mayr, W.R.; Parson, W.; Prinz, M.; Schneider, P.M.; Morling, N. ISFG: Recommendations regarding the use of non-human (animal) DNA in forensic genetic investigations. *Forensic Sci. Int. Genet.* **2011**, *5*, 501–505. [CrossRef]

71. Safer, M.A.; Murphy, R.P.; Wise, R.A.; Bussey, L.; Millett, C.; Holfeld, B. Educating jurors about eyewitness testimony in criminal cases with circumstantial and forensic evidence. *Int. J. Law Psychiatry* **2016**, *47*, 86–92. [CrossRef]
72. Albright, T.D. Why eyewitnesses fail. *Proc. Natl. Acad. Sci. USA* **2017**, *114*, 7758–7764. [CrossRef]
73. Wise, R.A.; Kehn, A. Can the effectiveness of eyewitness expert testimony be improved? *Psychiatry Psychol. Law* **2020**, *27*, 315–330. [CrossRef] [PubMed]
74. Wixted, J.T.; Wells, G.L. The Relationship between Eyewitness Confidence and Identification Accuracy: A New Synthesis. *Psychol. Sci. Public Interest* **2017**, *18*, 10–65. [CrossRef]
75. Berger, B.; Heinrich, J.; Niederstatter, H.; Hecht, W.; Morf, N.; Hellmann, A.; Rohleder, U.; Schleenbecker, U.; Berger, C.; Parson, W.; et al. Forensic characterization and statistical considerations of the CaDNAP 13-STR panel in 1184 domestic dogs from Germany, Austria, and Switzerland. *Forensic Sci. Int. Genet.* **2019**, *42*, 90–98. [CrossRef]
76. Evans, J.J.; Wictum, E.J.; Penedo, M.C.; Kanthaswamy, S. Real-time polymerase chain reaction quantification of canine DNA. *J. Forensic Sci.* **2007**, *52*, 93–96. [CrossRef]
77. Little, C.C. *The Inheritance of Coat Color in Dogs*; Comstock: Ithaca, NY, USA, 1957; Volume 118, p. 572.
78. Schmutz, S.M.; Melekhovets, Y. Coat color DNA testing in dogs: Theory meets practice. *Mol. Cell. Probes* **2012**, *26*, 238–242. [CrossRef]
79. Kaelin, C.B.; Barsh, G.S. Molecular genetics of coat colour, texture and length in the dog. In *The Genetics of the Dog*; Ostrander, E.A., Ruvinsky, A., Eds.; CABI: Wallingford, UK, 2012; pp. 57–82.
80. Kerns, J.A.; Cargill, E.J.; Clark, L.A.; Candille, S.I.; Berryere, T.G.; Olivier, M.; Lust, G.; Todhunter, R.J.; Schmutz, S.M.; Murphy, K.E.; et al. Linkage and segregation analysis of black and brindle coat color in domestic dogs. *Genetics* **2007**, *176*, 1679–1689. [CrossRef]
81. Kerns, J.A.; Newton, J.; Berryere, T.G.; Rubin, E.M.; Cheng, J.F.; Schmutz, S.M.; Barsh, G.S. Characterization of the dog Agouti gene and a nonagoutimutation in German Shepherd Dogs. *Mamm. Genome* **2004**, *15*, 798–808. [CrossRef]
82. Dreger, D.L.; Hooser, B.N.; Hughes, A.M.; Ganesan, B.; Donner, J.; Anderson, H.; Holtvoigt, L.; Ekenstedt, K.J. True Colors: Commercially-acquired morphological genotypes reveal hidden allele variation among dog breeds, informing both trait ancestry and breed potential. *PLoS ONE* **2019**, *14*, e0223995.
83. Schmutz, S.M.; Berryere, T.G.; Barta, J.L.; Reddick, K.D.; Schmutz, J.K. Agouti sequence polymorphisms in coyotes, wolves and dogs suggest hybridization. *J. Hered.* **2007**, *98*, 351–355. [CrossRef]
84. Philipp, U.; Quignon, P.; Scott, A.; Andre, C.; Breen, M.; Leeb, T. Chromosomal assignment of the canine melanophilin gene (MLPH): A candidate gene for coat color dilution in Pinschers. *J. Hered.* **2005**, *96*, 774–776. [CrossRef]
85. Schmutz, S.M.; Berryere, T.G.; Dreger, D.L. MITF and White Spotting in Dogs: A Population Study. *J. Hered.* **2009**, *100*, S66–S74. [CrossRef]
86. Langevin, M.; Synkova, H.; Jancuskova, T.; Pekova, S. Merle phenotypes in dogs-SILV SINE insertions from Mc to Mh. *PLoS ONE* **2018**, *13*, e0198536.
87. Parker, H.G.; Shearin, A.L.; Ostrander, E.A. Man's best friend becomes biology's best in show: Genome analyses in the domestic dog. *Annu. Rev. Genet.* **2010**, *44*, 309–336. [CrossRef]
88. Indrebo, A.; Langeland, M.; Juul, H.M.; Skogmo, H.K.; Rengmark, A.H.; Lingaas, F. A study of inherited short tail and taillessness in Pembroke Welsh corgi. *J. Small Anim. Pract.* **2008**, *49*, 220–224. [CrossRef]
89. Jones, P.; Chase, K.; Martin, A.; Davern, P.; Ostrander, E.A.; Lark, K.G. Single-nucleotide-polymorphism-based association mapping of dog stereotypes. *Genetics* **2008**, *179*, 1033–1044. [CrossRef]
90. Bannasch, D.; Young, A.; Myers, J.; Truve, K.; Dickinson, P.; Gregg, J.; Davis, R.; Bongcam-Rudloff, E.; Webster, M.T.; Lindblad-Toh, K.; et al. Localization of canine brachycephaly using an across breed mapping approach. *PLoS ONE* **2010**, *5*, e9632. [CrossRef]
91. Schoenebeck, J.J.; Hutchinson, S.A.; Byers, A.; Beale, H.C.; Carrington, B.; Faden, D.L.; Rimbault, M.; Decker, B.; Kidd, J.M.; Sood, R.; et al. Variation of BMP3 Contributes to Dog Breed Skull Diversity. *PLoS Genet.* **2012**, *8*, e1002849. [CrossRef]
92. Schoenebeck, J.J.; Ostrander, E.A. The genetics of canine skull shape variation. *Genetics* **2013**, *193*, 317–325. [CrossRef]
93. Rimbault, M.; Ostrander, E.A. So many doggone traits: Mapping genetics of multiple phenotypes in the domestic dog. *Hum. Mol. Genet.* **2012**, *21*, R52–R57. [CrossRef]
94. Dreger, D.L.; Parker, H.G.; Ostrander, E.A.; Schmutz, S.M. Identification of a Mutation that Is Associated with the Saddle Tan and Black-and-Tan Phenotypes in Basset Hounds and Pembroke Welsh Corgis. *J. Hered.* **2013**, *104*, 399–406. [CrossRef]
95. Wang, C.; Wallerman, O.; Arendt, M.L.; Sundstrom, E.; Karlsson, A.; Nordin, J.; Makelainen, S.; Pielberg, G.R.; Hanson, J.; Ohlsson, A.; et al. A novel canine reference genome resolves genomic architecture and uncovers transcript complexity. *Commun. Biol.* **2021**, *4*, 185. [CrossRef]
96. Hoeppner, M.P.; Lundquist, A.; Pirun, M.; Meadows, J.R.; Zamani, N.; Johnson, J.; Sundstrom, G.; Cook, A.; FitzGerald, M.G.; Swofford, R.; et al. An improved canine genome and a comprehensive catalogue of coding genes and non-coding transcripts. *PLoS ONE* **2014**, *9*, e91172. [CrossRef] [PubMed]
97. Schoenebeck, J.J.; Ostrander, E.A. Insights into morphology and disease from the dog genome project. *Annu. Rev. Cell. Dev. Biol.* **2014**, *30*, 535–560. [CrossRef] [PubMed]

98. Donner, J.; Anderson, H.; Davison, S.; Hughes, A.M.; Bouirmane, J.; Lindqvist, J.; Lytle, K.M.; Ganesan, B.; Ottka, C.; Ruotanen, P.; et al. Frequency and distribution of 152 genetic disease variants in over 100,000 mixed breed and purebred dogs. *PLoS Genet.* **2018**, *14*, e1007361. [CrossRef]

99. Anderson, H.; Honkanen, L.; Ruotanen, P.; Mathlin, J.; Donner, J. Comprehensive genetic testing combined with citizen science reveals a recently characterized ancient MC1R mutation associated with partial recessive red phenotypes in dog. *Canine Med. Genet.* **2020**, *7*, 16. [CrossRef] [PubMed]

100. Grubwieser, P.; Muhlmann, R.; Berger, B.; Niederstatter, H.; Pavlic, M.; Parson, W. A new "miniSTR-multiplex" displaying reduced amplicon lengths for the analysis of degraded DNA. *Int. J. Leg. Med.* **2006**, *120*, 115–120. [CrossRef] [PubMed]

101. Grubwieser, P.; Muhlmann, R.; Parson, W. New sensitive amplification primers for the STR locus D2S1338 for degraded casework DNA. *Int. J. Leg. Med.* **2003**, *117*, 185–188. [CrossRef]

102. Hughes-Stamm, S.R.; Ashton, K.J.; van Daal, A. Assessment of DNA degradation and the genotyping success of highly degraded samples. *Int. J. Leg. Med.* **2011**, *125*, 341–348. [CrossRef]

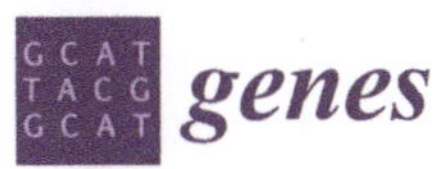

genes

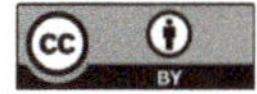

Review

A Review of Probabilistic Genotyping Systems: *EuroForMix, DNAStatistX* and *STRmix*™

Peter Gill [1,2,*], **Corina Benschop** [3], **John Buckleton** [4,5], **Øyvind Bleka** [1] and **Duncan Taylor** [6,7]

1   Forensic Genetics Research Group, Department of Forensic Sciences, Oslo University Hospital, 0372 Oslo, Norway; oeyble@ous-hf.no
2   Department of Forensic Medicine, Institute of Clinical Medicine, University of Oslo, 0315 Oslo, Norway
3   Division of Biological Traces, Netherlands Forensic Institute, P.O. Box 24044, 2490 AA The Hague, The Netherlands; c.benschop@nfi.nl
4   Department of Statistics, University of Auckland, Private Bag 92019, Auckland 1142, New Zealand; john.buckleton@esr.cri.nz
5   Institute of Environmental Science and Research Limited, Private Bag 92021, Auckland 1142, New Zealand
6   Forensic Science SA, GPO Box 2790, Adelaide, SA 5001, Australia; Duncan.Taylor@sa.gov.au
7   School of Biological Sciences, Flinders University, GPO Box 2100, Adelaide, SA 5001, Australia
*   Correspondence: peterd.gill@gmail.com

Abstract: Probabilistic genotyping has become widespread. *EuroForMix* and *DNAStatistX* are both based upon maximum likelihood estimation using a γ model, whereas *STRmix*™ is a Bayesian approach that specifies prior distributions on the unknown model parameters. A general overview is provided of the historical development of probabilistic genotyping. Some general principles of interpretation are described, including: the application to investigative vs. evaluative reporting; detection of contamination events; inter and intra laboratory studies; numbers of contributors; proposition setting and validation of software and its performance. This is followed by details of the evolution, utility, practice and adoption of the software discussed.

Keywords: probabilistic genotyping; *EuroForMix*; *DNAStatistX*; *STRmix*™

Citation: Gill, P.; Benschop, C.; Buckleton, J.; Bleka, Ø.; Taylor, D. A Review of Probabilistic Genotyping Systems: *EuroForMix, DNAStatistX* and *STRmix*™. *Genes* **2021**, *12*, 1559. https://doi.org/10.3390/genes12101559

Academic Editor: Emiliano Giardina

Received: 22 July 2021
Accepted: 28 September 2021
Published: 30 September 2021

1. Introduction

The use of software to evaluate DNA profile evidence is widespread in the forensic biology community. Since the late 1990 s software tools have been used to apply statistical evaluation models to observed DNA profile data. There are currently over a dozen different software applications that undertake this task. These can be grouped under the umbrella term 'probabilistic genotyping' (PG) systems. All evaluate DNA profile data within a probabilistic framework and provide a likelihood ratio (*LR*) to express the weight of evidence. The *LR* is the probability of the observed DNA profile data, given two competing propositions. Specifically, in the evaluation of DNA profile data within this framework, the *LR* is the ratio of the sum of weighted genotype sets that apply under each proposition.

In Section 2 we discuss some general, software-agnostic aspects of PG. We give an overview of available PG software and the class of modelling that each applies to carry out evaluation. An important aspect of any evaluation is the sensitivity of the *LR* to the data used to inform the model, and to the model choice itself (along with inherent underlying assumptions). Ideally, the *LR* would remain relatively stable regardless of the choices made within or between software (and therefore between models). There have been a number of validations for software individually, but also between laboratories using the same software, and between different software programs (Sections 2.4 and 3.6). User inputs are important to deal with uncertainty about the number of contributors to a DNA profile and to define propositions that are most appropriate to evaluate the value of the evidence.

In Sections 3 and 4 we review in detail three software applications; *EuroForMix, DNAStatistX* (these software utilise the same theory but have been independently prepared) and *STRmix™*. All are in regular use in multiple forensic biology laboratories around the world. These software applications utilise different models to describe DNA profile behaviour and have developed niche capabilities. There are also a number of support products, described in Sections 3 and 4, that add functionality for the user, either to perform additional analyses, or to display results in an interactive or more intuitive manner.

2. Probabilistic Genotyping in Generality

2.1. Probabilistic Genotyping Software

The recommended method for evaluation of DNA profile data in the forensic field is the *LR* [1–3]. It is assumed that autosomal markers are independent and in Hardy–Weinberg equilibrium. The *LR* seeks to determine the probability of obtaining some observed data (*O*) given a pair of competing propositions (H_1 and H_2), and any background information (*I*) about the framework of circumstances of the case that is relevant to the evaluation. Formulaically, the *LR* is expressed as:

$$LR = \frac{Pr(O|H_1, I)}{Pr(O|H_2, I)} \tag{1}$$

From this point on we omit the background information term, *I*, for visual clarity but note that it is ever present in the evaluation of any data. To calculate the *LR*, as shown in Equation (1), a number of nuisance parameters must be considered. The most fundamental of these (universal to any method of *LR* assignment) is the set of genotypes, *S*, that could belong to individuals whose DNA is present in the profile. Incorporating the *J* possible genotype sets into the *LR* from Equation (1) gives:

$$LR = \frac{\sum_{j=1}^{J} Pr(O|S_j)Pr(S_j|H_1)}{\sum_{j=1}^{J} Pr(O|S_j)Pr(S_j|H_2)} \tag{2}$$

The terms $Pr(S_j|H_x)$, $x \in \{1,2\}$, refer to the prior probability of observing the genotype set given a proposition. If the proposition specifies the presence of a particular individual, then any genotype set that does not contain the genotype corresponding to that individual (and depending on the model, the genotype of that individual in a specific component of the evidence profile) necessarily has a probability of 0. Any other genotype set has a prior probability that is assigned based on population genetic models and allele frequency databases. The terms $Pr(O|S_j)$ in Equation (2) are the probability of obtaining the observed data given a particular genotype set. These are often referred to as weights (and given the short-hand nomenclature of w_j) and are independent of propositions. The assignment of weights in the *LR* has been fundamental to much of the advancement that has occurred in probabilistic genotyping software used to interpret mixtures can be divided into three different groups;

Binary models

Qualitative, discrete or semi-continuous models

Quantitative, or continuous models

In early statistical models referred to as 'binary models', in which drop-out and drop-in were not considered, the weights were assigned values of 0 or 1, based on whether the genotype set accounted for the observed peaks (unconstrained combinatorial) and optionally on whether the peak balances were acceptable (constrained combinatorial). In essence binary models make yes/no decisions to associate genotypes with contributors, e.g., see the Clayton guidelines [4]. These early models were the precursors of more sophisticated methods that were introduced in later years. Whilst they perform calculations within a probabilistic framework, they are not probabilistic genotyping systems in nature as they do not treat the DNA profile information probabilistically, beyond specifying genotypes as being possible or impossible.

Later models referred to as qualitative ('discrete' or 'semi-continuous') [5–10] calculated weights as combinations of probabilities of drop-out and drop-in as required by the genotype set under consideration to describe the observed data. The qualitative models did not model peak heights directly but could use them to inform the nuisance parameter for the probability of drop-out or to infer a major donor genotype by applying different drop-out probabilities per contributor [11]. Whilst qualitative models do not use peaks heights directly, these systems do represent an advance over the binary model as they can take account of multiple contributors, low-template DNA and replicated samples.

Quantitative (or 'continuous') models [12–18] are the most complete because they take full account of the peak height information in order to assign numerical values to the weights. Using various statistical models these quantitative systems describe the expectation of peak behaviour in DNA profiles through a series of nuisance parameters that align with real-world properties such as DNA amount, DNA degradation, etc. A list of currently used PG software is provided in Supplement S1.

2.2. Investigative vs. Evaluative Forensic Genetics

The forensic scientist has a dual role as investigator and evaluator [3]. In conventional casework, a suspect is identified; the case-circumstances are reviewed, then the alternate propositions are formulated. This forms the basis of the court-case that the scientist will provide testimony. He/she is said to be in "evaluative mode" and the principles of interpretation apply as described, for example, by the ENFSI guideline [19].

Alternatively, a piece of evidence may be retrieved from a crime-scene, but there may not be a suspect available. In this instance the scientists will work in "investigation mode". To identify potential suspects for further investigation a national DNA database is typically searched.

Conventional database searches are usually restricted to searches of the person of interest (POI) from a crime-stain profile that has been deconvolved. This strategy is sufficient for single profiles and major/minor mixtures where the POI is represented in the former. However, if allele dropout has occurred and there are multiple contributors, then the POI may not be unambiguously resolved. The search is much more difficult, as many more candidates are possible, and it becomes much less likely to identify 'true-donor' candidates and more likely to obtain a long list of adventitious matches.

Probabilistic genotyping offers a much more complete way to search large databases. With a database of N individuals, each is considered as a possible candidate that is compared to the crime stain O. Consequently, a likelihood ratio can be generated for every individual in the database, where the propositions are:

H_1: Candidate n is a contributor to the evidence profile O

H_2: An unknown person is a contributor to the evidence profile O

Where all contributors to the profile not being considered as the candidate are designated as unknown and unrelated to the candidate. Consequently, for a well-represented DNA profile, the majority of candidates will return a low $LR < 1$, which means that they will be eliminated from the investigation; one or more may return $LR > 1$, and they are forwarded to the prosecuting authorities for further investigation. If the crime-stain is a low-template mixture of several contributors, the LRs will be lower and there may be numerous potential candidates, especially with searches of large databases of several million individuals. A list, ranked according to high→low LR, can be provided to investigators, but the extent of the investigation will be dependent upon the resources available. Lists may be shortened by prioritising candidates from a geographical location, or with known *modus operandi*. Once suspects are identified, they may become defendants and the scientist returns to evaluative mode reporting.

With complex cases, it may be of interest to identify individuals that may have contributed to multiple crime-stains. *STRmix*™ utilises the semi-continuous method of Slooten [20] to compare the alternative propositions:

The DNA profiles have a common contributor

The DNA profiles do not have any common contributors (it is assumed that contributors are unrelated)

The method does not depend upon a database search or direct reference profile comparison.

CaseSolver [21] is based upon *EuroForMix* and is designed to process complex cases with many reference samples and crime-stains. Here, mixtures are compared against reference samples only—however, mixtures can be deconvolved so that unknown contributors found in other samples may be cross-compared. *SmartRank* [22,23] (qualitative) and *DNAmatch2* [24] (quantitative) are used to search large databases and can also be used in contamination searches.

2.3. Probabilistic Genotyping to Detect Contamination Events

Investigative searches extend to comparisons of samples to detect potential contamination events [25,26] that may be propagated either by:

Contamination of reagents or consumables by laboratory staff or other laboratory employees, or at the crime scene, or in the examination room by investigators.

Sample to sample cross contamination during processing.

Type 1 contamination may be detected if each sample/mixture is compared to an elimination database of, e.g., crime scene investigators and laboratory staff.

Type 2 cross contamination, e.g., between capillary electrophoresis (CE) plates may occur. An extreme example is illustrated by the case of "wrongful arrest of Adam Scott" [27] pp. 21–31, where CE plates were accidentally reused by the laboratory. However, the biggest risk is with accidental carry-over of DNA on reusable tips or by capillary carry-over, where PCR products injected by a capillary are not completely removed during the cleaning process [25].

In much the same way that the improvement in PG systems has led to an increased ability to identify donors to profiles in a criminal context, so too has the power improved to identify contamination events. Additionally, with the continual drive for high-throughput capabilities, many contamination searching processes within PG systems are either automated, part of the laboratories information management system, or able to be set-up and run in bulk with minimal human effort. For further details about investigative searches with *STRmix*^{TM} refer to Section 4.5. *CaseSolver, DNAmatch2* and *SmartRank* are described in Section 3.4.

2.4. Inter and Intra-Laboratory Studies

The ultimate endpoint to a forensic biology evaluation is evidence presented in court. An expectation exists that information presented is reliable; one component of demonstrating reliability of PG systems, is to carry out studies on their practical use in casework. These studies can describe the performance of the PG systems in general (further details provided in Section 2.7), but also the consistency of their use in multiple laboratories by multiple people. Both inter- and intra-laboratory studies involve the distribution of mixtures with known ground truth, usually as electronic files after analysis, among forensic scientists within a laboratory and/or to a number of different laboratories. The compiled results give a measure of the variability in performance within and between laboratories [28–37]. At least two studies [38,39] (hereafter the GHEP-ISFG study and NIST studies) have appeared in courtroom discussion due to the wide range of results observed.

The GHEP-ISFG study applies various PG software to the same mixture and has been discussed in admissibility hearings. The results using *LRmix* varied from 2.6×10^3 to 3.2×10^{14}. This variability is based primarily upon human decision making and interpretation, e.g., choice of drop-in probability; drop-out probability and sub structuring population correction. It is further aggravated by the presence of three pairs of unresolved peaks. The variation is not intrinsic to the software but does emphasise that high reproducibility will only come by carefully considering the human element. We also note that much of the variation in human decision making comes from different actions intended to be conservative. In other studies using *LRmix*, such as [40], the results are comparable.

The NIST studies predate PG but have been subsequently reworked [41] using *STRmix™*, *EuroForMix* v1.10.0, *EuroForMix* v1.11.4, *Lab Retriever*, *LRmix*, and RMP (random match probability) [42]. The quantitative software, *STRmix* and *EuroForMix* (both versions), produced similar results with the exception of ref 5C for case 5. The qualitative software, *Lab Retriever* and *LRmix*, also produced results similar to each other. RMP was given as a benchmark.

Alladio et al. [43] compared *Lab Retriever*, *LRmix Studio*, DNA-VIEW®, *EuroForMix*, and *STRmix^{TM}*. In general, the quantitative software DNA-VIEW®, *EuroForMix*, and *STRmix^{TM}* performed similarly and the qualitative software *Lab Retriever* and *LRmix Studio* also performed similarly to each other, but differed from the quantitative methods. Alladio et al. concluded *"results provided by fully-continuous models proved similar and convergent to one another, with slightly higher within-software differences (i.e., approximatively 3–4 degrees of magnitude)"*. Iyer [44] has appealed to the community not to overlook the differences between software of the order of 3–4 orders of magnitude even in a pattern of overall similarity arguing that in some circumstances such differences could be crucial.

Alladio et al. suggested the use of a "statistic consensus approach [45]" which "consists in comparing likelihood ratio values provided by different software and, only if results turn out to be convergent, the most conservative likelihood ratio value is finally reported. On the contrary, if likelihood ratio results are not convergent, DNA interpretation is considered inconclusive." In the paper, convergent (a) and non-convergent (b) are defined as the two results both having (a) LR > 1 or LR < 1 and (b) one result LR > 1 and the other is LR < 1. Using such an approach would deem ref 5C for case 5 of the NIST study inconclusive using EuroForMix (LR about 10^3–10^6) and STRmix (LR about 0). The ground truth is that ref 5C is a non-donor, although it was an artificial construct based on resampling alleles from the profile [41] and consequently represents an outcome that would be rarely observed in actual case-work. However, from a recent collaborative study [46] we note that STRmix is more likely to report lower LRs when the alternative contributor has a high degree of shared alleles (as in cases of relatedness). In a much-discussed case in upstate New York (NY v Hillary) the result would also have been reported as inconclusive (STRmix LR about 10^5, TrueAllele LR not known but plausibly slightly less than 1). The ground truth in NY v Hillary is, of course, not known. Taylor et al. [47] take up the subject of the "statistic consensus approach" pointing out that either two quantitative or two qualitative systems should be used (this plausibly is also Alladio et al.'s view) and averaging might be better than taking the lowest. Furthermore, there is no particular reason to choose LR = 1 as a value to use in the definition of non-convergent. In fact, an LR that is the inverse of the, unknown, prior odds is more crucial from a decision theory perspective. To illustrate, suppose that the prior odds are 1:X, then it is not until the LR reaches X:1 that the posterior odds will begin to support a proposition that is potentially different from that supported by the prior odds. From a decision theory perspective, this is a threshold at which a switch may occur between two possible actions when making a decision.

Swaminathan et al. [48] create four variants of their *CEESIt* software and note some large differences in the resulting *LR*. This is relatively unsurprising as the underlying differences between their four versions are quite substantial and they analyse very low peak heights. For example, one large *LR* difference is driven by a peak at 6 rfu.

Whilst the *"statistic consensus approach"* is a rational approach to lack of consistency between different software we would add that it is vital to increase efforts to diagnose, and hopefully remedy, the inconsistency. It is a great pity that much larger efforts have not been made in this regard. Some of the authors are currently involved in such an exercise and results are already greatly promising.

A useful way to measure and compare the performance of models is with Receiver Operator Characteristics (ROC) plots [49]. These plots compare false positive support vs. false negative support rates relative to the observed *LR* (Figure 1). A good model simultaneously minimises the number of false positive and negative support for low values of *LR*. Figure 1 shows that the *LRmix* MLE and conservative qualitative models have lower true positive support rates compared to the quantitative *EuroForMix* MLE and conservative models, whereas false positive support rates are similar. This shows that the analysed quantitative models are more efficient; as discussed in the previous paragraph, this would not support a consensus approach between different classes (quantitative vs. qualitative) of models. For a given set of data, ROC plots are useful to compare performance of different models.

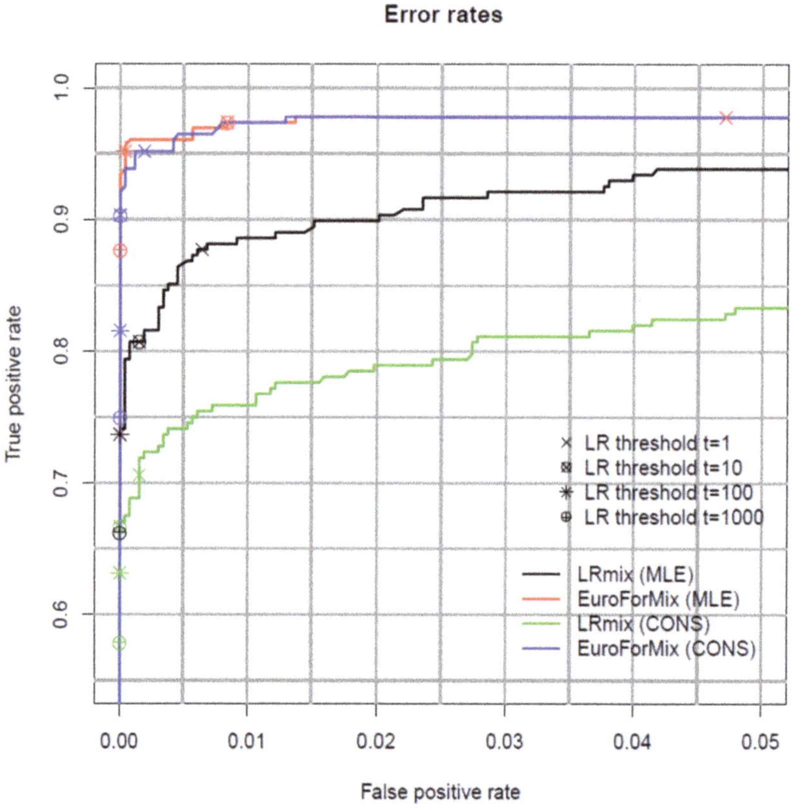

Figure 1. Receiver operating characteristic (ROC) plot where the rate of false positive support (FP) (horizontal axis) and true positives support (TP) (vertical axis) are plotted as a function of LR thresholds. The plot shows the results for the maximum likelihood estimation method (MLE) and the conservative method (CONS) for both *LRmix* and *EuroForMix*. The points on the curves show the FP and TP rates for different *LR* thresholds. Note that with this dataset, approximately 5% of samples were very low-level mixtures so that the POI was undetectable This caused the number of contributors to be underestimated, leading to very low (exclusionary) *LR*s. Therefore, the true positive rate does not reach 1.0 with the MLE method. Reprinted from [50], Copyright (2016), with permission from Elsevier.

You and Balding [51], also carried out ROC analysis to compare *EuroForMix* with *LikeLTD*. These are both γ models, with differing modelling assumptions; the overall results were similar. *LikeLTD* modelled forward $n + 1$ and complex $n - 2$ stutter and improvement was observed with some low template samples (since the version of *EuroForMix* used did not support these type of stutters). Manabe et al. [52] compared *Kongoh* with *EuroForMix*, both γ models, again finding strong similarities.

The first interlaboratory study with *STRmix* was reported by Cooper et al. [33]. In a subsequent enlargement of this exercise [53] two samples were examined. For one sample 176 responses were received with *LRs* ranging from $10^{28.3}$ to $10^{29.4}$. The bottom and top values were obtained by variation in human judgement elements such as dropping a locus (lowest *LR*) and a laboratory procedure that used a bespoke artefact handling process (top *LR*). For the 173 responses to the other sample, nine false exclusions were obtained by assigning numbers of contributors (NOC) as one fewer than the number used in construction of the sample. The remaining *LRs* reported varied from $10^{4.3}$ to $10^{6.6}$ with most of the variation attributable to *GeneMapper*® ID-X analysis settings used.

McNevin et al. [54] describe such variation as "extreme sensitivity" and set an expectation of much greater reproducibility in the reported statistic. This echoes a call, by for example the UK Forensic Science Regulator (pers. comm.) to obtain similar results regardless of the laboratory where the case is submitted. This would be dependent upon human factors, laboratory policy, and elements outside the province of the software, as well as the theory and application of the software itself.

Non-Contributor Tests and Calibration of the LR

Ramos and Gonzalez-Rodriguez [55] introduced the concept of "calibration of the likelihood ratio". Their purpose was to: "highlight that some desirable behaviour of *LR* values happens if they are well calibrated", meaning that the behaviour of the software is consistent with the expectations of a predefined model. Calibration applies a much more rigorous criterion than Turing expectation: the rate of non-contributor inclusionary support is at most the reciprocal of the *LR*, i.e., $\Pr(LR > x \mid H_2) \leq 1/x$ [56]. Calibration tests that *LRs* of any given magnitude are occurring at the expected rate. It has been applied to *STRmix*™ and *EuroForMix* [57,58].

It becomes increasingly difficult to test *LRs* as they become bigger as the number of samples needed becomes prohibitively large. Importance testing appears to be a remedy for this problem [59,60].

2.5. Number of Contributors (NOC)

In casework the number of contributors is unknown. This also holds for many mock samples, especially where at least one donor has left no detectable signal. When a parameter is unknown it is very useful to treat it as a nuisance parameter. We discuss some recently developed methods based on this principle.

For many years the assigned NOC to a DNA profile has been estimated by applying the maximum allele count (MAC) approach, often tempered by a human examination of peak heights. This approach uses the locus exhibiting the largest number of alleles at a locus, divided by two and rounded up to the nearest whole number [4,61] and ([62] chapter 7) and SWGDAM interpretation guidelines [63]. This method equates the NOC with the *minimum* number of contributors.

With such a method, the true NOC is uncertain, especially with high order mixtures (three or more) and/or low levels of DNA [64–66]. It is difficult to refer to the true NOC even in mock samples, but we will define it here as the number of donors that have left some signal above the analytical threshold.

Under- or over-estimating the NOC can affect the weight of evidence [67] with qualitative models [35,68,69].

With quantitative models, underestimating usually, but not always, leads to false negative support for the lowest template contributor. Overestimating tends to produce false positive support for non-donors, usually at relatively low *LRs*. The larger template donors are much more stable with respect to different NOC [70–73].

In some cases it is only possible to interpret the major contributor(s) of the DNA mixture. If minor contributors are not of interest, the NOC can be based upon the former, and this helps to simplify the model [72,74].

Increasing the number of loci, using those with a higher discriminatory power, or massively parallel sequencing (MPS) data of STR loci, resulted in fewer misinterpretations of the NOC compared to the MAC method [75–78].

Alternative methods using the total number of alleles (total allele count, TAC), the distribution of allele counts over the loci, the population's genotype frequencies, peak heights (PH), replicates, probability of allelic drop-out and stutter, or a Bayesian network approach have shown to yield improved NOC estimates [68,79–89].

The latest advances for estimating the NOC rely on machine learning approaches enabling optimal use of the available profile information. To date, a few models have been developed for use in forensic DNA casework [37,90–92]. These models make use of more information than the previously developed approaches since they are trained on a separate ground truth dataset. A big benefit of the machine learning approaches is that the estimation of the NOC can be performed in seconds, which is of importance in cases requiring rapid analyses. See Section 3.1.3 for a description of the NOC-tool used in *DNAxs*. The drawbacks of machine learning approaches are: (a) the requirement of large datasets that are specific to the laboratory that generated the data; (b) lack of transparency—the method of prediction may not be clear.

The need to assign the NOC for weight of evidence calculations is optimally treated by considering it as a nuisance parameter [71,92–98].

In an elegant mathematical development Slooten and Caliebe [94], making a few reasonable assumptions, show that the *LR* considering a reasonable range of NOC is the weighted average of the *LR* for each separate NOC. Specifically: $LR = \sum_i LR_i w_i$ where

$$LR_i = \frac{Pr(O_c, O_p | H_1, NOC = i)}{Pr(O_c, O_p | H_2, NOC = i)}$$

where $w_i = Pr(NOC = i | H_2, O_c, O_p)$ terms the weights, and O_c and O_p are the genotype of the crime profile and the POI, respectively. The weights are the probability of the number of contributors given the profile and assuming the POI is not a donor. This is the term that has been assessed subjectively for many years and can now be assigned as a probability distribution, sometimes with the assistance of software.

In an alternative approach, used with *EuroForMix*, the effective NOC is decided by maximizing the likelihood adjusted by application of the 'Akaike information criterion' (AIC) [99], which favours simpler models to explain the evidence. The smallest number of unknown contributors needed to explain the evidence usually maximises the respective likelihoods.

These approaches can be very useful since it is not necessary to define an absolute NOC and the field should move this way, though most of the current probabilistic genotyping systems still require that the user specifies the NOC [100]. *STRmix*™ v2.6 and higher treat NOC as a nuisance parameter but is currently only validated for taking into account two consecutive NOC values (say NOC = 3 or 4).

2.6. Proposition Setting/Hierarchy of Propositions

The application of Bayes' rule in odds form requires at least two propositions which are usually chosen to align with the prosecution position based upon the case circumstances and a reasonable alternative. The alternative will also be based on the case circumstances, ideally on information given by the defence (thus, the alternative is often referred to in the literature as the defence proposition).

There are at least two views of how the alternative should be set:

The scientist for the defence should assign this proposition, or in the absence of any meaningful consultation with the defense the scientist advising the prosecution assigns a reasonable alternative that is consistent with the best defense proposition and has a good approximation to exhaustiveness.

The concept of the hierarchy of propositions is well established [101,102]. Gittelson et al. [103] discussed this concept more recently; the ISFG DNA commission provides an extensive review [3], with recommendations for practitioners, also summarised by Gill et al. [62], chapter 12.

Propositions are classified into four levels: offence, activity, source, and sub-source.

Offence level propositions describe the issue for the fact finder which is one of guilt or innocence. This is a decision of the court; the forensic scientist does not offer opinions at this level.

Activity level propositions describe the activity that deposited the DNA. Provided that there is sufficient information, the forensic scientist may assist the court.

Source level refers to the origin of the body fluid or cell type examined. This is relatively straightforward if there is sufficient body fluid to test but may be challenging to address if there are low level mixtures of body-fluids.

Sub-source level refers to the origin of the DNA (i.e., donor).

It has proven useful to use a fifth level.

Sub-sub-source refers to the origin of part of the DNA, for example the major donor [104,105].

Probabilistic genotyping only provides information at sub-source and sub-sub-source levels. In order to make inferences at source and activity levels, separate calculations are required. If the distinction between levels in the hierarchy is not properly explained, it may lead to "carry-over" of the LR from one level to another which can lead to miscarriages of justice [3,27,106,107].

2.7. Validation of PG Systems

There are several publications that address 'validation' from scientific societies; for example: SWGDAM [108], ISFG [109], the AAFS Standards Board [110] and the UK Forensic Science Regulator [111]. Some laboratories have published validation studies—see Coble and Bright [100] for an excellent review and other guidance [108,109,112–117].

The purpose of validation is to define the scope and limitations of software. This is described in detail for *STRmix* (Section 4.6) and *EuroForMix/DNAStatistX* (Section 3.6) and Gill et al. [62] chapter 9.

George Box (a British statistician) famously stated: "Essentially, all models are wrong, but some are useful" [118]. All models are "wrong" in the sense that they are approximations of some unknown reality. However, so long as models demonstrate an empirical behaviour that conforms to expectations of a given reality, then they are "useful". The question that follows in relation to different PG software is whether models that are based upon different theories and assumptions are "equally reliable" or "equally useful"?

The terms "right" or "wrong" are two extremes. Probability is a numerical description, somewhere between 0 and 1, which describes how likely it is that an event will occur. Importantly, probability represents a personal belief about uncertainty, that is informed by available data. Provided scientists use the same or similar datasets and the same methods of analysis, then their personal beliefs should coincide. We never know if something is true or not, but probability is always conditioned upon some hypothesis/ proposition being true.

As an example, consider the probability assigned for an allele that has never been seen before in the population sample (hereafter "rare allele"), but is observed in this case. We can say for certain that the "true" probability of this allele is not 0, but we are uncertain exactly what it is. Whenever something is unknown and uncertain it is best to model the uncertainty with a probability density function. A workable option may be to insert a reasonable point estimate. Further, in forensic science, some aspects of utility are usually confounded into the probability assignment by deliberately biassing the assignment in a direction thought to be conservative. However, in mixture evaluation the conservative direction is very uncertain. For example, it is typically conservative to raise the sample allele probability for the alleles that correspond with the person of interest (POI), but for any other alleles the effect may be neutral or may vary either way. The use of a point estimate biased upwards (for example $5/2N$ or $3/2N$ where N is the number of alleles in the sample) is plausibly conservative on average, although we are unaware of any systematic investigation of this assumption. The use of a probability density distribution and resampling may enable the choice of a conservative quantile but requires assignment of a distribution. It would be very difficult, and be a matter of subjective judgement, to choose which of these methods is appropriately conservative.

In the context of PG software, where two software may implement two different models for the same process we can assess how well the models describe the empirical data, then we can have confidence in the result. This can readily be supplemented by varying the model within reasonable limits dictated by the data and thus creating a range of plausible outcomes. We are left with the uncertainty that small modelling and inferential errors accrue, or that the training data for the models are inappropriate.

There are various phases to a validation programme, originally described by Rykiel [119] in relation to ecological models:

Conceptual validation: verification of the mathematical formulae used in the software are correct.

Software validation: Verification and testing of the code, e.g., by running test scripts.

Operational validation: The output of the model is tested against a wide range of evidence types, representing a typical case, as well as extreme examples.

A validation programme can address the following:

(a)   Sensitivity (demonstrate the range of *LRs* that can be expected for true contributors)
(b)   Specificity (demonstrate the range of *LRs* that can be expected for non-contributors)
(c)   Precision (variation in *LRs* from repeated software analyses of the same input data)

Accuracy of statistical calculations and other results (comparison to an alternate statistical model or software program)

Determination of the limits of the software (either computational or conceptual, regarding for instance the number of unknown contributors or types of DNA profiles)

Steps towards internal validation, to enable a laboratory to adopt a given procedure, was described by [115] as an "accumulation of representative test data within the laboratory to demonstrate that the established parameters, software settings, formulae, algorithms and functions perform as expected"

In real casework, we do not know the ground truth. In validation, the model is tested against samples where the ground truth is usually known. This enables two kinds of tests to be carried out using the standard likelihood ratio formula: $LR = Pr(O \mid H_1)/Pr(O \mid H_2)$

(a) H_1 = true: where we know the POI is a contributor.
(b) H_2 = true: where we know that the POI is not a contributor

As a small word of caution: the ground truth is not known even for mock samples for very low level contributors. For these it can be unclear whether they are, in reality, a donor at all.

3. Evolution of *EuroForMix* and *DNAStatistX*

3.1. Evolution

An outline of the development and evolution of the software *EuroForMix* and *DNAStatistX*, including its predecessors and related modules is shown in Figure 2. These software will be discussed in the next sections.

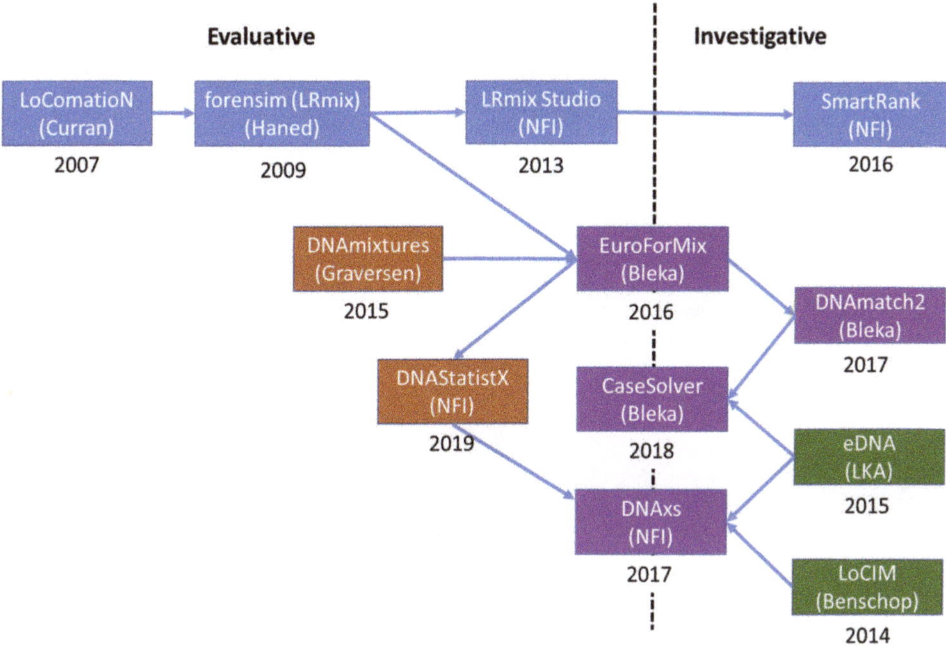

Figure 2. A diagram showing the evolution of probabilistic genotyping software developed by the NFI and Oslo University Hospital. Blue and orange boxes indicate qualitative and quantitative (γ) models, respectively. Green boxes are binary methods and purple boxes indicate software that include multiple types of methods.

3.1.1. Qualitative Software

The development of probabilistic genotyping undertaken by the authors began in 2007 with the development of qualitative software (discrete or semi-continuous) which took account of allele drop-out and drop-in, but peak heights were not modelled. The first software was the introduction of *LoComatioN* by James Curran [120], whilst at the Forensic Science Service (UK). The model was re-programmed by Hinda Haned [121,122], as part of her PhD at the University of Lyon: *LRmix* is written in R and the module is found in the *forensim* package: https://forensim.r-forge.r-project.org/ accessed on 28 September 2021. Four years later, in 2013, the Netherlands Forensic Institute (NFI) adopted *LRmix*, rewriting the code into Java and rebranding it as *LRmix* Studio: https://github.com/smartrank/lrmixstudio accessed on 28 September 2021. This software has been widely adopted in Europe and elsewhere. LRmix Studio was further developed by NFI to provide SmartRank: https://github.com/smartrank/smartrank accessed on 28 September 2021, a database search engine [23] which was shown to be more efficacious than the CODIS search engine [22]; it is still widely used by caseworkers (see collaborative study of Prieto et al. [40]).

For further details see Gill et al. [62] chapters 5 and 6. Exercises and presentations are available from: https://sites.google.com/view/dnabook/chapter-6?authuser=0 accessed on 28 September 2021.

3.1.2. Quantitative Software

Early models designed to explain variation in peak area observations were described in 1998 by *Evett* et al. [123] who defined an underlying normal distribution and in 2007 by *Cowell* et al. [18,124] who also defined a γ distribution (the γ model).

In 2013, Cowell, Graversen and colleagues released *DNAmixtures* which was based on the γ model [125,126]: http://dnamixtures.r-forge.r-project.org/ accessed on 28 September 2021, written in R code as open-source, but requires HUGIN (commercial software) to run it. Supported by the EU-funded EuroForGen-Network- of-Excellence: https://www.euroforgen.eu/ accessed on 28 September 2021, the γ model was re-written in R and C++ by Øyvind Bleka as *EuroForMix*: http://www.euroformix.com/ accessed on 28 September 2021. This program had enhanced capabilities compared to *DNAmixtures*, including degradation parameterisation and "theta-correction" (*Fst*).

EuroForMix was further utilized to provide the database search tool *DNAmatch2*, which also incorporated the *forensim LRmix* module, in order to carry out searches of large national DNA databases. Later, the same modules were integrated into a more user-friendly expert system called *CaseSolver* which is integrated into casework for analysing complex cases where there are multiple suspects and case-stains. *CaseSolver* includes many useful features for caseworkers: Visualization, automated comparison, deconvolution, weight-of-evidence evaluation and reporting (discussed in Section 3.4).

In 2019, the NFI implemented *DNAStatistX*, the statistical module based on the *EuroForMix* code which is further elucidated in Section 3.3.1. *DNAStatistX* can be used as a stand-alone application or within the DNA eXpert System, *DNAxs*. *DNAxs* is a software suite that was developed by the NFI, for the data management and (probabilistic) interpretation of DNA profiles. It was implemented in forensic casework in 2017 and is under continuous development to further advance the software, to improve the process of DNA casework and to broaden the scope of application. Further information on the *DNAxs* functionalities is provided in the following section.

3.1.3. DNAxs and Related Modules

Increased complexity of DNA profile comparisons and interpretation demands fast and automated software tools to assist DNA experts in routine casework. *eDNA* is one such application [127], whose functionalities were an inspiration for the development of *CaseSolver* [21] and the *DNA eXpert System DNAxs* [128].

Within *DNAxs*, profile comparisons can be achieved at various levels:

(1) By aggregating replicate profiles into one composite view (bar graphs)
(2) By viewing the trace profile as bar graphs underneath which alleles of reference profiles are comparedThrough the match matrix option
(3) By sending a DNA profile for a *SmartRank* search against the DNA database
(4) By calculating *LRs* using *DNAStatistX* for a comparison of a person of interest to a trace DNA profile [128]

DNAxs imports (pre-analyzed) DNA profiling data which is shown as the original electropherogram and is graphically represented as bar graphs with a color coding for reproduced and non-reproduced alleles in case of PCR replicates, and a color coding for alleles of the major component of a mixture through the *LoCIM* method (Locus Classification and Inference of the Major) [29]. This *LoCIM* method can be applied to one amplification of a DNA extract or to replicate DNA profiles. In the latter case, *LoCIM* first generates a consensus profile that includes alleles that are observed in at least half of the replicates [86]. Next, *LoCIM* classifies each locus as type I, II or III based on thresholds for peak height; ratio of major to minor contributors; and heterozygote balance. A Type I locus fulfils the most stringent criteria and will most likely be correctly inferred. Type II loci may have lower peak heights or a smaller difference in peak heights compared to minor donors. Type III loci do not meet one or more of the Type II criteria and are the most complex to infer a major contributor's genotype. Lastly, thresholds are used per locus type to infer the major component's alleles. It has been demonstrated that the *LoCIM* approach is successful regardless of the laboratory's STR typing kit and PCR and CE settings and the method is easy to implement (one only needs to specify the laboratory's stochastic threshold) [29,37].

The major contributor's genotype predicted by the deconvolution method of *EuroForMix* described in Section 3.3.4 (on loci with a probability that was at least twice as large as the second likeliest genotype possibility) was compared to that of *LoCIM* (on type I and II loci). Both methods are able to perform deconvolution by utilizing the peak height information, though *LoCIM* is threshold based while *EuroForMix* applies a statistical model which consists of a set of parameters which are inferred by maximizing the likelihood function [50]. *EuroForMix* applies a more comprehensive statistical model which calculates the uncertainty of different suggested genotype profiles extracted from the inferred uncertainty of the whole evidence profile. Therefore, these calculations are much more computationally intensive compared to the extremely fast *LoCIM* method. At the locus level, and as expected, the *EuroForMix* deconvolution showed improved performance compared to *LoCIM* [50]. Regardless, since *LoCIM* is extremely fast and was regarded useful to many cases, this approach was implemented in *DNAxs* [62], chapter 10 and [37].

DNAxs provides summary statistics for its comparisons, such as the number of mismatches or unseen alleles, and to help estimating the NOC- such as the maximum allele count (MAC) and the total allele count (TAC). Furthermore, *DNAxs* includes NOC tools based on a machine learning approach. These are designated as the RFC19 model that is specific to PowerPlex Fusion 6C (PPF6C) data as generated within NFI [89] and the generic RFC11 model which is laboratory independent [37]. The RFC19 model outperformed the MAC method and an in-house developed tool that utilised the TAC [89,91]. A drawback of such models is that it requires a large dataset for development and is specific to a laboratory's data. To that end, the generic model was developed, which only involves features of the 12 European Standard Set and U.S. core loci, and does not include features holding information on peak heights or fragment lengths. The generic RFC11 model overall showed improved NOC estimates for data of different laboratories when compared to the MAC method but performed less efficiently when compared to the PPF6C specific RFC19 model, since it uses less of the available information. However, in absence of a data specific machine learning NOC model, or in absence of data or too limited resources to develop such model, the generic RFC11 model was found to be a useful alternative that can serve as an addition to the reporting officer's toolbox to interpret mixed DNA profiles [37]. Another drawback of machine learning models is their lack of transparency; the model outputs a prediction but not how it obtained to the particular result. Therefore, in a study of Veldhuis et al. [129], eXplainable artificial intelligence (XAI) was introduced to help users understand why such predictions are made.

Lastly, through web APIs (Application Programming Interfaces) *DNAxs* can communicate with, for instance, CODIS, LIMS systems, *SmartRank*, and *Bonaparte* [128]. Additionally, as previously mentioned, for weight of evidence calculations, *DNAxs* implements *DNAStatistX*, which, alike *EuroForMix*, uses the γ distribution to model peak heights.

3.2. The γ Model

The model adopted by the authors is known as the "γ model" which was first described by Cowell et al. [124,130].

The γ distribution is defined by two parameters known as shape α and scale β. There is a different shape parameter per contributor in the *EuroForMix* model, but there is only one (universal) scale parameter that is applied. The observed peak height is given as y.

The probability density function of the γ distribution is:

$$f(y|\alpha,\beta) = \frac{1}{\beta^\alpha \Gamma(\alpha)} y^{\alpha-1} \exp(-\frac{y}{\beta}) = gamma(y|\alpha,\beta) \tag{3}$$

where α and β are the shape and scale parameters, respectively, and $\Gamma(x)$ is the γ function. The density function given in Equation (3) and provides the 'weightings' in *EuroForMix* and *DNAStatistX*.

The shape and scale parameters are calculated based on the following model parameters (for two donors):

M_x: the mixture proportion for contributor 1 and *1-Mx*, the mixture proportion for contributor 2

μ: the peak height expectation (close to the average peak heights)

ω: the coefficient of peak height variation (indicates variability)

An example is provided in Figure 3. Further details are in Supplement S2.

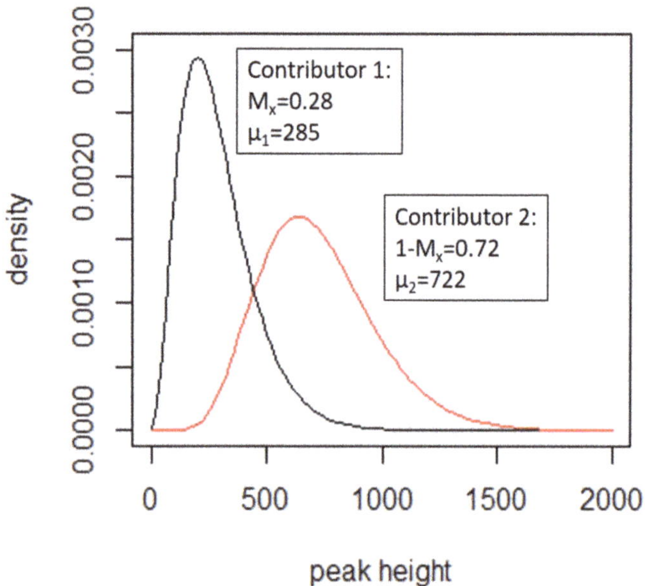

Figure 3. γ distributions for a simple case, where shape parameters = 3.312 and 8.381, respectively and the scale parameter is 86.2. The peak height expectation (μ) and *Mx* are shown for each contributor. The probability density function for the individual peak height contributions are derived from these curves. Reprinted from [62], chapter 7, Copyright (2020) with permission from Elsevier.

There is a detailed explanation of the model, in Gill et al. [62], chapter 7.

For a more detailed explanation, as applied to *EuroForMix* and *DNAStatistX*, see Gill et al. [62], chapter 7 and associated website where excel spreadsheets, tutorials and exercises can be downloaded: https://sites.google.com/view/dnabook/chapter-7?authuser=0 accessed on 28 September 2021.

The complexity of the γ model is increased by additional parameters: degradation, forward and backward stutter.

3.3. An Outline of the γ Model Incorporated into Euroformix and DNAStatistX

The aim is to quantify the value of evidence if a POI is a contributor to a crime-scene profile *O*. Two alternative propositions are specified and the likelihood ratio (*LR*) evaluates how many more times likely it is to observe the evidence given that H_1 is true compared to the alternative that H_2 is true.

3.3.1. Model Features

EuroForMix and *DNAStatistX* support multiple contributors, can condition upon any number of reference profiles and can specify any number of unknown individuals, although there is a practical limit of c. 4 due to computational time.

1. The software accommodates degradation, allele drop-out, allele drop-in, '$n-1$' and '$n+1$' stutters and sub-population structure (*Fst* correction). Note that stutters are not accommodated in the current version of *DNAStatistX*, but is under development for a future version.
2. Replicated samples can be analysed. Consensus or composite profiles, a feature of pre-PG software, are not used.
3. The model assumes same contributors and the same peak height properties for each replicate.

4. Optional Locus specific settings (*DNAStatistX* from v1, *EuroForMix* v3 onwards) are as follows:

   (a) Analytical threshold
   (b) Drop-in model
   (c) Fst correction

Although *EuroForMix* and *DNAStatistX* are based upon the same model, there are some differences. The software are programmed in different languages (*EuroForMix* in R and C++ and *DNAStatistX* in Java) and therefore not all of the numerical libraries *EuroForMix* uses were available when developing *DNAStatistX*. As a result, alternative methods for function optimization were explored and selected. Despite the differences in the choice of function optimizer, the two software yield *LRs* in the same order of magnitude when the same data and model options are used [128]. *DNAStatistX* is implemented within the overall software package, *DNAxs,* which supports parallel computing that can be delegated to a computer cluster and enables queuing of requested *LR* calculations. This feature can be extremely useful in a routine casework setting. Both software continue development though functionalities and options can be prioritized differently by their developers and users.

Whereas *DNAxs* parallelises over independent function optimizations (current version), *EuroForMix* applies parallelisation within the inner part of the algorithm, where genotype summation is performed (versions before v3 also parallelised over function optimizations).

3.3.2. Exploratory Data Analysis

The reported *LR* is critically dependent upon the assumptions applied in the model. The parameters that are fixed include: the population database including allele frequencies, the level of *Fst* and the drop-in parameters used to specify the drop-in model.

The variable parameters are mixture proportions (Mx), peak height variation (coefficient-of-variation), peak height expectation and the NOC. Decisions are needed whether to use a stutter and/or a degradation model: Real case examples typically employ degraded DNA causing a reduction in observed peak heights when the molecular fragment lengths increase. The stutter models are important to apply when stutter filters are not applied—nevertheless there may still be alleles present in the profile which could be explained as stutters. In addition, the number of contributors can have an impact—so this must be carefully decided (Section 2.5).

Finally, any model that is used for reporting must be a reasonable fit to the γ distribution. In order to highlight the principles of exploratory data analysis, details are described by Gill et al. [62] (chapter 8).

3.3.3. Relatedness

The defence may wish to put forward a proposition that a sibling (or another close relative) was the contributor to the crime stain, hence the defence alternative considered may be H_2: "The DNA is from a sibling of Mr. X".

The calculations are described using formulae described by Gill et al. [62], chapter 5.5.4 and appendix A.2; encoded into *LRmix Studio* and *EuroForMix*. Examples can be found from the "Relatedness" folder at: https://www.dropbox.com/home/Book/Data%20for%20website/Chapter8/Relatedness accessed on 28 September 2021.

This folder contains laboratory data from derived samples of three person mixtures using the 'PowerPlex® Fusion 6C' kit and Dutch database frequencies from a study by Benschop et al. [73]. To explore whether closely related individuals will give a high *LR* when Mr X is substituted by a sibling, we specify following propositions:

H_1: The DNA is from Mr. X
H_2: The DNA is from an unknown contributor

A total of 100 siblings were simulated. The majority provide a low *LR* (exclusionary: $LR < 1$). A total of six *LRs* were greater than 100, with two approximating $\log_{10}LR \approx 6$. However, if the propositions are altered to:

H_1: The DNA is from Mr. X
H_2: The DNA is from a sibling of Mr. X,

both *LR*s returned values less than one, favouring H_2. This exercise illustrated that (a) close relatives can occasionally provide high *LR*s when tested against the proposition of unrelatedness, but (b) if the proposition is altered to ask the question of relatedness, then the evidence can support H_2. This illustrates the importance of asking the right questions based upon the case-circumstances, i.e., when propositions are formulated, they must be reasonable and they must above all be based upon a clear understanding of the case circumstances.

3.3.4. Deconvolution

Deconvolution is used to predict the genotype of an 'unknown' contributor to a crime stain and it is typically undertaken to extract a profile in order to search a national DNA database. The method is described by Gill et al. [62], chapter 8.5.12, or in Section 4.3.1 for the specifics of the deconvolution model in *STRmix*™. There are several different ways to represent the data. The most common usage is to provide the 'top marginal' where the most likely genotype (for the unknown component) is extracted. Each genotype (per locus) is accompanied by 'the ratio to next genotype' which is the ratio of the top probability to the second highest probability. The larger the ratio, the greater the confidence in the genotype selected [50,131].

3.4. Investigative Forensic Genetics

Probabilistic Genotyping to Carry out Searches of National DNA Databases

SmartRank is based upon *LRmix Studio* [22,23], but was modified to enable searches of very large national DNA databases. A validation study [22] tested anonymised parts of the national DNA databases of Belgium, the Netherlands, Italy, France and Spain, along with a simulated DNA database. To each of the databases, 44 reference profiles were added. A total of 343 mixed DNA profiles were prepared from the reference samples, to act as the test set of data. Finally, the data were searched with both *SmartRank* and CODIS software.

Searches are most successfully employed when the mixtures are simple (major/minor) coupled with low levels of dropout. CODIS works by applying simple allele matching criteria whereas *SmartRank* takes account of allele drop-out, and was shown to be a more effective method to identify contributors for mixed profiles with low to moderate drop-out. *SmartRank* can be downloaded from https://github.com/smartrank/smartrank accessed on 28 September 2021 along with user guides; exercises are available at: https://www.dropbox.com/home/Book/Data%20for%20website/Chapter%2011/SmartRank_Exercises and chapter accessed on 28 September 2021 [62].

DNAmatch2 and CaseSolver are search engines which also adopt the quantitative model from *EuroForMix* [21,24]. A stepwise strategy is employed to search for matches, since a search using *EuroForMix* alone would be time-consuming. Consequently, the comparisons are filtered in a stepwise procedure. First, a simple matching allele count is carried out where for example, samples exceeding a defined drop-out level are rejected. The remaining comparisons are then searched using the qualitative *LRmix* model from *forensim* (similar to *SmartRank*). This step is very fast: samples providing *LR*s above a certain threshold are then re-tested using the quantitative *EuroForMix* model to provide a final list of ranked *LR*s. Studies show that quantitative models out-perform qualitative models [50,132]. DNAmatch2 is used both as a database search engine as well as providing a platform to carry out contamination searches during routine casework, whereas *CaseSolver* is mainly used for profile comparisons in casework. Importantly, both *CaseSolver* and *EuroForMix* can conduct (reference to evidence) database searches; with the main difference that *CaseSolver* can perform this with many evidence items at the same time, and it provides a more flexible interface for data integration.

Casesolver contains more functionalities than *DNAmatch2*, with the focus of being an effective and simple-to-use comparison tool for case officers (similar as *DNAxs*). This software is especially designed to cope with complex cases which have a large number of evidence profiles and multiple reference samples. An example with 119 evidence profiles and three references is described by Bleka et al. [21]. *CaseSolver* compares each reference sample with each evidence profile, identifying potential 'matches' qualified by an *LR*. The second step carries out cross-comparisons between case-stains to identify unknown contributors. These can be deconvolved and used in further searches as required. If it is known that contributors may be related to each other, then simple relatedness searches can also be carried out. *CaseSolver* offers various ways to visualise or export the data, even to a comprehensive report; for example, an informative graphical network can be displayed that summarises the connections between the case samples (Figure 4). The latest version of *CaseSolver* (v1.8) provides a weight-of-evidence module which offers conservative corrections of *LR* for evaluative purposes, and automated report generation.

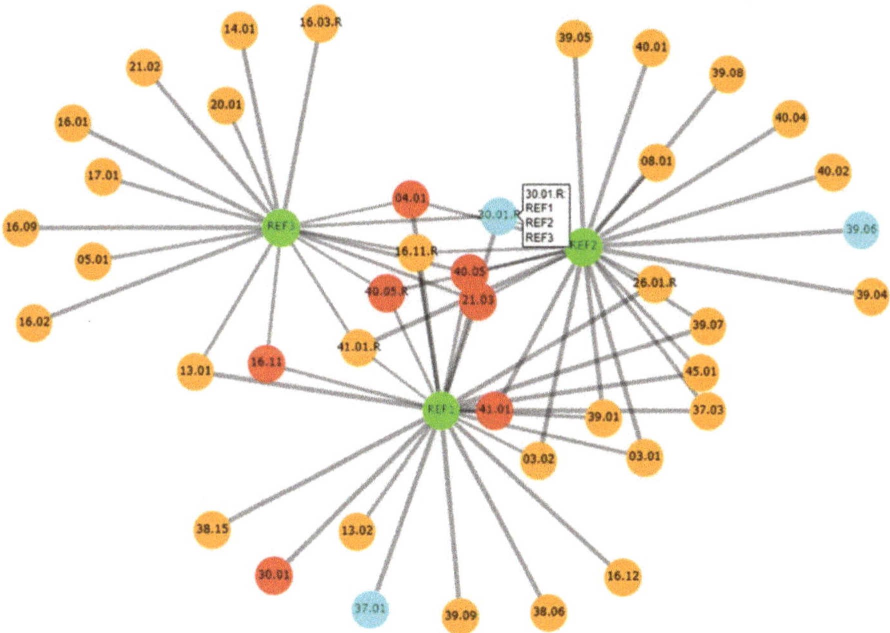

Figure 4. Graphical network summarizing the connections between case samples through *LR* calculations. The references are the green nodes. Single contributor evidences are in cyan; two contributors are in orange and three or more contributors are in red. If the 'plotly' function in R is used then the mouse can be hovered over a node and this displays a list of the matches, as shown for sample 30.01. The thickness of the edges between the nodes is inversely proportional to the size of the *LR* on a log10 scale. Reprinted from [62], chapter 11, Copyright (2020) with permission from Elsevier.

CaseSolver is available at: http://www.euroformix.com/casesolver accessed on 28 September 2021. Data and presentations are available at https://sites.google.com/view/dnabook/chapter-11?authuser=0 accessed on 28 September 2021.

3.5. Massively Parallel Sequencing (MPS)

Massive Parallel sequencing (MPS) is becoming increasingly used throughout the forensic community and may eventually supersede classic capillary gel (CE) methods [133]. MPS returns the entire sequence of a locus, not only the repeat region, but the flanking sequence as well; there is much more information to deal with compared to the standard repeat unit count used in classic CE. The main advantage of MPS is the potential to combine many more loci in multiplexes compared to CE. This results in much higher discriminating power. Shorter amplicon lengths should mean that more highly degraded DNA may be detected, but this will increase the potential to detect background DNA, as well as contamination. An additional challenge is that interpretation systems must be able to deal with profiles that are complicated by the presence of complex stutters.

Just and Irwin [134] developed a method of nomenclature of MPS-STRs that was based upon the longest uninterrupted sequence (LUS) and they used *LRmix Studio* to analyse mixtures. Later, the LUS nomenclature was extended to LUS+ [135], which is similar to that of Vilsen et al. [136], in order to identify as many different sequences as possible. They were able to identify 1050 out of 1059 sequences alleles. This system was adopted by Bleka et al. [137–139] who extended the analysis to the quantitative *EuroForMix* model. Instead of peak height (rfu), coverage (reads) are used to quantify allelic sequences. CE and MPS stutters are comparable [140]; '$n - 1$' stutters are the most common to be found, but '$n - 1$' and '$n + 2$' forms are also observed, though the latter have much lower coverage and can be removed by filtering. Stutters can arise from different blocks of sequences within the same allele. Software packages such as *FDSTools* [141] are able to predict stutters, both simple and complex, based upon the allelic sequence.

The *EuroForMix* implementation of MPS-STR interpretation is described by [138,139] and both '$n - 1$' and '$n + 1$' stutters are accommodated from version 3. In order to obtain data in LUS/LUS+ format, the R program *seq2lus* can be used to convert raw sequence data derived from the ForenSeq Verogen Universal Analysis (UAS) software: https://verogen. com/wp-content/uploads/2018/08/ForenSeq-Univ-Analysis-SW-Guide-VD2018007-A.pdf accessed on 28 September 2021. To carry out the conversion, a look-up table file is used: Table S5 from Just et al. [135]. Once the nomenclature conversions are made, the analysis can proceed. The tool and updated look-up files, together with a tutorial is provided at: http://euroformix.com/seq2lus accessed on 28 September 2021. A more general tool called lusSTR, written in python, has been developed to avoid the need of a lookup table (available at: https://github.com/bioforensics/lusSTR accessed on 28 September 2021).

Bleka et al. [138] explored the information gain, i.e., the LR increase, of the LUS vs. standard repeat unit (RU) nomenclature. Full profiles with the RU nomenclature provided an average log10LR = 37.04 whereas the LUS nomenclature returned log10LR = 43.3; the ratio is the theoretical information gain TIGRU→LUS = 1.17. However, the LRs are massive, and represent redundant information. Huge likelihood ratios have no benefit when presented in court. In practice any log10LR > 9 may be considered as providing redundant information because a greater LR has no impact upon a jury decision. Some jurisdictions e.g., UK have a reporting limit, upper threshold of 1 billion.

Therefore, the main benefit of MPS-STR is related to the analysis of low-level DNA profiles that may be highly degraded, so that the probability of successful amplification is low. If the number of loci is increased, then the chance of successful amplification of a given locus is also increased and this will be reflected in an expected increased *LR* (provided that H_1 is true). Doubling the number of loci from 27 loci to 54 loci will have an approximate proportionate doubling effect on the *LR* (log-scale). E.g., if log10*LR* = 2 for the former, it will return log10*LR* = 4 for the latter; if 128 loci are utilised then log10*LR* = 8, i.e., the more loci that are analysed, the more likely it is that reportable profiles can be achieved. We can summarise that the main advantage of MPS is the possibility to greatly increase the number of loci in the multiplex, the increased discrimination power per locus is secondary to this.

In addition, Benschop et al. [142] examined allele detection and *LR*s obtained from STR profiles generated by two different MPS systems that were analyzed with different settings. The *LR* results for the over 2000 sets of propositions were affected by the variation for the number of markers and analysis settings used in the three approaches tested. Nevertheless, trends for true and non-contributors, effects of replicates, assigned number of contributors, and model validation results were comparable for the different MPS approaches and were similar to the trends observed in CE data.

Even though sequence information from MPS technology provides higher data resolution, there is still a limitation in how mixture profiles, including major/minor components, are exported from MPS software. Two papers [138,142] point out that default analysis settings such as dynamic threshold potentially removes useful information forwarded for interpretation, weakening the ability to detect low-template components.

The above mentioned studies [142] demonstrate that probabilistic interpretation of MPS-STR data using the γ model in *EuroForMix* and *DNAStatistX* is fit for forensic DNA casework.

Probabilistic genotyping is not restricted to STRs, SNPs are also amenable [143,144]. Whereas STRs are multi-allelic, SNPs are generally di-allelic. This represents a particular challenge to assess the numbers of contributors because, with a maximum of two alleles in a population, we cannot use allele counting methods to ascertain this value.

Using a panel of 134 SNPs from Life Technologies' HID-Ion AmpliSeq™ Identity Panel v2.2: https://www.thermofisher.com/content/dam/LifeTech/Documents/PDFs/HID-Ion-AmpliSeq-Identity-Panel-Flyer.pdf accessed on 28 September 2021, Bleka et al. [143] compared the *LRmix* model with *EuroForMix* showing that the latter was much more efficient especially when there are more than two contributors. The effective NOC is decided by following exploratory data analysis, outlined for STRs in Section 2.5, where the likelihood is maximised under H_2. *LR*s obtained from overestimation of the actual NOC showed concordance with results compared to the actual NOC (from simulations up to six contributors). With the SNP panel tested, there is a limitation of that the mixture proportion (M_x) of the POI must exceed 0.2 in order to achieve an $LR > 100$, although this restriction would be removed with much larger SNP panels. More recently, the performance of *EuroForMix* was compared to machine learning approaches [145].

The data used in the MPS SNP and STR publications cited, along with presentations available online: https://sites.google.com/view/dnabook/chapter-13?authuser=0 accessed on 28 September 2021.

3.6. Validation, Guidelines for Best Practice and Quality

Developmental and internal validation of the probabilistic genotyping software *LRmix*, emphLRmix Studio, *SmartRank*, *EuroForMix*, *CaseSolver*, *DNAmatch2*, and *DNAxs/ DNAStatistX* is described in internal validation documents; much information has been published [22,23,62,113,128]. Furthermore, there has been much research effort to gain insights into trends and to characterize the various models, as well as to inform guidelines for best practice.

Using the qualitative model *LRmix Studio* research was carried out to show the effects of over- or under-assigning the NOC; the number of PCR replicates; the amount of DNA; and the drop-in rate [68,69,146–148].

The *SmartRank* output was compared to that of *LRmix Studio* in order to gain insight into the effects of model adaptations that enabled fast and efficient searching of voluminous databases [23]. In addition, the software was characterized in terms of the retrieval of true and non-donors; the effects of the size and composition of the DNA database; the number of contributors; the number of markers; and the level of drop-out [22,23]. As expected, positive effects on the retrieval of true donors were observed with: (1) a higher number of loci, (2) fewer contributors, (3) lower drop-out rates and/or (4) a higher discriminatory power. Retrieval of true donors was not influenced by the size of the DNA-databases used in this study (37,000–1.55 million). The size of the DNA-database, however, can have an effect on the retrieval of non-donors because of adventitious matches.

*LR*s generated from *EuroForMix* and *LRmix* were compared for true and non-donors to two- or three-person NGM DNA profiles [50] and to two- to four-person PPF6C DNA profiles [73]. This research demonstrated the effects of the NOC, over- or under-assigning the NOC; the number of PCR replicates; the amount of DNA; the level of unseen alleles for the person of interest; and the effect of increased PCR cycles. H_1-true tests and H_2-true tests were utilised. In the H_2-true tests, non-contributors were selected deliberately to a have large overlap with the alleles within the mixture and worst-case scenarios were examined where a simulated relative of one of the true donors was considered as the person of interest under the prosecution hypothesis [73]. A somewhat similar study was performed to compare MPS with CE-based DNA profiling data [142]. It was observed that the MPS read counts behaved in a similar manner to CE peak heights, and therefore similar results were obtained.

To summarize, the following overall trends were observed for CE and MPS profiles (note that exceptions can occur):

The lower the NOC and the lower the drop-out rate for the POI, the more often larger *LR*s were obtained.

The more donors and the more drop-out for the person of interest, the more often false-negative support was observed.

Using a lower NOC than designed yielded either equal results (predominantly with a true major donor as POI) or lower *LR*s.

Over assigning the NOC hardly affected *LR*s for true major donors.

An over-assigned NOC for H_2-true tests can have the effect of increasing the *LR* to around neutral evidence.

False-positive support, $LR > 1$, was observed more often and with larger *LR*s when the POI was a (simulated) relative of a true donor rather than if the POI was an unrelated non-donor to the DNA mixture.

The use of multiple, instead of one PCR replicate, often increased the *LR* for true minor donors and decreased the *LR* for non-donors.

Based on the outcomes of the above-mentioned research studies, guidelines for best practice in forensic casework were developed. For *LRmix (Studio)* this included the exploratory data analysis approach, in which the effect of model parameters (such as the probability of drop-out) on the *LR* is examined. Non-contributor tests provide an indication of the range of *LR*s obtained if H_2 is true. Although it is not mandatory, laboratories may find this a useful feature that can help to explain results in court. For *EuroForMix* and *DNAStatistX*, it is advised to perform model selection, to examine the model validation ('pp-plots') and iteration results and to report the *LR* only if defined criteria are met. Furthermore, for reasons of quality, efficiency and usefulness of performing weight of evidence calculations, guidelines for application of the *LR* models were developed by NFI. For *EuroForMix/DNAStatistX* these are presented in [128]; for instance there is an upper limit on the number of unseen alleles that a person of interest can have before an *LR* calculation is advised. Another quality aspect that relates to the use of the *DNAxs/DNAStatistX* software is the audit trail which automatically keeps track of who performed which action and when.

Apart from software validation, guidelines for best practice and an audit trail, NFI invests in (automated) software testing during development, prior to release and during validation. This is important to ensure that the software is robust and behaves as designed. With a growing number of features, software testing becomes a very time-consuming task if performed manually. To save time, improve the test coverage, increase ad hoc and exploratory testing, and, in the end, reduce costs and maintenance, automated tests were designed and built for *DNAxs*. In the first three years after implementation of the *DNAxs* software suite, a total of 521 bugs were reported by the software engineers during development, by testers during validation, by users in casework, or by users performing research. Software bugs are errors, flaws or faults causing the software to produce an incorrect or an unexpected result, or to behave in unintended ways. The majority of bugs were solved in major or minor software releases that were planned and a minority required the release of a bug fix version or occurred during the development of these version. This shows that bug detection and debugging is part of the developmental and validation process, but also occurs in validated and released software versions. The reported bugs are viewed from a software perspective and relate to the use of the software or functionalities thereof. The observed bugs did not have effects on the DNA profile interpretation and/or reported conclusions. Further information on code coverage by testing, bug detection and debugging, but also information on the use of *DNAxs* (including *DNAStatistX* and

SmartRank) and post-analytical errors in forensic casework can be found in [149]. Further details on the process of software testing can be found in [62], chapter 10.

4. STRmix™

4.1. History of STRmix™ Creation

STRmix™ is an Australian and New Zealand initiative that was jointly developed by Duncan Taylor from Forensic Science SA (FSSA) in Australia and John Buckleton and Jo-Anne Bright from the Institute of Environmental Science and Research (ESR) in New Zealand. *STRmix*™ was first introduced into casework at FSSA and ESR in August 2012, however the events that lead to its development occurred three years prior.

Prior to 2010 there was no focussed effort to drive standardisation in forensic biology between laboratories in Australasia (Australia and New Zealand). Each laboratory had accrued knowledge and developed policies in a siloed manner, which meant that in one state Random Man Not Excluded (RMNE) also known as Cumulative Probability of Inclusion (CPI) was being used, in others likelihood ratios (*LR*), and amongst those there was a variety of implementations. In 2009 the Victoria Police Forensic Science Laboratory (VPFSL) in Melbourne had been using a software program called *DNAmix* [150,151] for calculating *LR*s in situations where unresolvable mixtures were obtained. *DNAmix* had been created as a result of DNA profile evaluations in the OJ Simpson trial, and the models within *DNAmix* required that no dropout-out had occurred. The VPFSL came to realise that this assumption was not being met in the evaluations being carried out, which resulted in the DNA profile evaluations in a number of cases being redone and reports reissued. One result in particular, which shifted an *LR* from 550 billion to 3, concerned Victoria's police chief Simon Overland who ordered all DNA evidence be banned from court proceedings.

Following the laboratory shutdown, crisis talks were held with members of government forensic laboratories from across Australia and New Zealand. One of the outcomes was to form an Australasian forensic biology statistics working group in 2010 (with members from all government forensic laboratories from across Australia and New Zealand) with the overarching remit of standardisation across Australasia through the adoption of world leading evaluation and statistical practices. In this group were John Buckleton and Duncan Taylor, who started working on the ideas that would eventually become *STRmix*™ (Taylor and Buckleton thankfully acknowledge the technical input of David Balding and the vision of Ross Vining, Linzi Wilson-Wilde and Keith Bedford). In 2011 Buckleton and Taylor presented the idea of *STRmix*™ (initially to be called *DyNAmix*) to their member organisations, and the National Institute of Forensic Sciences (NIFS), and development was supported. Jo-Anne Bright joined the development team and by 2012 Taylor, Buckleton and Bright had completed development and validation on version 1.0 of *STRmix*™.

4.2. Probabilistic Genotyping and STRmix™

STRmix™ considers parameters that describe some observed fluorescent peak collectively as 'mass parameters', M. In essence probability of the observed data, given a genotype, treats these mass parameters as nuisance variables that are integrated across:

$$w_j = Pr(O\big|S_j) = \int p(O, M\big|S_j)p(M)dM$$

which assumes $p(M|S_j) = p(M)$.

In *STRmix*™ this integration is carried out using Markov Chain Monte Carlo (MCMC) sampling. The equation above applies across the whole profile. The locus terms (a superscript '*l*') are a product within the integral, across all loci in the profile with data. The model of *STRmix*™ then makes the assumption that the profile weight is approximated by the product of the integrals at each locus:

$$w_j = \int \prod_l p(O^l, M\big|S_j^l)p(M)dM = \prod_l \int p(O^l, M\big|S_j^l)p(M)dM$$

When tested, this assumption appears reasonable (see Figure 2 of [15]). As well as using weights to calculate the *LR*, having the weights themselves allows probing of the DNA profile data in powerful investigative ways, which we describe later.

Assumption 1 fulfils Slooten's [152] requirement that *"we will assume that the model … parameters are chosen independently of the hypotheses."* This allows the statement that the *"model cannot overstate the evidence very strongly very often for actual contributors: it cannot, averaged over all mixtures and contributors, happen with probability more than 1/t that the evidence is overstated by a factor t."*

We round out this claim by repeating Slooten's [152] statement in his Equation (5.2), which has a pedigree back to Turing (quoted in Good [153]), that the probability of obtaining an $LR \geq t$ from a non-donor is $\leq \frac{1}{t}$.

4.3. Capabilities of STRmix™

4.3.1. Deconvolution

The process of deconvolution is the assignment of weights to genotype sets. In other words, combinations of genotypes that could describe a profile(s) are considered, and a probability is assigned to them, proportional to how well they explain the observed peaks. In *STRmix™* this is achieved by integrating across a set of mass parameters using MCMC. The base model for *STRmix™* was described by Taylor et al. [15] and included parameters:

1. A template amount for each of the *n* contributors,
2. A degradation (described in [154]) which models the decay with respect to molecular weight (*m*) in the template for each of the contributors,
3. Amplification efficiency at each locus to allow for the observed amplification levels of each locus,
4. Replicate multipliers, which scales all peaks up or down between PCR replicates.

Later, Taylor et al. [155] extended the model to not only consider PCR replicates produced under the same system, but also DNA profiles from the sample produced under different conditions, i.e.,

Using the same DNA profiling kit, but with different laboratory processes (such as different PCR cycles or different models of laboratory hardware),

Using two different DNA profiling kits

which require the addition of mass parameter(s):

Kit multipliers, which scale all peaks in all replicates up or down between kits.

The expansion of the model for multiple kits/processes allowed various parameter freedoms between profiles produced by different processes. This was particularly useful for cold-cases where *STRmix™* could be used to combine the original profiling work with contemporary work in situations where technology had spanned multiple generations of profiling kit, and the DNA sample itself may have exhibited different degradation patterns between the generation of the two profiles.

Using a chosen set of values for the mass parameters allows the calculation of Total Allelic Product (TAP) [156], the total amount of fluorescence expected resulting from the amplification of an allele present in a DNA extract. As the PCR occurs, some of the fluorescence that was destined for the allele will shift to stutter positions on the EPG. The amount of the TAP that is expected to become stutter is based on the expected stutter ratios for each allele at each locus, either measured directly or regressed using the longest uninterrupted sequence (LUS) [156], or incorporating multiple repeat sequences of an interrupted STR in a multi-LUS model [136,157]. In reality, there are a number of stutter types that can occur, but the original *STRmix™* model (described in [15]) only included back stutter. This was later extended to include forward stutter (with modelling of forward stutter described in [157,158]), and then generalised so that any number of stutters (and with any size-based relationship to the parent peak), applied to any combination of specific loci, could be added by users with the mathematical framework automatically extending to incorporate them (generalised stutter modelling is described in [155]). The height of coincident peaks (either from multiple allele donations, or allele and stutter) are added [159,160] to produce the final expected peak heights.

The calculation of expected allele and stutter (of any combination thereof) peak heights using a set of mass parameters and expected stutter ratios ultimately results in a set of expected peaks and their heights, for each locus, in each PCR replicate and for each process or kit in which they have been generated. How well those mass parameter values explain the observed peak heights (or technically the probability of the observed data given the mass parameter values), depends on how well the observed and expected peak heights align.

Differences between an observed (O) and an expected (E) peak height are assigned a probability based on empirical models. These models take account of the magnitude of the difference and use a proxy for template to assess how tolerable such differences are. In order to determine how much to penalise stochastic effects in different types of fluorescence (i.e., allele, or stutter, or a combination), peak height variability models are used. An observed peak comprising a single fluorescence type, with peak height variability parameter value c^2 is modelled by a log-Normal distribution with mean and variance parameters:

$$O \sim LN\left(ln(E), \frac{c^2}{f(E)}\right) \text{ where } f(E) = \frac{b}{E} + E$$

and b is a constant that typically takes values around 1000. The variance is inversely proportional to the function of expected peak height (which is approximately equal to E when E is large), which describes the well-known phenomenon that the relative size of stochastic peak height imbalance tends to increase as peak height decrease. The function $f(E)$, deals with the fact that as the expected height decreases to very low levels the peak height variability starts to contract (see [161]). The constant b can be altered by the user from 0 (which turns off this low-level peak height variability contraction effect) to any arbitrarily high value.

A range of distributions were investigated for modelling stutter in Bright et al. [162]. The log-normal appeared to fit the empirical data adequately.

When a peak comprises different fluorescence types, the sum of log-normal random variables is approximated by a shifted-log-normal distribution using moment matching.

If a peak has an expected height, but is not observed, then it is modelled as a drop-out peak and a probability is used that is based on the integral of the probability of observing a peak between baseline and AT for a peak at expected height E. If a peak is not expected, but observed in the profile then it is modelled as a drop-in and a probability applied, based on the model of Puch-Solis [13].

The above process describes the generation of a set of expected peak heights and the probability for deviations of the expected heights from observed heights. The constant, 'b' in the variance term and the prior distribution parameters for c^2 are set during model calibration in a tool called 'Model Maker' (described in Section 4.4). The MCMC process within *STRmix*™ starts by assigning starting positions for all mass parameters, and randomly assigning genotype sets to each locus. This is the current set of parameters. Then, iteratively

(1)   Choose a locus at random and propose a genotype set at that locus.
(2)   Choose new values for all mass parameters by stepping a small distance from the values in the current set (known as a random walk, and with step size dictated by a Gaussian distribution). Propose these values.
(3)   Calculate the expected peak heights using the proposed sample values.
(4)   Calculate the likelihood value of the proposed sample values.
(5)   Use a Metropolis-Hastings algorithm to accept or reject the proposed sample. If the proposed sample is accepted, then the proposed set of parameter values becomes the current set. If the proposed sample is rejected, then the proposal is discarded.
(6)   Repeat steps 1 to 6 until a defined number of proposal accepts have been attained.

The first iterations of the MCMC are considered burn-in (the number of steps is set by the user) and discarded. After the burn-in the proportion of total iterations that a genotype set was the focus of the MCMC (called residence time) is the weight assigned to that genotype set.

A contributor that is assumed to be present under both H_1 and H_2 is described as a conditioning contributor. It is highly desirable to include as many contributors as possible as conditioning profiles. This is for practical reasons such as improving run time, but also for the much more important reason that any correctly assumed donor improves the ability of the system to differentiate between true and false donors [163]. Historically the use of conditioning contributors has been restricted to those situations where a donor is certain to correctly assumed, largely intimate samples. This underutilises the tool and is not in the interests of an innocent person accused of being a donor [95]. We recommend the extension of the use of conditioning to other evidential items such as assuming the presence of the habitual wearer of clothing and to any co-accused with a very high LR, especially if the POI is related to these persons [95,96]. Within a deconvolution, any number (up to the NOC from which the profile is designated as having originated) can be assumed as a conditioning profile, which during MCMC, locks their genotypes (known from their references) into any genotype set being considered.

Since *STRmix*™ V2.6 the analysis of a profile can proceed without a set single number assigned for a profile as *STRmix*™ has the ability to accept a range of contributors as the user input [164]. A range of contributors may be chosen if the user is unable to assign a single value due to the complexity or quality of the profile, or if different numbers may be required by the different parties in order for them to have their most probable explanations for the profile(s) [95,97]. The method works by carrying out a deconvolution of the evidence profile(s) given each NOC in the chosen range and then calculating the Bayes Factor (based on a method of Weinberg et al. [165,166]) to allow combination or contrast between the deconvolution. This is an alternative to the recent method described by Slooten et al. [94], but yields the same results under the same assumptions [71].

4.3.2. LR Calculation

Given the weights from a deconvolution, the calculation of an *LR* in *STRmix*™ is achieved by taking the ratio of the weighted sum of genotype set probabilities given two competing propositions. One or more references (some of which can have been assumed at the point deconvolution) are compared to the evidence profile(s) using propositions that are aligned with prosecution and a sensible alternative, in a way that best represents the strength of the evidence given the framework of circumstances of the case (see [3,71,95,103,167] for guidance documents on proposition setting). *STRmix*™ can compare individuals to specific combinations of contributor positions within the evidence profile(s), generating an *LR* considering sub-sub-source level propositions [104], or to the mixture as a whole (i.e., all components and all combinations) to generate an *LR* that considers sub-source level propositions. When considering sources of DNA under the H_2, *STRmix*™ can consider these to be unrelated to the POI or related to the POI [168] in various relationship types.

Following Balding [169,170] the different potential relationship types that the alternate donor could be to the POI can be assembled into one statistic. Writing $w_j = Pr(O|S_j)$ and introducing the different relationship types R_i, $i = 1, r$, where is the number of relationship types considered we obtain

$$LR = \frac{\sum_{j=1}^{J} w_j Pr(S_j|H_1)}{\sum_{i=1}^{r} Pr(R_i|H_2) \sum_{j=1}^{J} w_j Pr(S_j|H_2, R_i)}$$

The terms, $Pr(R_i|H_2)$, represent the prior probability that a person related to the POI by relationship R_i is the donor (given that the POI is not, H_2). The expected prior proportions that different relative types can make up in the population, $Pr(R_i|H_2)$, can either be set manually in *STRmix*™ or estimated using the number of individuals in the population and the average number of children per family in that population [171].

STRmix™ uses the sub-population model of Balding et al. [172], although the co-ancestry coefficient (F_{ST}, θ) can be set to 0 by the user if desired in order to revert the calculation to using the 'product rule'.

When assigning probabilities for an allele in the population the value is set using a Dirichlet distribution with a uniform prior. The posterior means of the allele probabilities are then obtained by updating the prior with the counts of alleles in a database (using a similar method as described in [173]). For allele 'A', the probability of occurrence in the population, given it has been seen x_A times out of N alleles is calculated by:

$$Pr(A) = \frac{x_A + k^{-1}}{N+1} \text{ in early } STRmix \text{ versions or } Pr(A) = \frac{x_A + (k+1)^{-1}}{N+1} \text{ in V2.8 and higher}$$

where k^{-1} is the prior allele probability [174], and k is the number of different allele states that have been observed in the population.

Multiple populations can be set up in *STRmix*™, each with their own allele frequency file, θ and population proportion in the local geographical region. This allows *STRmix*™ to calculate an *LR* considering the contributors to be from any of the set populations individually, or anyone in the local geographical region, by stratifying across all populations [175].

In addition to the point estimate *LR* *STRmix*™ also provides a credible interval [176] using the highest posterior density (HPD) method. While there has been justified debate over the provision of intervals for *LRs* [177–184], it is the preference for most practising forensic DNA laboratories to report a lower bound interval on the *LR* value. Within *STRmix*™ the HPD interval optionally takes into account any combination of:

(1)   sampling variation in allele frequency database
(2)   sampling variation in the iterations of the MCMC leading to the assignment of weights
(3)   uncertainty in the value of θ

The second of these factors intends to capture the amount of variability in the *LR* resulting from Monte Carlo resampling inherent within MCMC processes. More recently this process has been found to have variable coverage [185] although taken collectively with other aspects of conservative behaviours the coverage is good [186] The third of these factors is achieved by *STRmix*™ being able to take a point value for θ or a distribution described by a β distribution (see [187–189] for examples of θ distribution models).

The result of an *LR* calculation on *STRmix*™ is that the user can be provided with the *LRs* for the:

- sub-sub-source proposition pair,
- the sub-source proposition pair considering the alternate DNA donor as
    - unrelated,
    - sibling,
    - half-sibling,
    - parent/child,
    - aunt/uncle/niece/nephew,
    - grandparent,
    - cousin, or
    - unified across all relationship types,
- all of the above for:
    - each ethnic population in the local geographical region, and
    - stratified across all populations,
- all of the above for:
    - each NOC in a chosen range, and
    - stratified across the range (or with bespoke NOC choice for proposition),

and all with an associated HPD interval to account for uncertainty in allele frequencies, weights and θ. As well as generating *LR*s for the comparison of a reference to a deconvolution, *STRmix*™ can also compare a list of references in a database. Using an *LR* threshold provides a search capability [190]. This is not restricted to resolved genotypes of a single individual, but rather can be applied to any profile (single source or mixtures, resolved or unresolved). Using the *LR* calculation feature than considers a relative of a POI as a source of DNA, allows *STRmix*™ to carry out familial searches against any profile (again from complete single source to complex and unresolved mixtures) [168]. This lead to Australia's first conviction resulting from a familial search [191]. The ability to search any DNA profile against a database is also commonly used as a Quality Assurance tool to screen evidence profiles for potential contamination or assist in environmental monitoring [192].

STRmix™ has a profile sampling tool that can be used to generate profiles from a population and calculate *LR*s by comparison to a deconvolution. These profiles can either be generated using probabilities based on their probability of occurrence in a population [59] or using importance sampling [60] in order to build distributions of 'H_2 true' *LR*s and determine exceedance probabilities. Exceedance probabilities (sometimes called non-contributor performance tests [9]) provide the probability of randomly selecting someone from the population who would provide a particular level of support (typically for their inclusion to the profile, and typically the level of interest is that yielded by a *POI*). These probabilities, however, are fundamentally different from *LR*s and should not be confused with, or substituted for *LR*s in evaluations [193]. The LR itself provides an upper bound on exceedance probabilities (a simple proof was provided in [59] so that if LR_{POI} is produced by the comparison of a POI to an evidence profile the statement can be made:

> *The probability of observing a likelihood ratio of LR_{POI} or larger from an unrelated non-donor is less than or equal to 1 in LR_{POI}.*

Another database searching tool available in *STRmix*™ is to carry out a top-down analysis [74] in which only the main contributors to a highly complex profile are compared. In concept, a top-down analysis is similar to carrying out an evaluation on a major 'cluster' of peaks in a profile [194]. The process works by carrying out deconvolutions in steps, where in each step the AT is altered (on a per-locus basis) and only the peak information that meets or exceed the step-AT is used. Each deconvolution considers the profile as originating from N individuals (where N here represents the top N contributors in which you are interested, to the profile and not the total number of contributors to the profile). At the conclusion of each step's deconvolution the result is searched against a database and individuals that yield an LR that exceed a pre-determined LR threshold are flagged. The first step raises the AT (on a per-locus basis) to the height of the highest peaks and each step lowers the ATs by a proportion of the distance from the highest peak to the standard AT used. The steps stop when the profile can no longer be described by N individuals (due to excessive peaks that cannot be explained as allele, stutter or drop-in). The final database search report returns individuals flagged at any step, with the maximum LR attained across all steps in which they were flagged. This method has been extended to the quantitative model of *STRmix*™ and has been trialed on a set of complex mixtures (5+ contributors) from the no-suspect workflow of a forensic laboratory, showing an 80% link rate with someone on the local database [195].

4.4. Implementation of STRmix™

STRmix™ utilises general models to describe DNA profile behaviour, for example that peak height variability increases as peak heights decrease, or that loci can vary in their amplification efficiencies depending on the PCR micro-environment, or that stutters are expected to occur at a particular size (relative to their parent peak size) and height (dependent on their parent peak height). Each of these models have parameters that can be calibrated to the performance of DNA profile generation in a particular laboratory or for a particular process. A standard objective for a DNA profile analysis is to use the calibrated models, and the observed data in order to obtain weights. Figure 5 shows these three aspects diagrammatically, each connected to the other two.

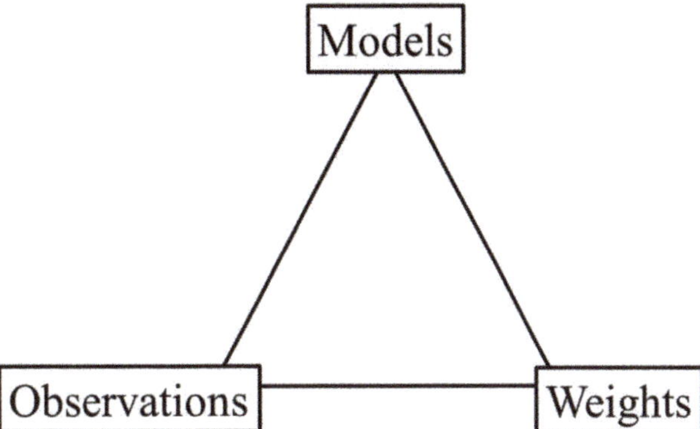

Figure 5. Representation of the components involved in the analysis of a DNA profile.

Using this relationship, if the weights are known for a set of observed profiles, then this information can be used to calibrate the models. Within *STRmix*™ there is a feature known as Model Maker [196], which takes sets of single source input profiles (whose donor references are known) to calibrate parameters in the *STRmix*™ models. The general process is carried out with a component-wise MCMC, whereby cycles of sampling mass parameters (on a per profile basis) followed by sampling of variance parameters (on a dataset wide basis) eventually reaches a steady-state for all parameters in the dataset. The variance parameter values are then attuned to the behaviour of profiles produced under the conditions tested and can be set in *STRmix*™ as the default values for casework use.

Some, parameters such as expected stutter ratios have been shown to be robust to laboratory effects [197], while others are more sensitive [196]. The most important factors for peak height variability have been found to be the number of PCR cycles carried out during amplification, the PCR kit used and the models of electrophoresis instrumentation [196]. The use of prior distributions rather than point values for parameters such as variances with the calibration setting the hyper-parameters of the prior distribution (using hierarchical Bayesian modelling) has shown that general settings can be applied and are robust to a wide range of factors [198]. Despite this robustness, it is standard practice (and the recommendation of the *STRmix*™ group, the SWGDAM 2015 [108] and the ASB guidelines (Standards for Validation Studies of DNA Mixtures, and Development and Verification of a Laboratory's Mixture Interpretation Protocol: http://asb.aafs.org/ accessed on 28 September 2021)) that each laboratory implementing *STRmix*™ undertakes a calibration prior to use on casework samples. In part this ensures the best alignment of the prior distributions for the input parameters to the validation data.

4.5. DBLR—A Companion Product to STRmix™

STRmix™ has closely aligned companion product *DBLR* (which stands for DataBase Likelihood Ratio, https://www.strmix.com/dblr/ accessed on 28 September 2021), which can take the results of a deconvolution and carry out interrogations of the results. An overview and developmental validation is given by Kelly at el [199]. It also has the flexibility and power to construct propositions that consider aspects of relatedness of contributors within a sample or between samples (including common DNA donorship). *DBLR* has databasing properties that allow automated, and auditable searching of deconvoluted mixtures against a reference DNA database.

The investigative properties of *DBLR* allow the user to probe the deconvolution to see what DNA profiles are the most supported by the data, to gauge the discrimination power of the analysis by producing distributions of *LR*s expected for contributor and non-contributors [200], or to calculate exceedance probabilities.

Two mixtures can be compared using *DBLR* in order to determine whether there is support for a common DNA donor, using the method described by Slooten [20]. Studies into this feature have found a high efficacy for identifying common donors [159]. The process has been shown to have use as a Quality Assurance tool to identify potential sample to sample contamination events [25].

Recently *DBLR* has implemented a general framework for the comparison of deconvoluted profiles or references. This general framework allows multiple deconvolutions, from different evidence samples that are believed to possess a common DNA donor, to be considered together in order to obtain better resolution in the genotypes of the donors to any (or multiple) of the profiles [201]. The distribution of probabilities across a number of potential genotypes (or genotype sets) can be thought of in similar ways whether considering a mixture deconvolution, or a kinship calculation [152]. Using this idea, the general framework in *DBLR* allows the setting-up of competing pedigrees within the evaluation [202]. The pedigrees can be linked to components of mixtures so that bespoke propositions can be set up to consider issues such as:

- How many common donors are in a mixture?
- Are any donors of the multiple mixtures related (see [203] for an investigation into the effect of not recognising relatedness in mixtures)?
- If I assume a relative of a POI to one mixture does that assist in resolving the other components?
- If I use multiple mixed samples from a disaster victim identification (DVI) together in a single analysis will that help to better resolve the genotypes of the donors?

The variation in potential propositions is virtually limitless. These types of questions, and the evaluations that follow, have applications to standard casework, but also DVI, or investigations looking into serial offenders, or offences involving multiple family members.

4.6. Validation of STRmix™

When *STRmix™* was first implemented into active casework in 2012, probabilistic genotyping was not as prevalent as it is in 2021. There were not yet the standards developed as there are now for the validation or use of such software [108,109,204]. In these guidance documents there are outlined various requirements for the development, validation, and implementation of probabilistic genotyping systems. One of the criteria mentioned is that the statistical and biological models used be published or otherwise generally accessible. In Table 1 we provide a list of publications that detail the models used within *STRmix™*.

The publications relating to *STRmix™* models (and some initial validation work) were initially all described in the Taylor et al. publication *"The interpretation of single source and mixed DNA profiles"* [15]. Since that publication, updates in models occurred over time and so by necessity have appeared in numerous publications. All information about modelling and validation are compiled in a single document in the *STRmix™* manuals, provided to users of the software and available to the defense under a non-disclosure agreement.

Table 1. Publications of conceptual components of *STRmix*™ modelling.

Algorithms, Scientific Principles and Methods	Version Introduced	Reference
Allele and stutter peak height variability as separate constants within the MCMC	V2.0	[15]
Peak height variability as random variables within the MCMC	V2.3	[196]
Model for calibrating laboratory peak height variability	V2.0	[196]
Application of a Gaussian random walk to the MCMC process	V2.3	[205]
Modelling of back stutter by regressing stutter ratio against allelic designation	V2.0	[156,197,206,207]
Modelling of back stutter by regressing stutter ratio against LUS	V2.3	[156,162,206,207]
Modelling of forward stutter	V2.4	[157]
Modelling of allelic drop-in using a simple exponential or uniform distribution	V2.0	[15]
Modelling of allelic drop-in using a γ distribution	V2.3	[13]
Modelling of degradation and dropout	V2.0	[154]
Modelling of the uncertainties in the allele frequencies using the HPD	V2.0	[208]
Modelling of the uncertainties in the MCMC	V2.3	[171,208,209]
Database searching of mixed DNA profiles	V2.0	[190]
Familial searching of mixed DNA profiles	V2.3	[168]
Relatives as alternate contributors under the defence proposition	V2.3	[168]
Modelling expected stutter peak heights in saturated data	V2.3	[157]
Taking into account the 'factor of two' in *LR* calculations	V2.3	[104]
Model for incorporating prior beliefs in mixture proportions	V2.3	[210]
Combining DNA profiles produced under different conditions into a single analysis	V2.5	[155]
Assigning a range for the number of contributors to a DNA profile	V2.6	[164]
Mixture-to-mixture comparison to identify common DNA donors	V2.7	[20]
A top-down DNA search approach	V2.8	[74]
The diagnostic outputs of *STRmix*™	V2.3	[211]

As well as detailing the machinations of the models, testing of their performance on data is required to show foundational validity and validity of application. There have been numerous such published validations of the performance of *STRmix*™ modelling either in part or as a whole and we provide a list of these in Table 2. Many of these validations have come from the desire of the developers (and more recently users) of *STRmix*™ to know the performance of the models, but some have come as responses to published perceptions of short-comings in validation efforts (for example the report of the President's Council of Advisors on Science and Technology [117]).

In a brief summary *STRmix*™ publications on validation work from Table 2 include data from profiling kits; Profiler Plus, Identifiler Plus, Fusion (5C, 6C), NGM SElect, GlobalFiler, PowerPlex (21, ESI17 Pro, 16 HS, ESI17 Fast), SGMPlus and MiniFiler (we are also aware of numerous other profiling kits that have been validated for use in casework, but do not have the work published). There have been hundreds of millions of 'H_2 true' tests, spanning over 3000 laboratory-produced profiles under a range of conditions (from 26 to 34 PCR cycles, and on multiple models of thermocycler or electrophoresis instrument) and of complexity spanning single source to six person mixtures.

Table 2. Publications of validation of *STRmix*™ models.

Focus of Validation	Reference
Ability of *STRmix*™ to deconvolute profiles and assign *LRs* that comport to manual interpretation and human expectation	[15]
Ability of *STRmix*™ to discriminate between donors and non-donors in database searches	[190]
Behaviour of *STRmix*™ to assign *LRs* when dealing with multiple replicates, different number of contributors, and assumed contributors	[163]
Sensitivity of *LR* produced by *STRmix*™ to different factors of uncertainty such as theta, relatedness of alternate DNA source and length of MCMC analysis	[171]
Tests to be performed when validating probabilistic genotyping, using *STRmix*™ as an example	[112]
Ability of individuals from different laboratories to standardise evaluations when using *STRmix*™	[33,53]
Ability of *STRmix*™ to reliably use peak height information in very low intensity profiles	[56,132,210]
Ability of *STRmix*™ to discriminate between donors and non-donors in large-scale Hd true tests, or using importance sampling	[59,60,190,200,212,213]
Sensitivity of *STRmix*™ model parameters to laboratory factors	[196,198]
Ability of *STRmix*™ to utilise information from profiles produced under different laboratory conditions within a single analysis	[155]
Effect of mixture complexity, allele sharing and contributor proportions on the ability *STRmix*™ to distinguish contributors from non-contributors	[54]
The ability of *STRmix*™ to identify common DNA donors in mixed samples	[25,159]
The sensitivity of *LRs* produced in *STRmix*™ to the choice of the number of contributors	[71,72,97]
Ability to use *STRmix*™ to resolve major components of mixtures	[72]
Testing the assumption of additivity of peak heights in *STRmix*™ models	[159,160]
Performance of the degradation model within *STRmix*™	[214]
The effect of relatedness of contributors to the *STRmix*™ analysis	[203,215]
Testing the calibration of *LRs* produced in *STRmix*™	[58]
Validation overviews of *STRmix*™	[205,216]
Comparison of *STRmix*™ to other probabilistic genotyping software	[41,43,112,217]

4.7. Growth of STRmix™

Since its introduction in 2012 in ESR and FSSA, *STRmix*™ has now been adopted throughout Australia and New Zealand and currently over 60 DNA forensic laboratories throughout the world, including the US army and the Federal Bureau of Investigation (FBI). Figure 6 shows the growth of *STRmix*™ between 2012 and 2020.

When last tallied, *STRmix*™ is believed to have been used in over 220,000 cases worldwide, available online: https://www.strmix.com/news/survey-shows-strmix-has-been-used-in-220000-cases-worldwide/ accessed 28 September 2021. For the past 6 years, users in the USA have organised a yearly *STRmix*™ workshop/conference, that had over 750 attending online presentations in 2020.

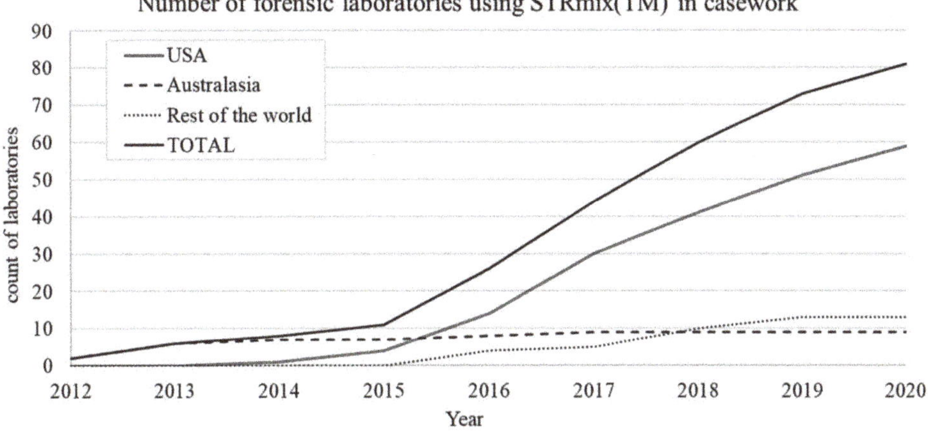

Figure 6. Growth of *STRmix*™ use over eight years.

The *STRmix*™ team has grown from an original three developers to employing over 20 individuals who work in training, support, validation, research and development, programming and quality assurance.

4.8. Admissibility Experiences with STRmix™

The *STRmix*™ group's experience with court and admissibility is mainly in the USA and Australia. In the, at least, 83 admissibility hearings to which *STRmix*™ has been subjected (as of 1 January 2021), a very wide range of issues have been raised but there are a few that recur. These can be divided into those specifically aimed at *STRmix*™, those aimed at PG in general, and those that relate more broadly to the use of *LRs* and especially understandability and the verbal scale. See information available online: https://johnbuckleton.wordpress.com/strmix/ accessed 28 September 2021, for a non-exhaustive list of admissibility hearings, most with attached rulings or transcripts

Recurrent issues that have been raised regarding *STRmix*™ include independence of validation, run to run variability, code access, code quality, and validation.

4.8.1. Independence of Validation

Perhaps the most recurrent complaint refers to the established fact that most publications on STRmix include one or more of the original developers. This is exemplified by two comments in the PCAST [117] report. PCAST @ pg 79 give: "*Appropriate evaluation of the proposed methods should consist of studies by multiple groups, not associated with the software developers, that investigate the performance and define the limitations of programs by testing them on a wide range of mixtures with different properties.*" PCAST @ pg 81 give: "*As noted above, such studies should be performed by or should include independent research groups not connected with the developers of the methods and with no stake in the outcome.*"

This argument has been taken further to suggest that even those labs separate from the developers but who have purchased *STRmix*™ have a vested interest and hence their publications should not be trusted.

Whilst we reject the suggestion that we, and the many professional collaborators that we have worked with, would distort our publications because of self-interest we acknowledge the desire to have further distance between the validators and the developers. The National Institute of Standards and Technology (NIST) is often suggested as a suitable organization for this purpose [218]. NIST has had STRmix since March 2014 initially as an evaluation copy but subsequently purchased. There is one publication from NIST [217] that represents a comparison of *STRmix™* and *EuroForMix* and both software perform well. There is desire for more independent work to be done and the developers would like to assist, at an appropriate distance, any efforts at independent validation.

4.8.2. Run to Run Variability

One complaint is that the MCMC means that the exact value reported for the *LR* could be different if the process were rerun. The argument is that the existence of variability raises doubts about whether any of the results should be accepted. This raises very significant questions about precision and accuracy that we will touch on briefly later. However, a full treatment is beyond the scope of this work. Here we simply note that *STRmix™* includes a partially successful attempt to give a lower bound to the MCMC variability [185]. In conjunction with other conservancies, it is almost certain that the *LR* is understated in the overwhelming majority of cases [186].

4.8.3. Code Access

The code for open source software is freely available on the internet. *STRmix*'s code is not open source but is available under an non-disclosure agreement (NDA) [219] This meets the ISFG guidelines [109] requirement *"However, if requested by the legal system, the code should be made available subject to the software provider's legitimate copyright or commercial interests being safeguarded. Supervised access to the code under a "no copy" policy is acceptable."* Objections to the use of an NDA have included that inconvenience of supervision and the risk presented by the sanctions agreed to in the NDA if the NDA is contravened.

4.8.4. Code Quality

The *STRmix™* code has been inspected three times by the same independent analyst under NDA. The comments made centre around coding practice, documentation, and adherence to software engineering standards [220]. At no stage has a coding fault been identified that affects the accuracy of the output although comments have been made that certain coding practices might increase the risk of, as yet undiscovered, miscodes. The *STRmix™* team maintain regularly updated specifications documentation, risk analysis, and a gap analysis. This latter specifies any gaps between current *STRmix* practice and various guidance documents. In summary *STRmix™* complies or very nearly complies with the SWGDAM [108], ISFG [109], Forensic Science Regulator [116] and IEEE requirements [221]. The *STRmix™* group is accredited to ISO 9001 standard.

4.8.5. Validation

Various aspects of *STRmix™* validation have been challenged in courts since 2012. The initial challenges related to the conceptual validation of the models used by *STRmix™* or the laboratory in-house validation of the software to show that it was performing to a high standard. Later challenges moved to the thoroughness of developmental validation, the adherence of developmental validation with published guidelines, or the validation of the computer coding (separately from the validation of the results produced by the computer code). This latter point was the focus of a multiple day defence challenge to *STRmix™* in R v Tuite [222] in Australia.

Supplementary Materials: The following are available online at https://www.mdpi.com/article/10.3390/genes12101559/s1, Supplement S1: Details of available software to carry out probabilistic genotyping, Supplement S2: Details of the gamma model.

Conflicts of Interest: The authors declare no conflict of interest.

References

1. Gill, P.; Brenner, C.; Buckleton, J.; Carracedo, A.; Krawczak, M.; Mayr, W.; Morling, N.; Prinz, M.; Schneider, P.M.; Weir, B. DNA commission of the International Society of Forensic Genetics: Recommendations on the interpretation of mixtures. *Forensic Sci. Int.* **2006**, *160*, 90–101. [CrossRef]
2. Gill, P.; Gusmão, L.; Haned, H.; Mayr, W.; Morling, N.; Parson, W.; Prieto, L.; Prinz, M.; Schneider, H.; Schneider, P.; et al. DNA commission of the International Society of Forensic Genetics: Recommendations on the evaluation of STR typing results that may include drop-out and/or drop-in using probabilistic methods. *Forensic Sci. Int. Genet.* **2012**, *6*, 679–688. [CrossRef]
3. Gill, P.; Hicks, T.; Butler, J.M.; Connolly, E.; Gusmão, L.; Kokshoorn, B.; Morling, N.; van Oorschot, R.A.; Parson, W.; Prinz, M.; et al. DNA commission of the International society for forensic genetics: Assessing the value of forensic biological evidence—Guidelines highlighting the importance of propositions. *Forensic Sci. Int. Genet.* **2018**, *36*, 189–202. [CrossRef] [PubMed]
4. Clayton, T.; Whitaker, J.; Sparkes, R.; Gill, P. Analysis and interpretation of mixed forensic stains using DNA STR profiling. *Forensic Sci. Int.* **1998**, *91*, 55–70. [CrossRef]
5. Gill, P.; Whitaker, J.; Flaxman, C.; Brown, N.; Buckleton, J. An investigation of the rigor of interpretation rules for STRs derived from less than 100 pg of DNA. *Forensic Sci. Int.* **2000**, *112*, 17–40. [CrossRef]
6. Balding, D. Evaluation of mixed-source, low-template DNA profiles in forensic science. *Proc. Natl. Acad. Sci. USA* **2013**, *110*, 12241–12246. [CrossRef]
7. Balding, J.D.; Buckleton, J. Interpreting low template DNA profiles. *Forensic Sci. Int. Genet.* **2009**, *4*, 1–10. [CrossRef]
8. Puch-Solis, R.; Clayton, T. Evidential evaluation of DNA profiles using a discrete statistical model implemented in the DNA LiRa software. *Forensic Sci. Int. Genet.* **2014**, *11*, 220–228. [CrossRef]
9. Gill, P.; Haned, H. A new methodological framework to interpret complex DNA profiles using likelihood ratios. *Forensic Sci. Int. Genet.* **2013**, *7*, 251–263. [CrossRef]
10. Curran, J.; Gill, P.; Bill, M. Interpretation of repeat measurement DNA evidence allowing for multiple contributors and population substructure. *Forensic Sci. Int.* **2005**, *148*, 47–53. [CrossRef]
11. Slooten, K. Accurate assessment of the weight of evidence for DNA mixtures by integrating the likelihood ratio. *Forensic Sci. Int. Genet.* **2017**, *27*, 1–16. [CrossRef]
12. Puch-Solis, R.; Rodgers, L.; Mazumder, A.; Pope, S.; Evett, I.; Curran, J.; Balding, D. Evaluating forensic DNA profiles using peak heights, allowing for multiple donors, allelic dropout and stutters. *Forensic Sci. Int. Genet.* **2013**, *7*, 555–563. [CrossRef]
13. Puch-Solis, R. A dropin peak height model. *Forensic Sci. Int. Genet.* **2014**, *11*, 80–84. [CrossRef] [PubMed]
14. Perlin, M.W.; Legler, M.W.; Spencer, C.E.; Smith, J.L.; Allan, W.P.; Belrose, J.L.; Duceman, B.W. Validating TrueAllele®DNA mixture interpretation. *J. Forensic Sci.* **2011**, *56*, 1430–1447. [CrossRef] [PubMed]
15. Taylor, D.; Bright, J.-A.; Buckleton, J. The interpretation of single source and mixed DNA profiles. *Forensic Sci. Int. Genet.* **2013**, *7*, 516–528. [CrossRef] [PubMed]
16. Robert, G.C. Validation of an STR peak area model. *Forensic Sci. Int. Genet.* **2009**, *3*, 193–199.
17. Bleka, Ø.; Storvik, G.O.; Gill, P. EuroForMix: An open source software based on a continuous model to evaluate STR DNA profiles from a mixture of contributors with artefacts. *Forensic Sci. Int. Genet.* **2016**, *21*, 35–44. [CrossRef]
18. Cowell, R.; Lauritzen, S.; Mortera, J. Probabilistic expert systems for handling artifacts in complex DNA mixtures. *Forensic Sci. Int. Genet.* **2011**, *5*, 202–209. [CrossRef]
19. ENFSI Guideline for Evaluative Reporting in Forensic Science. European Network of Forensic Science Institutes. 2015. Available online: https://enfsi.eu/wp-content/uploads/2016/09/m1_guideline.pdf (accessed on 28 September 2021).
20. Slooten, K. Identifying common donors in DNA mixtures, with applications to database searches. *Forensic Sci. Int. Genet.* **2017**, *26*, 40–47. [CrossRef]
21. Bleka, Ø.; Prieto, L.; Gill, P. CaseSolver: An investigative open source expert system based on EuroForMix. *Forensic Sci. Int. Genet.* **2019**, *41*, 83–92. [CrossRef]
22. Benschop, C.C.; van de Merwe, L.; de Jong, J.; Vanvooren, V.; Kempenaers, M.; van der Beek, C.; Barni, F.; Reyes, E.L.; Moulin, L.; Pene, L.; et al. Validation of SmartRank: A likelihood ratio software for searching national DNA databases with complex DNA profiles. *Forensic Sci. Int. Genet.* **2017**, *29*, 145–153. [CrossRef]
23. Benschop, C.; Jong, J.; Merwe, L.; Haned, H. Adapting a likelihood ratio model to enable searching DNA databases with complex STR DNA profiles. In Proceedings of the 2016 27th International Symposium on Human Identification, Nagoya, Japan, 28–30 November 2016. Available online: https://promega.media/-/media/files/products-and-services/genetic-identity/ishi-27-oral-abstracts/4-benschop.pdf (accessed on 28 September 2021).
24. Bleka, Ø.; Bouzga, M.; Fonneløp, A.; Gill, P. dnamatch2: An open source software to carry out large scale database searches of mixtures using qualitative and quantitative models. *Forensic Sci. Int. Genet. Suppl. Ser.* **2017**, *6*, e404–e406. [CrossRef]
25. Taylor, D.; Rowe, E.; Kruijver, M.; Abarno, D.; Bright, J.-A.; Buckleton, J. Inter-sample contamination detection using mixture deconvolution comparison. *Forensic Sci. Int. Genet.* **2019**, *40*, 160–167. [CrossRef]
26. Kloosterman, A.; Sjerps, M.; Quak, A. Error rates in forensic DNA analysis: Definition, numbers, impact and communication. *Forensic Sci. Int. Genet.* **2014**, *12*, 77–85. [CrossRef] [PubMed]
27. Gill, P. Misleading DNA Evidence: Reasons for Miscarriages of Justice. *Int. Comment. Évid.* **2012**, *10*, 55–71. [CrossRef]

28. Duewer, D.L.; Kline, M.C.; Redman, J.W.; Butler, J.M. NIST Mixed Stain Study 3: Signal Intensity Balance in Commercial Short Tandem Repeat Multiplexes. *Anal. Chem.* **2004**, *76*, 6928–6934. [CrossRef] [PubMed]

29. Benschop, C.C.; Sijen, T. LoCIM-tool: An expert's assistant for inferring the major contributor's alleles in mixed consensus DNA profiles. *Forensic Sci. Int. Genet.* **2014**, *11*, 154–165. [CrossRef] [PubMed]

30. Butler, J.M. Scientific Working Group on DNA Analysis Methods (SWGDAM) Mixture Interpretation Issues & Insights. 2007. Available online: https://strbase.nist.gov/pub_pres/SWGDAM_Jan2007_MixtureInterpretation.pdf (accessed on 28 September 2021).

31. Coble, M.D. MIX13: An Interlaboratory Study on the Present State of DNA Mixture Interpretation in the U.S. In Proceedings of the 5th Annual Prescription for Criminal Justice Forensics, New York, NY, USA, 6 June 2014. Available online: http://www.cstl.nist.gov/strbase/pub_pres/Coble-ABA2014-MIX13.pdf (accessed on 28 September 2021).

32. Crespillo, M.; Barrio, P.A.; Luque, J.A.; Alves, C.; Aler, M.; Alessandrini, F.; Andrade, L.; Barretto, R.; Bofarull, A.; Costa, S.; et al. GHEP-ISFG collaborative exercise on mixture profiles of autosomal STRs (GHEP-MIX01, GHEP-MIX02 and GHEP-MIX03): Results and evaluation. *Forensic Sci. Int. Genet.* **2014**, *10*, 64–72. [CrossRef]

33. Cooper, S.; McGovern, C.; Bright, J.-A.; Taylor, D.; Buckleton, J. Investigating a common approach to DNA profile interpretation using probabilistic software. *Forensic Sci. Int. Genet.* **2015**, *16*, 121–131. [CrossRef]

34. Torres, Y.; Flores, I.; Prieto, V.; López-Soto, M.; Farfán, M.J.; Carracedo, A.; Sanz, P. DNA mixtures in forensic casework: A 4-year retrospective study. *Forensic Sci. Int.* **2003**, *134*, 180–186. [CrossRef]

35. Benschop, C.C.; Haned, H.; de Blaeij, T.J.; Meulenbroek, A.J.; Sijen, T. Assessment of mock cases involving complex low template DNA mixtures: A descriptive study. *Forensic Sci. Int. Genet.* **2012**, *6*, 697–707. [CrossRef] [PubMed]

36. Benschop, C.C.G.; Connolly, E.; Ansell, R.; Kokshoorn, B. Results of an inter and intra laboratory exercise on the assessment of complex autosomal DNA pro-files. *Sci. Justice* **2017**, *57*, 21–27. [CrossRef] [PubMed]

37. Benschop, C.C.; Hoogenboom, J.; Bargeman, F.; Hovers, P.; Slagter, M.; van der Linden, J.; Parag, R.; Kruise, D.; Drobnic, K.; Klucevsek, G.; et al. Multi-laboratory validation of DNAxs including the statistical library DNAStatistX. *Forensic Sci. Int. Genet.* **2020**, *49*. [CrossRef] [PubMed]

38. Butler, J.M.; Kline, M.C.; Coble, M.D. NIST Interlaboratory Studies Involving DNA Mixtures (MIX05 and MIX13): Varia-tion Observed and Lessons Learned. *Forensic Sci. Int. Genet.* **2018**, *37*, 81–94. [CrossRef] [PubMed]

39. Barrio, P.A.; Crespillo, M.; Luque, J.; Aler, M.; Baeza-Richer, C.; Baldassarri, L.; Carnevali, E.; Coufalova, P.; Flores, I.; García, O.; et al. GHEP-ISFG collaborative exercise on mixture profiles (GHEP-MIX06). Reporting conclusions: Results and evaluation. *Forensic Sci. Int. Genet.* **2018**, *35*, 156–163. [CrossRef]

40. Prieto, L.; Haned, H.; Mosquera, A.; Crespillo, M.; Alemañ, M.; Aler, M.; Álvarez, F.; Baeza-Richer, C.; Dominguez, A.; Doutremepuich, C.; et al. Euroforgen-NoE collaborative exercise on LRmix to demonstrate standardization of the interpretation of complex DNA profiles. *Forensic Sci. Int. Genet.* **2014**, *9*, 47–54. [CrossRef] [PubMed]

41. Buckleton, J.S.; Bright, J.-A.; Cheng, K.; Budowle, B.; Coble, M.D. NIST interlaboratory studies involving DNA mixtures (MIX13): A modern analysis. *Forensic Sci. Int. Genet.* **2018**, *37*, 172–179. [CrossRef]

42. Bille, T.; Bright, J.-A.; Buckleton, J. Application of Random Match Probability Calculations to Mixed STR Profiles. *J. Forensic Sci.* **2013**, *58*, 474–485. [CrossRef]

43. Alladio, E.; Omedei, M.; Cisana, S.; D'Amico, G.; Caneparo, D.; Vincenti, M.; Garofano, P. DNA mixtures interpretation—A proof-of-concept multi-software comparison highlighting different proba-bilistic methods' performances on challenging samples. *Forensic Sci. Int. Genet.* **2018**, *37*, 143–150. [CrossRef]

44. Iyer, H.K. Validation Principles, Practices, Parameters, Performance Evaluations, and Protocols Reliability Assessment of LR Systems: General Concepts. In Proceedings of the ISHI 2020 Validation Workshop, Baltimore, MD, USA, 18 September 2020. Available online: https://strbase.nist.gov/pub_pres/5_W10-Hari.pdf (accessed on 28 September 2021).

45. Garofano, P.; Caneparo, D.; D'Amico, G.; Vincenti, M.; Alladio, E. An alternative application of the consensus method to DNA typing interpretation for Low Tem-plate-DNA mixtures. *FSI: Genet. Suppl. Ser.* **2015**, *5*, e422–e424.

46. Cheng, K.; Bleka, Ø.; Gill, P.; Curran, J.; Bright, J.; Taylor, D.; Buckleton, J. A comparison of likelihood ratios obtained from EuroForMix and STRmix™. *J. Forensic Sci.* **2021**. [CrossRef]

47. Taylor, D.A.; Buckleton, J.S.; Bright, J.-A. Comment on "DNA mixtures interpretation—A proof-of-concept multi-software comparison highlighting different probabilistic methods' performances on challenging samples" by Alladio et al. *Forensic Sci. Int. Genet.* **2019**, *40*, e248–e251. [CrossRef]

48. Swaminathan, H.; Qureshi, M.O.; Grgicak, C.M.; Duffy, K.; Lun, D.S. Four model variants within a continuous forensic DNA mixture interpretation framework: Effects on evidential inference and reporting. *PLoS ONE* **2018**, *13*, e0207599. [CrossRef]

49. Zweig, M.H.; Campbell, A.G. Receiver-operating characteristic (ROC) plots: A fundamental evaluation tool in clinical medi-cine. *Clin. Chem.* **1993**, *39*, 561–577. [CrossRef]

50. Bleka, Ø.; Benschop, C.C.; Storvik, G.O.; Gill, P. A comparative study of qualitative and quantitative models used to interpret complex STR DNA profiles. *Forensic Sci. Int. Genet.* **2016**, *25*, 85–96. [CrossRef]

51. You, Y.; Balding, D. A comparison of software for the evaluation of complex DNA profiles. *Forensic Sci. Int. Genet.* **2019**, *40*, 114–119. [CrossRef]

52. Manabe, S.; Morimoto, C.; Hamano, Y.; Fujimoto, S.; Tamaki, K. Development and validation of open-source software for DNA mixture interpretation based on a quantita-tive continuous model. *PLoS ONE* **2017**, *12*, e0188183. [CrossRef]

53. Bright, J.-A.; Cheng, K.; Kerr, Z.; McGovern, C.; Kelly, H.; Moretti, T.R.; Smith, M.A.; Bieber, F.R.; Budowle, B.; Coble, M.D.; et al. STRmix™ collaborative exercise on DNA mixture interpretation. *Forensic Sci. Int. Genet.* **2019**, *40*, 1–8. [CrossRef] [PubMed]

54. Bright, J.-A.; Richards, R.; Kruijver, M.; Kelly, H.; McGovern, C.; Magee, A.; McWhorter, A.; Ciecko, A.; Peck, B.; Baumgartner, C.; et al. Internal validation of STRmix™ – A multi laboratory response to PCAST, *Forensic Sci. Int. Genet.* **2019**, *34*, 11–24. *Forensic Sci. Int. Genet.* **2019**, *41*, e14–e17.

55. Ramos, D.; Gonzalez-Rodriguez, J. Reliable support: Measuring calibration of likelihood ratios. *Forensic Sci. Int.* **2013**, *230*, 156–169. [CrossRef] [PubMed]

56. Buckleton, J.S.; Pugh, S.N.; Bright, J.-A.; Taylor, D.A.; Curran, J.M.; Kruijver, M.; Gill, P.; Budowle, B.; Cheng, K. Are low LRs reliable? *Forensic Sci. Int. Genet.* **2020**, *49*, 102350. [CrossRef] [PubMed]

57. Hannig, J.; Riman, S.; Iyer, H.; Vallone, P.M. Are reported likelihood ratios well calibrated? *Forensic Sci. Int. Genet. Suppl. Ser.* **2019**, *7*, 572–574. [CrossRef]

58. Bright, J.-A.; Dukes, M.J.; Pugh, S.N.; Evett, I.W.; Buckleton, J.S. Applying calibration to LRs produced by a DNA interpretation software. *Aust. J. Forensic Sci.* **2019**, *53*, 147–153. [CrossRef]

59. Taylor, D.; Buckleton, J.; Evett, I. Testing likelihood ratios produced from complex DNA profiles. *Forensic Sci. Int. Genet.* **2015**, *16*, 165–171. [CrossRef]

60. Taylor, D.; Curran, J.M.; Buckleton, J. Importance sampling allows Hd true tests of highly discriminating DNA profiles. *Forensic Sci. Int. Genet.* **2017**, *27*, 74–81. [CrossRef]

61. Butler, J.M. *Advanced Topics in Forensic DNA Typing: Interpretation*; Academic Press: Cambridge, MA, USA, 2014. [CrossRef]

62. Gill, P.; Bleka, Ø.; Hansson, O.; Benschop, C.; Haned, H. *Forensic Practitioner's Guide to the Interpretation of Complex DNA Profiles*; Academic Press: London, UK, 2020. [CrossRef]

63. SWGDAM Interpretation Guidelines for Autosomal STR Typing by Forensic DNA Testing Laboratories. 2010. Available online: http://www.fbi.gov/about-us/lab/codis/swgdam-interpretation-guidelines (accessed on 28 September 2021).

64. Buckleton, J.S.; Curran, J.M.; Gill, P. Towards understanding the effect of uncertainty in the number of contributors to DNA stains. *Forensic Sci. Int. Genet.* **2007**, *1*, 20–28. [CrossRef]

65. Paoletti, D.R.; Doom, T.E.; Krane, C.M.; Raymer, M.L.; Krane, D.E. Empirical Analysis of the STR Profiles Resulting from Conceptual Mixtures. *J. Forensic Sci.* **2005**, *50*, 1–6. [CrossRef]

66. Norsworthy, S.; Lun, D.S.; Grgicak, C.M. Determining the number of contributors to DNA mixtures in the low-template regime: Exploring the impacts of sampling and detection effects. *Leg. Med.* **2018**, *32*, 1–8. [CrossRef]

67. Weir, B.S.; Triggs, C.M.; Starling, L.; Stowell, L.I.; Walsh, K.A.; Buckleton, J. Interpreting DNA mixtures. *J. Forensic Sci.* **1997**, *42*, 213–222. [CrossRef] [PubMed]

68. Benschop, C.C.; Haned, H.; Jeurissen, L.; Gill, P.D.; Sijen, T. The effect of varying the number of contributors on likelihood ratios for complex DNA mixtures. *Forensic Sci. Int. Genet.* **2015**, *19*, 92–99. [CrossRef] [PubMed]

69. Haned, H.; Benschop, C.C.; Gill, P.D.; Sijen, T. Complex DNA mixture analysis in a forensic context: Evaluating the probative value using a likelihood ratio model. *Forensic Sci. Int. Genet.* **2015**, *16*, 17–25. [CrossRef]

70. Bright, J.A.; Curran, J.M.; Buckleton, J.S. The effect of the uncertainty in the number of contributors to mixed DNA pro-files on profile interpretation. *Forensic Sci. Int. Genet.* **2014**, *12*, 208–214. [CrossRef] [PubMed]

71. Buckleton, J.S.; Bright, J.-A.; Cheng, K.; Kelly, H.; Taylor, D.A. The effect of varying the number of contributors in the prosecution and alternate propositions. *Forensic Sci. Int. Genet.* **2018**, *38*, 225–231. [CrossRef]

72. Bille, T.; Weitz, S.; Buckleton, J.S.; Bright, J.-A. Interpreting a major component from a mixed DNA profile with an unknown number of minor contributors. *Forensic Sci. Int. Genet.* **2019**, *40*, 150–159. [CrossRef] [PubMed]

73. Benschop, C.C.; Nijveld, A.; Duijs, F.E.; Sijen, T. An assessment of the performance of the probabilistic genotyping software EuroForMix: Trends in likelihood ratios and analysis of Type I & II errors. *Forensic Sci. Int. Genet.* **2019**, *42*, 31–38. [CrossRef] [PubMed]

74. Slooten, K. A top-down approach to DNA mixtures. *Forensic Sci. Int. Genet.* **2020**, *46*, 102250. [CrossRef] [PubMed]

75. Coble, M.D.; Bright, J.-A.; Buckleton, J.S.; Curran, J.M. Uncertainty in the number of contributors in the proposed new CODIS set. *Forensic Sci. Int. Genet.* **2015**, *19*, 207–211. [CrossRef]

76. Curran, J.M.; Buckleton, J. Uncertainty in the number of contributors for the European Standard Set of loci. *Forensic Sci. Int. Genet.* **2014**, *11*, 205–206. [CrossRef]

77. Dembinski, G.M.; Sobieralski, C.; Picard, C.J. Estimation of the number of contributors of theoretical mixture profiles based on allele counting: Does increasing the number of loci increase success rate of estimates? *Forensic Sci. Int. Genet.* **2018**, *33*, 24–32. [CrossRef]

78. Young, B.A.; Gettings, K.B.; McCord, B.; Vallone, P.M. Estimating number of contributors in massively parallel sequencing data of STR loci. *Forensic Sci. Int. Genet.* **2019**, *38*, 15–22. [CrossRef]

79. Haned, H.; Pène, L.; Lobry, J.R.; Dufour, A.B.; Pontier, D. Estimating the Number of Contributors to Forensic DNA Mixtures: Does Maximum Likelihood Perform Better Than Maximum Allele Count? *J. Forensic Sci.* **2011**, *56*, 23–28. [CrossRef] [PubMed]

80. Haned, H.; Pène, L.; Sauvage, F.; Pontier, D. The predictive value of the maximum likelihood estimator of the number of contributors to a DNA mixture. *Forensic Sci. Int. Genet.* **2011**, *5*, 281–284. [CrossRef]

81. Biedermann, A.; Bozza, S.; Konis, K.; Taroni, F. Inference about the number of contributors to a DNA mixture: Comparative analyses of a Bayesian network approach and the maximum allele count method. *Forensic Sci. Int. Genet.* **2012**, *6*, 689–696. [CrossRef]

82. Tvedebrink, T. On the exact distribution of the numbers of alleles in DNA mixtures. *Int. J. Leg. Med.* **2013**, *128*, 427–437. [CrossRef]

83. Benschop, C.; Haned, H.; Sijen, T. Consensus and pool profiles to assist in the analysis and interpretation of complex low template DNA mixtures. *Int. J. Leg. Med.* **2011**, *127*, 11–23. [CrossRef]

84. Paoletti, D.R.; Krane, D.E.; Raymer, M.L.; Doom, T.E. Inferring the Number of Contributors to Mixed DNA Profiles. *IEEE/ACM Trans. Comput. Biol. Bioinform.* **2011**, *9*, 113–122. [CrossRef]

85. Perez, J.; Mitchell, A.A.; Ducasse, N.; Tamariz, J.; Caragine, T. Estimating the number of contributors to two-, three-, and four-person mixtures containing DNA in high template and low template amounts. *Croat. Med. J.* **2011**, *52*, 314–326. [CrossRef]

86. Benschop, C.C.; van der Beek, C.P.; Meiland, H.C.; van Gorp, A.G.; Westen, A.A.; Sijen, T. Low template STR typing: Effect of replicate number and consensus method on genotyping reliability and DNA database search results. *Forensic Sci. Int. Genet.* **2011**, *5*, 316–328. [CrossRef] [PubMed]

87. Alfonse, L.; Tejada, G.; Swaminathan, H.; Lun, D.S.; Grgicak, C.M. Inferring the Number of Contributors to Complex DNA Mixtures Using Three Methods: Exploring the Limits of Low-Template DNA Interpretation. *J. Forensic Sci.* **2016**, *62*, 308–316. [CrossRef]

88. Swaminathan, H.; Grgicak, C.M.; Medard, M.; Lun, D.S. NOCIt: A computational method to infer the number of contributors to DNA samples analyzed by STR genotyping. *Forensic Sci. Int. Genet.* **2015**, *16*, 172–180. [CrossRef] [PubMed]

89. Benschop, C.; Backx, A.; Sijen, T. Automated estimation of the number of contributors in autosomal STR profiles. *Forensic Sci. Int. Genet. Suppl. Ser.* **2019**, *7*, 7–8. [CrossRef]

90. Marciano, M.A.; Adelman, J.D. PACE: Probabilistic Assessment for Contributor Estimation—A machine learning-based assessment of the number of contributors in DNA mixtures. *Forensic Sci. Int. Genet.* **2017**, *27*, 82–91. [CrossRef] [PubMed]

91. Benschop, C.C.; van der Linden, J.; Hoogenboom, J.; Ypma, R.; Haned, H. Automated estimation of the number of contributors in autosomal short tandem repeat profiles using a machine learning approach. *Forensic Sci. Int. Genet.* **2019**, *43*, 102150. [CrossRef] [PubMed]

92. Kruijver, M.; Kelly, H.; Cheng, K.; Lin, M.-H.; Morawitz, J.; Russell, L.; Buckleton, J.; Bright, J.-A. Estimating the number of contributors to a DNA profile using decision trees. *Forensic Sci. Int. Genet.* **2020**, *50*, 102407. [CrossRef] [PubMed]

93. Taylor, D.; Bright, J.A.; Buckleton, J. Interpreting forensic DNA profiling evidence without specifying the number of con-tribuors. *Forensic Sci. Int. Genet.* **2014**, *13*, 269–280. [CrossRef]

94. Slooten, K.; Caliebe, A. Contributors are a nuisance (parameter) for DNA mixture evidence evaluation. *Forensic Sci. Int. Genet.* **2018**, *37*, 116–125. [CrossRef]

95. Buckleton, J.; Taylor, D.; Bright, J.A.; Hicks, T.; Curran, J. When evaluating DNA evidence within a likelihood ratio framework, should the propositions be exhaustive? *Forensic Sci. Int. Genet.* **2021**, *50*, 102406. [CrossRef]

96. Hicks, T.; Kerr, Z.; Pugh, S.; Bright, J.-A.; Curran, J.; Taylor, D.; Buckleton, J. Comparing multiple POI to DNA mixtures. *Forensic Sci. Int. Genet.* **2021**, *52*, 102481. [CrossRef]

97. Kelly, H. The effect of user defined number of contributors within the LR assignment. *Aust. J. Forensic Sci.* **2021**, 1–14. [CrossRef]

98. McGovern, C.; Cheng, K.; Kelly, H.; Ciecko, A.; Taylor, D.; Buckleton, J.S.; Bright, J.A. Performance of a method for weighting a range in the number of contributors in probabilistic genotyping. *Forensic Sci. Int. Genet.* **2020**, *48*, 102352. [CrossRef]

99. Akaike, H. A new look at the statistical model identification. *IEEE Trans. Autom. Control.* **1974**, *19*, 716–723. [CrossRef]

100. Coble, M.D.; Bright, J.-A. Probabilistic genotyping software: An overview. *Forensic Sci. Int. Genet.* **2018**, *38*, 219–224. [CrossRef]

101. Cook, R.; Evett, I.; Jackson, G.; Jones, P.; Lambert, J. A hierarchy of propositions: Deciding which level to address in casework. *Sci. Justice* **1998**, *38*, 231–239. [CrossRef]

102. Evett, I.W.; Jackson, G.; Lambert, J.A. More on the hierarchy of propositions: Exploring the distinction between explana-tions and propositions. *Sci. Justice* **2000**, *40*, 3–10. [CrossRef]

103. Gittelson, S.; Kalafut, T.; Myers, S.; Taylor, D.; Hicks, T.; Taroni, F.; Buckleton, J. A Practical Guide for the Formulation of Propositions in the Bayesian Approach to DNA Evidence Inter-pretation in an Adversarial Environment. *J. Forensic Sci.* **2016**, *61*, 186–195. [CrossRef] [PubMed]

104. Taylor, D.A.; Bright, J.-A.; Buckleton, J.S. The 'factor of two' issue in mixed DNA profiles. *J. Theor. Biol.* **2014**, *363*, 300–306. [CrossRef] [PubMed]

105. Evett, I. On meaningful questions: A two-trace transfer problem. *J. Forensic Sci. Soc.* **1987**, *27*, 375–381. [CrossRef]

106. Gill, P. Analysis and implications of the miscarriages of justice of Amanda Knox and Raffaele Sollecito. *Forensic Sci. Int. Genet.* **2016**, *23*, 9–18. [CrossRef] [PubMed]

107. Foreman, L.; Smith, A.F.M.; Evett, I.W.; Aitken, C.G.G.; Taroni, A.F. Comment on Foreman L., Smith A.F.M., Evett I.W., Bayesian analysis of DNA profiling data in forensic identification applications. *J. R. Stat. Soc.* **1997**, *160*, 463. [CrossRef]

108. Scientific Working Group on DNA Analysis Methods (SWGDAM): Guidelines for the Validation of Probabilistic Genotyping Systems. 2015. Available online: https://1ecb9588-ea6f-4feb-971a-73265dbf079c.filesusr.com/ugd/4344b0_22776006b67c4a3 2a5ffc04fe3b56515.pdf (accessed on 25 September 2021).

109. Coble, M.; Buckleton, J.; Butler, J.; Egeland, T.; Fimmers, R.; Gill, P.; Gusmão, L.; Guttman, B.; Krawczak, M.; Morling, N.; et al. DNA Commission of the International Society for Forensic Genetics: Recommendations on the validation of software programs performing biostatistical calculations for forensic genetics applications. *Forensic Sci. Int. Genet.* **2016**, *25*, 191–197. [CrossRef]

110. ANSI/ASB Standard 018, First Edition. 2020: Standard for Validation of Probabilistic Genotyping Systems. Available online: http://www.asbstandardsboard.org/wp-content/uploads/2020/07/018_Std_e1.pdf (accessed on 28 September 2021).

111. Ballim, A.; Wilks, A.Y. Beliefs, stereotypes and dynamic agent modeling. *User Model. User-Adapt. Interact.* **1991**, *1*, 33–65. [CrossRef]

112. Bright, J.-A.; Evett, I.W.; Taylor, D.; Curran, J.M.; Buckleton, J. A series of recommended tests when validating probabilistic DNA profile interpretation software. *Forensic Sci. Int. Genet.* **2015**, *14*, 125–131. [CrossRef]

113. Haned, H.; Gill, P.; Lohmueller, K.; Inman, K.; Rudin, N. Validation of probabilistic genotyping software for use in forensic DNA casework: Definitions and illustra-tions. *Sci. Justice* **2016**, *56*, 104–108. [CrossRef] [PubMed]

114. Ropero-Miller, J.; Melton, P.; Ferrara, L.; Hall, J. Landscape Study of DNA Mixture Interpretation Software. National Institute of Justice, Forensic Technology Centre of Excellence. 2015. Available online: https://nij.ojp.gov/library/publications/landscape-study-dna-mixture-interpretation-software (accessed on 28 September 2021).

115. European Network of Forensic Science Institutes (ENFSI). Best Practice Manual for the Internal Validation of Probabilistic Software to Undertake DNA Mixture Interpretation ENFSI-BPM-DNA-01 issue 001. 17 May 2017. Available online: https://enfsi.eu/wp-content/uploads/2017/09/Best-Practice-Manual-for-the-internal-validation-of-probabilistic-software-to-undertake-DNA-mixture-interpretation-v1.docx.pdf (accessed on 28 September 2021).

116. Forensic Science Regulator, Software Validation for DNA Mixture Interpretation, FSR-G-223 (2). 2018. Available online: https://www.gov.uk/government/publications/software-validation-for-dna-mixture-interpretation-fsr-g-223 (accessed on 28 September 2021).

117. PCAST, Forensic Science in Criminal Courts: Ensuring Scientific Validity of Feature Comparison Methods, US President's Council of Advisors on Science and Technology. 2016. Available online: https://obamawhitehouse.archives.gov/sites/default/files/microsites/ostp/PCAST/pcast_forensic_science_report_final.pdf (accessed on 28 September 2021).

118. Box, G.E.P.; Draper, N.R. *Empirical Model-Building and Response Surfaces*; Wiley: New York, NY, USA, 1987.

119. Rykiel, E.J., Jr. Testing ecological models: The meaning of validation. *Ecol. Model.* **1996**, *90*, 229–244. [CrossRef]

120. Gill, P.; Kirkham, A.; Curran, J. LoComatioN: A software tool for the analysis of low copy number DNA profiles. *Forensic Sci. Int.* **2007**, *166*, 128–138. [CrossRef] [PubMed]

121. Haned, H. Forensim: An open-source initiative for the evaluation of statistical methods in forensic genetics. *Forensic Sci. Int. Genet.* **2011**, *5*, 265–268. [CrossRef]

122. Haned, H.; Gill, P. Analysis of complex DNA mixtures using the Forensim package. *Forensic Sci. Int. Genet. Suppl. Ser.* **2011**, *3*, e79–e80. [CrossRef]

123. Evett, I.W.; Gill, P.D.; Lambert, J.A. Taking account of peak areas when interpreting mixed DNA profiles. *J. Forensic Sci.* **1998**, *43*, 62–69. [CrossRef]

124. Cowell, R.G.; Lauritzen, S.L.; Mortera, J. A γ model for {DNA} mixture analyses. *Bayesian Anal.* **2007**, *2*, 333–348. [CrossRef]

125. Graversen, T.; Lauritzen, S. Estimation of parameters in DNA mixture analysis. *J. Appl. Stat.* **2013**, *40*, 2423–2436. [CrossRef]

126. Graversen, T.; Lauritzen, S. Computational aspects of DNA mixture analysis. *Stat. Comput.* **2014**, *25*, 527–541. [CrossRef]

127. Haldemann, B.; Dornseifer, S.; Heylen, T.; Aelbrecht, C.; Bleka, O.; Larsen, H.J.; Neuhaus-Steinmetz, U. eDNA—An expert software system for comparison and evaluation of DNA profiles in forensic case-work. *Forensic Sci. Int. Genet. Suppl. Ser.* **2015**, *5*, e400–e402. [CrossRef]

128. Benschop, C.C.; Hoogenboom, J.; Hovers, P.; Slagter, M.; Kruise, D.; Parag, R.; Steensma, K.; Slooten, K.; Nagel, J.H.; Dieltjes, P.; et al. DNAxs/DNAStatistX: Development and validation of a software suite for the data management and probabilistic interpretation of DNA profiles. *Forensic Sci. Int. Genet.* **2019**, *42*, 81–89. [CrossRef] [PubMed]

129. Veldhuis, M. Explainable artificial intelligence in forensics: Realistic explanations for number of contributor predictions of DNA profiles. *Forensic Sci. Int. Genet.* **2021**, submitted.

130. Cowell, R.G.; Graversen, T.; Lauritzen, S.L.; Mortera, J. Analysis of forensic DNA mixtures with artefacts. *J. R. Stat. Soc. Ser. C Appl. Stat.* **2015**, *64*, 1–48. [CrossRef]

131. Duijs, F.E.; Hoogenboom, J.; Sijen, T.; Benschop, C. Performance of EuroForMix deconvolution on PowerPlex®Fusion 6C profiles. *Forensic Sci. Int. Genet. Suppl. Ser.* **2019**, *7*, 5–6. [CrossRef]

132. Taylor, D.; Buckleton, J. Do low template DNA profiles have useful quantitative data? *Forensic Sci. Int. Genet.* **2015**, *16*, 13–16. [CrossRef]

133. Bruijns, B.; Tiggelaar, R.M.; Gardeniers, J. Massively parallel sequencing techniques for forensics: A review. *Electrophoresis* **2018**, *39*, 2642–2654. [CrossRef]

134. Just, R.S.; Irwin, J.A. Use of the LUS in sequence allele designations to facilitate probabilistic genotyping of NGS-based STR typing results. *Forensic Sci. Int. Genet.* **2018**, *34*, 197–205. [CrossRef]

135. Just, R.S.; Le, J.; Irwin, J.A. LUS+: Extension of the LUS designator concept to differentiate most sequence alleles for 27 STR loci. *Forensic Sci. Int. Rep.* **2020**, *2*, 100059. [CrossRef]

136. Vilsen, S.B.; Tvedebrink, T.; Eriksen, P.S.; Bøsting, C.; Hussing, C.; Mogensen, H.S.; Morling, N. Stutter analysis of complex STR MPS data. *Forensic Sci. Int. Genet.* **2018**, *35*, 107–112. [CrossRef]

137. Bleka, Ø.; Just, R.; Le, J.; Gill, P. Automation of high volume MPS mixture interpretation using CaseSolver. *Forensic Sci. Int. Genet. Suppl. Ser.* **2019**, *7*, 14–15. [CrossRef]

138. Bleka, Ø.; Just, R.; Le, J.; Gill, P. An examination of STR nomenclatures, filters and models for MPS mixture interpretation. *Forensic Sci. Int. Genet.* **2020**, *48*, 102319. [CrossRef]

139. Gill, P.; Just, R.; Parson, W.; Phillips, C.; Bleka, Ø. Interpretation of complex DNA profiles generated by Massively Parallel Sequencing. In *Forensic Practitioner's Guide to the Interpretation of Complex DNA Profiles*; Gill, P., Bleka, O., Hansson, O., Benschop, C., Haned, H., Eds.; Academic Press: Cambridge, MA, USA; Elsevier: Amsterdam, The Netherlands, 2020; pp. 419–451. [CrossRef]

140. van der Gaag, K.J.; de Leeuw, R.H.; Hoogenboom, J.; Patel, J.; Storts, D.R.; Laros, J.F.; de Knijff, P. Massively parallel sequencing of short tandem re-peats-Population data and mixture analysis results for the PowerSeq system. *Forensic Sci. Int. Genet.* **2016**, *24*, 86–96. [CrossRef]

141. Hoogenboom, J.; van der Gaag, K.J.; de Leeuw, R.H.; Sijen, T.; de Knijff, P.; Laros, J.F. FDSTools: A software package for analysis of massively parallel sequencing data with the ability to recognise and correct STR stutter and other PCR or sequencing noise. *Forensic Sci. Int. Genet.* **2016**, *27*, 27–40. [CrossRef] [PubMed]

142. Benschop, C.C.; van der Gaag, K.J.; de Vreede, J.; Backx, A.J.; de Leeuw, R.H.; Zuñiga, S.; Hoogenboom, J.; de Knijff, P.; Sijen, T. Application of a probabilistic genotyping software to MPS mixture STR data is supported by similar trends in LRs compared with CE data. *Forensic Sci. Int. Genet.* **2021**, *52*, 102489. [CrossRef] [PubMed]

143. Bleka, Ø.; Eduardoff, M.; Santos, C.; Phillips, C.; Parson, W.; Gill, P. Open source software EuroForMix can be used to analyse complex SNP mixtures. *Forensic Sci. Int. Genet.* **2017**, *31*, 105–110. [CrossRef] [PubMed]

144. Bleka, Ø.; Eduardoff, M.; Santos, C.; Phillips, C.; Parson, W.; Gill, P. Using EuroForMix to analyse complex SNP mixtures, up to six contributors. *Forensic Sci. Int. Genet. Suppl. Ser.* **2017**, *6*, e277–e279. [CrossRef]

145. Yang, T.-W.; Li, Y.-H.; Chou, C.-F.; Lai, F.-P.; Chien, Y.-H.; Yin, H.-I.; Lee, T.-T.; Hwa, H.-L. DNA mixture interpretation using linear regression and neural networks on massively parallel sequencing data of single nucleotide polymorphisms. *Aust. J. Forensic Sci.* **2021**, 1–13. [CrossRef]

146. Benschop, C.C.; Haned, H.; Yoo, S.Y.; Sijen, T. Evaluation of samples comprising minute amounts of DNA. *Sci. Justice* **2015**, *55*, 316–322. [CrossRef] [PubMed]

147. Benschop, C.C.; Yoo, S.Y.; Sijen, T. Split DNA over replicates or perform one amplification? *Forensic Sci. Int. Genet. Suppl. Ser.* **2015**, *5*, e532–e533. [CrossRef]

148. Benschop, C.C.; Graaf, E.S.; Sijen, T. Is an increased drop-in rate appropriate with enhanced DNA profiling? *Forensic Sci. Int. Genet. Suppl. Ser.* **2015**, *5*, e71–e72. [CrossRef]

149. Slagter, M.; Kruise, D.; van Ommen, L.; Hoogenboom, J.; Steensma, K.; de Jong, J.; Hovers, P.; Parag, R.; van der Linden, J.; Kneppers, A.L.; et al. The DNAxs software suite: A three-year retrospective study on the development, architecture, testing and implementation in forensic casework. *Forensic Sci. Int. Rep.* **2021**, *3*, 100212. [CrossRef]

150. Beecham, G.W.; Weir, B.S. Confidence interval of the likelihood ratio associated with mixed stain DNA evidence. *J. Forensic Sci.* **2010**, *56*, S166–S171. [CrossRef]

151. Curran, J.M.; Triggs, C.M.; Buckleton, J.; Weir, B.S. Interpreting DNA mixtures in structured populations. *J. Forensic Sci.* **1999**, *44*, 12028J. [CrossRef]

152. Slooten, K. The analogy between DNA kinship and DNA mixture evaluation, with applications for the interpretation of like-lihood ratios produced by possibly imperfect models. *Forensic Sci. Int. Genet.* **2021**, *52*, 102449. [CrossRef]

153. Good, I.J. *Probability and the Weighing of Evidence*; Charles Griffin & Company Limited: London, UK, 1950.

154. Bright, J.A.; Taylor, D.; Curran, J.M.; Buckleton, J.S. Degradation of forensic DNA profiles. *Aust. J. Forensic Sci.* **2013**, *45*, 445–449. [CrossRef]

155. Taylor, D.; Bright, J.-A.; Kelly, H.; Lin, M.-H.; Buckleton, J. A fully continuous system of DNA profile evidence evaluation that can utilise STR profile data produced under different conditions within a single analysis. *Forensic Sci. Int. Genet.* **2017**, *31*, 149–154. [CrossRef]

156. Bright, J.-A.; Taylor, D.; Curran, J.M.; Buckleton, J.S. Developing allelic and stutter peak height models for a continuous method of DNA interpretation. *Forensic Sci. Int. Genet.* **2013**, *7*, 296–304. [CrossRef]

157. Taylor, D.; Bright, J.-A.; McGovern, C.; Hefford, C.; Kalafut, T.; Buckleton, J. Validating multiplexes for use in conjunction with modern interpretation strategies. *Forensic Sci. Int. Genet.* **2016**, *20*, 6–19. [CrossRef]

158. Bright, J.-A.; Buckleton, J.S.; Taylor, D.; Fernando, M.A.C.S.S.; Curran, J.M. Modeling forward stutter: Toward increased objectivity in forensic DNA interpretation. *Electrophoresis* **2014**, *35*, 3152–3157. [CrossRef]

159. Bright, J.-A.; Taylor, D.; Kerr, Z.; Buckleton, J.; Kruijver, M. The efficacy of DNA mixture to mixture matching. *Forensic Sci. Int. Genet.* **2019**, *41*, 64–71. [CrossRef]

160. Cheng, K.; Bright, J.-A.; Kerr, Z.; Taylor, D.; Ciecko, A.; Curran, J.; Buckleton, J. Examining the additivity of peak heights in forensic DNA profiles. *Aust. J. Forensic Sci.* **2020**, 1–15. [CrossRef]

161. Hansson, O.; Egeland, T.; Gill, P. Characterization of degradation and heterozygote balance by simulation of the forensic DNA analysis process. *Int. J. Leg. Med.* **2016**, *131*, 303–317. [CrossRef] [PubMed]

162. Bright, J.-A.; Curran, J.M.; Buckleton, J.S. Investigation into the performance of different models for predicting stutter. *Forensic Sci. Int. Genet.* **2013**, *7*, 422–427. [CrossRef] [PubMed]

163. Taylor, D. Using continuous DNA interpretation methods to revisit likelihood ratio behaviour. *Forensic Sci. Int. Genet.* **2014**, *11*, 144–153. [CrossRef] [PubMed]
164. Taylor, D.A.; Bright, J.-A.; Buckleton, J.S. The effect of varying the number of contributors in the prosecution and alternate propositions. *Forensic Sci. Int. Genet.* **2019**, *13*, 269–280. [CrossRef] [PubMed]
165. Weinberg, M. Computing the Bayes Factor from a Markov Chain Monte Carlo Simulation of the Posterior Distribution. *Bayesian Anal.* **2012**, *7*, 737–770. [CrossRef]
166. Weinberg, M.D.; Yoon, I.; Katz, N. A remarkably simple and accurate method for computing the Bayes Factor from a Markov chain Monte Carlo Simulation of the Posterior Distribution in high dimension. *arXiv* **2013**, arXiv:1301.3156v1.
167. Buckleton, J.; Bright, J.-A.; Taylor, D.; Evett, I.; Hicks, T.; Jackson, G.; Curran, J.M. Helping formulate propositions in forensic DNA analysis. *Sci. Justice* **2014**, *54*, 258–261. [CrossRef]
168. Taylor, D.; Bright, J.-A.; Buckleton, J. Considering relatives when assessing the evidential strength of mixed DNA profiles. *Forensic Sci. Int. Genet.* **2014**, *13*, 259–263. [CrossRef]
169. Balding, D.J. *Weight-of-Evidence for Forensic DNA Profiles*; John Wiley and Sons: Chichester, UK, 2005.
170. Buckleton, J.; Triggs, C. Relatedness and DNA: Are we taking it seriously enough? *Forensic Sci. Int.* **2005**, *152*, 115–119. [CrossRef] [PubMed]
171. Taylor, D.; Bright, J.-A.; Buckleton, J.; Curran, J. An illustration of the effect of various sources of uncertainty on DNA likelihood ratio calculations. *Forensic Sci. Int. Genet.* **2014**, *11*, 56–63. [CrossRef] [PubMed]
172. Balding, D.; Nichols, R.A. DNA profile match probability calculation: How to allow for population stratification, relatedness, database selection and single bands. *Forensic Sci. Int.* **1994**, *64*, 125–140. [CrossRef]
173. Balding, D.J. Estimating products in forensic identification using DNA profiles. *J. Am. Stat. Assoc.* **1995**, *90*, 839–844. [CrossRef]
174. Curran, J.M.; Buckleton, J.S. An investigation into the performance of methods for adjusting for sampling uncertainty in DNA likelihood ratio calculations. *Forensic Sci. Int. Genet.* **2011**, *5*, 512–516. [CrossRef] [PubMed]
175. Triggs, C.; Harbison, S.; Buckleton, J. The calculation of DNA match probabilities in mixed race populations. *Sci. Justice* **2000**, *40*, 33–38. [CrossRef]
176. Curran, J.M. An introduction to Bayesian credible intervals for sampling error in DNA profiles. *Law Probab. Risk* **2005**, *4*, 115–126. [CrossRef]
177. Morrison, G.S. Special issue on measuring and reporting the precision of forensic likelihood ratios: Introduction to the debate. *Sci. Justice* **2016**, *56*, 371–373. [CrossRef] [PubMed]
178. Morrison, G.; Enzinger, E. What should a forensic practitioner's likelihood ratio be? *Sci. Justice* **2016**, *5*, 374–379. [CrossRef]
179. Curran, J.M. Admitting to uncertainty in the LR. *Sci. Justice* **2016**, *56*, 380–382. [CrossRef]
180. Ommen, D.M.; Saunders, C.P.; Neumann, C. An argument against presenting interval quantifications as a surrogate for the value of evidence. *Sci. Justice* **2016**, *56*, 383–387. [CrossRef]
181. Berger, C.E.; Slooten, K. The LR does not exist. *Sci. Justice* **2016**, *56*, 388–391. [CrossRef] [PubMed]
182. Biedermann, A.; Bozza, S.; Taroni, F.; Aitken, C. Reframing the debate: A question of probability, not of likelihood ratio. *Sci. Justice* **2016**, *56*, 392–396. [CrossRef] [PubMed]
183. Hout, A.v.d.; Alberink, I. Posterior distribution for likelihood ratios in forensic science. *Sci. Justice* **2016**, *5*, 397–401. [CrossRef] [PubMed]
184. Taylor, D.; Hicks, T.; Champod, C. Using sensitivity analyses in Bayesian networks to highlight the impact of data pauci-ty and direct future analyses: A contribution to the debate on measuring and reporting the precision of likelihood ratios. *Sci. Justice* **2016**, *56*, 402–410. [CrossRef] [PubMed]
185. Bright, J.-A. *Testing Methods for Quantifying Monte Carlo Variation for Categorical Variables in Probabilistic Genotyping*; Report; Institute of Environmental Science and Research: Wellington, New Zealand, 2020. [CrossRef]
186. Bright, J.-A. *Revisiting the STRmix™ Likelihood Ratio Probability Interval Coverage Considering Multiple Factors*; Report; Institute of Environmental Science and Research: Wellington, New Zealand, 2021.
187. Buckleton, J.; Curran, J.; Goudet, J.; Taylor, D.; Thiery, A.; Weir, B.S. Population-specific FST values for forensic STR markers: A worldwide survey. *Forensic Sci. Int. Genet.* **2016**, *23*, 126–133.
188. Steele, C.D.; Court, D.S.; Balding, D.J. Worldwide F(ST) estimates relative to five continental-scale populations. *Ann. Hum. Genet.* **2014**, *78*, 468–477. [CrossRef]
189. Weir, B.S.; Cockerham, C.C. Estimating F-statistics for the analysis of population structure. *Evolution* **1984**, *38*, 1358–1370.
190. Bright, J.-A.; Taylor, D.; Curran, J.; Buckleton, J. Searching mixed DNA profiles directly against profile databases. *Forensic Sci. Int. Genet.* **2014**, *9*, 102–110. [CrossRef]
191. Abarno, D.; Sobieraj, T.; Summers, C.; Taylor, D. The first Australian conviction resulting from a familial search. *Aust. J. Forensic Sci.* **2019**, *51*, S56–S59. [CrossRef]
192. Taylor, D.; Abarno, D.; Rowe, E.; Rask-Nielsen, L. Observations of DNA transfer within an operational Forensic Biology Laboratory. *Forensic Int. Genet.* **2016**, *23*, 33–49. [CrossRef] [PubMed]
193. Kruijver, M.; Meester, R.; Slooten, K. p-Values should not be used for evaluating the strength of DNA evidence. *Forensic Sci. Int. Genet.* **2015**, *16*, 226–231. [CrossRef] [PubMed]

194. Budowle, B.; Onorato, A.J.; Callaghan, T.F.; Della Manna, A.; Gross, A.M.; Guerrieri, R.A.; Luttman, J.C.; McClure, D.L. Mixture Interpretation: Defining the Relevant Features for Guidelines for the Assessment of Mixed DNA Profiles in Forensic Casework. *J. Forensic Sci.* **2009**, *54*, 810–821. [CrossRef] [PubMed]

195. Taylor, D.; Bright, J.-A.; Scandrett, L.; Abarno, D.; Lee, S.-I.; Wivell, R.; Kelly, H.; Buckleton, J. Validation of a top-down DNA profile analysis for database searching using a fully continuous probabilistic genotyping model. *Forensic Sci. Int. Genet.* **2021**, *52*, 102479. [CrossRef] [PubMed]

196. Taylor, D.; Buckleton, J.; Bright, J.-A. Factors affecting peak height variability for short tandem repeat data. *Forensic Sci. Int. Genet.* **2015**, *21*, 126–133. [CrossRef] [PubMed]

197. Bright, J.-A.; Curran, J.M. Investigation into stutter ratio variability between different laboratories. *Forensic Sci. Int. Genet.* **2014**, *13*, 79–81. [CrossRef]

198. Kelly, H.; Bright, J.-A.; Kruijver, M.; Cooper, S.; Taylor, D.; Duke, K.; Strong, M.; Beamer, V.; Buettner, C.; Buckleton, J. A sensitivity analysis to determine the robustness of STRmix™ with respect to laboratory calibration. *Forensic Sci. Int. Genet.* **2018**, *35*, 113–122. [CrossRef]

199. Kelly, H. Developmental validation of a software implementation of a flexible framework for the assignment of likeli-hood ratios for forensic investigations. *Forensic Sci. Int. Rep.* **2021**, 100231. [CrossRef]

200. Kruijver, M.; Bright, J.-A.; Kelly, H.; Buckleton, J. Exploring the probative value of mixed DNA profiles. *Forensic Sci. Int. Genet.* **2019**, *41*, 1–10. [CrossRef]

201. Taylor, D.; Kruijver, M. Combining evidence across multiple mixed DNA profiles for improved resolution of a donor when a common contributor can be assumed. *Forensic Sci. Int. Genet.* **2020**, *49*. [CrossRef]

202. Kruijver, M.; Taylor, D.; Bright, J.-A. Evaluating DNA evidence possibly involving multiple (mixed) samples, common donors and related contributors. *Forensic Sci. Int. Genet.* **2021**, *54*, 102532. [CrossRef]

203. Allen, P.S.; Pugh, S.N.; Bright, J.-A.; Taylor, D.A.; Curran, J.M.; Kerr, Z.; Buckleton, J.S. Relaxing the assumption of unrelatedness in the numerator and denominator of likelihood ratios for DNA mixtures. *Forensic Sci. Int. Genet.* **2020**, *51*, 102434. [CrossRef] [PubMed]

204. Regulator, F.S. *The Forensic Science Regulator Guidance on DNA Mixture Interpretation FSR-G-222*; The Forensic Science Regulator: Birmingham, UK, 2018; pp. 1–63.

205. Bright, J.-A.; Taylor, D.; McGovern, C.; Cooper, S.; Russell, L.; Abarno, D.; Buckleton, J. Developmental validation of STRmix™, expert software for the interpretation of forensic DNA profiles. *Forensic Sci. Int. Genet.* **2016**, *23*, 226–239. [CrossRef] [PubMed]

206. Brookes, C.; Bright, J.-A.; Harbison, S.; Buckleton, J. Characterising stutter in forensic STR multiplexes. *Forensic Sci. Int. Genet.* **2012**, *6*, 58–63. [CrossRef]

207. Kelly, H.; Bright, J.-A.; Buckleton, J.S.; Curran, J.M. Identifying and modelling the drivers of stutter in forensic DNA profiles. *Aust. J. Forensic Sci.* **2013**, *46*, 194–203. [CrossRef]

208. Triggs, C.; Curran, J. The sensitivity of the Bayesian HPD method to the choice of prior. *Sci. Justice* **2006**, *46*, 169–178. [CrossRef]

209. Bright, J.-A.; Stevenson, K.; Curran, J.M.; Buckleton, J.S. The variability in likelihood ratios due to different mechanisms. *Forensic Sci. Int. Genet.* **2015**, *14*, 187–190. [CrossRef]

210. Taylor, D.; Buckleton, J.; Bright, J.-A. Does the use of probabilistic genotyping change the way we should view sub-threshold data? *Aust. J. Forensic Sci.* **2017**, *49*, 78–92. [CrossRef]

211. Russell, L.; Cooper, S.; Wivell, R.; Kerr, Z.; Taylor, D.; Buckleton, J.; Bright, J. A guide to results and diagnostics within a STRmix™ report. *Wiley Interdiscip. Rev. Forensic Sci.* **2019**, *1*, e1354. [CrossRef]

212. Moretti, T.; Just, R.S.; Kehl, S.C.; Willis, L.E.; Buckleton, J.S.; Bright, J.-A.; Taylor, D..; Onorato, A.J. Internal validation of STRmix for the interpetation of single source and mixed DNA profiles. *Forensic Sci. Int. Genet.* **2017**, *29*, 126–144. [CrossRef]

213. Noël, S.; Noël, J.; Granger, D.; Lefebvre, J.-F.; Séguin, D. STRmix™ put to the test: 300,000 non-contributor profiles compared to four-contributor DNA mixtures and the impact of replicates. *Forensic Sci. Int. Genet.* **2019**, *41*, 24–31. [CrossRef]

214. Duke, K.R.; Myers, S.P. Systematic evaluation of STRmix™ performance on degraded DNA profile data. *Forensic Sci. Int. Genet.* **2019**, *44*, 102174. [CrossRef]

215. Lin, M.-H.; Bright, J.-A.; Pugh, S.N.; Buckleton, J.S. The interpretation of mixed DNA profiles from a mother, father, and child trio. *Forensic Sci. Int. Genet.* **2019**, *44*, 102175. [CrossRef] [PubMed]

216. Buckleton, J.S.; Bright, J.-A.; Gittelson, S.; Moretti, T.R.; Onorato, A.J.; Bieber, F.R.; Budowle, B.; Taylor, D.A. The Probabilistic Genotyping SoftwareSTRmix: Utility and Evidence for its Validity. *J. Forensic Sci.* **2018**, *64*, 393–405. [CrossRef] [PubMed]

217. Riman, S.; Iyer, H.; Vallone, P. Exploring DNA interpretation software using the PROVEDIt dataset. *Forensic Sci. Int. Genet. Suppl. Ser.* **2019**, *7*, 724–726. [CrossRef]

218. Takano, M.H. *R.4368—Justice in Forensic ALGORITHMS Act of 2019*; 2019.

219. *Access to STRmix™ Software by Defence Legal Teams ("Access Policy")*; 2020. [CrossRef]

220. Adams, N.; Koppl, R.; Krane, D.; Thompson, W.; Zabell, S. Letter to the Editor-Appropriate Standards for Verification and Validation of Probabilistic Genotyping Systems. *J. Forensic Sci.* **2018**, *63*, 339–340. [CrossRef] [PubMed]

221. Software and Systems Engineering Standards Committee of the IEEE Computer Society. *IEEE Standard for System, Software, and Hardware Verification and Validation IEEE Std 1012™-2016*; IEEE: New York, NY, USA, 2017.

222. The Queen v. Clinton James Tuite. *S CR 2014 007*, 23 October 2017.

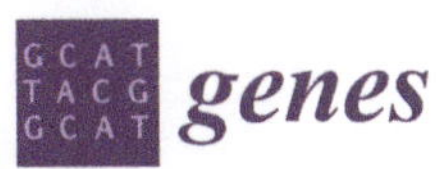

genes

MDPI

Review

A Logical Framework for Forensic DNA Interpretation

Tacha Hicks [1,2,*], **John Buckleton** [3,4], **Vincent Castella** [1], **Ian Evett** [5] and **Graham Jackson** [6,7]

[1] Forensic Genetics Unit, University Center of Legal Medicine, Lausanne—Geneva, Lausanne University Hospital and University of Lausanne, 1000 Lausanne 25, Switzerland; vincent.castella@chuv.ch

[2] Fondation pour la Formation Continue Universitaire Lausannoise (UNIL-EPFL) & School of Criminal Justice, Batochime, 1015 Lausanne, Switzerland

[3] Department of Statistics, University of Auckland, Private Bag 92019, Auckland 1142, New Zealand; john.buckleton@esr.cri.nz

[4] Institute of Environmental Science and Research Limited, Private Bag 92021, Auckland 1142, New Zealand

[5] Principal Forensic Services Ltd., Bromley BR1 2EB, UK; ianevett@btinternet.com

[6] Advance Forensic Science, St. Andrews KY16 0NA, UK; advanceforensicscience@gmail.com

[7] School of Applied Sciences, Division of Psychology and Forensic Science, Abertay University, Bell Street, Dundee DD1 1HG, UK

* Correspondence: tacha.hickschampod@unil.ch

Abstract: The forensic community has devoted much effort over the last decades to the development of a logical framework for forensic interpretation, which is essential for the safe administration of justice. We review the research and guidelines that have been published and provide examples of how to implement them in casework. After a discussion on uncertainty in the criminal trial and the roles that the DNA scientist may take, we present the principles of interpretation for evaluative reporting. We show how their application helps to avoid a common fallacy and present strategies that DNA scientists can apply so that they do not transpose the conditional. We then discuss the hierarchy of propositions and explain why it is considered a fundamental concept for the evaluation of biological results and the differences between assessing results given propositions that are at the source level or the activity level. We show the importance of pre-assessment, especially when the questions relate to the alleged activities, and when transfer and persistence need to be considered by the scientists to guide the court. We conclude with a discussion on statement writing and testimony. This provides guidance on how DNA scientists can report in a balanced, transparent, and logical way.

Keywords: DNA; forensic; principles of interpretation; investigative; evaluative; reporting; LR; propositions; activity issues; transfer

Citation: Hicks, T.; Buckleton, J.; Castella, V.; Evett, I.; Jackson, G. A Logical Framework for Forensic DNA Interpretation. *Genes* **2022**, *13*, 957. https://doi.org/10.3390/genes13060957

Academic Editor: Fulvio Cruciani

Received: 2 May 2022
Accepted: 20 May 2022
Published: 27 May 2022

Publisher's Note: MDPI stays neutral with regard to jurisdictional claims in published maps and institutional affiliations.

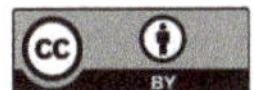

1. Introduction

In this article we discuss a framework that has been established by forensic scientists (and by extension, forensic DNA scientists) to help them reason about, and convey, their findings in a balanced, robust, logical, and transparent way. This form of reasoning was applied as early as the end of the 19th century [1]. It was formalised by the Case Assessment and Interpretation team of the former Forensic Science Service of England and Wales in the 1990's [2]. The approach is a paradigm for reasoning in the face of uncertainty, whatever the forensic discipline, although here we focus on DNA. This paradigm, which we consider to be the fundamental basis for reasoning in all forensic science disciplines, is discussed in numerous books [3–8] and interpretation guidelines [9–12].

2. Uncertainty in the Criminal Trial

In the context of a criminal trial, there are few elements that are known unequivocally to be true: the court is uncertain about key disputed events but needs to give a verdict. Disputed events could be, for example, whether "Mr Smith is the father of the child", or if "Ms Jones is the source of the blood that has been recovered from the crime scene". In those cases, the court will seek the help of DNA scientists. Very often, the court will have high expectations and expect definitive answers. Because of the CSI effect [13], they might believe that DNA is unique and, as such, will allow the identification of the person who is the father of the child or is the origin of the blood/DNA found at a crime scene. However, things are not that simple: the approach that is used does not allow the formal identification of the person who is the father of the child or who is the origin of the trace. There are very few forensic results that can be presented as "facts" and where one can be categorical. Is this problematic? We argue that it is not: uncertainty exists and, as explained by Dennis Lindley [14], rather than neglecting it or wanting to suppress it, the best approach is to find a logical way to manage it. As we will see, this is done by invoking the notion of probability, which provides a coherent logical basis for reasoning in the face of uncertainty.

3. Roles of the DNA Scientist and Different Type of Reporting (Factual, Investigative, Evaluative)

Information given by DNA scientists may be factual or may be in the form of an opinion. (Here, we refer to opinions based on knowledge and professional judgement (i.e., inferences drawn on the basis of forensic observations)).

A factual report describes what has been done and the observations obtained. The scientist makes no inference based on these observations and offers no opinion on the meaning of the results. Factual reporting is appropriate when conclusions are straightforward. A typical example would be a report where the DNA profile of a person is described so that it can be entered into a national DNA database. If expert knowledge is needed to draw a conclusion from the observations, then it would be misleading to present only the observations without offering a professional opinion. An example would be if the scientist only reported the description of the results of a presumptive test for blood. Simply stating that the item was tested for the presence of blood and that the result was positive could be misleading. Indeed, one cannot assume that a positive presumptive test for blood demonstrates unequivocally that the material is blood, even in the investigation stage [15]. Similarly, reporting in a paternity case that the child and the alleged father share one allele in common for all but one locus, without offering an opinion, could be easily misunderstood.

It has been suggested that the opinions given by forensic scientists can be classified broadly into two types—"investigative" and "evaluative" [16]. This should not be taken to mean that forensic scientists conduct police investigation or that they work as investigators. The point of this distinction is to underline that the questions encountered during the investigation and the court proceedings generally are of a different form. This leads to a difference in the inferential process [16,17] used in the generation of the opinion that then contributes to addressing these questions. Examples of the different activities that typify the two different roles that DNA scientists can take is shown in Table 1. It must be stressed that sometimes it may be difficult to separate these roles unequivocally.

Table 1. Differences between investigative and evaluative roles.

Investigative Role	Evaluative Role
Tends to be crime-focused.	Tends to be suspect-focused.
Tends to be at the beginning of the criminal justice process.	Tends to be at the culmination of the criminal justice process.
Helps the investigator make decisions.	Helps the court take decisions.
Type of questions: What happened? What is this? Who could be involved?	Type of questions: Is Mr Smith the source of the DNA or is it someone else? Did Mr Smith drive the car or was he a passenger?
Suggests explanations for the observations and gives guidance.	Evaluates the observations (i.e., results) given at least two mutually exclusive propositions.
Open-ended process.	More formal and structured.
Explanations need to encompass all realistic possibilities to avoid bias and avoid potentially misleading the inquiry.	Assigned probabilities should be calibrated; rates of misleading opinions should be low and documented.

An investigative opinion arises when explanations are generated to account for the observations. They are generally, but not exclusively, made in the absence of a person of interest (POI). An investigative opinion could be given in a case where a victim of a possible rape does not have a clear recollection of what happened and where no semen is recovered. Possible explanations for the absence of sperm could be that a condom was worn, or that there was no ejaculation or that all trace of sperm was lost, or that the victim used a vaginal douche or that there was no sexual intercourse. The list of explanations offered by the scientist may not be exhaustive—there may be other possible explanations that the scientist has not considered or has not been able to generate, and they are not necessarily mutually exclusive (i.e., several explanations might be true [18], for example maybe a condom was worn and the victim used a vaginal douche). Another example of an investigative opinion could be a case where a DNA analysis of an athlete's urine is performed in the context of possible doping. Imagine that the single DNA profile derived from the urine does not align with the DNA profile of the athlete, but that many alleles are shared between both DNA profiles. In such a case, provided no error has been made, the athlete cannot be the source of the urine. A possible explanation for the findings would be that a close relative is the source of the urine. This could be suggested as a possible avenue of investigation.

As mentioned, the separation of the roles and the types of opinion provided by forensic scientists is not always straightforward. There is nothing wrong in assessing the value of a DNA comparison for investigative purposes, for example. This is typically the case where a database search is carried out, when there is no suspect associated with the scene. Here, the aim is to provide investigative leads and information on who could be the source of the DNA. The main difference is that in the initial stages of a case, there might be no suspect/defendant. When there is, if the results are meant to be used in court, the scientist will need to take into account at least one alternative, for example, the defence's perspective of events. This may be based on what the defendant says, but as there is no obligation for the defence to provide information, this can also be grounded in case information gathered during the investigation (e.g., the defendant works at the same place as the victim) and/or in what appears to be a reasonable alternative (i.e., a proposition that would be amenable to a reasoned assignment of credibility by a judicial body). In a case in which there is a defendant, scientists should offer an evaluative opinion on their results, based upon a pair of case-specific propositions (sometimes also called "allegations" or "hypotheses") and the framework of circumstances. According to Willis et al. [9], evaluative reports for use in court should be produced when two conditions are met:

1. The forensic practitioner has been asked by a mandating authority or party to examine and/or compare material (typically recovered trace material with reference material from known potential sources).
2. The forensic practitioner seeks to evaluate the results with respect to particular competing propositions set by the specific case circumstances or as indicated by the mandating authority.

4. Desiderata and Principles of Interpretation for Evaluative Reporting

When choosing the approach for the evaluation of forensic findings, there is a need to first define what the desired properties of the interpretation framework are [16,19]. The desiderata of any approach to interpretation have been proposed as: balance, logic, transparency, and robustness. Not unsurprisingly, these have since been included in several guidelines on evaluative reporting [9,10,12,20]. This is not to say that investigative opinions do not have these properties. However, the principles of interpretation [4,21,22] apply mainly for forming evaluative opinions. This is because in the early stages of an investigation, there may be very little case information, little in the way of suggestions for what happened, and no suspect. In that case, it would not be possible to consider alternatives put forward by, for example, a defence team. Below, we consider only the principles for evaluative reporting as applied to issues relating to a POI when their case proceeds to court.

4.1. First Principle of Evaluative Reporting: Importance of Case Information

The first principle for forming evaluative opinions tells us that interpretation takes place in a framework of circumstances. Note that this is also true for our choice regarding the methods of analysis: we would need to know what the issue is. One can distinguish between aspects of the circumstances that are task-pertinent and task-irrelevant. The role of the forensic scientist can be divided in two parts: (1) understanding the uncertainties facing the fact finder and (2) helping the fact finder to resolve them. They will thus first need information to identify the issue(s) with which forensic science can help. Then, the scientist should devise and agree on an effective case strategy, including an assessment of the possible outcomes and their value, to help address the issue. Once the examinations have been completed and observations have been made, scientists will assign a probability to the specific observations, given propositions that are meaningful in the case and given the available information (task-pertinent case circumstances, but also expert knowledge). The probability they assign will be personal and conditional in the sense that it depends on what the individual knows, is told, and what is assumed. For a DNA scientist, case circumstances such as whether the persons of interest have legitimate access to the objects/persons/premises, what they say about the alleged incident in question, the activities that are alleged to have taken place, and the timelines, are all examples of task-pertinent information that will impact the value of the results. Examples of information that is not relevant for the DNA scientist and is potentially harmful because of bias could include (1) there is eyewitness evidence that points toward the POI, (2) there is a partial finger-mark that supports the proposition that a specified person touched the object, or (3) the POI had first confessed to the offence but later retracted that admission. As task-pertinent case information impacts the value of the findings, it is essential to give a signal that should the framework of circumstances change, it will be necessary to review the interpretation. We discuss examples of caveats in Section 12.

4.2. Second Principle of Evaluative Reporting: Two or More Competing Propositions Should Be Considered

To be balanced, when assessing the value of biological results, one must consider at least two propositions (i.e., statements that are either true or false, and that can be affirmed or denied). They will be formulated in pairs based on the case information (we discuss proposition formulation in Section 7) and should represent the views of the two parties as understood at the time of the writing of the report.

Propositions need to be mutually exclusive (if one is true, the other is not) and, if possible, exhaustive in the context of the case (i.e., one should not consider all propositions as default, but only those that are of interest to the court [23]). It is not feasible nor desirable to consider absolute exhaustiveness, and practice can proceed with an acceptable coverage, that is without the omission of a relevant proposition [24]. It is important to ensure that the propositions to be considered are based on case information. If, the case information changes and it is shown that the propositions considered are not meaningful anymore, a new evaluation will need to be performed and a new written statement issued.

4.3. Third Principle of Evaluative Reporting: Scientists Need to Assign Their Probability of the Findings, Not Their Probability of the (Alleged) Facts

To respect logic, forensic scientists shall assign the probability of their findings given the truth of propositions, not the probability of the propositions given the findings. It may seem obvious that scientists need to focus on the value of the findings. However, it is not a straightforward endeavour, and many scientists are tempted to give an opinion on propositions. An example could be the doping case discussed earlier: while the DNA scientist is in a position to assign the probability of the results given the urine is from the athlete's sister, it is not possible—based on the results only—to assign the probability that the urine is from the athlete's sister. To do so, one would need to consider all the information in the case (for example that the athlete has a sister).

4.4. Forth Principle of Evaluative Reporting: The Value of the Findings Is Expressed by the Ratio of the Probability of the Scientific Observations Given the Case Information and Given That Each, in Turn, of the Propositions Are True

To measure how the new evidence (e.g., DNA results) affects one's uncertainty about the proposition (e.g., the urine is from the sister) considering conditioning information, one can use a model which is known as Bayes' rule. It is a mathematical idealisation that the belief about a set of propositions is updated based on the (weight of the) evidence [25]. Note that Bayes' rule is seldom used in court (except maybe for paternity cases). Generally, the different pieces of evidence are combined intuitively by the fact finder without assigning any figure. This is done, for instance, when referring to "corroborating evidence". Notwithstanding, Bayes' rule provides a very useful framework for understanding how DNA results may be presented in a logical, transparent, and impartial way in legal proceedings.

Bayes' rule may be depicted in a format known as the odds form of Bayes' rule (Equation (1)). Odds are the ratio of the probability of the proposition being true divided by the probability of it being false.

$$\underbrace{\frac{\Pr(H_p|I)}{\Pr(H_d|I)}}_{\text{prior odds}} \times \underbrace{\frac{\Pr(E|H_p,I)}{\Pr(E|H_d,I)}}_{\text{likelihood ratio}} = \underbrace{\frac{\Pr(H_p|E,I)}{\Pr(H_d|E,I)}}_{\text{posterior odds}} \tag{1}$$

where "Pr" denotes probability, "H_p" the proposition summarising the prosecution's point of view, and "H_d" the proposition summarising the defence's point of view. The letter "I" stands for the information mentioned in the section on the first principle of interpretation, and "E" (for evidence) represents the scientific observations (i.e., results or findings). The vertical bar " | " is called the conditioning bar and can be read as "given" or "assuming that".

One of the most important lessons that can be learned from Bayes' rule, as depicted in this form, is the nature of the roles played by different actors in the judicial process. It can be seen there are three terms in the equation, and the important question is: who takes responsibility for each of these three?

The first term represents prior odds, where the probability of each proposition given the information is considered. Assessing the allegations or the facts in issue is, without doubt, the duty of the fact finders. The last term also represents odds, which again relate to the probability of the propositions, but this time considering in addition the DNA results (or other forensic observations). These are said to be posterior odds, as they represent one's updated belief after knowing the results (or the evidence) "E".

The second term is the likelihood ratio (LR for short), which is a measure of the value of the findings. It is defined in terms of the ratio of two conditional probabilities: (i) the probability of the findings given that one proposition is true and given the conditioning information; and (ii) the probability of the findings given that the other proposition is true and given the conditioning information. The two conditional probabilities forming the LR may be assigned either on the basis of (published) data and/or the general knowledge (base) of the forensic practitioner. It is a measure of the relative strength of support that particular findings give to one proposition against a stated alternative [3,4,7,26,27]. A LR is a ratio of probabilities; thus, by definition, it is a number (as probabilities are numbers between 0 and 1). If the LR is 1, results are uninformative, and they do not support one proposition over the other. If the LR is larger than one, results support the first proposition compared to the alternative. If the LR is smaller than 1 (e.g., 0.001), then results support the alternative proposition over the first proposition. (It is sometimes reported that LRs can be negative, that is smaller than 0. This is incorrect. LRs theoretically can range between 0 and infinity. Log(LR) can be negative, but not LRs).

The focus of the LR is always on the findings, never on the proposition. It should be seen as a reinforcing or weakening factor in the perception of the truth of propositions that existed without the technical findings. This factor measures the change produced by the findings on the odds of the fact in issue being true. (In the literature, this factor is also more generally called a Bayes Factor (BF). With simple propositions, a BF reduces to a LR, as discussed in [28]. However, when multiple propositions are used, the BF does not reduce to the LR: it is a ratio of weighted likelihoods). Because the focus of the LR is on the scientific result, it is clearly in the domain and remit of the scientists. It allows them to provide assistance through the use of their expertise to assign probabilities for their observations given the truth of the competing propositions.

In addition, without considering Bayes' rule, it appears quite sensible to say that scientists must give their opinion on the results and not on the disputed facts in issue. It is for the factfinder to render opinions on facts, and for DNA scientists to give the value of their results. When DNA scientists give their opinion on the alleged facts (or propositions) based only on the value of their results (i.e., LR), then they are said to transpose the conditional [26,27]. This is a very common error of logic and appears in many forms [29]. It has been called the "prosecutor's fallacy" [30], but it is just as frequently to be found on the lips of defenders, judges, and journalists. It is more properly known as the "fallacy of the transposed conditional" because it is a matter of confusion between two conditional probabilities: the probability of the findings given the propositions and the probability of the propositions given the findings. One can erroneously transpose the conditional when giving an opinion on a single probability or on a ratio of probabilities.

5. Avoiding the Transposed Conditional

Not transposing the conditional is difficult, and it would be satisfying if one could avoid it just by knowing about Bayes' rule and reporting a LR. It is so natural for the human mind to want an opinion on (alleged) facts, that it takes time and training to avoid this fallacy. There are several strategies that one can adopt to avoid this error of logic. Some of these were developed at the time when the Case Assessment Interpretation team from the former Forensic Science Service of England and Wales was training all their reporting officers; these are outlined in [6] and summarised below.

The first thing to investigate is whether the opinion pertains to the DNA results or to the proposition. The second aspect to check is that the sentence contains a word such as "if" or "given" and that these are associated with the propositions. If one has pen and paper, it is always a good idea to use notation, as spotting an error is then easier. Another coping strategy is to memorise correct and incorrect statements. When in doubt, one should re-phrase the statement of opinion along the lines of the correct format. Another strategy to ensure that there is no transposed conditional is to begin one's sentence with the term "The DNA results" and add the probabilistic statement and the conditioning.

A lot of practice is needed to avoid inadvertently transposing the conditional: we discuss examples of incorrect formulations in Table 2. One should remember to state both propositions, as a LR is relative.

Table 2. Statements with transposed conditionals and their associated correct statement.

	Incorrect or Ambiguous Statement (A)	Correct Statement (B)	Notation
1.	Given the DNA results, it is a billion times more likely that the DNA is from Ms Jones than from an unknown unrelated person.	The results are a billion times more probable if the DNA is from Ms Jones rather than if it is from an unknown unrelated person.	A: $\mathrm{Pr}(H_p\,\vert\,E,I)/\mathrm{Pr}(H_d\,\vert\,E,I)$ B: $\mathrm{Pr}(E\,\vert\,H_p,I)/\mathrm{Pr}(E\,\vert\,H_d,I)$ Note: In A, the use of the term "that" is always suspicious.
2.	The likelihood ratio calculated the probability that the DNA evidence observed in the profile originated from the applicant, rather than another person chosen at random from the Australian Caucasian population. (Sometimes, scientists will write "the probability that a randomly selected person would have this DNA profile is 1 in a billion.". However, the alternative source of the DNA is not "selected at random", but rather an unknown person, related or not to the persons of interest depending on the case).	The likelihood ratio represents the ratio of two probabilities: the probability of the result given that the DNA is from the applicant and the probability of the result given the DNA is from an unknown person from the Australian Caucasian population.	A: $\mathrm{Pr}(H_p\,\vert\,E,I)/\mathrm{Pr}(H_d\,\vert\,E,I)$ B: $\mathrm{Pr}(E\,\vert\,H_p,I)/\mathrm{Pr}(E\,\vert\,H_d,I)$ Note: a word such as « if » or « given » should always be present when using conditional probabilities.

Table 2. *Cont.*

	Incorrect or Ambiguous Statement (A)	Correct Statement (B)	Notation
3.	Participants of the proficiency test were asked whether their DNA results more probably originated due to the disputed activity or social interactions. (In the exercise, it read as "Participants were required to consider each DNA profile separately and assess whether they originated either due to primary or secondary transfer" however, it is best not to put the word transfer in the propositions as transfer/persistence and recovery are factors that scientists will take into account in their evaluation.)	Participants of the proficiency test were asked whether their DNA results were more probable given the disputed activity than given social interactions.	A: $\Pr(H_p\,\|\,E,I)/\Pr(H_d\,\|\,E,I)$ B: $\Pr(E\,\|\,H_p,I)/\Pr(E\,\|\,H_d,I)$ Note: In A, the absence of the term "if [the proposition]"or "given [the proposition]"is a clue that the statement needs review.
4.	The probability that the DNA comes from a random unrelated person is one in a million.	The probability of the results if the DNA comes from a random unrelated person is one in a million.	A: $\Pr(H_d\,\|\,I)$ B: $\Pr(E\,\|\,H_d,I)$ Note: statement B is correct (not transposed) but not balanced since $\Pr(E\,\|\,H_p,I)$ is missing.
5.	Considering the genetic characteristics of the trace, it is a million times more likely that Mr S is the source of the DNA rather than his uncle.	The genetic characteristics of the trace are a million times more likely if Mr S is the source of the DNA rather than his uncle.	A: $\Pr(H_p\,\|\,E,I)/\Pr(H_d\,\|\,E,I)$ B: $\Pr(E\,\|\,H_p,I)/\Pr(E\,\|\,H_d,I)$ Note: in statement A, the phrase "considering the genetic characteristics of the trace" implies that the DNA characteristics represent the conditioning information (thus are present behind the conditional bar). However, the conditioning information should be the propositions and the information; the term "given" should be associated with the propositions and information, not with the results.
6.	As explained by this Court in Tuite [No 1] for each DNA sample where the suspect cannot be excluded as a contributor, a ratio was calculated which shows how much more likely it is <u>that</u> the suspect was the source of the DNA (or a contributor to it) than that some other person chosen at random from the population was the source (or a contributor).	As explained by this Court in Tuite [No 1] for each DNA sample where the suspect cannot be excluded as a contributor, a ratio was calculated which shows how much more likely the DNA results would be given the suspect were the source of the DNA (or a contributor to it) than given an unknown person from the population were the source (or a contributor).	A: LR defined incorrectly as $\Pr(H_p\,\|\,E,I)/\Pr(H_d\,\|\,E,I)$ B: LR is defined as $LR = \Pr(E\,\|\,H_p,I)/\Pr(E\,\|\,H_d,I)$
7.	The most favoured proposition is that S is the source of the DNA rather than an unknown unrelated person.	The DNA results strongly support the proposition that S, rather than an unknown unrelated person, is the source of the DNA.	Note: in A the use the term favour could be read as saying the first proposition is most likely. The term "support" is more appropriate.

All incorrect/ambiguous statements originate from statements, judgements [31], or scientific communications. The last statement "The most favoured proposition is that S is the source of the DNA" is ambiguous: it could lead the reader to think that the proposition which is the most favoured is the most probable. This is not the case, as depending on prior odds, the most probable proposition might not be the one that is the most supported by the results. An example is shown in Table 3 using Bayes' rule. One can see that with a LR of 1 million and very low prior odds of 1 to 10 million, the posterior probability of the first proposition would be 9% (or 0.09); the most favoured or most likely proposition would be the alternative.

One can note that, if the prior probability of the first proposition is zero, then whatever the LR, the posterior probability is zero as well. It would be rare to have this situation. According to [14], when assigning our probabilities, we should admit the possibility that we might be wrong. If we do, this rule denies probabilities of 1 or 0. (This rule is called Cromwell's rule, named after Oliver Cromwell, who said to the Church of Scotland, "I beseech you, in the bowels of Christ, think it possible you may be mistaken". Calling it Cromwell's rule is attributed to Dennis Lindley). The probability of an event given K is 1 if, and only if, K logically implies the truth of E (and of zero if K implies the falsity of E). To provide an illustration where there can be a prior probability of zero, we revisit the case where the issue was whether the urine was from the athlete or not. You will remember that the DNA was different from the athlete's DNA, but that the donor and the athlete shared many alleles. In that case, it was reported that the DNA profile comparison was of the order of a billion times more likely if the person's sister was the source of the urine, rather than if an unrelated person was. The DNA scientist reported that the probability that the urine originated from the sister was 99.9999999%. In those conditions, they conclude that it was practically proven that the urine was from the sister. This prompted the athlete's lawyer to write a letter to say that there was only a minor problem in that reasoning: the athlete did not have a sister (but she did have a half-sister). In this case, the probability of the proposition is zero. This also shows why it is best for scientists to give an opinion on the results, however large their LR. It is generally not considered the scientists' remit to give an opinion on facts (except, as mentioned earlier, in some countries for paternity cases), which is the case if they give posterior probabilities.

Table 3. Posterior probabilities with the same LR of a million, but different prior odds. In the first case, although results support the first proposition, the most favoured proposition is the alternative, with a probability of 91%. When prior odds are equal to the LR, the probability of the proposition is 50%. If prior odds are 1:1, then posterior odds are equal to the LR.

Prior Odds	LR	Posterior Odds	Posterior Probability of the First Proposition	Posterior Probability of the Alternative
1 to 10 million	1×10^6	1 to 10	9%	91%
1 to 1 million	1×10^6	1 to 1	50%	50%
1 to 10,000	1×10^6	100 to 1	99%	1%

To calculate posterior probabilities using Bayes' rule in odds form (Equation (1)), one multiplies the prior odds by the LR. This gives us posterior odds. If the odds are a to b, to obtain the probability of the first proposition, one divides a by (a + b). If the odds are, for example, 1:1, the probability of the proposition is 1 divided by 2, thus 0.50 (or 50%, as probabilities can also be expressed as percentages).

It should be noted that, when being extra careful about not transposing the conditional, some think that it is incorrect to say "the results support the first proposition rather than the second". The use of the word "support" in this context was proposed in a manner analogous to H. Jeffreys [32]. It does not indicate that one proposition is more likely than the other, only that the results are more probable if the first proposition is true than if the alternative is. Because it is important to indicate what our results mean and do not mean, we recommend outlining this point in our statements.

6. Hierarchy of Propositions

The concept of a hierarchy of propositions [33] applies to all forensic disciplines. It was developed initially for evaluative rather than investigative opinions, and one will note that the examples of propositions given in the early Case Assessment and Interpretation (CAI) publications were generally suspect-focused. Over time, the CAI development team found that the concept of a hierarchy of issues and propositions was equally applicable to investigative issues [16]. The classification of propositions into three main levels (source, activity, and offence) allows forensic scientists to contextualise the results, to consider the factors in their evaluation and to communicate to the client the purpose of the proposed examinations. The demarcation between the levels is not meant to be rigid, and it is recognised that sometimes levels will be difficult to distinguish. The levels simply provide a model framework that helps scientists to organise their thinking, actions, and decisions. The important point to stress to practitioners is: do not try to force all the issues you will encounter into one of the levels of the framework. Instead, just specify clearly in words the issue, and hence the propositions to consider. If the issue and propositions then fall neatly into one of the categories (i.e., one of the levels), so much the better, but do not worry if the issue/propositions do not seem to fit one of the categories. The important thing is that you have clearly specified the issue, with which the examinations can help, both for yourself and for the factfinders.

The hierarchy of propositions is generally presented from source to offence (see examples in Table 4). It is structured in a hierarchy as scientists will need more case information and more knowledge to assess their results given offence- or activity-level propositions, compared to those of the source level. It is important to outline that when identifying the level in the hierarchy where they can be the most helpful, experts shall not stray outside the bounds of their expertise, and value must be added. This is done by bringing knowledge that is needed for understanding the meaning of the results in the context of the case and that otherwise would remain unavailable to the court.

Table 4. Evaluative examples of pairs of mutually exclusive propositions at different levels in the hierarchy that DNA scientists could contribute to addressing provided they have knowledge that is needed but which otherwise would be unavailable to the court.

Level	Question/Issue	Results	Example of Pairs of Propositions
Source	Is the POI the source of the body fluid?		Mr A is the source of the blood. An unknown unrelated person is the source of the blood.
Sub-source	Is the POI the source of the DNA?	DNA profiling comparison.	Mr A is the source of the DNA. An unknown unrelated person is the source of the DNA.
Sub-sub-source	Is the POI the source of the part of the mixture?		Mr A is the major contributor of the DNA mixture. An unknown unrelated person is the major contributor of the DNA mixture.
Activity	Did the POI do the activity?	Presence/absence of DNA at different locations. Quantity/quality of the DNA. (DNA profiling comparison) *. Presumptive tests. Multiple traces from same activity.	Mr A and Ms B had penile-vaginal intercourse Mr A and Ms B only had social activities as described in the case information. Mr Smith was the driver and Mr Jones the passenger at the relevant time. Mr Jones was the driver and Mr Smith the passenger at the relevant time.
Offence	Is the POI the offender?	Multiple traces possibly resulting from different activities compared to Mr A. Presence/absence of DNA. Quantity/quality of the DNA. (DNA profiling comparison) *. Presumptive tests.	Mr A is the burglar (in the sense of "Mr A did the specified activities that the burglar has allegedly done, as specified in the paragraph on case information"). Mr A has nothing to do with the burglary.

* In some cases, considering whether or not the DNA is from the POI can have an impact on the evaluation.

6.1. Issue with Which the Forensic Scientist Can Help: Is Mr Smith's the Source of the DNA/Biological Material?

When the hierarchy of propositions was first suggested, it was only possible to obtain a DNA profile from biological fluids present in relatively large quantities. In such cases, one could reasonably assume that the DNA profile was derived from a known biological fluid (e.g., blood). This assumption became questionable with the advent of more sensitive techniques. This led to new levels (still contributing to answering the question of the source): the DNA level (or sub-source level) and the DNA contributor level (or sub-sub-source level [34]), for situations where the issue is whether a person is the source of part of the DNA mixture (e.g., a major component). We discuss below when it is meaningful to choose source-level propositions or their associated sub-levels.

6.1.1. Source-Level Propositions

Source-level propositions are adequate given two conditions: first, the issue should be whether a given person is the source of the material. Second, there should be no risk for the court to misinterpret the findings in the context of the alleged activities. This would typically be the case when the material is found in such a quantity that there is (i) no need to consider its presence for reasons other than the alleged activity (i.e., it will be accepted by the fact finder that the material is relevant), and (ii) that the nature of the material can be safely assumed. The following example is adapted from [9], illustrating when considering the results of a DNA comparison given source-level propositions is not misleading:

"A large pool of fresh red bloodlike material is recovered at the point of entry at a burglary scene and the circumstances suggest it has originated from the offender(s), whomever they may be. A sample is delivered to the laboratory for DNA analysis. Combination of a positive presumptive test, large quantity and appearance allows the scientist to safely assume that it would be agreed that the stain is blood. The defendant, Mr D., says that he has never been in the premises and denies that the blood at the scene is from him. The set of propositions can be (1) the bloodstain came from the defendant and (2) the bloodstain came from an unknown individual." Assuming that the nature of the material will not be contested, the same term, "bloodstain", can be used in both propositions. It is sometimes believed that source-level propositions can be formulated when the nature of the material (e.g., blood, semen, saliva, cellular material) is disputed and that this accommodates consideration of the probability of presumptive tests. However, it does not as the probability of observing a positive (or a negative) result for the presumptive test would be equivalent whether the blood is from Mr D or from someone else. Therefore, if the nature of the material is disputed, it is, in general, more meaningful to consider activity-level propositions [11]: these will take into account the results of presumptive tests as well as the transfer, persistence, and the presence of the material as background (i.e., material from an unknown source present for unknown reasons).

6.1.2. Sub-Source-Level Propositions

The advent of highly sensitive methods has made it possible to produce DNA profiles from very small quantities of biological material [35]. With invisible or small stains, the nature of the material from which the DNA profile is produced is often unknown. In such cases, if the issue is who is the source of the DNA, one can assess the results of a DNA comparison given sub-source propositions (i.e., the source of the DNA, not of a given body fluid). These are especially useful for producing investigative leads. As mentioned in [10], one can use a LR in both the investigative and the evaluative phase. The main difference is that in the evaluation phase, there will generally be a suspect/defendant around whom the issues and propositions will be defined. In this situation, it will be necessary to take into account an alternative proposition, typically the defence's view of events, if that has been communicated to the scientist. This person may, for example, mention that they know the victim. Again, in such cases, assessing the results given activity-level propositions will generally be more meaningful. However, the DNA scientist operates in "investigative mode" where, for example, a database search is carried out because there is no suspect for the crime. Here, in the initial phase, what is of interest is to provide information about who could be the source of the DNA. An example of sub-source propositions would be: "The DNA is from candidate X" or "The DNA is from an unknown person". If the aim is to produce a useful lead, the person will not have been arrested yet, and de facto, the scientist will have been provided with no alternative proposition or information. The person making the investigative decision (here, for example, to arrest the candidate or not) will not be the court but, in some jurisdictions, an investigating magistrate, or in others, a police investigator. When there is very little case information, the value of the comparison needs to be much higher for the person making the decision (e.g., to arrest the candidate or not). In addition, for cost effectiveness, one may also want to avoid investigating many false leads. This explains why larger LRs will often be needed for investigative purposes.

6.1.3. Sub-Sub-Source-Level Propositions

If the issue is whether a POI is the major (or minor) contributor of a DNA mixture, then one can consider sub-sub-source propositions [34]. An example of sub-sub-source propositions would be: "Mr A is the major contributor to the DNA mixture" or "An unknown person is the major contributor to the DNA mixture". If it is important that the POI is compatible with the major component, then this generally is an indication that the issue lies in the activities and that scientists can add value by considering activity-level propositions. If the relative quantity is not an important factor, then sub-source propositions are generally preferred to sub-sub-source, as the former allow accounting for all the results (and not only part of the mixture).

6.2. Issue with Which the Forensic Scientist Can Help: Did Mr Smith Perform the Activities Alleged by the Prosecution or Those Alleged by the Defence?

The next level in the hierarchy of propositions is the activity level. The evaluation of given activity-level propositions generally involves assessment of the extrinsic characteristics (e.g., quality of the DNA profile, relative quantity of DNA, where the DNA was sampled from) and should be considered when transfer, persistence, or background have a significant impact on the understanding of the value of the findings in the context of relevant case circumstances and the alleged activities [9,11,36]. Depending on the case and the information content of the profile, the source of the DNA might be contested or agreed. When the source of the DNA is not contested, but the activities leading to the deposition of the DNA are, one does not necessarily need to consider the source of the DNA anymore For investigative purposes, the DNA profile of the trace and of the person still need to be compared. To determine the value of this comparison, one will assign a LR given sub-source-level propositions. However, if there is no dispute and thus only one proposition (i.e., the DNA is from the POI), this LR value is not relevant. It is the LR given activity-level propositions that is meaningful. It is sometimes believed that to consider activity-level propositions, one needs to agree on the source of the DNA. This is not true: in this type of evaluation, one can consider both possibilities (i.e., that the DNA is from the POI or not). If so, one has associated sub-source propositions. However, depending on the rarity of the DNA profile, this consideration will have little impact on the value of the findings given activity-level propositions. Indeed, as indicated by the England and Wales Court of Appeal [37]: "It makes the task of the jury so much easier if they do not have to plough through and listen to evidence that is simply not in dispute." Let us look at an example where the issue is one of activity. Assume a stolen car crashed into a group of pedestrians, killing one and injuring others. Two people escaped from inside the car and ran away. Acting on information, the police quickly arrested two men, Mr Smith and Mr Jones. Both admitted to being in the car at the time of the collision, but both denied being the driver, instead accusing the other of being the driver. The issue would be: "Did Mr Smith or Mr Jones drive the car at the relevant time?". The activity-level propositions would be: "Mr Smith drove the car at the relevant time and Mr Jones was the passenger." The alternative would be the reverse: "Mr Jones was the driver and Mr Smith the passenger.". As both the driver's and the passenger's airbags were activated at the time of the collision, an examination of the airbags for biological material could help to address the issue. Another typical case where sub-source-level propositions might not be meaningful, would be when a person has legitimate access to the object or person on which examinations have been performed (e.g., a gun found in the POI's car). In such cases, the source of the DNA (i.e., the person) may well not be contested (which does not mean that the DNA does not need to be analysed, only that, depending on the results, these may not need to be assessed). It is worth noting that activity-level propositions allow for the assessment of the absence of evidence [33,38]. The saying "The absence of (matching) evidence is not evidence of absence" is not always true. To know when it is, formal evaluation is needed. (As much as possible we try and avoid the term match for two reasons: first, laypersons believe that saying there is a match means that the DNA is from the person; second, scientists can at best state they were unable to see any difference they judge relevant. This does not mean that the two profiles are identical: indeed, two separate identities cannot be identical because, given sufficient resolution, all distinct entities are distinguishable from each other, even when two items come from the same source). Activity-level propositions also facilitate the combination of DNA results from different items that were touched because of the same activity (e.g., the two airbags, and possibly the steering wheel, in the example above). Finally, one should note that sometimes it may be difficult to distinguish offence from activity. As an example, a proposition such as "Mr A stabbed Mr B." or "Ms A shot Mr B." may be considered either as an offence and/or an activity-level proposition. Remember, as indicated previously, the lines of demarcation in the hierarchy should not be seen as rigid: it is meant to organise thinking, actions, and decisions.

6.3. Issue with Which the Forensic Scientist Can Help: Is Mr Smith the Offender or Does He Have Nothing to Do with the Offence?

The issue for the court is always the offence, which is at the top level of the hierarchy. An example of a pair of competing offence-level propositions could be: "Mr Smith committed the burglary" and "Mr Smith had nothing to do with the burglary". It should be remembered that propositions and case information are closely entwined so that in the case information, more detail would be given indicating, for example, that Mr Smith visited the jewellery store 3 days prior to the burglary. It is sometimes cautioned that offence-level propositions are not the domain of the scientist but of the court. Although this is true, this statement applies to all levels of propositions, as scientists offer their opinion on the results and not on propositions (or else, they would transpose the conditional). This is valid whatever the level, and offence level is not special in that sense. However, the evaluation of findings given offence-level propositions is special in the sense that it is rare that forensic scientists add value by considering propositions at the offence level, compared to a level lower in the hierarchy. Indeed, in many cases, the difference between activities and offence lies in the intent or consent, and in that case, obviously, biological results cannot help discriminating between these two levels. A typical case where DNA scientists cannot add value would be if they considered "rape" instead of "vaginal/penile penetration or consensual sex" [39]. Biological results do not give any information on the issue of consent, pre-meditation, nor intent, thus DNA scientists cannot help the court address those issues. In these situations, DNA scientists should not rise in the hierarchy, as they would not use any specialised knowledge, nor add value, when considering the offence rather than the activities.

However, the consideration of offence-level propositions allows adding value when there are multiple forensic findings that need to be combined by a forensic scientist. Such a case could be a burglary implying multiple activities: for example, breaking glass, jumping out of window, opening a safe. In this situation, offence-level propositions would enable combining the different results (e.g., shoe-marks, fibres, and DNA profile comparisons). The list of the activities would be very similar to what constitutes an offence in that case. Offence-level propositions have also been proposed to explore the impact of other factors such as relevance [40,41].

7. Formulation of Propositions

Within a forensic case, people (e.g., the police, the defence, or witnesses) will make various claims or statements. These are either true or false and can be affirmed or refuted. It is once they are formalised by the scientist that these claims will be referred to as propositions.

(Some people use the term hypothesis to designate propositions used for the evaluation of findings. We prefer to keep this term for situations where scientific experiments are performed to "test" a hypothesis. As discussed in [3], this enables distinguishing between both concepts, and it is only when a proposition is formulated for empirical testing that we will call it a hypothesis). As described in [33], propositions need to be mutually exclusive (if one is true, the other is false) and formulated in pairs (e.g., views put forward by the parties to the cases) against a background of information and assumptions. They should also be amenable to a reasoned assignment of credibility by a judicial body [9]. There may be more than two propositions, but in the context of a criminal trial there will be two views. For the formalisation of propositions, the basic criterion is that they should be formulated in such a way that it is reasonable for the scientist to address a question of the form: "What is the probability of the observations given this proposition and given the framework of circumstances?" [12]. There are other important criteria to keep in mind when formulating propositions. For example, propositions are about causes and as such will be assessed by the decision maker (e.g., factfinder). If propositions contain factors that are to be considered in the evaluation, these factors cannot be assessed by the scientists anymore: being part of the proposition, they will be assessed by the decision maker. Formulation of propositions needs to adhere to specific criteria and appropriate phrasing. As it is a difficult task that requires expertise, the DNA scientist is in the best position to formalise the propositions, and one cannot expect that prosecution or defence formally define the so-called "Prosecution or Defence propositions" themselves. (The defence proposition may be compound. For example, if the alternative is that the DNA is from an unknown person, this unknown person may be unrelated or a sibling or a cousin). These terms are used to indicate that the propositions represent the views of these two parties as understood from the case information available (i.e., that the propositions were formulated against the background of information available from the parties). However, should one of these not accept the propositions considered by the scientist, a new evaluation will be needed. Ideally the formulation of propositions should be discussed between the parties and the DNA scientist before doing the work.

There have been many publications on the formulation of propositions [10,11,18,23,33,42–46]. In Table 5, we give the criteria to which they should adhere and examples of poorly worded propositions, and their corresponding, more meaningful formulations are discussed in Table 6. It is important to emphasise that case information and propositions are entwined and will both appear in a statement. What goes in the information and the proposition will depend on the case. However, because we repeat propositions in our statements and in court, it is preferable to keep them short and snappy.

Table 5. Criteria that help spotting whether propositions are formulated in a meaningful way.

Criteria for Propositions	Basis of the Criteria
They come in pairs, so there are at least two propositions.	To ensure a balanced view representing both parties.
They are based on the views of the parties and contextual information.	So that the evaluation is relevant to the case.
They are formal and relate to inductive inference.	To allow scientists logically to assess their findings
They are mutually exclusive.	If not, a LR cannot be used.
They represent the positions that prosecution and defence respectively would be expected to take at court.	So that there is one value of the findings and not several values (one LR, not several).
Propositions are about "causes", not results.	To enable the scientists to add value and expertise that is needed for the understanding the case.

Table 6. Examples of propositions that should be avoided and how to formulate them in a more meaningful way.

	Examples to Avoid	More Meaningful Examples	Comments
1.	Mr Smith was not the passenger.	Mr Smith was the driver.	If propositions are vague, it is difficult to assign a probability, unless this is specified in the paragraph summarising task-pertinent information.
2.	The DNA is from someone other than Mr Smith.	The DNA is from an unknown person.	
3.	Mr Smith was in recent contact with the victim.	Mr Smith visited the victim's house as described in the case information.	
4.	The matching profile comes from Mr Smith.	The DNA is from Mr Smith.	"Matching profile" is a result: it should not be included in the proposition.
5.	The male DNA is from Mr Smith or someone of his paternal lineage.	The male DNA is from Mr Smith.	Here, it is Mr Smith who would be on trial, not his paternal lineage. If one needs to consider a person from the paternal lineage, this should be done in the alternative. It is the methods that depend on the issue and not the reverse (i.e., propositions do not depend on methods).
6.	Mr A's DNA was transferred on the drug package via Officer B.	Officer B arrested Mr A before seizing the drug package.	As written, the statement says that "DNA was transferred". This is essentially an explanation for the observations. The probability of the findings given this explanation is approaching 1. The probability of DNA being transferred needs to be taken into account by the scientist when evaluating results given activity-level propositions and the case information. That transfer has occurred cannot be included in the proposition for evaluation.

In the evaluative stage, propositions should not be findings-led, and thus, ideally, the formulation of propositions should be made without knowing the results. This is an essential, early component of the recommended process of Case Assessment and Interpretation (mentioned later in Section 11 on Pre-assessment). In DNA casework—especially for investigative purposes—when considering sub-source propositions, the alternative source is generally by default an unknown person. If the propositions are standard and if knowing the findings does not impact the value of the comparison, then it is acceptable. However, if there is an impact, it is more problematic. An example, of a findings-led proposition could be "Mr A is the minor contributor of the DNA mixture", because Mr A happens to be compatible with the minor contributor. Another could be to change the number of contributors because there is one exclusion at a locus if the mixture is considered as a two-person mixture, but not if it is assigned as a three-person mixture. Regarding the number of contributors to a mixture, one should note that there is no need to consider a specific number. It is sensible in some cases to consider a variable number of contributors [44,47]. A last example of findings-led propositions would be the situation where there are two candidates for the same mixture. If one chooses a different set of propositions based on whether they explain the mixture together or not, then the propositions could be findings-led. In such cases, a suggested solution is again to consider multiple propositions [48].

8. Formulation of the Alternative in the Absence of Information from the Person(s) of Interest

A POI is under no obligation to provide information and may give a no-comment interview. In such a case, scientists will formulate an alternative that appears the most reasonable based on what they know [9,12]. The investigation might provide information, for example that the victim and defendant visit the same gym, suggesting that activity-level propositions might be appropriate. One can also suggest the negation of the first proposition (e.g., Mr Smith is not the source of the DNA), provided we are explicit on what is meant by "not" [46]. This ought to be explained in the paragraph describing the case information. The implication of adopting such a negation should be set out clearly for the receivers and users of the opinion—it tends to maximise the value of the observations in support of the main proposition over the alternative. Some scientists do point this out in their reports. The important considerations regarding, for example, from whom the DNA comes (e.g., if not from Mr Smith) will be clearly disclosed. A caveat should indicate that should these assumptions not be relevant to the case, a new interpretation and perhaps further analysis will be necessary based on the new case information and new alternative.

9. Distinction between Explanations and Propositions

It is particularly important to distinguish propositions from explanations when the issue is activity, as these explanations are more and more commonly offered by the parties. In the context of the Case Assessment and Interpretation model [2,18], explanations have been recognised as intermediate considerations when exploring less formal alternatives. Explanations can be very useful in the investigative stage: they provide new leads and outline what information is needed. Explanations will be generated based on the observations and generally do not qualify as formal propositions for the evaluative stage. If the explanation is prescriptive, the probability of the observations given this explanation will be one. Examples of prescriptive explanations could be "The trace has been contaminated with the suspect's DNA", "The persons were in contact recently and transferred DNA directly," or if we want to state the obvious, "The stain came from someone with the same DNA profile". Explanations may be speculative or fanciful. Contrary to propositions, they do not depend on case information and are not necessarily mutually exclusive. Examples of various types of explanations are given in Table 7.

Table 7. Examples of explanations that can be given as investigative opinions, but not evaluative.

Observations	Explanations
DNA profile of Mr Smith is compatible with the DNA profile of the trace.	The DNA was planted by the police. The real offender has the same DNA profile His DNA was transported from his beer can to the door by the wind. The government synthesised a DNA profile with the same allelic designations as him. The DNA is from his lost twin. There was contamination. The DNA was secondarily transferred. The person was recently in contact with the object.
No semen.	There was no ejaculation. A condom was used. There was no intercourse. There was intercourse but all trace of semen was lost following a vaginal douche. The swab taken did not recover the material that was present because of bad procedures.

In the context of DNA, especially when the issue is how the DNA was deposited, one should avoid, or at least outline the limitations of, considering explanations in court: in this process the scientist cannot assign the value of the results which then could easily be misunderstood. As indicated in [49], "'bare' explanations are likely to be of limited assistance to fact-finders, and might even be regarded as potentially misleading and, sometimes, pernicious." We will revisit this aspect in the section on communication and reporting.

10. A Note on Multiple Propositions

While it is not feasible to achieve absolute exhaustiveness, it is important that all the relevant case information is considered when formulating the propositions. This can imply having two main propositions, but several sub-propositions. Indeed, if the scientist omits a proposition that is relevant, it is possible to have results that support a proposition that would not be supported if all pertinent information had been considered. In the context of mixtures, one may have to consider different numbers of contributors [44,47], different persons of interest [48], or different degrees of relatedness between the POI and the alternative source and/or different populations [50,51]. It has also been shown that for close relatives, considering multiple propositions (but two views) achieves better sensitivity and specificity [52]. An example of multiple propositions (two main propositions and associate sub-propositions) with two persons of interest—Mr A and Mr B—could be for the evaluation of the comparison of Mr A's DNA profile with a two-person DNA mixture:

- Mr A is a contributor

    - Mr A and Mr B are the source of the DNA mixture.
    - Mr A and an unknown are the source of the DNA mixture.

- Mr A is NOT a contributor

    - Mr B and an unknown are the source of the DNA mixture.
    - Two unknown persons are the source of the DNA mixture.

11. Pre-Assessment

With the segmentation of forensic science and the use of DNA databases for investigation, it is not always realised how crucial case information is for devising an appropriate case strategy and for giving meaningful answers. One important outcome of the Case Assessment and Interpretation project was to formalise what is known as case pre-assessment [49,53,54]. Most of the stages described imply thinking and communicating about the problem before proceeding to examinations and the commitment of resources; one can argue that it just reflects good forensic practice.

11.1. Revisiting Good Forensic Practices for Evaluative Reporting

To deliver the best service, the first stage will be to define the needs in the case and explore how one can help with the issue. Once the questions have been clearly identified and discussed with the mandating authority, an effective examination strategy can be devised and agreed to with the client, the work can be performed, and the results and subsequent interpretation reported. This process appears straightforward, but it can be difficult to apply in practice. First, because the police will not always be taught how important case information is to help define the best examination strategy, they might not be aware of some limitations. Moreover, in many cases, the work will first be performed to provide an investigative lead. Once the lead has been produced, the criminal justice system might not always be aware that the case information provided by the POI can drastically change the value of the results.

Efficient case management cannot proceed without task-pertinent information, such as the allegations that are contested and those that are not, what the persons of interest say (if available), or where and how the items were recovered (e.g., inside the car of the POI). The case circumstances help the scientist to understand the issues and identify what types of opinion (investigative or evaluative) they should offer. Administrative information, such as the deadline and the budget, will inform the choice of the examination strategy. Thinking of the case and of one's expectations before doing the actual work has many advantages, including ensuring (i) that the work done is meaningful and cost-effective, (ii) that the scientist thinks and writes down the expected results given the truth of each proposition, helping to mitigate post-hoc rationalisation (or bias). Indeed, even the most logical of scientists, once confronted with the results, will tend to rationalise their expectations; these will appear more likely once they are observed. Having to think of the range of different outcomes also ensures that the probabilities assigned are coherent. Pre-assessment is particularly valuable when DNA scientists need to consider phenomena such as transfer and persistence.

11.2. An Example of Post-Hoc Rationalisation That Can Be Avoided Using Pre-Assessment

Let us imagine that we have a case where it is alleged by prosecution that Mr S digitally penetrated Ms J's vagina. Mr S says that he only spent the night taking care of Ms J as she had drunk too much alcohol. DNA swabs are taken from Mr S's nails 3 h after the events. Assume we did not carry out any case pre-assessment (i.e., we did not set out, broadly, all the potential outcomes of the examination and, more importantly, their probabilities). Assume that we now know that a full female DNA profile was produced from the swab from the right hand, we could be tempted to say that this was an expected outcome (i.e., there was a high probability that we would have obtained this outcome if the prosecution proposition were true) or "within the range of our expectations". However, if a partial female profile had been obtained, we could be tempted to say that one needs to consider the possibility that Mr S has washed his hands. If that were true, then we would have expected a partial profile. So, whatever the outcome, there is a temptation to rationalise it. Had we not known the outcome, then we could not be biased by it. The same can be said for the POI—once confronted with the results, they might be tempted to rationalise the findings. For this reason, one should ideally: (i) assign the probability of the possible outcomes without any knowledge of the actual results (this can be done by another scientist unaware of the findings, or using a previously built Bayesian Network [55]), (ii) ask the parties their version of events, without mentioning the results. This should theoretically not be problematic, as the alleged facts should not depend on the results.

12. Communication, Reporting, and Testimony

To exchange information, the messenger (e.g., the DNA scientist) needs to convey the value of the findings clearly, and the recipient of information (e.g., judiciary, police investigator) needs to understand the message in the intended manner. This implies that DNA scientists explain their reasoning and the meaning of the results in an accessible way to a large audience, who will have different education, backgrounds, languages, and expectations. As discussed in [56], more research is needed to address the effective presentation of forensic findings. In this section, we briefly explore the topic, but are of the opinion that, to tackle this challenge, DNA scientists should master the key concepts of interpretation. This will be easier if they have received formal education in forensic interpretation.

For efficient communication, it is also important to adapt to the audience. As alluded to earlier, the recipient of forensic information does not come without preconceived ideas: in one case, they may have the impression that DNA is unique; science is exact, precise, and gives answers that are independent of human judgement. In another case, they may think that DNA is too complex and cannot be helpful. There can easily be a disconnection between prior (mis) knowledge and the reality of forensic DNA interpretation. Another point is that, if communication takes place in the context of a given case, then according to [57], "the audience's pre-existing beliefs or attitudes towards the communicator, topic or object of uncertainty might influence or change the effects of uncertainty communication". Thus, not only will the communicator have a bearing on how the value of the evidence is perceived, but so will the other case information available to the recipient of information. For these reasons, formal education outside the courtroom is certainly the best means to ensure that the nature of forensic opinions is well communicated and understood. Having forensic interpretation courses in the curriculum of law degrees, as is the case in some universities (e.g., Lausanne, Switzerland), helps ensure that the future judiciary and advocates understand key concepts such as uncertainty, probability, and likelihood ratios.

The provision of a common language contributes to the improvement of communication: explaining what we mean (with the use of a glossary) as well as what we do not mean is key. Moreover, one needs to acknowledge that some words (e.g., guess, subjective, match, assumption) come with a strong connotation and are prone to misunderstandings: as such, they should be avoided whenever possible or be explained.

12.1. Reporting: General Desiderata

The desiderata, as well as the principles of interpretation, that have been proposed for evaluation of the results apply to reporting (orally or in writing). In addition, it has been proposed that the goals of communication should be truthfulness, candour, and comprehensibility [23]. The pursuit of one goal often requires the sacrifice of the others. The tension between these three goals can be illustrated by a triangle where each goal represents an angle (see Figure 1, Buckleton, personal communication). Candour implies that experts adhere to a code of conduct and only report in their area of expertise.

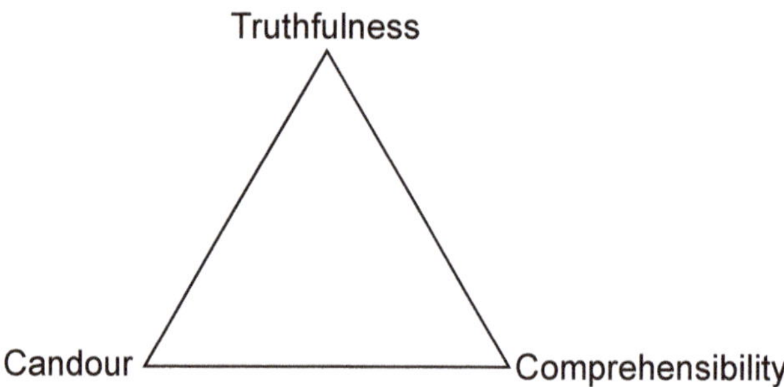

Figure 1. Triangle representing the tensions between the goals of communication.

12.2. Statement Writing

The exact requirements for statement writing will depend on the jurisdiction, but guidelines for good practice [9,21] should be followed. These provide suggestions regarding the content of the statement and caution the reader against certain words and phrases still in use today (e.g., consistent with, association, link, contact, support or refute. Because refute is a categorical statement, it is not considered as the converse of support. There are degrees of support, but not of refutation. Instead of writing "whether the results support or refute", one could say "whether the results support one proposition compared to the alternative or neither proposition".) Because of their nebulous meaning, these terms generally poorly convey the value of the findings.

Because the value of the results depends on the scientific knowledge of the DNA scientist and the task-pertinent case circumstances, statements should include a specific paragraph describing the information that was provided, as well as the assumptions made. The issue should be clearly identified, propositions formulated, and scientists should state their willingness to help address other alternative propositions if the framework of circumstances changes or if it has been misunderstood. As the case information is not a collection of "facts", it is important to indicate that should the case information change, it will be necessary to review the interpretation. Following the description of the items, methodological aspects sometimes referred to as "Technical issues" (e.g., methods of analysis and interpretation, aspects regarding transfer, persistence, and recovery of DNA) will be described. The results of the analysis will be presented and evaluated. In complex situations (e.g., when assigning the value of the findings given activity-level propositions) a paragraph pertaining to the probability of the results given the case information and given each proposition will allow the reader to understand the basis of the reasoning and the source of the data. Reporting what a LR is and what it is not should help convey the difference between the probability of the findings (given the propositions and information) and the probability of the propositions (given the findings and the information). The limitations of the interpretation and the issues considered should also be clearly stated. In Table 8, we suggest examples of useful caveats.

Table 8. Examples of useful caveats in written statements.

Reason for the Caveat	Example
Underline the importance of case information and propositions.	The evaluation presented in this report is crucially dependent on the information provided to the examiner and on the propositions addressed. Any change in the framework of circumstances or in either of the propositions should be seen as sufficient reason for a new evaluation. If some information were found to be incorrect, or if new information were made available, I would need to re-evaluate the value of the findings. Re-evaluation will be more effective if performed in advance of a trial.
Explain what a LR is and is not.	A likelihood ratio indicates if and to what extent the DNA analysis results support one proposition over another. It is not possible, on this basis alone, to determine which is the most probable proposition. To assign the probability of a proposition, the DNA analysis results should be combined with other information in the case. This is generally not considered to be the remit of the DNA scientist.
Alert on the difference between source and activity issues.	This report does not provide any information on the mechanisms or actions that led to the deposition of the recovered biological material. It only provides information regarding its origin (e.g., who is the source of the DNA). Should there be any issue regarding the transfer mechanisms that led to the detection of this material, the results should be evaluated given the alleged activities.
Delineate the meaning of a verbal scale.	The likelihood ratio is a numerical value. Words can be assigned to brackets of numerical values and used as a descriptor of the results' support for a proposition. Several verbal equivalence tables have been published, and it is above all a convention.

12.3. The Use of Verbal Equivalents

To communicate the meaning of the LR, verbal equivalents (or verbal scales) have been suggested [4,58,59]. If a quantitative LR is presented, the LR value shall come first [9] and can be accompanied by a verbal equivalent [56,59,60]. An example could be: "A likelihood ratio of the order of 1000 has been assigned, which means that the DNA results are 1000 times more probable if Mr Smith is the source of the DNA rather than if his unavailable brother is the source. Therefore, the DNA findings support the proposition that Mr Smith is the source of the DNA rather than his unavailable brother. The level of support can be qualified as strong.". If one understands what a LR is, verbal equivalents are superfluous. To show how beliefs should be theoretically updated based on the DNA results, it might be more efficient to include a table with a few examples of prior odds and the effect of the results (i.e., the LR obtained) on posterior odds. (For persons who are unfamiliar with odds, it is also possible to transform odds into probabilities.) This also has the advantage of showing the difference between LRs, prior odds, and posterior odds.

It is sometimes believed that one needs different verbal scales for DNA (more precisely, for autosomal DNA) because LRs are much larger than those of say mtDNA or another discipline such as fibres. This is not the case: an explanation of why some DNA scientists believe that a DNA comparison with a LR of 1000 is uninformative is that DNA scientists nowadays work mainly in the investigation phase. In such a situation, larger LRs are generally needed to avoid having too many candidates from the national DNA database (and too many false leads). In addition, if there is little additional case information, then the authority may need more discriminative results to decide if a person should be arrested or not. Another (non-mutually exclusive explanation) could be that DNA scientists are so used to having very large LRs that they are like billionaires: 1000 could thus be perceived as "pocket money". As outlined by several authors [4,9,61], one should adopt the same verbal equivalents whatever the discipline and whatever the results (autosomal DNA, Y-STR, or mtDNA comparisons). It follows that one needs the same verbal scale whether reporting results given activity- or sub-source-level propositions and whether the results are to be used for missing persons, paternity, or sibling cases. There has been much discussion on verbal scales [21,58–60,62,63]. There are three points where there seems to be a consensus: (1) If the LR value is "one", then results must be considered as uninformative (it is the results and not the LR that is uninformative. Similarly, it is the results and not the LR that provide support for one proposition compared to the other. The LR indicates the magnitude of the support given by the results to one or the other of the propositions). Therefore, the observations provide no assistance in addressing the stated propositions. (2) If LRs are larger than one, the results support the first proposition. (3) When LRs are smaller than one, the results support the alternative. Because verbal scales are based on a convention, it is difficult to achieve standardisation: different scales have been proposed with different resolutions (number of intervals) and terminology. Although verbal equivalents are unsatisfactory, concentrating on the LR value alone does not look very promising either, and it has been shown that people have difficulties understanding the concept of LRs in isolation. While no one has yet identified the ideal method for the presentation of the value of scientific findings, this does not mean we should change the method of evaluation (we would not change the methods of analysis because people do not understand DNA analysis). However, until there is more widespread understanding of the concepts of LR and probability, if the DNA scientist thinks it is desirable to add a verbal equivalent, this is not harmful provided that the LR value is given first.

12.4. Testimony

Questions in court relate more and more as to how the DNA was deposited. However, few DNA experts will prepare a report on this topic and some are tempted to wait and answer questions in court. This is not ideal [12,64], because evaluation of biological results is difficult. As such, it should be submitted to the same criteria as any other evaluation (i.e., be the subject of a written statement that has been peer reviewed and is available to the defence).

In court, DNA scientists may be asked to report the value of the results given sub-source propositions, and then answer hypothetical questions, which generally are explanations rather than propositions. An example could be: "What if the defendant had shaken hands with the real offender, would it not be possible to recover in such a case DNA from my client?". One might be tempted to say, yes, this is possible. However, as stated in [65] "if at the end of the expert's evidence, the fact-finder is left with, on the one hand, an impressive big number (the LR given sub-source propositions) and on the other hand, a list of possible explanations for the transfer (as a result of specific activities), how do they decide what the DNA evidence means, and how does the evidence impact their decision?".

Questions about the possibilities of DNA transfer require a more subtle answer. In general, when a case comes to court, DNA scientists will help the triers of fact in a more meaningful way if they assess the value of the DNA results in the context of the case. One must also be aware that if answering questions such as "Is it possible that there was secondary transfer?", one would be giving an opinion on the alleged activities implying secondary transfer. Similarly, if one comments on the origin of the DNA and says that "The most likely source of the DNA is the vagina" [37], then if one does not specify how prior odds were assigned, it is unclear if it is a transposed conditional or a posterior probability. If the nature of the fluid implies an activity (as would be the case for vaginal cells), this is problematic, as the nature of the material relates directly to the issue that is of the remit of the court.

If the questions regarding how DNA was transferred appear reasonable to the court, it is recommended to ask for a recess [12,25] and perform a proper evaluation of the results given what is alleged.

If DNA scientists cannot assess the value of the observations, for example, in light of the proposed activities, because there is no time, a lack of case information, or a lack of knowledge, then, provided the person is qualified, they should outline that without further information, the findings should be considered uninterpretable (thus uninformative) and presumably inadmissible, because of the risk of their being prejudicial.

13. A Discussion on Likelihood Ratios

Now that you are familiar with the main concepts of interpretation, we would like to discuss aspects relating to what LRs are, if they can be estimated, how precise they should be, and whether it is problematic to transpose the conditional when LRs are very large.

13.1. Likelihood Ratio and Probability

Scientists should know how to explain what a likelihood ratio is. As described earlier, a LR is a ratio of two conditional probabilities given competing propositions and conditioning information. However, what is a probability? A probability is a number between zero and one that represents our uncertainty with regard to the truth of some aspect of the universe in the past, present, or future. All probabilities are conditional: they depend on what you know, what you are told, and what you assume. In some simple situations, such as coin-tossing, there might be little disagreement between people about the truth of a statement such as "the coin will land showing a head". In general, though, the central component of knowledge means that different people will have different probabilities for the same thing. We say that probability is *personal*. In relation to any uncertain event there is no "correct" probability, so we say that probabilities are "assigned" rather than "estimated".

Because a likelihood ratio is the ratio of two probabilities, it necessarily follows that a LR is personal also. Thus, in relation to any particular pair of propositions in a DNA case, there is no "correct" LR: different scientists will bring different levels of knowledge (and understanding) to bear. What we require is that the scientist to whom we pay attention is *well calibrated*: that is, we expect that the scientist can be relied upon to assign large values to the LR in cases where the prosecution proposition is actually true and to assign small values to the LR in cases where the defence proposition is actually true. This concept of calibration is critical to software systems that are created to assist scientists in assigning LRs and to the publications supporting advanced DNA probabilistic genotyping calculations, include extensive studies of *ground truth* cases. A ground truth case is one that has been artificially created; in its simplest form, it will consist of two sets of data and the truth with regard to whether the two are from the same original source (H_p true) or not (H_d true) is known without doubt. The distribution of LRs from H_p-true ground truth cases should peak at high values (greater than one); the distribution from H_d-true ground truth cases should peak at small values (less than one). If considering, for example, the source of a DNA mixture recovered on a scene, because people can share part of their DNA, it is expected that some non-donors will share alleles adventitiously and have a LR larger than one fortuitously. This is even more true when comparing mixed/partial DNA profile with individuals who are closely related to contributors or due to co-ancestry effects [52]. There are sophisticated measures for assessing calibration experiments quantitatively, but one simple one is known as "Turing's rule". This follows from a theorem, attributed by IJ Good to Alan Turing [66,67], that shows that the "expected value of a LR in favour of a wrong proposition is one". This implies that the average value of the LR in a large H_d-true calibration experiment should be approximately one: in practice, this means a highly skewed distribution, with most LRs close to zero and the odd one or two substantially greater than one. For example, suppose that a LR of a million is computed given sub-source propositions. It follows that if we simulated profiles of millions of non-donors, we would expect roughly 1 in every million non-donor DNA profiles to yield a LR of 1 million when compared to the DNA profile of the trace. We would also expect 999,999 out of every million non-donor profiles to yield a LR of 0 when compared to the DNA profile of the trace. The average LR of these ground truth comparisons is then 1.

Good (ibid) also showed how he and Turing regarded the logarithm of the LR as a measure of evidential weight, and this view appears highly relevant to the forensic field. This notion contributes to the idea of expressing verbal conventions in rough correspondence to orders of magnitude of the LR [58]. It also suggests the notion that precise values of the LR are not needed for effective communication of evidential weight to jurors. Hence, our suggestion is to report LRs to one significant figure. If a LR of 10,256.32 were computed, we would conclude that the findings are of the order of 10,000 more probable if . . . than if . . . This allows us to convey that it is the order of magnitude that is important.

For LRs smaller than one (i.e., when results support the alternative), it has been suggested to reverse the propositions and adopt the same rounding rules. Indeed, numbers smaller than one are difficult to understand: for example, if our LR is 0.01, shall we say results are 0.01 times less (or more?) likely if the first proposition were true rather than if the alternative were true? It is easier to report that results are 100 times more likely if the alternative proposition were true rather than if the first proposition were true.

Current population genetic models condone the multiplying together of genotype probabilities across many loci, and this in turn leads to extremely large LRs—billions, trillions, quadrillions, and still further. When this issue first arose in the UK, Foreman and Evett [68] argued that the extent of investigations into the independence assumptions implicit in this process was insufficient to justify the robustness of LRs in excess of one billion. So, when the Forensic Science Service introduced the ten locus STR system into casework, the largest magnitude of LR quoted was one billion. This was expected to be a temporary expedient, but to this day, there still seems to be little in the way of large-scale between-locus dependence effects. This seems to cause little embarrassment, and it is common to see LRs of the order 10^{20} reported in DNA cases (It should be noted that with very small numbers, there are some analogies that are misleading. An example is the "several planets earth" or the "galaxy" argument used, for example, in the Jama Case [69]. "The range, it was said, within which the calculation was made was between 1 in 45 billion and 1 in 14 trillion. [. . .] In other words, it would appear to be necessary to search well beyond this planet and conceivably this galaxy to find a match". This argument leads the layperson to think that DNA is sufficient for individualisation, when it is not [70]). In some countries, for example, the UK [71], it is still current practice to report all LRs that are computed as greater than 10^9 to be "of the order of one billion", even though the number of loci in routine use is much greater than the original 10 at the time of the Foreman and Evett study. This seems to cause no problem, but it is a peculiar state of affairs.

In addition, it has been advocated that one should consider the possibility of an error, [72] as DNA analysis is not error free [73]. When we do, the value of the results will be largely dominated by this probability [3,7,74].

13.2. With High LRs, Does It Really Matter if One Transposes the Conditional?

Some might advocate that we should not split hairs and that if the LR is very high, then the effect of prior odds is washed away and it is not a real issue if the scientist transposes the conditional. Reporting and testimony represent the end-product of the scientist's job. Whether or not it would be acceptable in some cases to let the court believe that the results allow the scientist to assign a posterior probability, is a matter of ethics and code of conduct. The scientist's remit is scientific results and their value in the context of the alleged facts, not the facts themselves. It is the duty of factfinders to consider both the results and the alleged facts.

14. Conclusions

Understanding and conveying uncertainty is a difficult endeavour. As we cannot suppress uncertainty, we need to face it and include it in our actions [14]. For DNA scientists, this involves putting measures in place to ensure that results are appropriately interpreted and their value well communicated. Identifying the issue with which forensic science can help and using the framework we presented is the first step: it allows scientists to rationally assess and present the value of their results in a transparent way. It ensures that the LRs assigned given sub-source-level propositions are not carried over to activity-level propositions [75]. It is important to acknowledge that DNA, although extremely useful, is not the magic bullet. There will be situations where DNA comparisons alone will not be helpful. If the person involved has legitimate access to the object or person, and one can safely assume that the DNA comes from this person, then it does not make much sense to consider the probability of the results given the DNA is from an unknown person, as this is not what is alleged. Another example could be a case where the issue is not the person from whom the DNA comes from, but the activities that led to the deposition of the material: if the activities alleged by both parties are very similar to each other, the DNA outcome will not allow discrimination of the propositions. These points need to be conveyed to the trier of facts.

To help communication, harmonisation, and to raise the standards of interpretation, several measures could be taken: (1) invest in the formal education of the key players (i.e., the messenger and the recipient of the information), (2) provide the forensic community with appropriate tools and knowledge, and (3) make interpretation part of the scope of accreditation. Having technical assessors and adequate proficiency tests would allow for the monitoring of the evaluation of DNA results given both sub-source and activity-level propositions. It would ensure DNA scientists adhere to the principles of interpretation as advocated in the Forensic Science Regulator of England and Wales codes of practice and conduct for evaluative opinions [12]. We note also that in some countries, such as the Netherlands, there have been initiatives by The Netherlands Register of Court Experts [76,77] to guarantee and promote the quality of the contribution made by court experts to the legal process. This is an avenue other countries could pursue to ensure that experts are fully qualified and certified for both types of reporting.

Author Contributions: Conceptualisation, T.H.; writing—original draft preparation, T.H., J.B., V.C., I.E. and G.J.; writing—review and editing, T.H., J.B., V.C., I.E. and G.J.; project administration, T.H.; All authors have read and agreed to the published version of the manuscript.

Funding: This research received no external funding.

Institutional Review Board Statement: Not applicable.

Informed Consent Statement: Not applicable.

Data Availability Statement: Not applicable.

Conflicts of Interest: The authors declare no conflict of interest.

References

1. Taroni, F.; Champod, C.; Margot, P. Forerunners of Bayesianism in early forensic science. *J. Forensic Identif.* **1999**, *49*, 285–310.
2. Jackson, G. The Development of Case Assessment and Interpretation (CAI) in Forensic Science. Ph.D. Thesis, University of Abertay, Dundee, UK, 2011.
3. Aitken, C.; Taroni, F.; Bozza, S. *Statistics and the Evaluation of Evidence for Forensic Scientists*, 3rd ed.; John Wiley & Sons: Chichester, UK, 2021.
4. Evett, I.W.; Weir, B.S. *Interpreting DNA Evidence—Statistical Genetics for Forensic Scientists*; Sinauer Associates, Inc.: Sunderland, MA, USA, 1998.
5. Kaye, D.H. *The Double Helix and the Law of Evidence*; Harvard University Press: Cambridge, MA, USA, 2010.
6. Buckleton, J.S.; Bright, J.-A.; Taylor, D. *Forensic DNA Evidence Interpretation*, 2nd ed.; CRC Press: Boca Raton, FL, USA, 2016.
7. Robertson, B.; Vignaux, G.A.; Berger, C.E.H. *Interpreting Evidence*, 2nd ed.; Wiley & Sons: Chichester, UK, 2016.
8. Aitken, C.G.G.; Stoney, D.A. *The Use of Statistics in Forensic Science*, 1st ed.; Ellis Horwood Series in Forensic Science; CRC Press: Boca Raton, FL, USA, 1991.
9. Willis, S.M.; McKenna, L.; McDermott, S.D.; O'Donnell, G.; Barrett, A.; Rasmusson, B.; Höglund, T.; Berger, C.E.H.; Sierps, M.J.; Lucena-Molina, J.J.; et al. ENFSI Guideline for Evaluative Reporting in Forensic Science: Strengthening the Evaluation of Forensic Results Across Europe (STEOFRAE). 2015. Available online: http://enfsi.eu/wp-content/uploads/2016/09/m1_guideline.pdf (accessed on 14 May 2022).

10. Gill, P.; Hicks, T.; Butler, J.M.; Connolly, E.; Gusmao, L.; Kokshoorn, B.; Morling, N.; van Oorschot, R.A.H.; Parson, W.; Prinz, M.; et al. DNA commission of the International society for forensic genetics: Assessing the value of forensic biological evidence—Guidelines highlighting the importance of propositions: Part I: Evaluation of DNA profiling comparisons given (sub-)source propositions. *Forensic Sci. Int. Genet.* **2018**, *36*, 189–202. [CrossRef] [PubMed]

11. Gill, P.; Hicks, T.; Butler, J.M.; Connolly, E.; Gusmão, L.; Kokshoorn, B.; Morling, N.; van Oorschot, R.A.H.; Parson, W.; Prinz, M.; et al. DNA commission of the International society for forensic genetics: Assessing the value of forensic biological evidence—Guidelines highlighting the importance of propositions. Part II: Evaluation of biological traces considering activity level propositions. *Forensic Sci. Int. Genet.* **2020**, *44*, 102186. [CrossRef] [PubMed]

12. Forensic Science Regulator. Development of Evaluative Opinion. FSR-C-118; 2021. Available online: https://assets.publishing. service.gov.uk/government/uploads/system/uploads/attachment_data/file/960051/FSR-C-118_Interpretation_Appendix_ Issue_1__002_.pdf (accessed on 14 May 2022).

13. Edmond, G.; Cole, S.A. Legal aspects of forensic science. In *Encyclopedia of Forensic Sciences, Second ed.*; Siegel, J.A., Saukko, P.J., Houck, M.M., Eds.; Academic Press: Waltham, MA, USA, 2013; pp. 466–470.

14. Lindley, D.V. *Understanding Uncertainty*; John Wiley & Sons, Ltd.: Hoboken, NJ, USA, 2006.

15. Samie, L.; Champod, C.; Delemont, S.; Basset, P.; Hicks, T.; Castella, V. Use of Bayesian Networks for the investigation of the nature of biological material in casework. *Forensic Sci. Int.* **2022**, *331*, 111174. [CrossRef] [PubMed]

16. Jackson, G.; Jones, S.; Booth, G.; Champod, C.; Evett, I.W. The nature of forensic science opinion—A possible framework to guide thinking and practice in investigations and in court proceedings. *Sci. Justice* **2006**, *46*, 33–44. [CrossRef]

17. Nordby, J.J. *Dead Reckoning: The Art of Forensic Detection*; CRC Press LLC.: Boca Raton, FL, USA, 2000.

18. Evett, I.W.; Jackson, G.; Lambert, J.A. More on the hierarchy of propositions: Exploring the distinction between explanations and propositions. *Sci. Justice* **2000**, *40*, 3–10. [CrossRef]

19. Jackson, G. The scientist and the scales of justice. *Sci. Justice* **2000**, *40*, 81–85. [CrossRef]

20. Association of Forensic Science Providers. Standards for the formulation of evaluative forensic science expert opinion. *Sci. Justice* **2009**, *49*, 161–164. [CrossRef]

21. Evett, I.W.; Jackson, G.; Lambert, J.A.; McCrossan, S. The impact of the principles of evidence interpretation on the structure and content of statements. *Sci. Justice* **2000**, *40*, 233–239. [CrossRef]

22. Berger, C.E.H.; Buckleton, J.; Champod, C.; Evett, I.W.; Jackson, G. Evidence evaluation: A response to the court of appeal judgment in R v T. *Sci. Justice* **2011**, *51*, 43–49. [CrossRef]

23. Gittelson, S.; Kalafut, T.; Myers, S.; Taylor, D.; Hicks, T.; Taroni, F.; Evett, I.W.; Bright, J.A.; Buckleton, J. A practical guide for the formulation of propositions in the Bayesian approach to DNA evidence interpretation in an adversarial environment. *J. Forensic Sci.* **2016**, *61*, 186–195. [CrossRef] [PubMed]

24. Biedermann, A.; Hicks, T.; Taroni, F.; Champod, C.; Aitken, C. On the use of the likelihood ratio for forensic evaluation: Response to Fenton et al. *Sci. Justice* **2014**, *54*, 316–318. [CrossRef] [PubMed]

25. OSAC. Best Practice Recommendation for Evaluative Forensic DNA Testimony OPEN COMMENT VERSION (2022-S-0024). Draft OSAC Proposed Standard; 2022. Available online: www.nist.gov/system/files/documents/2022/01/04/OSAC%202022-S-0024%20BPR%20for%20Evaluative%20Forensic%20DNA%20Testimony.OPEN%20COMMENT%20VERSION.pdf (accessed on 14 May 2022).

26. Evett, I.W. Avoiding the transposed conditional. *Sci. Justice* **1995**, *35*, 127–131. [CrossRef]

27. Aitken, C.G.G.; Roberts, P.; Jackson, G. Fundamentals of Probability and Statistical Evidence in Criminal Proceedings; Working Group on Statistics the Law of the Royal Statistical Society: 2011; Volume Practitioner Guide No.1. Available online: https://www.maths.ed.ac.uk/~{}cgga/Guide-1-WEB.pdf (accessed on 14 May 2022).

28. Taroni, F.; Marquis, R.; Schmittbuhl, M.; Biedermann, A.; Thiéry, A.; Bozza, S. Bayes factor for investigative assessment of selected handwriting features. *Forensic Sci. Int.* **2014**, *242*, 266–273. [CrossRef]

29. Koehler, J.J. Forensic fallacies and a famous judge. *Jurimetrics* **2014**, *54*, 211–219.

30. Thompson, W.C.; Schumann, E.L. Interpretation of statistical evidence in criminal trials: The prosecutor's fallacy and the defence attorney's fallacy. *Law Hum. Behav.* **1987**, *11*, 167–187. [CrossRef]

31. Supreme Court of Victoria (Australia)—Court of Appeal. Tuite v The Queen 49 VR 196, 200 2015 Maxwell ACJ, Redlich and Weinberg JJA. Available online: https://jade.io/article/397203 (accessed on 19 May 2022).

32. Jeffreys, H. *Theory of Probability*, 3rd ed.; Clarendon Press: Oxford, UK, 1983.

33. Cook, R.; Evett, I.W.; Jackson, G.; Jones, P.J.; Lambert, J.A. A hierarchy of propositions: Deciding which level to address in casework. *Sci. Justice* **1998**, *38*, 231–240. [CrossRef]

34. Taylor, D.; Bright, J.A.; Buckleton, J. The 'factor of two' issue in mixed DNA profiles. *J. Theor. Biol.* **2014**, *363*, 300–306. [CrossRef]

35. Evett, I.W.; Gill, P.D.; Jackson, G.; Whitaker, J.; Champod, C. Interpreting small quantities of DNA: The hierarchy of propositions and the use of Bayesian networks. *J. Forensic Sci.* **2002**, *47*, 520–530. [CrossRef]

36. Taroni, F.; Biedermann, A.; Vuille, J.; Morling, N. Whose DNA is this? How relevant a question? (A note for forensic scientists). *Forensic Sci. Int. Genet.* **2013**, *7*, 467–470. [CrossRef]

37. England and Wales Court of Appeal (Criminal Division) Decisions, Weller, R. v [2010] EWCA Crim 1085 (04 March 2010). Available online: http://www.bailii.org/ew/cases/EWCA/Crim/2010/1085.html (accessed on 19 May 2022).

38. Taroni, F.; Bozza, S.; Hicks, T.; Garbolino, P. More on the question 'When does absence of evidence constitute evidence of absence?' How Bayesian confirmation theory can logically support the answer. *Forensic Sci. Int.* **2019**, *301*, e59–e63. [CrossRef] [PubMed]
39. Taylor, D.; Kokshoorn, B.; Biedermann, A. Evaluation of forensic genetics findings given activity level propositions: A review. *Forensic Sci. Int. Genet.* **2018**, *36*, 34–49. [CrossRef] [PubMed]
40. Evett, I.W. Establishing the evidential value of a small quantity of material found at a crime scene. *J. Forensic Sci. Soc.* **1993**, *33*, 83–86. [CrossRef]
41. Stoney, D.A. Transfer Evidence. In *The Use of Statistics in Forensic Science*, 1st ed.; Ellis Horwood Series in Forensic Science; Aitken, C.G.G., Stoney, D.A., Eds.; CRC Press: Boca Raton, FL, USA, 1991; pp. 107–138.
42. Biedermann, A.; Hicks, T. The importance of critically examining the level of propositions when evaluating forensic DNA results. *Front. Genet.* **2016**, *7*, 8. [CrossRef]
43. Buckleton, J.; Bright, J.-A.; Taylor, D.; Evett, I.; Hicks, T.; Jackson, G.; Curran, J.M. Helping formulate propositions in forensic DNA analysis. *Sci. Justice* **2014**, *54*, 258–261. [CrossRef]
44. Buckleton, J.; Taylor, D.; Bright, J.A.; Hicks, T.; Curran, J. When evaluating DNA evidence within a likelihood ratio framework, should the propositions be exhaustive? *Forensic Sci. Int. Genet.* **2021**, *50*, 102406. [CrossRef]
45. Hicks, T.; Biedermann, A.; de Koeijer, J.A.; Taroni, F.; Champod, C.; Evett, I.W. The importance of distinguishing information from evidence/observations when formulating propositions. *Sci. Justice* **2015**, *55*, 520–525. [CrossRef]
46. Taylor, D.; Kokshoorn, B.; Hicks, T. Structuring cases into propositions, assumptions, and undisputed case information. *Forensic Sci. Int. Genet.* **2020**, *44*, 102199. [CrossRef]
47. Taylor, D.; Bright, J.A.; Buckleton, J. Interpreting forensic DNA profiling evidence without specifying the number of contributors. *Forensic Sci. Int. Genet.* **2014**, *13*, 269–280. [CrossRef]
48. Hicks, T.; Kerr, Z.; Pugh, S.; Bright, J.A.; Curran, J.; Taylor, D.; Buckleton, J. Comparing multiple POI to DNA mixtures. *Forensic Sci. Int. Genet.* **2021**, *52*, 102481. [CrossRef]
49. Jackson, G.; Roberts, P.; Aitken, C. Guidance for Judges, Lawyers, Forensic Scientists and Expert Witnesses. 4. Case Assessment and Interpretation of Expert Evidence. 2015. Available online: https://rss.org.uk/RSS/media/File-library/Publications/rss-case-assessment-interpretation-expert-evidence.pdf (accessed on 14 May 2022).
50. Buckleton, J.S.; Walsh, K.A.J.; Evett, I.W. Who is "Random Man"? *J. Forensic Sci. Soc.* **1991**, *31*, 463–468. [CrossRef]
51. Balding, D.J. *Weight-of-Evidence for Forensic DNA Profiles*; Wiley: Chichester, UK, 2005.
52. Kalafut, T.; Pugh, S.; Gill, P.; Abbas, S.; Semaan, M.; Mansour, I.; Curran, J.; Bright, J.A.; Hicks, T.; Wivell, R.; et al. A mixed DNA profile controversy revisited. *J. Forensic Sci.* **2021**, *67*, 128–135. [CrossRef] [PubMed]
53. Cook, R.; Evett, I.W.; Jackson, G.; Jones, P.J.; Lambert, J.A. A model for case assessment and interpretation. *Sci. Justice* **1998**, *38*, 151–156. [CrossRef]
54. Jackson, G.; Jones, P. Case Assessment and Interpretation. In *Encyclopedia of Forensic Science*; Jamieson, A., Moenssens, A., Eds.; John Wiley & Sons, Ltd.: Chichester, UK, 2009; pp. 483–497.
55. Taroni, F.; Aitken, C.; Bozza, S.; Garbolino, P.; Biedermann, A. *Bayesian Networks and Probabilistic Inference in Forensic Science*, 2nd ed.; John Wiley & Sons, Ltd.: Chichester, UK, 2014.
56. Neumann, C.; Kaye, D.; Jackson, G.; Reyna, V.; Ranadive, A. Presenting Quantitative and Qualitative Information on Forensic Science Evidence in the Courtroom. *Chance* **2016**, *29*, 37–43. [CrossRef]
57. van der Bles, A.M.; van der Linden, S.; Freeman, A.L.J.; Mitchell, J.; Galvao, A.B.; Zaval, L.; Spiegelhalter, D.J. Communicating uncertainty about facts, numbers and science. *R. Soc. Open Sci.* **2019**, *6*, 181870. [CrossRef]
58. Aitken, C.G.G.; Taroni, F. A verbal scale for the interpretation of evidence. *Sci. Justice* **1998**, *38*, 279–281. [CrossRef]
59. Marquis, R.; Biedermann, A.; Cadola, L.; Champod, C.; Gueissaz, L.; Massonnet, G.; Mazzella, W.D.; Taroni, F.; Hicks, T. Discussion on how to implement a verbal scale in a forensic laboratory: Benefits, pitfalls and suggestions to avoid misunderstandings. *Sci. Justice* **2016**, *56*, 364–370. [CrossRef]
60. Martire, K.A.; Watkins, I. Perception problems of the verbal scale: A reanalysis and application of a membership function approach. *Sci. Justice* **2015**, *55*, 264–273. [CrossRef]
61. Nordgaard, A.; Ansell, R.; Drotz, W.; Jaeger, L. Scale of conclusions for the value of evidence. *Law Probab. Risk* **2011**, *11*, 1–24. [CrossRef]
62. Eldridge, H. Juror comprehension of forensic expert testimony: A literature review and gap analysis. *Forensic Sci. Int. Synerg.* **2019**, *1*, 24–34. [CrossRef]
63. Sjerps, M.; Biesheuvel, D.B. The interpretation of conventional and 'Bayesian' verbal scales for expressing expert opinion: A small experiment among jurists. *Forensic Linguist.* **1999**, *6*, 214–227. [CrossRef]
64. Hicks, T.; Biedermann, A.; Taroni, F.; Champod, C. Problematic reporting in DNA cases: The need for accredited formats and certified reporting competence. *Forensic Sci. Int. Genet. Suppl. Ser.* **2019**, *7*, 205–207. [CrossRef]
65. Jackson, G.; Biedermann, A. "Source" or "activity". What is the level of issue in a criminal trial? *Significance* **2019**, *16*, 36–39. [CrossRef]
66. Good, I.J. *Probability and the Weighing of Evidence*; Charles Griffin & Company Limited: London, UK, 1950.
67. Taylor, D.; Buckleton, J.; Evett, I. Testing likelihood ratios produced from complex DNA profiles. *Forensic Sci. Int. Genet.* **2015**, *16*, 165–171. [CrossRef] [PubMed]

68. Foreman, L.A.; Evett, I.W. Statistical Analysis to Support Forensic Interpretation of a New Ten-Locus STR Profiling System. *Int. J. Leg. Med.* **2001**, *114*, 147–155. [CrossRef]

69. Vincent, F.H.R. Report: Inquiry into the Circumstances That Led to the Conviction of Mr Farah Abdulkadir Jama. 2010. Available online: https://www.parliament.vic.gov.au/papers/govpub/VPARL2006-10No301.pdf (accessed on 14 May 2022).

70. Biedermann, A.; Vuille, J. Understanding the logic of forensic identification decisions (without numbers). *Sui Generis* **2018**, *83*, 397–413. [CrossRef]

71. Hopwood, A.J.; Puch-Solis, R.; Tucker, V.C.; Curran, J.M.; Skerrett, J.; Pope, S.; Tully, G. Consideration of the probative value of single donor 15-plex STR profiles in UK populations and its presentation in UK courts. *Sci. Justice* **2012**, *52*, 185–190. [CrossRef]

72. Koehler, J.J.; Chia, A.; Lindsey, S. The random match probability in DNA evidence: Irrelevant and prejudicial? *Jurimetr. J.* **1995**, *35*, 201–219.

73. Kloosterman, A.; Sjerps, M.; Quak, A. Error rates in forensic DNA analysis: Definition, numbers, impact and communication. *Forensic. Sci. Int. Genet.* **2014**, *12*, 77–85. [CrossRef]

74. Coquoz, R.; Comte, J.; Hall, D.; Hicks, T.; Taroni, F. *Preuve Par l'ADN-la Génétique au Service de la Justice*, 3rd ed.; Presses Polytechniques et Universitaires Romandes: Lausanne, Switzerland, 2013.

75. Biedermann, A.; Champod, C.; Jackson, G.; Gill, P.; Taylor, D.; Butler, J.; Morling, N.; Hicks, T.; Vuille, J.; Taroni, F. Evaluation of forensic DNA traces when propositions of interest relate to activities: Analysis and discussion of recurrent concerns. *Front. Genet.* **2016**, *7*, 215. [CrossRef]

76. Doyle, S. *Quality Management in Forensic Science*, 1st ed.; Academic Press: London, UK, 2018.

77. van Oorschot, R.A.H.; Meakin, G.E.; Kokshoorn, B.; Goray, M.; Szkuta, B. DNA transfer in forensic science: Recent progress towards meeting challenges. *Genes* **2021**, *12*, 1766. [CrossRef] [PubMed]

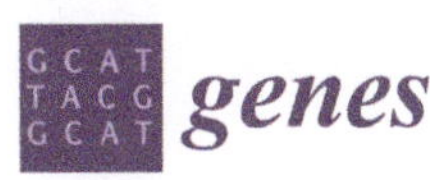

Review

An Introductory Overview of Open-Source and Commercial Software Options for the Analysis of Forensic Sequencing Data

Tunde I. Huszar *, Katherine B. Gettings and Peter M. Vallone

National Institute of Standards and Technology (NIST), Gaithersburg, MD 20899, USA; katherine.gettings@nist.gov (K.B.G.); peter.vallone@nist.gov (P.M.V.)
* Correspondence: tuende.huszar@nist.gov

Abstract: The top challenges of adopting new methods to forensic DNA analysis in routine laboratories are often the capital investment and the expertise required to implement and validate such methods locally. In the case of next-generation sequencing, in the last decade, several specifically forensic commercial options became available, offering reliable and validated solutions. Despite this, the readily available expertise to analyze, interpret and understand such data is still perceived to be lagging behind. This review gives an introductory overview for the forensic scientists who are at the beginning of their journey with implementing next-generation sequencing locally and because most in the field do not have a bioinformatics background may find it difficult to navigate the new terms and analysis options available. The currently available open-source and commercial software for forensic sequencing data analysis are summarized here to provide an accessible starting point for those fairly new to the forensic application of massively parallel sequencing.

Keywords: massively parallel sequencing (MPS); next-generation sequencing (NGS); short tandem repeat (STR); sequence analysis; software

Citation: Huszar, T.I.; Gettings, K.B.; Vallone, P.M. An Introductory Overview of Open-Source and Commercial Software Options for the Analysis of Forensic Sequencing Data. *Genes* **2021**, *12*, 1739. https://doi.org/10.3390/genes12111739

Academic Editor: Niels Morling

Received: 15 October 2021
Accepted: 27 October 2021
Published: 29 October 2021

Publisher's Note: MDPI stays neutral with regard to jurisdictional claims in published maps and institutional affiliations.

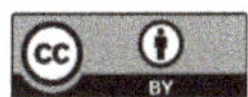

1. Introduction

Next-generation sequencing (NGS) technologies transformed the field of genetics in the past decade. Descriptively referred to also as massively parallel sequencing (MPS), this high-throughput genomics method developed on various platforms provides genome-scale insights from data for the fields of medical diagnostics [1], epidemiology [2], population genetics [3], and more recently for forensic genetics [4–7] as well. The generation of massive datasets creates new challenges in data storage and security, analysis, interpretation, and comparable reporting, which is required to be consistent with traditional forensic genetics standards.

The field of forensic genetics often requires its scientists to have widespread knowledge in related fields such as general genetics, chemistry, physics, physiology, and pathology; however, bioinformatics was rarely among the skills in demand previously. With the introduction of MPS to the field came the generation of a greater amount of data. Due to the lack of readily available user-friendly software, such scarce skills became not just desirable but necessary for early adopters. In the beginning, software to interpret the sequencing data was only developed by research laboratories, naturally with none of the usual emphasis on an attractive graphical user interface (GUI) but focused on functionality and required the users to comfortably navigate the command line. Most analysts working in the forensic DNA laboratories are familiar with running software on the Windows operating system; even those using their Macintosh with the Unix-based operating system rarely would open their terminals and engage in command line operations. Suddenly, the need for data analysis required skills in navigating a whole new world of software running on Unix- and Linux-based computers, and while purchasing such computers was simple enough, gaining the skills to use the software may seem more challenging [8]. Such limitations were recognized and, with time, more software options were developed from research laboratories for the needs of the forensic community, some even offering versions run on Windows or more accessible web-based software. To date, several commercial options also entered the arena, offering to close the gap by providing visual, easy to use and ready-to-export solutions, which would satisfy those in need of quick answers and no particular desire to look 'under the hood'.

Some forensic laboratories already established analysis of the mitochondrial DNA (mtDNA) using Sanger sequencing, and for those laboratories the introduction of MPS brings benefits mostly from the upscaling of the sequencing processes, lowering costs and manual workload, speeding up and automating the analyses. Furthermore, MPS of mtDNA may allow insight into more nuanced phenomena, such as low-level heteroplasmy, length heteroplasmy, and better detection of low-level mixtures. Short tandem repeat (STR) typing, however, had never used sequencing as a standard for forensic analysis, therefore the analysis of this new type of data introduces challenges. DNA analysts are familiar with interpreting STR data from capillary electrophoresis (CE) electropherograms from the last two decades, and many of the CE features are transferable to sequencing, e.g., the length-based allele names, the electrophoretic peaks, and the stutter artifacts. The application of sequencing offers an extra dimension of information for the markers, which drives the ongoing efforts to standardize the nomenclature of the sequence-level data, with the requirement to be back-compatible with the length-based allele names. Software solutions developed individual reporting formats that are sometimes difficult to reliably compare; however, most of these also provide a visual representation of the data, comparable to the already familiar electropherograms, and detailed counts of coverage read depth, similar to CE relative fluorescence unit (RFU) values. Despite the variable formats, these efforts aim to provide a human-readable sequence structure, as well as a sequence string format for universal comparison of the detected sequence variants. One area of non-consensus is the degree or range of reporting of the flanking regions surrounding the markers. While this is mostly influenced by the chemistry used, interpretation of these regions may be optional, dependent on settings, or may even be omitted; therefore becoming a potential source of discrepancy between analysis methods. Similar to reporting from CE data, the analysts will be required to report which kit they used, supplemented with the genomic range of reporting to avoid such discrepancies. While adjustments to reporting will become straightforward with nomenclature standardization and the available software options are increasingly user-friendly, the most critical adaptation for the analysis of STR sequencing data is reaching a comfort level with this data type, developing some basic bioinformatic skills to process data and interpret sequence variants routinely or in challenging cases.

Here we provide a short compendium of the various software and algorithm options available for sequencing data analysis to date with a focus on the forensic context. We aim to provide an accessible guide for forensic professionals starting to implement these novel sequencing methods into their standard forensic DNA analysis workflows.

2. Rationale of Massively Parallel Sequencing Data Analysis Methods for STRs

True to the proverbial concept of bioinformatics, that 'there is more than one way to solve a problem', individual algorithms indeed differ, but regardless of which programming language they use, on which operating systems they run or which sequencing data type, or platform they can process, the general approach is broadly similar and summarized on the schematic graph in Figure 1.

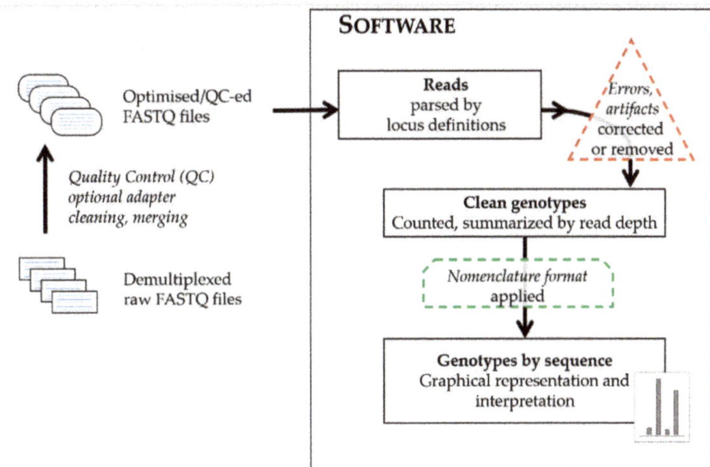

Figure 1. Schematic representation of general forensic MPS data processing steps.

The input files are text files containing sequence data in different formats generated by the sequencing platforms: files of sequence data with or without quality values for each base call in each read (FASTQ or FASTA), or sequence alignment files and their indices (BAM and BAI). The sequencing reads from the input files are parsed by using a defined set of attributes with characteristics of the targeted markers by which to filter. The terminology of the software describing these attributes significantly differ, therefore Table 1 compares not just the software themselves, but the verbiage for the files providing locus definitions and names for the landmarks of the targeted loci. These files provide configurations for the analyses in respect to the range and specificity of sequence targeted, by allowing strict or flexible matching to the short sequences landmarking the targeted loci and their immediate flanking regions. These landmark sequences anchor the reads to the selected loci, and often coincide with known or presumed primer regions of the amplicons. The targeted markers are also described by their repeat motifs and/or structure, which increases the locus-specificity and allows for the precise recognition of allele variants. Approaches differ as to whether software only recognizes a predefined set of allele variants aligning reads to these references, or could recognize and call undefined, novel variants, and furthermore, capable of creating various possible combinations of expected alleles just from the provided repeat blocks of the array. Regardless of the approach, the reads of each marker are tallied and summarized in the form of a read depth value (or coverage) for each allele. The recognition of a group of reads as alleles are also facilitated by adjustable analytical thresholds separating signal from noise. The relationship between observed sequences is often used to categorize calls as true alleles or their derivatives (stutter or reads with errors). Some software offers options to flag, remove, and/or correct potential artifacts and errors from sequencing. At the end of the process, allele calls are designated based on adequate coverage surpassing thresholds for interpretation and being excluded as artifacts. The common denominator of any software approach is the generation of sequence strings as the ultimate comparable form of sequence alleles, a requirement [9,10] for publishing population study sequence variants that allow for concordance checking between methods; with the caveat of different analysis ranges may still generate discrepancies between different methods. While such sequence strings are easily comparable by computer programs, this is not true for human analysts, therefore the software also reports a human-friendly format of the sequence alleles in their preferred nomenclature. These usually are presented in a 'bracketed' form with the counts of the repeat blocks summarized using brackets (e.g., [GATA]8); furthermore, these formats could address the marker, genomic location analyzed, the length equivalent of the allele and may also include any flanking region variation observed when compared to the human reference genome (usually the most recent version, GRCh38). Most software, apart from the standard outputs of the sequence strings, read depths and a form of bracketed nomenclature, also provide a visual output: a graphical representation of the detected alleles in a familiar histogram format, which being similar to the electropherogram peaks aids the transition of analysts from STR typing by CE to sequencing.

Table 1. Summary of characteristics of software for the interpretation of MPS data of forensic markers.

Software	Versions	Author/Vendor	Year	Accessibility	Runs on	Locus Definition	Landmarks for Loci
STRait Razor	v1.0	Warshauer et al. [11]	2013	free	Unix/Linux	config file	'anchor'
	v2.0	Warshauer et al. [12]	2015	free	Unix/Linux		
	v2s	King et al. [13]	2017	free	Unix/Linux		
	v3.0	Woerner et al. [14]	2017	free	all platforms		
	Online	King et al. [15]	2021	free	online/ all platforms		
FDSTools	TSSV	Anvar et al. [16]	2014	free	Unix/Linux	library file	'flank'
	v1.0	van der Gaag et al. [17]	2016	free	Unix/Linux		
	v1.1.1	Hoogenboom et al. [18]	2017	free	Unix/Linux		
	v2.0	Hoogenboom et al. [19]	2021	free	all platforms	STRNaming	
STRinNGS	v1.0	Friis et al. [20]	2016	on request	Unix/Linux	configuration file	'flanking sequences'
	v2.0	Jonck et al. [21]	2020	free	Unix/Linux		
MyFLq	v1.1	Van Neste et al. [22,23]	2014	free	online/Unix/Linux	panels	'recognition elements'
toaSTR	v1.0	Ganschow et al. [24]	2018	free	online	allele database	'primer'
Altius	Cloud	Bailey et al. [25]	2017	on request	online	lookup table	'target regions'
ExactID	v2.0	Battelle [26]	2015	commercial	Windows	config file	default
GeneMarker HTS	v1.0	SoftGenetics [27]	2017	commercial	Windows	default	default
MixtureAce	v1.0	NicheVision [28]	2018	commercial	Windows	default	default
CLC Genomics Workbench	AQME	Sturk-Andreaggi et al. [29]	2017	commercial	all platforms	non STR	non STR
Universal Analysis Software	v2.3	Verogen [30]	2021	commercial	Windows	default	default
Converge Forensic Analysis Software	v2.2	Thermo Fisher [31]	2019	commercial	Windows	BED files	default

A new phenomenon introduced by using bioinformatic software for forensic DNA analysis is the occasional appearance of bioinformatic null alleles. These are the bioinformatic equivalents of null alleles in CE where sequence variation underneath the primer binding sites could impair or prevent amplification of the actual alleles. In the case of bioinformatic nulls, the amplification is not compromised and the sequencing reads are present in the raw data files, but there is an unexpected sequence variation underneath the landmark regions of a locus that a software uses to recognize locus-specific reads. While most software allows for 'wobble' or approximate matching in these landmark regions, this sequence variation can be significant enough for the software to fail to recognize and analyze the true reads in the filtering process, thus resulting in a null allele. The best prevention of bioinformatic nulls being reported in profiles is the use of a secondary data analysis method, which can be particularly useful in forensic validations or population studies. Using a sequencing platform-specific software in combination with another commercial, free or open-source software can largely eliminate the chance of bioinformatic nulls remaining unrecognized. In the case of the custom loci set developed in-house, where only open-source software can be used, it is good practice to use multiple software to call alleles, or at least use the same software with different settings in their locus definition files specifying different landmark regions, to avoid the occasional bioinformatic nulls.

Analysis of sequencing data requires access to adequate storage and safeguarding of the generated data. Local protocols need to be developed for the long-term maintenance and expansion of these resources, considering the size of the data files is not comparable to those originating from CE, often measured in gigabytes per run. Most of the following tools can be run on a standard laptop or desktop, but high-performance computing resources can be beneficial when processing a lot of samples.

3. Freely Available Software

In the early stages of the application of massively parallel sequencing to the forensic field, most solutions were developed in academic settings as a necessary research tool to be able to characterize and analyze data generated by sequencing platforms [11,16,20,22]. These approaches often focused on STR markers, occasionally offering options to analyze mtDNA data as well [18]. These software are freely available but assume the users have a basic level of bioinformatics skills allowing them to navigate and operate through the command line. Such basic skills can be obtained either through professional training [32] or self-taught courses via one of the several available online tutorials on 'how to Linux' [33]. Once the basic command-line skills are comfortably obtained, the following software can be run just as confidently through a terminal window as clicking an icon in a GUI. While there are a few software options available through web-based interfaces [23–25], some developers offer [21,34] or transition to [35] providing a version of their software that can be downloaded as a 'Docker image'. This is a 'ready to use' packet of the program and all its dependencies required to run the application successfully, regardless of the underlying resources available locally [36]. A program, the Docker engine, facilitates the use of such packets on both Linux and Windows-based applications. While similar to virtual machines, this solution is more flexible and portable, as the isolated environment does not require a part of the hardware to be closed off, but rather creates such containers on a software level. This form of software availability improves not only data security, satisfying those who cannot allow data file exchange outside of their local laboratory but can also make these applications more accessible for those who are just beginning their journey with software operated through the command line.

3.1. STRait Razor

This software, designed to analyze reads from sequenced amplicons targeting STRs, was first published in 2013. Its evolution went through iterations from STRait Razor [11], v2.0 [12], v2s [13], v3.0 [14], and STRait Razor Online (SRO) [15] improving its processing speeds and output files, extending its analysis to the flanking regions and providing secondary analysis tools, such as additional workbooks for visual interpretation of the data using histograms and reporting sequence alleles following the International Society for Forensic Genetics (ISFG) early considerations [37].

The software uses FASTQ files as an input and versions prior to SRO required command line navigation. Detailed help files and guides are available, instructing users how to run an analysis by entering a command with the desired options. The file that sets the locus definitions is referred to as the 'config file' and the landmarks on each side of the loci are called the 'anchors'. These modifiable config files are included for the currently available main sequencing kits, or custom files can be generated by the user. The output are simple text files, which can be processed further either by the provided Excel workbooks, the online platform, or custom scripts for the advanced users. These additional processes can summarize the results in a tabular and a visual format and facilitate additional insights such as allele nomenclature, stutter analysis, or sequencing error profiles. While previous versions could be run on the command line (using a Mac or a Linux computer), the v3.0 of this software can also run using the Command Prompt in Windows. The latest version (SRO) introduces the main functionality of the software in an online tool format, suitable for quick analysis of individual files, without the use of a Unix or Linux environment. The online format significantly decreases the need for bioinformatics skills; however, for batch processing a large number of files or for the use of custom settings running the downloaded command-line version of SRO is more practical.

The software includes config files for the commercially available sequencing kits and a default set of predefined alleles to call theses from the sequencing reads it analyzes, therefore any undefined sequence allele by default would require the user to establish an appropriate nomenclature. In such cases, the software may label the unrecognized variant as 'novel' by default, however, the variant may have been reported in more up-to-date literature or increasingly available databases [38–40].

The software is a general starting point for those interested in exploring their data further, specifically to be able to provide an unrestricted reporting of the flanking region variants [41]. It has proven useful in providing a secondary analysis to commercial software outputs as a means for eliminating bioinformatic null alleles [42].

3.2. FDSTools

This software is also designed to analyze reads from amplified STRs, with later versions offering the capability to analyze mtDNA results [43] from sequencing data. The evolution of the software through its iterations starts with the standalone TSSV tool [16] recognizing repetitive motifs in the reads, which was integrated into the FDSTools bundles v1.0, later v1.1.1 [17,18]. The latest version (v2.0) was expanded by an integrated nomenclature package STRNaming [19]. The software is a bundle of several tools to be used in the analyses of sequencing data from raw FASTQ files. Analyzed loci and their analysis attributes are defined by a 'library file', including their landmark regions referred to as 'flanks'. Results include coverage values with options for different outputs including bracketed and string formats. The package includes several additional tools for stutter analysis and correction, databasing, and visualizations as well. The addition of the STR-Naming module eliminates the need for user input on the locus definition files. Instead, the program now automatically recognizes repetitive sequences in the reference sequence using these as the preset preferences for bracketing interpretation of the sequence reads and, as such, automates nomenclature classification of the called alleles. The addition of this module facilitates the ongoing efforts to reach a unified nomenclature for the standard human forensic STR markers [37,44,45].

The software is a good starting point as a secondary analysis option with additional flexibility for those interested in building custom solutions for their more specific needs beyond standard reports [17,46,47]. The offered modular tools and customization are ideal for stutter analysis or the visualization of stutter restoration to the respective parent allele [48]. Those who appreciate graphics generated in a report-ready format will find the graphical HTML outputs useful [17]. Beyond the standard or custom niche sets of STR markers of human forensics, the software is an ideal tool for those developing wildlife forensic markers with the need for flexible software adaptable to species identification from novel STR multiplexes [49].

3.3. STRinNGS

The software STRinNGS v1.0 [20] was one of the early approaches available on request developed by researchers. This tool required command-line skills to analyze the data and use the output files in further scripts to summarize stutter and error profiles observed. The recently released v2.0. [21] is openly available to download for local use and has been updated to provide a more refined set of criteria for improved reliability in allele calling including error filtering, identifying stutter reads, and flagging unusual sequences for manual review. STRinNGS accepts FASTQ files as input and runs the settings via its locus definition file which is referred to as the 'configuration file' where it defines the marker landmarks as 'flanking sequences'. To accommodate the need for quality control (QC), the software offers an output format that can be used directly for submission to STRidER [9]. This site (https://strider.online/) is dedicated to the QC of autosomal STR population data sets, providing unique identification numbers as proof of data passing their checks.

The software is a good alternative as a secondary analysis to eliminate bioinformatic nulls in the analysis and is now an improved tool that helps the analyst with the manual review by providing several optional flags and settings. The software reports a format in line with guidance from the forensic community [9,10,37] as well as its own developed format for allele nomenclature which is easily comparable with other free software outputs for concordance. It provides clear indications of the genomic locations, the length-based alleles, the sequence structures, and the flanking variations [50] and, for the convenience of the user, includes the sequence strings analyzed.

3.4. MyFLq

One of the earliest software solutions for forensic STR data analysis from MPS was developed [22] in a form of a web-based user-friendly application using FASTA or FASTQ files for input. In the past, this was also available as an integrated online tool on BaseSpace [23], for use with Illumina sequencing data output. For the practicality of analyzing sensitive data locally, a desktop version of the software is also available to download [22] or provided as a Docker-container file [34] to be downloaded as a functional package and run locally. To help recognize non-predefined true alleles, MyFLq can estimate whether an unrecognized allele is truly a novel allele or a result of errors. The landmarks defining the loci analyzed are referred to as 'primers', however, this does not necessarily mean that they completely overlap with the primers in the amplification reaction. The approach uses a dynamic calculation of the flanking regions and the region of interest (ROI), rather than a static definition of repeat region and flanking regions. The ROI, the variable part of the sequence, is compared to the reference alleles and allows an easy interpretation of SNPs as well as STR length polymorphisms within the analyzed region. The output is a report of the sequences with their sequence and the derived length alleles as well, including visualization of the results.

The use of this software can be interesting for those who want an alternative analysis when comparing methods and those who are interested in viewing their data in a simple, non-bracketed nomenclature format. MyFLq has the potential to work with SNP and mtDNA data as well. This approach could also be useful for working with new STRs or non-human STRs, capitalizing on the flexible approach of locus analysis which can adjust to a dynamically growing reference allele database.

3.5. ToaSTR

This software offers a user-friendly graphical web-based solution for the analysis of STR data from sequencing. It does not require bioinformatics expertise from the users as it provides an intuitive GUI to analyze data from FASTQ or FASTA files. Web-based software options often face questions about data security and laboratories may be restricted from uploading sensitive data to the web, therefore the developers currently provide access to this secure web-based tool upon request [24]. Those who require further assurance will welcome the recent update that will move the web-based application at the end of 2021 to a Docker-based format [35], allowing the software to be downloaded as a functional unit operating securely locally.

ToaSTR defines the analyzed loci together as a 'panel' and refers to the landmark sequences as 'recognition elements'. The panels to be analyzed are customizable and therefore independent of the sequencing platforms and kits [51]. The software includes predictive stutter modeling allowing an automatic classification of the observed sequences and the differentiation of artifacts. The reporting nomenclature format of ToaSTR is aligned to the ISFG considerations [37] and includes graphical visualization of the results.

Until the introduction of the new format of the software, the web-based version can still prove to be useful for analyzing training data and experiments or mobile demonstrations that require quick, visually appealing outputs.

3.6. Altius

Altius was developed as an independent secure Cloud-based software optimized for high-throughput data processing from FASTQ files. As users access this intuitive GUI through a web browser, it requires no bioinformatic expertise. The software is capable of processing MPS data of a predefined set of STRs (autosomal, X- and Y-STRs) [52,53] generated by different platforms, including the MinION. The analysis is robust and is ready to accommodate batch data processing [25]. The target regions for locus identification parameters are adapted from STRaitRazor v2.0 [12] and locus definitions are collated in a lookup table for the software to identify the targeted loci. The results are output to a MySQL database and exportable reports are provided for the sequences, including full sequence strings, a visual output of the results, and a format of nomenclature in line with the considerations of ISFG [37]. Data security for this software is provided by the resources of Amazon Web Services, allowing users to set their locally required level of access-control measures. Because Altius is using the secure cloud system, access is provided upon request and after authentication.

4. Commercial Software

Apart from the freely available academic software, there are several options offered by commercial companies. These are either provided as a supplement to the vendors' own sequencing chemistry and platform or developed as standalone solutions for analyzing raw data output from various sequencers.

In general, these are user-friendly programs with visually appealing graphical interfaces and with limited options to customize processes, all designed to provide a streamlined process of hassle-free analysis, familiar graphical output, and presentation-ready results. Many of these offer options for mtDNA analysis as well as STR data analysis, both generated on the sequencing platforms. Commercial software is designed to make the introduction of MPS easier to any new user, building confidence working with sequence data; however, there is less control of the algorithms and occasional troubleshooting requires the assistance of the companies. For high-throughput routine laboratories, these qualities are attractive and the reliable convenience offered by these programs could justify the cost.

4.1. GeneMarker HTS (SoftGenetics, State Collage, PA)

GeneMarker HTS [27] offers an integrated solution for analyzing sequencing data from mtDNA, STRs, and SNPs generated on either Illumina or Ion Torrent platforms. The software is validated for mtDNA data analysis [54,55]. It can be used to analyze the mtDNA control region or the whole mtDNA genome, as required [56]. The STR analysis utilizes an in-built panel for the Promega PowerSeq 46GY kit (Promega, Madison, WI, USA), using FASTQ files generated from an Illumina MiSeq (Illumina, San Diego, CA, USA), alternatively, a panel for custom chemistries can be used for analyzing data from other kits. MtDNA and STR analysis (including flanking region variations) can be performed individually or simultaneously. GeneMarker HTS reports the length-equivalent of the sequence alleles, provides sequence strings and a visual interpretation of the results using histograms. An audit trail of changes and analysis settings are logged, and user access rights are controlled by its database. Demo and trial versions, training materials, and product support are available. GeneMarker HTS operates under Windows.

4.2. ExactID (Battelle, Colombus, OH)

Battelle's ExactID [26] offers another fully integrated agnostic software solution designed for professional use in government agencies and crime laboratories. The sequencing platform-independent software analyzes data from FASTQ files generated from various chemistries targeting forensic markers, such as autosomal, X- and Y-STRs [57,58], SNPs, microhaplotypes, and mtDNA. The analysis settings are defined in 'config files' for the various marker panels. The user-friendly GUI offers a familiar display of the observed alleles in a histogram format along with the length-equivalent alleles and the bracketed sequence alleles in line with the ISFG considerations [37] for STRs. The software can recognize previously undefined alleles and to report flanking region variation. The results can be exported in multiple formats: .pdf file with tabular and graphical summaries, .csv files for further external analysis, and an additional .sef file format for evidence preservation. Furthermore, ExactID offers additional intelligence leads by interpreting data relating to phenotypic markers and biogeographical ancestry using the Battelle Avatar plugin. Audit trail and user access control are provided by the software. ExactID operates under Windows.

4.3. MixtureAce (NicheVision, Akron, OH)

MixtureAce [28] the plugin tool for the ArmedXpert software offers a user-friendly option to analyze MPS data from FASTQ files for STR (autosomal, X- and Y-STR) markers [59,60] with the benefit of the integrated hash-based Sequence Identifier (SID) nomenclature [61], a unique abbreviated format of sequence-based alleles designed to identify the relationships between sequences. MixtureAce uses the SIDs to recognize reads of stutter or other predefined artifacts using customizable thresholds and thus facilitates the recognition of reads not filtered out as true alleles. Undefined artifacts still need to be manually curated [60]. The software reports within the ranges of sequences encompassing the STRs following the UAS flanking region report [44]. This ready-to-use solution can report from a single source or interpret mixed samples using another ArmedXpert plugin: Mixture Interpretation. MixtureAce operates under Windows.

4.4. CLC Genomics Workbench (QIAGEN, Hilden, Germany)

CLC Genomics Workbench [62] is a genomic bioinformatic tool collection developed by and offered from Qiagen for comprehensive sequencing data analysis in general. This tool allows customization of its collection with plugins, such as the AQME [29], the toolbox specifically developed in collaboration with AFDIL to accommodate forensic-specific mtDNA sequence analysis for data generated from any MPS platform. AQME also includes haplogroup estimation and phylogenetically consistent nomenclature to facilitate reporting of the results. This specific plugin can be applied within the CLC Workbench framework.

4.5. Universal Analysis Software (Verogen, San Diego, CA)

Universal Analysis Software (UAS) [30] is the custom software of the MiSeq FGx sequencing platform that can analyze sequencing data from forensic markers using specific modules for the ForenSeq line of kits. Currently available chemistries target STRs (autosomal, X- and Y-STRs), SNPs, and mtDNA. Raw data is directly processed from the sequencer to generate demultiplexed raw sequence output FASTQ files. This is then further analyzed within the software using alignment to the human reference sequence and variant calling from the sequences at the range reported by the software. To extend the reported range outside of the repeat region an additional flanking region report is also available in the form of an excel file. To further analyze variation outside of expected flanking region variations, the raw FASTQ files can also be exported and processed by external software for independent analysis and concordance. The software is validated together with the platform and chemistry as the MiSeq Forensic Genomics System [63,64] supported by training and direct product support from the vendor.

The GUI is designed to be intuitive and user-friendly and with default and additional modules for different forensic genomic applications for the FGx platform, such as the STR analysis module or the data analysis for mtDNA sequencing chemistries. A supplementary analysis generates investigative leads, such as the estimation of phenotypic markers (hair and eye color) and biogeographical ancestry estimation of the samples [65,66]. Furthermore, genomic applications can analyze data generated from dedicated SNP panels for SNP-based identification of degraded remains; or can pre-format the generated data for downstream use in databases specific to the application of forensic genetic genealogy (FGG). FGG is an investigative tool for identifying distant kinship of a sample using databases built from 'direct-to-consumer' (DTC) genealogy DNA test results, data volunteered by citizen scientists. The generated data is formatted to be comparable with the markers in the database allowing to facilitate the investigation of serious crimes or to identify unidentified human remains [67].

4.6. Converge Forensic Analysis Software (Thermo Fisher, Waltham, MA)

Converge Forensic Analysis Software [31] is the comprehensive validated software customized to the HID Ion S5 sequencing platforms of Thermo Fisher. Converge is designed for this specific sequencing platform and visualizes the analyzed results obtained from the Torrent Server via the HID Genotyper plugin. It has modules specific to workflows of the offered chemistries targeting specific forensic markers: STRs including multiple markers for sex-determination [68], mtDNA control region, or the full mitochondrial genome [69]. Additional modules beyond STR analysis include those interpreting data from kits targeting selected SNP sets, which can establish identity from degraded samples [70,71] or can provide investigative leads and estimate biogeographic ancestry [72]. Data organization in Converge is optimized and streamlined around case management. The software and chemistries are validated for mtDNA analysis [73] and the users are supported by training and documentation from the vendor.

Via the HID Genotyper plugin, the generated sequencing reads are demultiplexed and aligned to the default reference sequence in regions specified by the BED file. The BED files are specific to the chemistries targeting different marker sets. Both the chosen reference and the BED files can be customized. The generated data can be downloaded as alignment files (BAM and BAI) or alternatively can also be generated as FASTQ files to download for independent analysis and concordance analysis.

The GUI is designed to be intuitive for the sequence-based data and follows the familiar look of the vendor's CE-based software (GeneMapper ID-X, Thermo fisher, Waltham, MA, USA) and it can integrate and compare the two data types for casework, paternity, and kinship calculations. For markers that are not currently supported by the offered kits and the software (for example chemistry targeting multiple Y chromosomal markers), sequencing can be performed using a custom set of amplicons [74,75]. The generated raw data then can be downloaded and analyzed with the available independent software options.

5. Other Software Options for Whole Genome Sequencing (WGS) Data

Without exhausting the list there are other software options available [76,77], and many were designed to identify and analyze STR markers from genome-wide sequencing data without a forensic focus. STRs, in general, may be medically relevant or used as markers for population genetics, and specific software has also been designed to identify other relevant tandem repeats to facilitate medical diagnosis or genotype of these markers [78–83]. Recent reviews [84,85] also provided an overview of several alternative software that can generate STR profiles from whole-genome sequencing data [86–94].

While these may not be the immediate focus of forensic analysts mainly interested in reporting the sequencing data from the targeted amplification of markers specifically curated for forensic purposes, WGS data analysis methods could prove useful in exploring alternative approaches with already available data sources or in research projects.

6. Tips, Tricks, and More Tools

Despite the evolution of software solutions for forensic MPS data, occasionally data analysis can come to a halt if suspicious results are observed. This could be an unexpected null or supernumerary allele, unreasonably low coverage, or confusing sequence structure. In case of concern, there are always a few options to investigate the reason for discrepancies. For example, one can investigate the observed coverage values in relation to the expected inter-locus balance, which can indicate failure to detect an allele in heterozygotes interpreted falsely as homozygotes (bioinformatic null alleles). Any software can potentially generate bioinformatic null calls, i.e., the inability to recognize and report a specific variant. The best approach to confirm any unexpected instances is to use multiple software (or at least multiple settings) for the analysis and perform a concordance check-in between analysis methods.

In-built software of the sequencing platforms (UAS and Converge) can offer investigative leads using SNP data from some of their chemistries. Additionally, the user can harvest the relevant SNP data and independently verify certain phenotypic traits: eye and hair color using the constantly updated and freely available tools (https://hirisplex.erasmusmc.nl/) hosted at the Erasmus MC University. The website offers options for a manual or automated upload of the SNP genotype data to verify the prediction of these phenotypic traits using the established results from relevant studies (IrisPlex [95], HIrisPlex [96], HIRISPlex-S [97–99]).

Visualizing variants often helps to understand how some nucleotide changes create unusual sequence structures. A useful tool for visualization is the Integrative Genomics Viewer (IGV) [100], where alignment and variant calling files can be viewed manually compared to the reference sequence. If the consensus sequence of the reads is not obvious by manual revision another tool, VisCoSe, may be of interest that can calculate and compare consensus sequences of multiple datasets [101].

It is a good practice to perform independent Quality Control of the raw data prior to analysis, starting by monitoring the main characteristics of the dataset before and after any additional clean-up steps, which can be done, for example, using the FastQC program [102]. The additional steps of detailed adapter trimming using additional software (for example Trimmomatic [103], Cutadapt [104], seqtk [105]) or the merging of paired-end reads (using FLASH [106], BBMerge [107], CASPER [108]) may improve the analysis downstream. There are instances where using additional clean-up tools on raw data can improve the analysis. For example, removing erroneous reads and/or low-quality parts of reads specific to chemistry and platform can lead to unambiguous allele calls and can even improve retrieved coverage values for the dataset.

Available open datasets are a valuable resource for those not yet engaged in massively parallel sequencing but interested to learn more about data analysis ahead of establishing a workflow locally. One such source is the Forensic DNA Open Dataset, published by the NIST Applied Genetics Group [109] at https://doi.org/10.18434/M32157. Open datasets for WGS data are also available at the 1000 Genomes Project data portal, the International Genome Sample Resource (IGSR) [110–112] (https://www.internationalgenome.org/home), and the variants found in these projects can be viewed at the 1000 Genome Browsers hosted at NCBI [113] (https://www.ncbi.nlm.nih.gov/variation/tools/1000genomes/).

7. Summary

In this review, the aim was to provide a short, digestible overview of the currently available software options, acknowledging the challenges for the bioinformatically non-specialist reporting forensic professionals of this field. DNA analysts already familiar with the CE-based analysis and software, but inexperienced in high-throughput sequencing, or those planning to generate sequencing data in the future, would benefit from this review.

All the presented software options perform well and selecting one (or as suggested here: more) over others may be due to personal preference, financial limits or the compatibility to already available equipment. If routine forensic casework laboratories engage in exploring these various options, the DNA analysts will better understand the sequence-level variation of the forensic markers and the advantages of incorporating sequence data analysis into their workflows. An increased comfort level with basic bioinformatics is a key step to utilizing the new possibilities introduced by MPS to the field.

Author Contributions: Conceptualization, T.I.H. and P.M.V.; resources, P.M.V.; writing—original draft preparation, T.I.H.; writing—review and editing, T.I.H., P.M.V. and K.B.G.; visualization, T.I.H.; supervision, P.M.V. and K.B.G.; project administration, P.M.V.; funding acquisition, P.M.V. and K.B.G. All authors have read and agreed to the published version of the manuscript.

Funding: This research was funded by the NIST Special Programs Office (Forensic Genetics Focus Area).

Institutional Review Board Statement: Not applicable.

Informed Consent Statement: Not applicable.

Data Availability Statement: Not applicable.

Acknowledgments: The authors wish to thank Lisa A. Borsuk, Kevin M. Kiesler, and Nathanael Olson for their review of the manuscript. Points of view in this document are those of the authors and do not necessarily represent the official position or policies of the National Institute of Standards and Technology or the U.S. Department of Commerce. Certain commercial equipment, instruments, and materials are identified. In no case does such identification imply a recommendation or endorsement by NIST, nor does it imply that any of the materials, instruments, or equipment identified are necessarily the best available for the purpose.

Conflicts of Interest: The authors declare no conflict of interest. The funders had no role in the design of the study; in the collection, analyses, or interpretation of data; in the writing of the manuscript, or in the decision to publish the results.

References

1. Chen, M.; Zhao, H. Next-generation sequencing in liquid biopsy: Cancer screening and early detection. *Hum. Genom.* **2019**, *13*, 34. [CrossRef]
2. John, G.; Sahajpal, N.S.; Mondal, A.K.; Ananth, S.; Williams, C.; Chaubey, A.; Rojiani, A.M.; Kolhe, R. Next-Generation Sequencing (NGS) in COVID-19: A Tool for SARS-CoV-2 Diagnosis, Monitoring New Strains and Phylodynamic Modeling in Molecular Epidemiology. *Curr. Issues Mol. Biol.* **2021**, *43*, 845–867. [CrossRef]
3. Gonzalez-Quezada, B.A.; Creary, L.E.; Munguia-Saldana, A.J.; Flores-Aguilar, H.; Fernandez-Vina, M.A.; Gorodezky, C. Exploring the ancestry and admixture of Mexican Oaxaca Mestizos from Southeast Mexico using next-generation sequencing of 11 HLA loci. *Hum. Immunol.* **2019**, *80*, 157–162. [CrossRef]
4. Borsting, C.; Morling, N. Next generation sequencing and its applications in forensic genetics. *Forensic Sci. Int. Genet.* **2015**, *18*, 78–89. [CrossRef] [PubMed]
5. Bruijns, B.; Tiggelaar, R.; Gardeniers, H. Massively parallel sequencing techniques for forensics: A review. *Electrophoresis* **2018**, *39*, 2642–2654. [CrossRef] [PubMed]
6. Alonso, A.; Barrio, P.A.; Muller, P.; Kocher, S.; Berger, B.; Martin, P.; Bodner, M.; Willuweit, S.; Parson, W.; Roewer, L.; et al. Current state-of-art of STR sequencing in forensic genetics. *Electrophoresis* **2018**, *39*, 2655–2668. [CrossRef]
7. Ballard, D.; Winkler-Galicki, J.; Wesoly, J. Massive parallel sequencing in forensics: Advantages, issues, technicalities, and prospects. *Int. J. Legal Med.* **2020**, *134*, 1291–1303. [CrossRef]
8. Alonso, A.; Muller, P.; Roewer, L.; Willuweit, S.; Budowle, B.; Parson, W. European survey on forensic applications of massively parallel sequencing. *Forensic Sci. Int. Genet.* **2017**, *29*, e23–e25. [CrossRef] [PubMed]
9. Bodner, M.; Bastisch, I.; Butler, J.M.; Fimmers, R.; Gill, P.; Gusmao, L.; Morling, N.; Phillips, C.; Prinz, M.; Schneider, P.M.; et al. Recommendations of the DNA Commission of the International Society for Forensic Genetics (ISFG) on quality control of autosomal Short Tandem Repeat allele frequency databasing (STRidER). *Forensic Sci. Int. Genet.* **2016**, *24*, 97–102. [CrossRef]
10. Gusmao, L.; Butler, J.M.; Linacre, A.; Parson, W.; Roewer, L.; Schneider, P.M.; Carracedo, A. Revised guidelines for the publication of genetic population data. *Forensic Sci. Int. Genet.* **2017**, *30*, 160–163. [CrossRef]
11. Warshauer, D.H.; Lin, D.; Hari, K.; Jain, R.; Davis, C.; Larue, B.; King, J.L.; Budowle, B. STRait Razor: A length-based forensic STR allele-calling tool for use with second generation sequencing data. *Forensic Sci. Int. Genet.* **2013**, *7*, 409–417. [CrossRef]
12. Warshauer, D.H.; King, J.L.; Budowle, B. STRait Razor v2.0: The improved STR Allele Identification Tool–Razor. *Forensic Sci. Int. Genet.* **2015**, *14*, 182–186. [CrossRef] [PubMed]
13. King, J.L.; Wendt, F.R.; Sun, J.; Budowle, B. STRait Razor v2s: Advancing sequence-based STR allele reporting and beyond to other marker systems. *Forensic Sci. Int. Genet.* **2017**, *29*, 21–28. [CrossRef]

14. Woerner, A.E.; King, J.L.; Budowle, B. Fast STR allele identification with STRait Razor 3.0. *Forensic Sci. Int. Genet.* **2017**, *30*, 18–23. [CrossRef] [PubMed]

15. King, J.L.; Woerner, A.E.; Mandape, S.N.; Kapema, K.B.; Moura-Neto, R.S.; Silva, R.; Budowle, B. STRait Razor Online: An enhanced user interface to facilitate interpretation of MPS data. *Forensic Sci. Int. Genet.* **2021**, *52*, 102463. [CrossRef] [PubMed]

16. Anvar, S.Y.; van der Gaag, K.J.; van der Heijden, J.W.; Veltrop, M.H.; Vossen, R.H.; de Leeuw, R.H.; Breukel, C.; Buermans, H.P.; Verbeek, J.S.; de Knijff, P.; et al. TSSV: A tool for characterization of complex allelic variants in pure and mixed genomes. *Bioinformatics* **2014**, *30*, 1651–1659. [CrossRef]

17. van der Gaag, K.J.; de Leeuw, R.H.; Hoogenboom, J.; Patel, J.; Storts, D.R.; Laros, J.F.J.; de Knijff, P. Massively parallel sequencing of short tandem repeats-Population data and mixture analysis results for the PowerSeq system. *Forensic Sci. Int. Genet.* **2016**, *24*, 86–96. [CrossRef]

18. Hoogenboom, J.; van der Gaag, K.J.; de Leeuw, R.H.; Sijen, T.; de Knijff, P.; Laros, J.F. FDSTools: A software package for analysis of massively parallel sequencing data with the ability to recognise and correct STR stutter and other PCR or sequencing noise. *Forensic Sci. Int. Genet.* **2017**, *27*, 27–40. [CrossRef]

19. Hoogenboom, J.; Sijen, T.; van der Gaag, K.J. STRNaming: Generating simple, informative names for sequenced STR alleles in a standardised and automated manner. *Forensic Sci. Int. Genet.* **2021**, *52*, 102473. [CrossRef] [PubMed]

20. Friis, S.L.; Buchard, A.; Rockenbauer, E.; Borsting, C.; Morling, N. Introduction of the Python script STRinNGS for analysis of STR regions in FASTQ or BAM files and expansion of the Danish STR sequence database to 11 STRs. *Forensic Sci. Int. Genet.* **2016**, *21*, 68–75. [CrossRef] [PubMed]

21. Jonck, C.G.; Qian, X.; Simayijiang, H.; Borsting, C. STRinNGS v2.0: Improved tool for analysis and reporting of STR sequencing data. *Forensic Sci. Int. Genet.* **2020**, *48*, 102331. [CrossRef]

22. Van Neste, C.; Vandewoestyne, M.; Van Criekinge, W.; Deforce, D.; Van Nieuwerburgh, F. My-Forensic-Loci-queries (MyFLq) framework for analysis of forensic STR data generated by massive parallel sequencing. *Forensic Sci. Int. Genet.* **2014**, *9*, 1–8. [CrossRef] [PubMed]

23. Van Neste, C.; Gansemans, Y.; De Coninck, D.; Van Hoofstat, D.; Van Criekinge, W.; Deforce, D.; Van Nieuwerburgh, F. Forensic massively parallel sequencing data analysis tool: Implementation of MyFLq as a standalone web- and Illumina BaseSpace((R))-application. *Forensic Sci. Int. Genet.* **2015**, *15*, 2–7. [CrossRef] [PubMed]

24. Ganschow, S.; Silvery, J.; Kalinowski, J.; Tiemann, C. toaSTR: A web application for forensic STR genotyping by massively parallel sequencing. *Forensic Sci. Int. Genet.* **2018**, *37*, 21–28. [CrossRef]

25. Bailey, S.F.; Scheible, M.K.; Williams, C.; Silva, D.; Hoggan, M.; Eichman, C.; Faith, S.A. Secure and robust cloud computing for high-throughput forensic microsatellite sequence analysis and databasing. *Forensic Sci. Int. Genet.* **2017**, *31*, 40–47. [CrossRef]

26. Battelle. ExactID®. Available online: https://www.battelle.org/government-offerings/homeland-security-public-safety/security-law-enforcement/forensic-genomics/exactid (accessed on 1 October 2021).

27. SoftGenetics. GeneMarker®HTS. Available online: https://softgenetics.com/GeneMarkerHTS.php (accessed on 1 October 2021).

28. NicheVision. ArmedXpert™ MixtureAce™. Available online: https://nichevision.com/mixtureace/ (accessed on 1 October 2021).

29. Sturk-Andreaggi, K.; Peck, M.A.; Boysen, C.; Dekker, P.; McMahon, T.P.; Marshall, C.K. AQME: A forensic mitochondrial DNA analysis tool for next-generation sequencing data. *Forensic Sci. Int. Genet.* **2017**, *31*, 189–197. [CrossRef]

30. Verogen. Universal Analysis Software v2.0 Reference Guide (VD2019002). Available online: https://verogen.com/wp-content/uploads/2021/05/universal-analysis-software-v2-0-reference-guide-vd2019002-d.pdf (accessed on 1 October 2021).

31. ThermoFisher. User Guide: Converge Software v2.2—Setup and Reference (100039539E). Available online: https://assets.thermofisher.com/TFS-Assets/LSG/manuals/100039539_ConvergeSftwre_UG.pdf (accessed on 1 October 2021).

32. EBI. EMBL-EBI Training Courses. Available online: https://www.ebi.ac.uk/training/ (accessed on 1 October 2021).

33. The Linux Foundation. Introduction to Linux (Free Course). Available online: https://training.linuxfoundation.org/training/introduction-to-linux/ (accessed on 1 October 2021).

34. Van Neste, C. MyFLq Site on GitHub—Docker Container. Available online: https://github.com/beukueb/myflq (accessed on 1 October 2015).

35. LABCON-OWL. toaSTR—Announcement: Transition to a Docker-Based Application. Available online: https://www.toastr.de/ (accessed on 1 October 2021).

36. Docker. Docker Containers. Available online: https://www.docker.com/resources/what-container (accessed on 1 October 2021).

37. Parson, W.; Ballard, D.; Budowle, B.; Butler, J.M.; Gettings, K.B.; Gill, P.; Gusmao, L.; Hares, D.R.; Irwin, J.A.; King, J.L.; et al. Massively parallel sequencing of forensic STRs: Considerations of the DNA commission of the International Society for Forensic Genetics (ISFG) on minimal nomenclature requirements. *Forensic Sci. Int. Genet.* **2016**, *22*, 54–63. [CrossRef] [PubMed]

38. Gettings, K.B.; Borsuk, L.A.; Ballard, D.; Bodner, M.; Budowle, B.; Devesse, L.; King, J.; Parson, W.; Phillips, C.; Vallone, P.M. STRSeq: A catalog of sequence diversity at human identification Short Tandem Repeat loci. *Forensic Sci. Int. Genet.* **2017**, *31*, 111–117. [CrossRef]

39. Van Neste, C.; Van Criekinge, W.; Deforce, D.; Van Nieuwerburgh, F. Forensic Loci Allele Database (FLAD): Automatically generated, permanent identifiers for sequenced forensic alleles. *Forensic Sci. Int. Genet.* **2016**, *20*, e1–e3. [CrossRef]

40. Willuweit, S. *Challenges and Paradigm Shifts by the Adoption of MPS in Forensic Casework—Lessons Learned from the Collaborative DNASeqEx Project So Far*; HIDS: Vienna, Austria, 2017.

41. Wendt, F.R.; King, J.L.; Novroski, N.M.M.; Churchill, J.D.; Ng, J.; Oldt, R.F.; McCulloh, K.L.; Weise, J.A.; Smith, D.G.; Kanthaswamy, S.; et al. Flanking region variation of ForenSeq DNA Signature Prep Kit STR and SNP loci in Yavapai Native Americans. *Forensic Sci. Int. Genet.* **2017**, *28*, 146–154. [CrossRef]

42. Gettings, K.B.; Borsuk, L.A.; Steffen, C.R.; Kiesler, K.M.; Vallone, P.M. Sequence-based U.S. population data for 27 autosomal STR loci. *Forensic Sci. Int. Genet.* **2018**, *37*, 106–115. [CrossRef] [PubMed]

43. van der Gaag, K.J.; Desmyter, S.; Smit, S.; Prieto, L.; Sijen, T. Reducing the Number of Mismatches between Hairs and Buccal References When Analysing mtDNA Heteroplasmic Variation by Massively Parallel Sequencing. *Genes* **2020**, *11*, 1355. [CrossRef]

44. Gettings, K.B.; Ballard, D.; Bodner, M.; Borsuk, L.A.; King, J.L.; Parson, W.; Phillips, C. Report from the STRAND Working Group on the 2019 STR sequence nomenclature meeting. *Forensic Sci. Int. Genet.* **2019**, *43*, 102165. [CrossRef]

45. Phillips, C.; Gettings, K.B.; King, J.L.; Ballard, D.; Bodner, M.; Borsuk, L.; Parson, W. "The devil's in the detail": Release of an expanded, enhanced and dynamically revised forensic STR Sequence Guide. *Forensic Sci. Int. Genet.* **2018**, *34*, 162–169. [CrossRef] [PubMed]

46. Huszar, T.I.; Jobling, M.A.; Wetton, J.H. A phylogenetic framework facilitates Y-STR variant discovery and classification via massively parallel sequencing. *Forensic Sci. Int. Genet.* **2018**, *35*, 97–106. [CrossRef]

47. Claerhout, S.; Verstraete, P.; Warnez, L.; Vanpaemel, S.; Larmuseau, M.; Decorte, R. CSYseq: The first Y-chromosome sequencing tool typing a large number of Y-SNPs and Y-STRs to unravel worldwide human population genetics. *PLoS Genet.* **2021**, *17*, e1009758. [CrossRef]

48. de Leeuw, R.H.; Garnier, D.; Kroon, R.; Horlings, C.G.C.; de Meijer, E.; Buermans, H.; van Engelen, B.G.M.; de Knijff, P.; Raz, V. Diagnostics of short tandem repeat expansion variants using massively parallel sequencing and componential tools. *Eur. J. Hum. Genet.* **2019**, *27*, 400–407. [CrossRef]

49. Beasley, J.; Shorrock, G.; Neumann, R.; May, C.A.; Wetton, J.H. Massively parallel sequencing and capillary electrophoresis of a novel panel of falcon STRs: Concordance with minisatellite DNA profiles from historical wildlife crime. *Forensic Sci. Int. Genet.* **2021**, *54*, 102550. [CrossRef] [PubMed]

50. Hussing, C.; Huber, C.; Bytyci, R.; Mogensen, H.S.; Morling, N.; Borsting, C. Sequencing of 231 forensic genetic markers using the MiSeq FGx forensic genomics system—an evaluation of the assay and software. *Forensic Sci. Res.* **2018**, *3*, 111–123. [CrossRef]

51. Silvery, J.; Ganschow, S.; Wiegand, P.; Tiemann, C. Developmental validation of the monSTR identity panel, a forensic STR multiplex assay for massively parallel sequencing. *Forensic Sci. Int. Genet.* **2020**, *46*, 102236. [CrossRef]

52. Silva, D.; Sawitzki, F.R.; Scheible, M.K.R.; Bailey, S.F.; Alho, C.S.; Faith, S.A. Genetic analysis of Southern Brazil subjects using the PowerSeq AUTO/Y system for short tandem repeat sequencing. *Forensic Sci. Int. Genet.* **2018**, *33*, 129–135. [CrossRef] [PubMed]

53. Silva, D.; Scheible, M.K.; Bailey, S.F.; Williams, C.L.; Allwood, J.S.; Just, R.S.; Schuetter, J.; Skomrock, N.; Minard-Smith, A.; Barker-Scoggins, N.; et al. Sequence-based autosomal STR characterization in four US populations using PowerSeq Auto/Y system. *Forensic Sci. Int. Genet.* **2020**, *48*, 102311. [CrossRef]

54. Holland, M.M.; Pack, E.D.; McElhoe, J.A. Evaluation of GeneMarker® HTS for improved alignment of mtDNA MPS data, haplotype determination, and heteroplasmy assessment. *Forensic Sci. Int. Genet.* **2017**, *28*, 90–98. [CrossRef] [PubMed]

55. Brandhagen, M.D.; Just, R.S.; Irwin, J.A. Validation of NGS for mitochondrial DNA casework at the FBI Laboratory. *Forensic Sci. Int. Genet.* **2020**, *44*, 102151. [CrossRef] [PubMed]

56. Wisner, M.; Erlich, H.; Shih, S.; Calloway, C. Resolution of mitochondrial DNA mixtures using a probe capture next generation sequencing system and phylogenetic-based software. *Forensic Sci. Int. Genet.* **2021**, *53*, 102531. [CrossRef] [PubMed]

57. Gettings, K.B.; Kiesler, K.M.; Faith, S.A.; Montano, E.; Baker, C.H.; Young, B.A.; Guerrieri, R.A.; Vallone, P.M. Sequence variation of 22 autosomal STR loci detected by next generation sequencing. *Forensic Sci. Int. Genet.* **2016**, *21*, 15–21. [CrossRef] [PubMed]

58. Montano, E.A.; Bush, J.M.; Garver, A.M.; Larijani, M.M.; Wiechman, S.M.; Baker, C.H.; Wilson, M.R.; Guerrieri, R.A.; Benzinger, E.A.; Gehres, D.N.; et al. Optimization of the Promega PowerSeq Auto/Y system for efficient integration within a forensic DNA laboratory. *Forensic Sci. Int. Genet.* **2018**, *32*, 26–32. [CrossRef] [PubMed]

59. Young, B.A.; Gettings, K.B.; McCord, B.; Vallone, P.M. Estimating number of contributors in massively parallel sequencing data of STR loci. *Forensic Sci. Int. Genet.* **2019**, *38*, 15–22. [CrossRef]

60. Sharma, V.; Young, B.; Armogida, L.; Khan, A.; Wurmbach, E. Evaluation of ArmedXpert software tools, MixtureAce and Mixture Interpretation, to analyze MPS-STR data. *Forensic Sci. Int. Genet.* **2021**, *56*, 102603. [CrossRef]

61. Young, B.; Faris, T.; Armogida, L. A nomenclature for sequence-based forensic DNA analysis. *Forensic Sci. Int. Genet.* **2019**, *42*, 14–20. [CrossRef]

62. QIAGEN. CLC Genomics Workbench. Available online: https://digitalinsights.qiagen.com/products-overview/discovery-insights-portfolio/analysis-and-visualization/qiagen-clc-genomics-workbench/ (accessed on 1 October 2021).

63. Jager, A.C.; Alvarez, M.L.; Davis, C.P.; Guzman, E.; Han, Y.; Way, L.; Walichiewicz, P.; Silva, D.; Pham, N.; Caves, G.; et al. Developmental validation of the MiSeq FGx Forensic Genomics System for Targeted Next Generation Sequencing in Forensic DNA Casework and Database Laboratories. *Forensic Sci. Int. Genet.* **2017**, *28*, 52–70. [CrossRef]

64. Hollard, C.; Ausset, L.; Chantrel, Y.; Jullien, S.; Clot, M.; Faivre, M.; Suzanne, E.; Pene, L.; Laurent, F.X. Automation and developmental validation of the ForenSeq() DNA Signature Preparation kit for high-throughput analysis in forensic laboratories. *Forensic Sci. Int. Genet.* **2019**, *40*, 37–45. [CrossRef]

65. Sharma, V.; Jani, K.; Khosla, P.; Butler, E.; Siegel, D.; Wurmbach, E. Evaluation of ForenSeq Signature Prep Kit B on predicting eye and hair coloration as well as biogeographical ancestry by using Universal Analysis Software (UAS) and available web-tools. *Electrophoresis* **2019**, *40*, 1353–1364. [CrossRef]
66. Fregeau, C.J. Validation of the Verogen ForenSeq DNA Signature Prep kit/Primer Mix B for phenotypic and biogeographical ancestry predictions using the Micro MiSeq(R) Flow Cells. *Forensic Sci. Int. Genet.* **2021**, *53*, 102533. [CrossRef]
67. Kling, D.; Phillips, C.; Kennett, D.; Tillmar, A. Investigative genetic genealogy: Current methods, knowledge and practice. *Forensic Sci. Int. Genet.* **2021**, *52*, 102474. [CrossRef]
68. Barrio, P.A.; Martin, P.; Alonso, A.; Muller, P.; Bodner, M.; Berger, B.; Parson, W.; Budowle, B.; Consortium, D. Massively parallel sequence data of 31 autosomal STR loci from 496 Spanish individuals revealed concordance with CE-STR technology and enhanced discrimination power. *Forensic Sci. Int. Genet.* **2019**, *42*, 49–55. [CrossRef] [PubMed]
69. Strobl, C.; Eduardoff, M.; Bus, M.M.; Allen, M.; Parson, W. Evaluation of the precision ID whole MtDNA genome panel for forensic analyses. *Forensic Sci. Int. Genet.* **2018**, *35*, 21–25. [CrossRef]
70. Avila, E.; Felkl, A.B.; Graebin, P.; Nunes, C.P.; Alho, C.S. Forensic characterization of Brazilian regional populations through massive parallel sequencing of 124 SNPs included in HID ion Ampliseq Identity Panel. *Forensic Sci. Int. Genet.* **2019**, *40*, 74–84. [CrossRef] [PubMed]
71. Turchi, C.; Previdere, C.; Bini, C.; Carnevali, E.; Grignani, P.; Manfredi, A.; Melchionda, F.; Onofri, V.; Pelotti, S.; Robino, C.; et al. Assessment of the Precision ID Identity Panel kit on challenging forensic samples. *Forensic Sci. Int. Genet.* **2020**, *49*, 102400. [CrossRef]
72. Pereira, V.; Mogensen, H.S.; Borsting, C.; Morling, N. Evaluation of the Precision ID Ancestry Panel for crime case work: A SNP typing assay developed for typing of 165 ancestral informative markers. *Forensic Sci. Int. Genet.* **2017**, *28*, 138–145. [CrossRef] [PubMed]
73. Cihlar, J.C.; Amory, C.; Lagace, R.; Roth, C.; Parson, W.; Budowle, B. Developmental Validation of a MPS Workflow with a PCR-Based Short Amplicon Whole Mitochondrial Genome Panel. *Genes* **2020**, *11*, 1345. [CrossRef] [PubMed]
74. Ralf, A.; van Oven, M.; Montiel Gonzalez, D.; de Knijff, P.; van der Beek, K.; Wootton, S.; Lagace, R.; Kayser, M. Forensic Y-SNP analysis beyond SNaPshot: High-resolution Y-chromosomal haplogrouping from low quality and quantity DNA using Ion AmpliSeq and targeted massively parallel sequencing. *Forensic Sci. Int. Genet.* **2019**, *41*, 93–106. [CrossRef]
75. de la Puente, M.; Phillips, C.; Xavier, C.; Amigo, J.; Carracedo, A.; Parson, W.; Lareu, M.V. Building a custom large-scale panel of novel microhaplotypes for forensic identification using MiSeq and Ion S5 massively parallel sequencing systems. *Forensic Sci. Int. Genet.* **2020**, *45*, 102213. [CrossRef]
76. Wang, D.; Tao, R.; Li, Z.; Pan, D.; Wang, Z.; Li, C.; Shi, Y. STRsearch: A new pipeline for targeted profiling of short tandem repeats in massively parallel sequencing data. *Hereditas* **2020**, *157*, 8. [CrossRef]
77. Lee, J.C.; Tseng, B.; Chang, L.K.; Linacre, A. SEQ Mapper: A DNA sequence searching tool for massively parallel sequencing data. *Forensic Sci. Int. Genet.* **2017**, *26*, 66–69. [CrossRef]
78. Budis, J.; Kucharik, M.; Duris, F.; Gazdarica, J.; Zrubcova, M.; Ficek, A.; Szemes, T.; Brejova, B.; Radvanszky, J. Dante: Genotyping of known complex and expanded short tandem repeats. *Bioinformatics* **2019**, *35*, 1310–1317. [CrossRef]
79. Costa, I.P.D.; Almeida, B.C.; Sequeiros, J.; Amorim, A.; Martins, S. A Pipeline to Assess Disease-Associated Haplotypes in Repeat Expansion Disorders: The Example of MJD/SCA3 Locus. *Front. Genet.* **2019**, *10*, 38. [CrossRef] [PubMed]
80. Holtgrewe, M.; Stolpe, O.; Nieminen, M.; Mundlos, S.; Knaus, A.; Kornak, U.; Seelow, D.; Segebrecht, L.; Spielmann, M.; Fischer-Zirnsak, B.; et al. VarFish: Comprehensive DNA variant analysis for diagnostics and research. *Nucleic Acids Res.* **2020**, *48*, W162–W169. [CrossRef] [PubMed]
81. Liu, Q.; Tong, Y.; Wang, K. Genome-wide detection of short tandem repeat expansions by long-read sequencing. *BMC Bioinform.* **2020**, *21* (Suppl. 21), 542. [CrossRef]
82. Tang, H.; Kirkness, E.F.; Lippert, C.; Biggs, W.H.; Fabani, M.; Guzman, E.; Ramakrishnan, S.; Lavrenko, V.; Kakaradov, B.; Hou, C.; et al. Profiling of Short-Tandem-Repeat Disease Alleles in 12,632 Human Whole Genomes. *Am. J. Hum. Genet.* **2017**, *101*, 700–715. [CrossRef] [PubMed]
83. Dashnow, H.; Lek, M.; Phipson, B.; Halman, A.; Sadedin, S.; Lonsdale, A.; Davis, M.; Lamont, P.; Clayton, J.S.; Laing, N.G.; et al. STRetch: Detecting and discovering pathogenic short tandem repeat expansions. *Genome Biol.* **2018**, *19*, 121. [CrossRef]
84. Liu, Y.Y.; Harbison, S. A review of bioinformatic methods for forensic DNA analyses. *Forensic Sci. Int. Genet.* **2018**, *33*, 117–128. [CrossRef]
85. Halman, A.; Oshlack, A. Accuracy of short tandem repeats genotyping tools in whole exome sequencing data. *F1000Research* **2020**, *9*, 200. [CrossRef]
86. Gymrek, M.; Golan, D.; Rosset, S.; Erlich, Y. lobSTR: A short tandem repeat profiler for personal genomes. *Genome Res.* **2012**, *22*, 1154–1162. [CrossRef] [PubMed]
87. Highnam, G.; Franck, C.; Martin, A.; Stephens, C.; Puthige, A.; Mittelman, D. Accurate human microsatellite genotypes from high-throughput resequencing data using informed error profiles. *Nucleic Acids Res.* **2013**, *41*, e32. [CrossRef] [PubMed]
88. Fungtammasan, A.; Ananda, G.; Hile, S.E.; Su, M.S.; Sun, C.; Harris, R.; Medvedev, P.; Eckert, K.; Makova, K.D. Accurate typing of short tandem repeats from genome-wide sequencing data and its applications. *Genome Res.* **2015**, *25*, 736–749. [CrossRef]
89. Willems, T.; Zielinski, D.; Yuan, J.; Gordon, A.; Gymrek, M.; Erlich, Y. Genome-wide profiling of heritable and de novo STR variations. *Nat. Methods* **2017**, *14*, 590–592. [CrossRef] [PubMed]

90. Tang, H.; Nzabarushimana, E. STRScan: Targeted profiling of short tandem repeats in whole-genome sequencing data. *BMC Bioinform.* **2017**, *18* (Suppl. 11), 398. [CrossRef]

91. Mousavi, N.; Margoliash, J.; Pusarla, N.; Saini, S.; Yanicky, R.; Gymrek, M. TRTools: A toolkit for genome-wide analysis of tandem repeats. *Bioinformatics* **2020**, *37*, 731–733. [CrossRef] [PubMed]

92. Kojima, K.; Kawai, Y.; Misawa, K.; Mimori, T.; Nagasaki, M. STR-realigner: A realignment method for short tandem repeat regions. *BMC Genom.* **2016**, *17*, 991. [CrossRef]

93. Kristmundsdottir, S.; Sigurpalsdottir, B.D.; Kehr, B.; Halldorsson, B.V. popSTR: Population-scale detection of STR variants. *Bioinformatics* **2017**, *33*, 4041–4048. [CrossRef]

94. Bolognini, D.; Magi, A.; Benes, V.; Korbel, J.O.; Rausch, T. TRiCoLOR: Tandem repeat profiling using whole-genome long-read sequencing data. *Gigascience* **2020**, *9*, giaa101. [CrossRef]

95. Walsh, S.; Liu, F.; Ballantyne, K.N.; van Oven, M.; Lao, O.; Kayser, M. IrisPlex: A sensitive DNA tool for accurate prediction of blue and brown eye colour in the absence of ancestry information. *Forensic Sci. Int. Genet.* **2011**, *5*, 170–180. [CrossRef]

96. Walsh, S.; Liu, F.; Wollstein, A.; Kovatsi, L.; Ralf, A.; Kosiniak-Kamysz, A.; Branicki, W.; Kayser, M. The HIrisPlex system for simultaneous prediction of hair and eye colour from DNA. *Forensic Sci. Int. Genet.* **2013**, *7*, 98–115. [CrossRef] [PubMed]

97. Walsh, S.; Chaitanya, L.; Clarisse, L.; Wirken, L.; Draus-Barini, J.; Kovatsi, L.; Maeda, H.; Ishikawa, T.; Sijen, T.; de Knijff, P.; et al. Developmental validation of the HIrisPlex system: DNA-based eye and hair colour prediction for forensic and anthropological usage. *Forensic Sci. Int. Genet.* **2014**, *9*, 150–161. [CrossRef]

98. Walsh, S.; Chaitanya, L.; Breslin, K.; Muralidharan, C.; Bronikowska, A.; Pospiech, E.; Koller, J.; Kovatsi, L.; Wollstein, A.; Branicki, W.; et al. Global skin colour prediction from DNA. *Hum. Genet.* **2017**, *136*, 847–863. [CrossRef]

99. Chaitanya, L.; Breslin, K.; Zuniga, S.; Wirken, L.; Pospiech, E.; Kukla-Bartoszek, M.; Sijen, T.; Knijff, P.; Liu, F.; Branicki, W.; et al. The HIrisPlex-S system for eye, hair and skin colour prediction from DNA: Introduction and forensic developmental validation. *Forensic Sci. Int. Genet.* **2018**, *35*, 123–135. [CrossRef]

100. Robinson, J.T.; Thorvaldsdottir, H.; Winckler, W.; Guttman, M.; Lander, E.S.; Getz, G.; Mesirov, J.P. Integrative genomics viewer. *Nat. Biotechnol.* **2011**, *29*, 24–26. [CrossRef] [PubMed]

101. Spitzer, M.; Fuellen, G.; Cullen, P.; Lorkowski, S. VisCoSe: Visualization and comparison of consensus sequences. *Bioinformatics* **2004**, *20*, 433–435. [CrossRef]

102. BabrahamBioinformatics. FastQC: A Quality Control Tool for High Throughput Sequence Data. Available online: http://www.bioinformatics.babraham.ac.uk/projects/fastqc/ (accessed on 1 October 2010).

103. Bolger, A.M.; Lohse, M.; Usadel, B. Trimmomatic: A flexible trimmer for Illumina sequence data. *Bioinformatics* **2014**, *30*, 2114–2120. [CrossRef] [PubMed]

104. Martin, M. Cutadapt removes adapter sequences from high-throughput sequencing reads. *EMBnet. J.* **2011**, *17*, 10–12. [CrossRef]

105. Li, H. Seqtk: A Fast and Lightweight Tool for Processing FASTA or FASTQ Sequences. Available online: https://github.com/lh3/seqtk (accessed on 1 October 2013).

106. Magoc, T.; Salzberg, S.L. FLASH: Fast length adjustment of short reads to improve genome assemblies. *Bioinformatics* **2011**, *27*, 2957–2963. [CrossRef] [PubMed]

107. Bushnell, B.; Rood, J.; Singer, E. BBMerge—Accurate paired shotgun read merging via overlap. *PLoS ONE* **2017**, *12*, e0185056. [CrossRef]

108. Kwon, S.; Lee, B.; Yoon, S. CASPER: Context-aware scheme for paired-end reads from high-throughput amplicon sequencing. *BMC Bioinform.* **2014**, *15* (Suppl. 9), S10. [CrossRef] [PubMed]

109. NIST Applied Genetics Group. Forensic DNA Open Dataset. Available online: https://data.nist.gov/od/id/mds2-2157 (accessed on 1 October 2019). [CrossRef]

110. 1000 Genomes Project. The International Genome Sample Resource (IGSR) Data Portal. Available online: https://www.internationalgenome.org/data-portal/data-collection (accessed on 1 October 2017).

111. Clarke, L.; Fairley, S.; Zheng-Bradley, X.; Streeter, I.; Perry, E.; Lowy, E.; Tasse, A.M.; Flicek, P. The international Genome sample resource (IGSR): A worldwide collection of genome variation incorporating the 1000 Genomes Project data. *Nucleic Acids Res.* **2017**, *45*, D854–D859. [CrossRef]

112. Fairley, S.; Lowy-Gallego, E.; Perry, E.; Flicek, P. The International Genome Sample Resource (IGSR) collection of open human genomic variation resources. *Nucleic Acids Res.* **2020**, *48*, D941–D947. [CrossRef] [PubMed]

113. NCBI. 1000 Genomes Browser. Available online: https://www.ncbi.nlm.nih.gov/variation/tools/1000genomes/ (accessed on 1 October 2019).

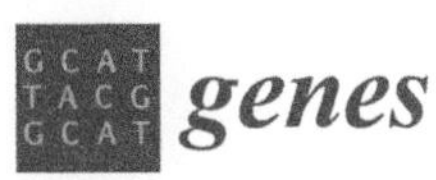

genes

Review

Animal Forensic Genetics

Adrian Linacre

College of Science & Engineering, Flinders University, Adelaide, SA 5042, Australia;
adrian.linacre@flinders.edu.au

Abstract: Animal forensic genetics, where the focus is on non-human species, is broadly divided in two: domestic species and wildlife. When traces of a domestic species are relevant to a forensic investigation the question of species identification is less important, as the material comes from either a dog or a cat for instance, but more relevant may be the identification of the actual pet. Identification of a specific animal draws on similar methods to those used in human identification by using microsatellite markers. The use of cat short tandem repeats to link a cat hair to a particular cat paved the way for similar identification of dogs. Wildlife forensic science is becoming accepted as a recognised discipline. There is growing acceptance that the illegal trade in wildlife is having devasting effects on the numbers of iconic species. Loci on the mitochondrial genome are used to identify the most likely species present. Sequencing the whole locus may not be needed if specific bases can be targeted. There can be benefits of increased sensitivity using mitochondrial loci for species testing, but occasionally there is an issue if hybrids are present. The use of massively parallel DNA sequencing has a role in the identification of the ingredients of traditional medicines where studies found protected species to be present, and a potential role in future species assignments. Non-human animal forensic testing can play a key role in investigations provided that it is performed to the same standards as all other DNA profiling processes.

Keywords: animal forensics; wildlife forensics; cat STRs; dog STRs; cyt *b*; COI

Citation: Linacre, A. Animal Forensic Genetics. *Genes* **2021**, *12*, 515. https://doi.org/10.3390/genes 12040515

Academic Editor: Emiliano Giardina

Received: 16 March 2021
Accepted: 29 March 2021
Published: 1 April 2021

Publisher's Note: MDPI stays neutral with regard to jurisdictional claims in published maps and institutional affiliations.

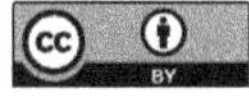

1. Introduction

The plight of endangered iconic species, such as tigers, rhino, and elephants, gains much media attention. Additionally, the affectionate bonds that humans have with domestic pets, particularly dogs and cats, is such that maltreatment of pets ranks highly in the human psyche. It may therefore seem contrary that the forensic investigation and prosecution of alleged cases involving animals (non-human) has always had a lower priority compared to human identification. As a further example regarding research in this area, there are often only a few talks in a miscellaneous section of the ISFG congress on DNA in wildlife crime and non-human DNA profiling compared to many days devoted to human identification. The reason for this low priority is many-fold, but a prime reason is that in the past it was perceived that investigations where the focus was on non-human material required lower standards than those accepted as the norm in human identification. It was the case that so much of non-human DNA typing has traditionally been performed in non-accredited laboratories, often at academic institutes, although this is now starting to change with a number of laboratories gaining full ISO17025 accreditation.

The fact that a review was requested as part of a Special Issue is further evidence of the continuing acceptance of including non-human DNA typing as a tool in forensic investigations. This review is in two main sections: section one looks at the parallels with identification of individual dogs and cats using processes akin to those used in human DNA profiling; the second section discusses the more traditional wildlife forensic testing where the key question is what species is present and hence the focus is on mitochondrial DNA sequence analyses.

2. Wildlife Forensic Laboratories

Genetic testing to enforce national legislation is rarely performed by the same operational laboratories that undertake human identification. This is primarily attributable to time and cost constraints, and the fact that most operational laboratories are accredited to undertake standard operating procedures relevant to human identification only. Most wildlife forensic investigations are undertaken by universities on an ad hoc basis and performed by university academics who may not routinely undertake work for the criminal justice system. Good laboratory practice has been encouraged, and guidelines have been suggested for Quality Control and Quality Assurance within an academic-based wildlife forensic laboratory [1]. There are notable exceptions. These include the US Fish & Wildlife Laboratory in Ashland, Oregon (https://www.fws.gov/lab/ (accessed on 12 March 2021)), the Scotland-based Wildlife DNA Forensics Laboratory (http://www.sasa.gov.uk/ (accessed on 12 March 2021)) and the Australian Museum in Sydney (http://www.Australianmuseum.com (accessed on 12 March 2021)); these laboratories have attained ISO17025 accreditation.

3. Short Tandem Repeat (STR) Analyses in Animal Forensic Science

Dogs and cats are two pet species that are commonly in close contact with humans. According to the North American Pet Insurance Association (NAPHIA), 65% of households in the USA, or 85 million homes, have a dog (https://www.iii.org/fact-statistic/facts-statistics-pet-statistics (accessed on 12 March 2021)). Equally over 9 million dogs and 8 million cats are owned in the UK (according to statista.com), this is about 25% of all homes. It is not surprising therefore that hairs from either dogs or cats are found associated with forensic evidence such as clothing, car seats, and household soft furnishing, an example is shown in Figure 1.

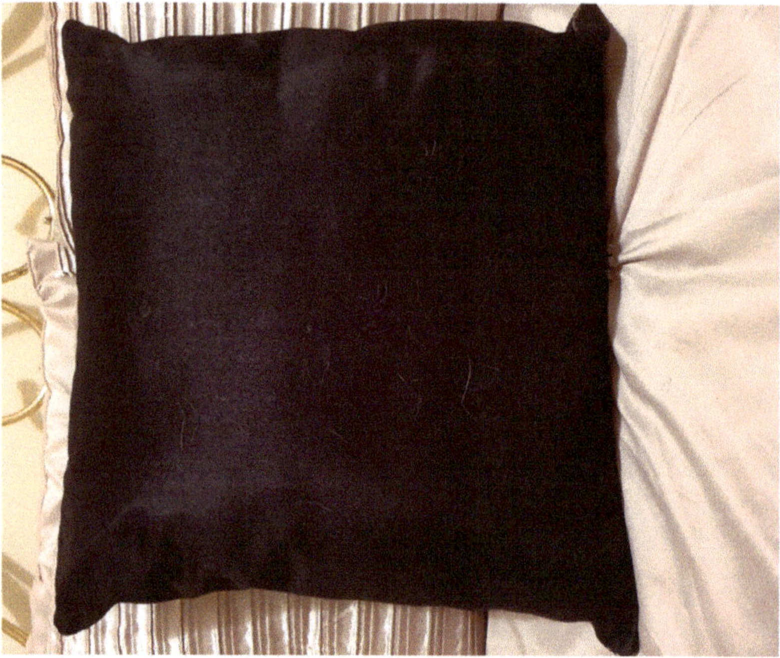

Figure 1. Showing how easy it is for cat hairs to transfer onto soft furnishing, in this case a cushion. These cat hairs can be valuable associative forensic evidence. Note also that these hairs can be transferred to another substrate by secondary transfer.

Such items onto which cat or dog hairs can be transferred, may themselves be associative evidence or be a substrate for secondary transfer to further items that may be of forensic relevance in an investigation. Therefore, it was with the first case of cat hairs to identify a person of interest and lead to a conviction.

3.1. Feline STR Typing

Snowball the cat became famous in arena of forensic DNA profiling for aiding in the resolution of an alleged homicide [2]. The work was initiated by the Royal Canadian Mounted Police (RCMP) after a 32-year-old woman from Prince Edward Island, Canada, was reported missing on 3 October 1994. This occurred in a remote wooded area. A man's jacket was found close to the abandoned car of the missing person, along with other items. White hairs clinging to the lining of the jacket were identified by the RCMP's laboratory to be from a cat. The only suspect in the case happened to own a white cat called Snowball.

Ten dinucleotide STR loci were used in a comparison of the DNA profiles from the hairs taken from the jacket to a hair samples that had been taken from Snowball; these ten loci were found to match. Now the issue was to determine the probability of this match and therefore a population genetic database was generated from cats in Prince Edward Island. In addition, a second database was generated from outbred cats from the Eastern United States [3]. The resulting match probabilities were 2.2×10^{-8} and 6.9×10^{-7} for the Prince Edward Island and the U.S. population databases, respectively [3].

The cat DNA evidence was accepted by the court, and in combination with additional human DNA evidence, was presented to the jury at the Supreme Court of Prince Edward Island. On 19 July 1996, the jury convicted the defendant of second-degree murder [2].

This first case was ground-breaking and showed the real potential of such evidence. The case required a number of steps: developing microsatellite markers, ensuring that the loci were variable, developing primer sets, ensuring the loci were not linked, testing to confirm that they could be co-amplified, developing an allelic database that was representative to allow for the use of robust statistics to support any matching DNA types. These steps are all part of the characterisation of hypervariable STR loci used in human identification, although the use of commercially available products circumvents this massive undertaking.

The first uses of STR loci used dinucleotide repeat markers, but these suffer from a number of stochastic effects, particularly increase in stutter peaks. Feline STR testing was developed further by a group in Germany who characterised 14 hypervariable STR markers, predominantly tetranucleotide repeats, and developed and allelic ladder [4]. These work adhered to the recommendations of the International Society for Forensic Genetics [1]. To allow initial use of these 14 STRs in casework, the authors surveyed 122 unrelated cats in the local area and created an allelic database. Another key point to this work is that, with careful primer design, all 14 STR loci produced amplicons smaller than 260 bases; an important point when working on DNA from hairs and therefore likely to be degraded. An important aspect of this work is that the authors isolated and sequenced each locus to report on the underlying repeat structure. This type of work not only shows a model for the future, but also allowed interlaboratory testing to be performed.

Since this first case, there has been extensive research into increasing the number of hypervariable loci for both cats and dogs.

3.2. Canine STR Typing

A group based in Portugal characterised nine STR loci, all of which were tetranucleotide repeats, which were combined into one multiplex PCR [5]. The primer design ensured that the largest allele was still smaller than 350 bases. The authors had also isolated and characterised each of the nine loci so that the repeat sequence could be reported accurately. The authors had access to 113 dog samples to test the multiplex for all the standard conditions as expected in human identification. In combination, and based on the 113 sample set, the authors reported a very high discriminating power (matching probability = $1.63/10^{10}$). This type of work was the foundation for further canine studies.

This assay was extended by two more loci and used in the identification of wolves (*Canis lupus*) [6]. Dogs (*Canis lupus familiaris*) are a subspecies of the grey wolf and therefore the authors surmised rightly that the same primers would work effectively on wolf as on dogs. Wolves in European come into conflict with humans and are frequently blamed for killing livestock or attacking humans. A case study looked at one such case where a male had received many injuries to the body and claimed to been attacked by a wolf [7]. DNA typing showed conclusively that the man was attacked by a guard dog and not a wolf, or wolf/dog hybrid, as claim; the male later confessed that this was the case [7].

The International Society for Animal Genetics (ISAG) had published a list of putative dog STRs: these comprised 21 dinucleotide loci and 3 tetra repeats. Due to the issues of increased stutters with dinucleotide repeats, and that tetra repeats were recommended by the ISFG [1], a group at UC Davies developed a canine STR test that used 15 unlinked STR loci combined into one multiplex, entitled DogFiler [8]. A full validation was performed in accordance with the recommendations of the Scientific Working Group for DNA Analysis Methods (SGDAM). The authors of this study sequenced alleles to characterise fully the repeat motifs and also created allelic ladders to allow genotyping. The publication of DogFiler set a precedent as to how to create an STR multiplex that meets the same standards as commercially available kits used in human identification.

Often only shed dog hairs are available for analyses. In such instances, amplification of all the loci to generate a full STR profile might not be possible. To overcome this problem, the same group developed three mini multiplexes by moving the primers closer to the amplicons, thus shortening the length of any allele amplified [9]. The result is that no locus is greater than 205 bases in length. Therefore, called Mini-DogFiler met the same standards as the full multiplex.

The CaDNAP group based at the Medical University of Innsbruck separately developed 13 hypervariable microsatellite loci into a multiplex and analysed 1184 dogs [10]. All the dogs were from either Germany, Austria or Switzerland (the so called DACH countries). CaDNAP is a working group of the ISFG and members of the CaDNAP group have extensive experience in human identification and very familiar with the requirements for full validation prior to publication and use in the criminal justice system. The equipment required is also that used in any operational forensic science laboratory performing human identification. The inclusion of such a large number of individual dogs from many breeds allowed the construction of a dog population sample database. The chance of two dogs sharing an allele identical by decent could be calculated allowing the same statistics to be used as performed in human identification.

3.3. Livestock

Cats and dogs are the predominant domestic pets. Livestock such as cattle, horses, sheep and camel, are also sometimes the subject of forensic investigation. The ISAG is prominent in standardising genetic testing for parentage (stud or pedigree analyses) that can also be used in criminal cases if required. Two examples are provided below where case reports have been published.

There are currently 16 cattle (*Bos taurus*) STR loci listed on a prominent website (https://strbase.nist.gov//cattleSTRs.htm (accessed on 15 March 2021)), all of which are dinucleotide repeats. There is a StockMarks® available from ThermoFisher Scientific (Waltham, MA, USA) that includes 11 loci. A recent report extended the panel of STRs to 30 [11]. This is largely for parentage studies where many loci are needed for confidence in associating a bull with calves, but also highly useful in confirming meat in the food industry.

Sheep (*Ovis aries*) are the most commonly grazed species and breeds such as merino and mouflon are either highly prized, or protected. A case report used 16 STR loci, that there amplified in four separate multiplex reactions, to link a carcass of a mouflon to items sized from a vehicle [12]. This case occurred on the island of Sardinia, used Bayesian assignment modelling to support this genetic linkage.

3.4. Wildlife STR Typing

The trade in ivory is leading to the extinction of elephants from many countries in Africa. An elephant tusk is an over-grown tooth and therefore a potential source of trace DNA. Linking ivory seizures by DNA typing from this genetic material opens the possibility to identify the number of elephants slaughtered in any seizure of ivory samples; such knowledge will aid in forensic investigations, or at least in highlighting the extent of the illegal trade. A group at the University of Washington led by Professor Sam Wasser developed a series of STRs from the two species of African elephant [13,14]: the savannah species (*Loxodonta Africana*) and the forest dwelling species (*Loxodonta cyclotis*). The concept behind the study was to identify the geographic location from which the elephants were poached. It would be expected that elephants with shared recent ancestors (i.e., distant family groups), will have more alleles in common at the STR loci tested than individual elephants with a more distant genetic heritage. Knowledge of the way in which matriarchal herds roam over either the savannahs or forests of Africa aid in understanding clusters of STR alleles within a broad geographic area. This pioneering work not only had to overcome the problems in creating a multiplex of STR loci, but also in being able to isolate sufficient quality DNA from tusks, particularly when the tusks may have been stored in poor conditions such that bacterial action might degrade the trace DNA present.

RhODIS® is a comparable system for the linkage of rhino horns to that of elephants [15]. The RhODIS® test is promoted by the University of Pretoria and is comprised of 12 STR loci plus a gender test. It was developed for the two species of rhino that still live in Africa: the white rhino (*Ceratotherium simum*) and the black rhino (*Diceros bicornis*). A potential for RhODIS® is that samples from members of the last remaining white and black rhino in wildlife parks such as Kruger can be collected and then later matched to seized horns taken from poached rhino. The author of this review was a guest of a World Bank and TRAFFIC supported visit to Kruger national park in eastern South Africa to witness RhODIS® in action. Figure 2 is an image of the author attending the poaching of a mother rhino, nearby was the corpse of the offspring; both killed for their horns.

A panel of STR markers have also been created for the one horned Indian rhino (*Rhinocerosunicornis*) [16], as this species has also suffered extreme loss of numbers due to poaching for their horns. This work is part of the official RhODIS-India program. The authors of this paper used 14 STR markers—these were all dinucleotide repeats and far from ideal but had been characterised previously and therefore saved time and resources rather than trying to find and characterise new tetra-repeats [16].

As is likely to be the case for any species that has suffered a loss in numbers and is now breeding from a small set of individuals, the frequency of some alleles starts to either increase as homozygosity increases, and conversely some alleles will decrease or be lost. As reported in the paper on the Indian rhino, many of the STR loci only have 3 or 4 alleles. Despite this, a power of discrimination was reported as 1.4×10^{-9} [16].

Elephant and rhino are iconic mammalian species whose body parts are highly traded internationally. Other mammalian species for which STR multiplexes have been developed include bears, wolves and badgers. As populations increase in the USA there is greater encroachment onto territories of the American black bear (*Ursus americanus*). Such human bear interactions can lead to injury, and on very rare occasions, death of the human, so tracking down the bear responsible is needed so that an innocent bear is not shot. Eleven tetra-nucleotide repeats were selected along with a sex test and made into one multiplex [17]. The test worked on trace amounts of DNA, down to 78 pg, so it is possible using this method to generate profiles from hairs and scat. A further example is that of STR typing for the European badger (*Meles meles*) [18]. Badgers are still hunted illegally and therefore the need to link samples from dead badgers or badger parts to items found in the cars, homes or persons of interest is needed.

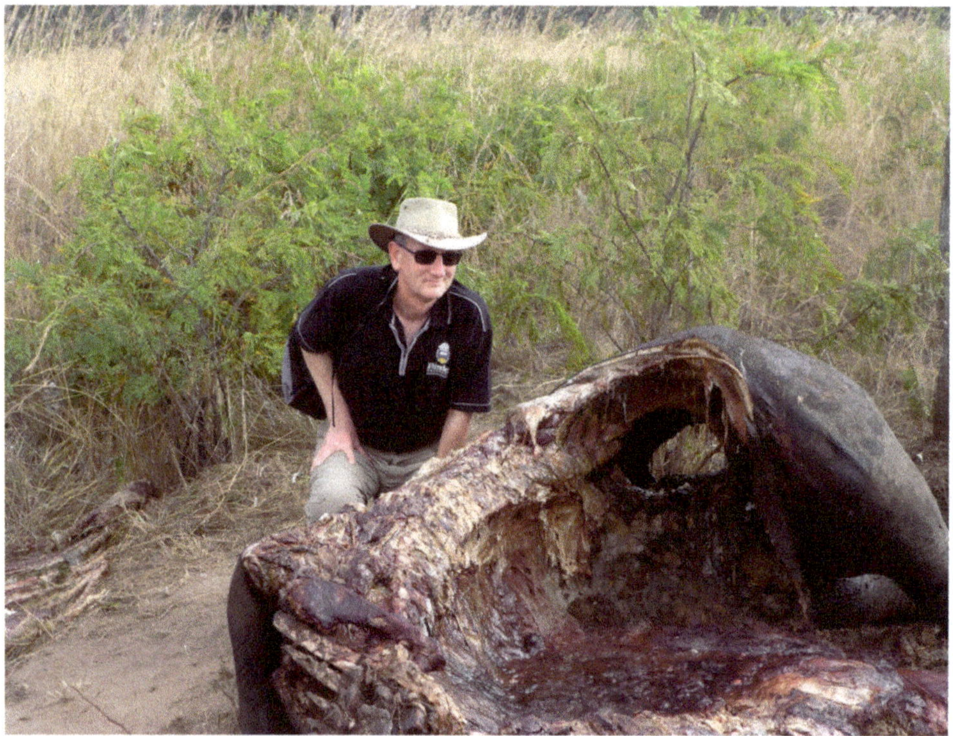

Figure 2. Showing the author at the site of a recently (within 4 days of taking the image) poached mother rhino. The rhino had been shot and then the horn removed with a chain saw. The image was taken in Kruger National Park, South Africa, and is one of around 34 poached rhino recorded in the park every month.

Bird species are traded illegally for their use in the pet trade, i.e., parrots and cockatoos, or persecuted as perceived threats to livestock, i.e., eagles, harriers and hawks. Cockatoos can be brightly coloured and are also known to be birds that can be caged and then kept as pets. As so happens, a criminal case spurred this research as there was a need to analyse the parentage of seized cockatoos, resulting in the application of 20 STR loci to aid in resolving a dispute as to whether eggs in possession of a person of interest had been taken from a nest illegally [19]. Hen harriers (*Circus cyaneus*) were once a very common sight over northern European moorlands, but now they are extremely rare due to habitat loss and being shot or poisoned as a perceived threat to grouse and other game birds. In response to the need to link carcasses of dead birds to biological material (blood and feathers) on seized items (such as traps and snares) a multiplex of 8 STR markers was created (tetra-repeats with one tri-repeat locus) and validated for use [20]. A sex test based on the CHD 1 gene (male birds are Z,Z and females are W,Z) was included and an allelic ladder created.

Reptiles and amphibians have also been the subject of development of STR panels. The carpet python (*Morelia spilota*) is common in the pet trade and can be kept in captivity if bred from pairs that were also captive (i.e., not taken from the wild). However, the number of known captive snakes appears greater than the expected captive bred population and therefore it is likely that snakes are collected illegally from the wild. In response to a need to test this, three separate multiplexes that covered a total of 24 loci, plus allelic ladders for each locus, was created and called OzPythonPlex [21].

The illegal collection of animals from the wild to fuel the pet trade extends to tortoise. The slow-moving reptiles are commonly kept as pets as they are easy to look after. A result, along with habitat loss, is that the number of tortoises in the wild has fallen dramatically.

An example is Herman's tortoise (*Testudo hermanni*), that used to span much of the northern Mediterranean countries. To ensure that seized tortoise are correctly relocated to their correct geographical range, a panel of STR markers were applied for geographical provenance [22].

3.5. Finding, Characterising and Applying Short Tandem Repeat Loci

In all the above reports using STRs, there was an extensive amount of research required to develop a multiplex STR test. For those from the forensic community whose experience is solely in human identification, the arduous steps to develop such a multiplex assay are unlikely to be known. The author of this review is from a time when the first STR test was reported, using four STR loci [23], which then to six STRs plus amelogenin in what was called 'second generation multiplex (or SGM) [24]; SGM was made in-house by the UK Forensic Science Service.

The use of STRs from dogs, elephant, rhino and hen harriers as examples, is based on previously reported putative loci. More recently, such as from pythons, the entire genome of the animal was sequenced using massively parallel DNA sequencing (MPS) technology [21]. From the mass of genetic sequence data, there are software programs to locate repetitive DNA, then provide a list of putative primers [25]. Having ordered primer sequences, these need to be tested on DNA from multiple members of the species to ensure reproducibility and variability at the locus. If still suitable, then homozygotes at each locus need to be sequenced to confirm the repeat motif. Ideally the primers should have similar binding temperatures (termed TMs) so that they can all the amplified in the same reaction. By characterising the loci, an allelic window can be created to determine the smallest and largest alleles likely to be encountered; this is needed to ensure that the alleles do not overlap and fit within a size limit using up to 5 dyes. Sampling many members of the population leads to the creation of allelic ladders, essential for accurate genotyping. This sample set might form the basis of a frequency data set (typically need up to 200 individuals from a population). Standard population genetic calculations need to be undertaken: examining loci for Hardy–Weinberg equilibrium, checking if there is any genetic linkage, and examining for power of discrimination. Validation steps, akin to those provided by SGDAM, include: specificity testing to ensure the primers only amplify from the species/genus for which they were designed; sensitivity tests to determine the limit of detection and effect of adding sub-optimal mass of DNA; stability to see the effects of environmental factors; reproducibility to see the effect of running multiple samples for instance down a column by capillary electrophoresis; interlaboratory testing to ensure the test works on varying equipment and by different operators; blind trial testing to ensure the results are not biased by the inadvertent selection of samples; and perhaps finally publishing the data, as was the case for so many of the papers cited in this review. It is clear reading the above, that this is not something achieved in a matter of weeks and also the reason why so few complex multiplex assays exist for species other than humans and domesticated species such as dogs and cats.

4. Species Assignment in Wildlife Forensic Science

A question raised in wildlife forensic science is *'which species is this?'*. This is because legislation at a national level is many countries prohibits the trade or ownership products originating from legally protected species. The illegal trade in protected species is central to much of wildlife forensic science as tools employed by forensic practitioners can be applied when called on to determine whether something is, or is not, legal to trade or own.

Interpol recognized wildlife crime as the second most prevalent crime worldwide after drug trafficking [26]. The value of the trade is often quoted as $20 billion (USD) per year [26,27] although the exact figure is unknown as very little illegal trade is ever detected. It is only from intercepting seizures that the true scale be estimated. Furthermore, the low penalties and potential large financial gain lead to extensive and lucrative trade in endangered species [28–30]. This figure of USD 20 billion is also only the estimated illegal revenue from international trade and does not include the illegal trade within countries.

The scope and range of wildlife crime is wide and encompasses a variety of criminal activities such as poaching and illegal hunting of mammals [31,32], birds [20,33] and reptiles [21,34,35], and the use of animal derivatives in traditional medicines [36,37].

Forensic investigations can only be undertaken if it is alleged that legislation has been breached. Further, the willingness to conduct DNA profiling of suspected illegally traded/owned samples requires: Approval from prosecuting authorities, availability of persons competent to conduct the work, and funds to compensate that laboratory performing any wildlife investigation.

4.1. Legislation Covering Wildlife Trade

The international trade in endangered species is monitored and regulated through recommendations made by Convention on International Trade in Endangered Species of Wild Fauna and Flora (CITES) [38]. These recommendations are enforced at a national level by legislation. Normally, this legislation stipulates the names of the species that are protected. It is for these reasons that much interest at a research level has focused on methods of species identification [38,39].

Many countries have legislation covering the collection from the wild, breeding, ownership or international trade in animal parts or whole organisms. An example repository of information detailing the federal law in the USA can be found at https://www.animallaw.info/article/federal-wildlife-law-20th-century (accessed on 15 March 2021). The US Endangered Species Act (ESA) of 1973 is a key piece of legislation for both domestic (USA), and international conservation. The act aims to provide a framework to conserve and protect endangered and threatened species and their habitats. Additionally, in the USA, the Lacey Act is central to conservation of wildlife and dates from 1900 when it became the first federal law protecting wildlife. The Act makes it unlawful to import, export, sell, acquire, or purchase fish, wildlife or plants that are taken, possessed, transported, or sold: 1) in violation of U.S. or Indian law, or 2) in interstate or foreign commerce involving any fish, wildlife, or plants taken possessed or sold in violation of State or foreign law. The Lacey Act covers all fish and wildlife and their parts or products, plants protected by CITES and those protected by State law; thus regulating international trade of protected species.

The EU, comprised currently of 27 countries, has the free movement of goods across internal borders as a core value. It is only therefore trade across the first border of a member state that is an issue. The EU Council Regulation (EC) No 338/97 deals with the protection of species of wild fauna and flora by regulating trade of any species covered by this regulation. It lays down the provisions for import, export and re-export as well as internal EU trade in specimens of species listed in its four Annexes.

In the UK, the Wildlife and Countryside act of 1981 gave protection to native species, controlled the release of non-native species, protected sites of special scientific interest, and made provision for rights-of-way. A devolved Scotland and separately administered Northern Ireland and Wales resulted in local legislation to protect the environment.

4.2. mtDNA in Species Testing

It may be that the seized material has been processed to create a sculpture, ornament, item of clothing, food, or supposed medicinal product. DNA can be obtained at trace levels from ivory [40] where ivory is made into statues, or rhino horn is proceesed into knife handles [32]. The most traded mammalian species currently is one of the members of the pangolin family. Pangolins are the only mammals to have scales on the outer surface and are one of eight species: three of which are critically endangered (*Manis culionensis*, *Manis pentadactyla* and *Manis javanica*), three are endangered (*Phataginus tricuspis*, *Manis crassicaudata* and *Smutsia gigantea*) and two (*Phataginus tetradactyla* and *Smutsia temminckii*) are recorded as being 'vulnerable' on the Red List of Threatened Species of the International Union for Conservation of Nature. The threat to pangolins is their misguided use in traditional medicines, specifically when the scales are used as bogus remedies. DNA can be obtained from pangolin scales, even when processed as a soup [41,42]. Performing mtDNA sequencing can link seizures of pangolins, but also indicates the geographical origin from where they were taken from the wild to inform authorities about hotspots of poaching.

Ivory, rhino horn and pangolin scales are examples of evidential material where DNA is at trace levels. This is typical of much of the seizures encountered in the illegal wildlife trade such that mtDNA is the only genetic material available [28]. Human identification has centered on a small section of mtDNA that does not encode; termed the hypervariable regions that constitute less than 1000 of the 16,569 bases that make up the human mitochondrial genome. Vertebrate mtDNA has two strands of different densities: the heavy (or H-strand) and the light (or L-strand). The mitochondrial genome in eukaryotes encodes a total of 37 genes, 22 of which encode tRNA molecules, two encode rRNA molecules, and the other 13 encode proteins involved primarily with the process of oxidative respiration [39]. While the number of these genes on the mitochondrial genome does not vary within all vertebrate mitochondrial genomes decoded to-date, the order of the genes may alter [39]. As an example, the order is different between avian and mammalian mitochondrial genomes.

Although the use of mitochondrial loci in species testing has many benefits, there are a few disadvantages as well. Part of the benefit of mitochondrial loci is that they are inherited maternally and as a haplotype with no recombination. Maternal inheritance can be a problem if hybrid species occur, particularly if the mother is from a nonprotected species and the father is from a species that is protected [43,44] (see Section 4.5).

4.3. Species Identification Using Loci on Mitochondrial Genome

A classic characteristic for a locus used in species identification is that it should exhibit very little variation for any member of the same species such that all members of that species have the same, or very nearly the same, sequence; this is referred to as intraspecies variation. The second characteristic is that this same locus should exhibit sufficient differences from any member of the next closest species, being interspecies DNA sequence variation.

The main locus used in taxonomic and phylogenetic studies until recently was cytochrome *b* (cyt *b*) [45,46]. This occurs between bases 14,747 and 15,887 in human mtDNA and encodes a protein 380 amino acids in length. The cyt *b* locus has been used extensively in taxonomic and forensic studies [32,34,35,47].

The cytochrome *c* oxidase I (COI) mitochondrial gene locus was adopted by the Barcode for Life Consortium (BOLD) (www.boldsystems.org (accessed on 15 March 2021)) [48–50]. COI is found between bases 5904 and 7445 in human mtDNA and at a similar position for all other mammals. COI was used initially in the identification of invertebrate species [51,52] and became the locus of choice in forensic entomology [53] before being adopted by BOLD.

Currently, there is no standardized locus in species testing, hence a divergence between cyt *b*, COI and other locus such as ND5. The Commission for the International Society for Forensic Genetics (ISFG) recommended that there should be some rationale behind the choice of the locus used in any analysis [1]. It is most likely that different loci will exhibit varying inter- and intraspecies similarity depending on whether examining insects, other invertebrates, fish, reptiles, birds, or mammals. Mammals are the only taxonomic group where a detailed study has been performed to determine whether cyt *b* or COI have fewer false positive and false negative identifications [54]; in this study, cyt *b* was found to outperform COI.

It may often be the case, such as for ivory and rhino horn, that the DNA is highly fragmented and therefore not possible to examine the entire locus of either COI or cyt *b*; rather, sections of the loci are used. The first 400 bases section of the cyt *b* gene is typically used [46]. For the COI the first 645 bp are used as part of BOLD [48]. The use of either section of the cyt *b* or COI loci is aided by the design of universal primers; these are primers that can be used in PCR to amplify a section of a gene from all the species from which the specific primers are designed. For instance, up-stream from the cyt *b* gene is a gene for a tRNA molecule, and this sequence is highly conserved such that the primers will bind to any mammalian species. This is a real benefit if the material is single source and not contaminated with DNA from another species; as an example, it is all too easy to amplify human DNA due to external contamination.

4.4. Mitochondrial Sequence Analysis

The standard workflow for species identification is to: (1) isolate DNA; (2) then quantify the amount of DNA isolated; (3) amplify the section of mtDNA chosen; (4) confirm that a PCR product has been generated; (5) purify the PCR amplicon; (6) DNA sequence the amplicon (in both directions); (7) compare the sequence data to a reference data base such as GenBank or ForCyt [55]. ForCyt was established to remove errors that do exist in GenBank [56]. When publishing the reference DNA sequence from a species to which comparisons of unknown material can be made, it is essential that this known sample comes from a voucher specimen; this is recommended by the ISFG Commission [1]. Software such as the Basic Local Alignment Search Tool (BLAST) compares the target sequence fragment to the data deposited on the database (GenBank) and produces a similarity score of the 100 most closely matched sequences. These are listed with the closest similarity at the top of the list. The ideal is a similarity score of 100% to a known species, with the next closest being less than a similarity of 95%. This situation rarely occurs with a similarity score of 98% between the sequence tested and the nearest sequence being more typical. There is no consensus on how many differences and over what number of bases is either due to intra- or interspecies variation. It was reported that one base variation per 400 bp sequence is acceptable intraspecies variation [39].

4.5. SNP Testing

Performing a complete DNA sequence analysis from a section of DNA provides the maximum amount of genetic information. It may be that only a few DNA bases that differ (are polymorphic), and that much of the DNA sequence is of little value as the species being considered share much of their DNA. In such instances, if the polymorphic DNA bases are known, these bases can be targeted specifically. A recent example of this is the identification of SNPs within the mitochondrial genome of tigers [57]. In this instance, small parts of the tiger mitochondrial genome are amplified in one reaction using primers specific for the genus *Panthera*. The assay is based on SNaPshot®, a process used in ancestry assignments of human populations [58–60]. As the sections amplified in the first instance are short, no more than 300 bases, this type of DNA testing works very effectively on highly degraded DNA, with a recent example being the species assignment from ivory [61]. In this paper the authors were able to differentiate ivory taken from Asian elephants (*Elephas maximus*) compared to either of the African elephants with a 99.92% reported accuracy based on an impressive 140 samples of ivory. The paper targeted SNPs in either the cyt *b* gene or ND5 gene. Additionally, because the SNP detection can be species-specific, the test works well even when there is a complex mixture of other species. An example was to identify up to 18 European mammalian species by using universal primers in the cyt *b* gene in combination with species specific primers [62]. The size of the resulting species-specific amplicon is itself specific for each species and with 3 amplicons per species there is redundancy to cope with one of the tests not working.

4.6. Hybrids

Sequence comparison using regions of the mitochondrial genome has a tremendous advantage over nuclear markers for sensitivity; this is due to the multiple copy number of mitochondrial genomes per cell. A potential disadvantage in species testing is the maternal inheritance of mitochondrial DNA. When the male is from a protected species, but the female is from species not protected, and viable young are produced, due to the maternal of inheritance of mtDNA, the offspring will not be recognised as a protected species. This issue was highlighted in a recent report [43], which is based on a talk at the ISFG congress in 2019 in Prague. There are in reality only a few examples where hybrids are the result of this type of mating as the majority of examples include species that are geographically isolated, or of little forensic relevance: examples of geographical separation are mating between an African lion (*Panthera leo*) and Indian tiger (*Panthera tigris tigris*) resulting in either a tigon or liger; and of limited forensic relevance between a horse (*Equus caballus*) and a donkey (*Equus asinus*) to produce a hinny or mule.

An example where hybrids are an issue was highlighted in a case report on the alleged poaching of protected South American camelids: llamas (*Lama glama*), vicuñas (*Vicugna vicugna*), alpacas (*Vicugna pacos*) and guanaco (*Lama guanicoe*) [44]. Wild (vicuña and guanaco) and domesticated (llama and alpaca) animals roam within Chile freely and can mate to produce viable young capable of themselves producing young. In Chile it is illegal to hunt and kill guanaco and llama but hybrids are not protected; this leads to the potential to sell meat from protected species as from a legally killed animal. The colour of the coats of the domestic and hybrids are different and specific to the variants. This led to the group in Chile, who were faced with this problem, to use in addition to cyt *b* sequence data, a diagnostic base in the melanocortin 1 receptor (*MC1R*). The combination of species assignment with a marker for coat colour resolved this case.

4.7. Traditional Medicines

Seizures of rhino horn, ivory and pangolins usually are of either identifiable using morphology or by DNA as will be from only one species. An example where multiple protected species are found in a complex mix, along with other plant and animal derivatives, is the trade in traditional medicines. Here, the ingredients might not be listed, rather the spurious cure for while they are taken can be prominent. An example is shown in Figure 3.

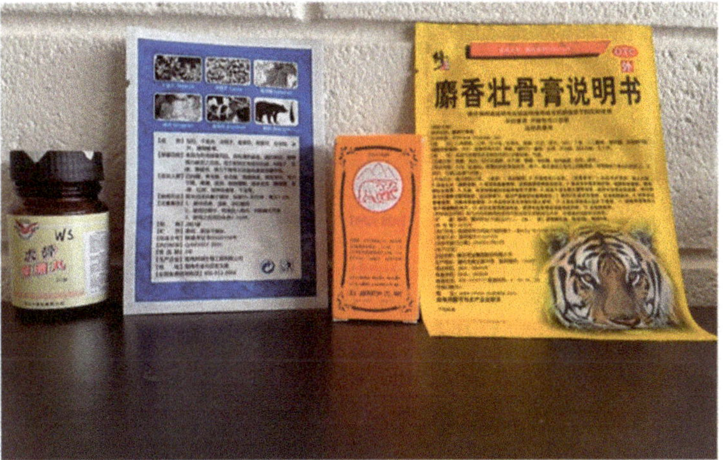

Figure 3. Showing examples of a traditional east Asian medicine that was seized by Border Force officials. The items were later show to contain traces of DNA from endangered species.

These plasters and pills list bear and tiger on the packaging, which is an offence in many countries, breaching CITES agreements, even if there is no tiger or bear present. It is likely that the amounts of any genetic material would be at extremely low amounts, and in a complex mix with potentially other species. This makes standard species testing problematic. Using universal primers and then amplifying using standard Sanger sequencing of part of the mtDNA will result in unreadable DNA sequence data. Undoubtedly the application of massively parallel DNA sequence technology overcomes the issue of any complex mixtures. The first example of this work on seized traditional medicines identified a number of protected species along with large numbers of other plant and animal species not listed on the packaging but with poor health outcomes [37]. A more recent study found protected species in traditional medicine products that could be bought in Australia [36], yet no prosecutions were undertaken even though there is clear evidence of breaching federal law.

5. Conclusions on Animal Forensic Profiling

This review clearly identifies the need, and the growing use of, non-human animal DNA for a range of forensic applications. There are a few laboratories dedicated to this type of analyses and can demonstrate that they work to the same exacting standards required in human identification. More such facilities are needed and, when it comes to wildlife forensic science, in countries closer to where seizures happen. The STR typing of non-human animals, with cats and dogs being prime examples, uses the same equipment as in human identification and therefore creating Standard Operating Procedures and adopting the STR typing of dog for example into use in mainstream accredited laboratories is therefore possible.

There remains no standard locus for species testing. A wealth of data exists on GenBank for sections of cyt *b*, COI and other mtDNA regions such as ND5 from a wide range of animal species. It may be that one locus has fewer false negatives and false positives than another for different taxonomic Orders, although data only exist in some mammalian species as a comparison. Intraspecies variation needs to be known for many more species as currently there are very little data available. One answer would be to use the power of MPS and analyse multiple loci in one reaction. The common use of MPS is on the near horizon as prices for consumables and the use of this equipment decreases. MPS is also seeing acceptance in other areas of non-human DNA typing such as in analyses of bacteria for post mortem interval [63,64] and now in tracking microbiomes [65,66] and was the subject of a recent review [67]. If the use of MPS is growing a profile in bacterial work, then there is every reason to expect the same acceptance and profile from eukaryotic and in particular vertebrate species.

The application of non-human DNA, now with examples of now bacterial DNA typing, can add an extra dimension to a forensic investigation. The use of DNA from species other than humans can add a further dimension to a forensic investigation. It is for those working in the non-human arena to ensure that their standards meet those expected and can provide a valuable service to the criminal justice system.

Funding: The author's research is supported by the Attorney General's Department of South Australia, through a grant supported by Forensic Science South Australia.

Conflicts of Interest: The author declares no conflict of interest.

References

1. Linacre, A.; Gusmão, L.; Hecht, W.; Hellmann, A.; Mayr, W.; Parson, W.; Prinz, M.; Schneider, P.; Morling, N. ISFG: Recommendations regarding the use of non-human (animal) DNA in forensic genetic investigations. *Forensic Sci. Int. Genet.* **2011**, *5*, 501–505. [CrossRef] [PubMed]
2. Menotti-Raymond, M.A.; David, V.A.; O'Brien, S.J. Pet car hair implicates murder suspect. *Nature* **1997**, *386*, 774. [CrossRef] [PubMed]
3. Menotti-Raymond, M.; David, V.A.; Stephens, J.C.; Lyons, L.A.; O'Brien, S.J. Genetic individualization of domestic cats using feline STR loci for forensic applications. *J. Forensic Sci.* **1997**, *42*, 14258J. [CrossRef]
4. Schury, N.; Schleenbecker, U.; Hellmann, A. Forensic animal DNA typing: Allele nomenclature and standardization of 14 feline STR markers. *Forensic Sci. Int. Genet.* **2014**, *12*, 42–59. [CrossRef]
5. van Asch, B.; Alves, C.; Gusmão, L.; Pereira, V.; Pereira, F.; Amorim, A. A new autosomal STR nineplex for canine identification and parentage testing. *Electrophoresis* **2009**, *30*, 417–423. [CrossRef]
6. van Asch, B.; Alves, C.; Santos, L.; Pinheiro, R.; Pereira, F.; Gusmão, L.; Amorim, A. Genetic profiles and sex identification of found-dead wolves determined by the use of an 11-loci PCR multiplex. *Forensic Sci. Int. Genet.* **2010**, *4*, 68–72. [CrossRef]
7. Caniglia, R.; Galaverni, M.; Delogu, M.; Fabbri, E.; Musto, C.; Randi, E. Big bad wolf or man's best friend? Unmasking a false wolf aggression on humans. *Forensic Sci. Int. Genet.* **2016**, *24*, e4–e6. [CrossRef]
8. Wictum, E.J.; Kun, T.; Lindquist, C.; Malvick, J.; Vankan, D.; Sacks, B. Developmental validation of DogFiler, a novel multiplex for canine DNA profiling in forensic casework. *Forensic Sci. Int. Genet.* **2013**, *7*, 82–91. [CrossRef]

9.   Kun, T.; Lyons, L.A.; Sacks, B.N.; Ballard, R.E.; Lindquist, C.; Wictum, E.J. Developmental validation of Mini-DogFiler for degraded canine DNA. *Forensic Sci. Int. Genet.* **2013**, *7*, 151–158. [CrossRef]

10. Berger, B.; Heinrich, J.; Niederstätter, H.; Hecht, W.; Morf, N.; Hellmann, A.; Rohleder, U.; Schleenbecker, U.; Berger, C.; Parson, W. Forensic characterization and statistical considerations of the CaDNAP 13-STR panel in 1184 domestic dogs from Germany, Austria, and Switzerland. *Forensic Sci. Int. Genet.* **2019**, *42*, 90–98. [CrossRef]

11. Gamarra, D.; Taniguchi, M.; Aldai, N.; Arakawa, A.; Lopez-Oceja, A.; De Pancorbo, M.M. Genetic Characterization of the Local Pirenaica Cattle for Parentage and Traceability Purposes. *Animals* **2020**, *10*, 1584. [CrossRef]

12. Lorenzini, R.; Cabras, P.; Fanelli, R.; Carboni, G.L. Wildlife molecular forensics: Identification of the Sardinian mouflon using STR profiling and the Bayesian assignment test. *Forensic Sci. Int. Genet.* **2011**, *5*, 345–349. [CrossRef]

13. Wasser, S.K.; Mailand, C.; Booth, R.; Mutayoba, B.; Kisamo, E.; Clark, B.; Stephens, M. Using DNA to track the origin of the largest ivory seizure since the 1989 trade ban. *Proc. Natl. Acad. Sci. USA* **2007**, *104*, 4228–4233. [CrossRef]

14. Wasser, S.K.; Shedlock, A.M.; Comstock, K.; Ostrander, E.A.; Mutayoba, B.; Stephens, M. Assigning African elephant DNA to geographic region of origin: Applications to the ivory trade. *Proc. Natl. Acad. Sci. USA* **2004**, *101*, 14847–14852. [CrossRef]

15. Harper, C.K.; Vermeulen, G.J.; Clarke, A.B.; de Wet, J.I.; Guthrie, A.J. Extraction of nuclear DNA from rhinoceros horn and characterization of DNA profiling systems for white (*Ceratotherium simum*) and black (*Diceros bicornis*) rhinoceros. *Forensic Sci. Int. Genet.* **2013**, *7*, 428–433. [CrossRef]

16. Ghosh, T.; Sharma, A.; Mondol, S. Optimisation and application of a forensic microsatellite panel to combat Greater-one horned rhinoceros (*Rhinoceros unicornis*) poaching in India. *Forensic Sci. Int. Genet.* **2021**, *52*, 102472. [CrossRef]

17. Meredith, E.P.; Adkins, J.K.; Rodzen, J.A. UrsaPlex: An STR multiplex for forensic identification of North American black bear (*Ursus americanus*). *Forensic Sci. Int. Genet.* **2020**, *44*, 102161. [CrossRef]

18. Dawnay, N.; Ogden, R.; Thorpe, R.S.; Pope, L.C.; Dawson, D.A.; McEwing, R. A forensic STR profiling system for the Eurasian badger: A framework for developing profiling systems for wildlife species. *Forensic Sci. Int. Genet.* **2008**, *2*, 47–53. [CrossRef]

19. White, N.E.; Dawson, R.; Coghlan, M.L.; Tridico, S.R.; Mawson, P.R.; Haile, J.; Bunce, M. Application of STR markers in wildlife forensic casework involving Australian black-cockatoos (*Calyptorhynchus* spp.). *Forensic Sci. Int. Genet.* **2012**, *6*, 664–670. [CrossRef]

20. van Hoppe, M.J.C.; Dy, M.A.V.; van den Einden, M.; Iyenga, A. SkydancerPlex: A novel STR multiplex validated for forensic use in the hen harrier (*Circus cyaneus*). *Forensic Sci. Int. Genet.* **2016**, *22*, 100–109. [CrossRef]

21. Ciavaglia, S.; Linacre, A. OzPythonPlex: An optimised forensic STR multiplex assay set for the Australasian carpet python (*Morelia spilota*). *Forensic Sci. Int. Genet.* **2018**, *34*, 231–248. [CrossRef] [PubMed]

22. Biello, R.; Zampiglia, M.; Corti, C.; Deli, G.; Biaggini, M.; Crestanello, B.; Delaugerre, M.; Di Tizio, L.; Francesco, L.L.; Stefano, C.; et al. Mapping the geographic origin of captive and confiscated Hermann's tortoises: A genetic toolkit for conservation and forensic analyses. *Forensic Sci. Int. Genet.* **2021**, *51*, 102447. [CrossRef]

23. Kimpton, C.; Fisher, D.; Watson, S.; Adams, M.; Urquhart, A.; Lygo, J.; Gill, P. Evaluation of an automated DNA profiling system employing multiplex amplification of four tetrameric STR loci. *Int. J. Leg. Med.* **1994**, *106*, 302–311. [CrossRef]

24. Sparkes, R.; Kimpton, C.; Gilbard, S.; Carne, P.; Andersen, J.; Oldroyd, N.; Thomas, D.; Urquhart, A.; Gill, P. The validation of a 7-locus multiplex STR test for use in forensic casework. (II), Artefacts, casework studies and success rates. *Int. J. Legal Med.* **1996**, *109*, 195–204. [CrossRef] [PubMed]

25. Lee, J.C.-I.; Tseng, B.; Ho, B.-C.; Linacre, A. pSTR Finder: A rapid method to discover polymorphic short tandem repeat markers from whole-genome sequences. *Investig. Genet.* **2015**, *6*, 10. [CrossRef] [PubMed]

26. Linacre, A. Wildlife crime in Australia. *Emerg. Top. Life Sci.* **2021**. [CrossRef] [PubMed]

27. Alacs, E.; Georges, A. Wildlife across our borders: A review of the illegal trade in Australia. *Aust. J. Forensic Sci.* **2008**, *40*, 147–160. [CrossRef]

28. Linacre, A.; Ciavaglia, S.A. Wildlife Forensic Science. In *Handbook of Forensic Genetics*; Amorin, A., Budowle, B., Eds.; World Scientific Publishing: London, UK, 2017; pp. 449–772.

29. Wilson-Wilde, L.; Norman, J.; Robertson, J.; Sarre, S.; Georges, A. Current issues in species identification for forensic science and the validity of using the cytochrome oxidase I (COI) gene. *Forensic Sci. Med. Pathol.* **2010**, *6*, 233–241. [CrossRef]

30. Johnson, R.N.; Wilson-Wilde, L.; Linacre, A. Current and future directions of DNA in wildlife forensic science. *Forensic Sci. Int. Genet.* **2014**, *10*, 1–11. [CrossRef]

31. Zhang, H.; Ades, G.; Miller, M.P.; Yang, F.; Lai, K.-W.; Fischer, G.A. Genetic identification of African pangolins and their origin in illegal trade. *Glob. Ecol. Conserv.* **2020**, *23*, e01119. [CrossRef]

32. Ewart, K.M.; Frankham, G.J.; McEwing, R.; Webster, L.M.; Ciavaglia, S.A.; Linacre, A.M.; The, D.T.; Ovouthan, K.; Johnson, R.N. An internationally standardized species identification test for use on suspected seized rhinoceros horn in the illegal wildlife trade. *Forensic Sci. Int. Genet.* **2018**, *32*, 33–39. [CrossRef]

33. Coghlan, M.L.; White, N.E.; Parkinson, L.; Haile, J.; Spencer, P.B.; Bunce, M. Egg forensics: An appraisal of DNA sequencing to assist in species identification of illegally smuggled eggs. *Forensic Sci. Int. Genet.* **2012**, *6*, 268–273. [CrossRef]

34. Meganathan, P.R.; Dubey, B.; Jogayya, K.N.; Whitaker, N.; Haque, I. A novel multiplex PCR assay for the identification of Indian crocodiles. *Mol. Ecol. Resour.* **2010**, *10*, 744–747. [CrossRef]

35. Lee, J.C.-I.; Tsai, L.-C.; Liao, S.-P.; Linacre, A.; Hsieh, H.-M. Species identification using the cytochrome b gene of commercial turtle shells. *Forensic Sci. Int. Genet.* **2009**, *3*, 67–73. [CrossRef]

36. Byard, R.W. Traditional medicines and species extinction: Another side to forensic wildlife investigation. *Forensic Sci. Med. Pathol.* **2016**, *12*, 125–127. [CrossRef]

37. Coghlan, M.L.; Haile, J.; Houston, J.; Murray, D.C.; White, N.E.; Moolhuijzen, P.; Bellgard, M.I.; Bunce, M. Deep Sequencing of Plant and Animal DNA Contained within Traditional Chinese Medicines Reveals Legality Issues and Health Safety Concerns. *PLoS Genet.* **2012**, *8*, e1002657. [CrossRef]

38. Sellar, J. Illegal Trade and the Convention on International Trade in Endangered Wild Species of Fauna and Flora. In *Forensic Science in Wildlife Investigations*; Linacre, A., Ed.; CRC Press, Taylor Francis Group: Boca Raton, FL, USA, 2009; pp. 11–18.

39. Linacre, A.; Tobe, S. *Wildlife DNA Analysis: Applications in Forensic Science*; John Wiley & Co.: Chichester, UK, 2013.

40. Ewart, K.M.; Lightson, A.L.; Sitam, F.T.; Rovie-Ryan, J.J.; Mather, N.; McEwing, R. Expediting the sampling, decalcification, and forensic DNA analysis of large elephant ivory seizures to aid investigations and prosecutions. *Forensic Sci. Int. Genet.* **2020**, *44*, 102187. [CrossRef]

41. Mwale, M.; Dalton, D.L.; Jansen, R.; De Bruyn, M.; Pietersen, D.; Mokgokong, P.S.; Kotzé, A. Forensic application of DNA barcoding for identification of illegally traded African pangolin scales. *Genome* **2017**, *60*, 272–284. [CrossRef]

42. Hsieh, H.-M.; Lee, J.C.-I.; Wu, J.-H.; Chen, C.-A.; Chen, Y.-J.; Wang, G.-B.; Chin, S.-C.; Wang, L.-C.; Linacre, A.; Tsai, L.-C. Establishing the pangolin mitochondrial D-loop sequences from the confiscated scales. *Forensic Sci. Int. Genet.* **2011**, *5*, 303–307. [CrossRef]

43. Amorim, A.; Pereira, F.; Alves, C.; García, O. Species assignment in forensics and the challenge of hybrids. *Forensic Sci. Int. Genet.* **2020**, *48*, 102333. [CrossRef]

44. González, B.A.; Agapito, A.M.; Novoa-Muñoz, F.; Vianna, J.; Johnson, W.E.; Marín, J.C. Utility of genetic variation in coat color genes to distinguish wild, domestic and hybrid South American camelids for forensic and judicial applications. *Forensic Sci. Int. Genet.* **2020**, *45*, 102226. [CrossRef] [PubMed]

45. Kocher, T.D.; Thomas, W.K.; Meyer, A.; Edwards, S.V.; Paabo, S.; Villablanca, F.X.; Wilson, A.C. Dynamics of mitochondrial DNA evolution in animals: Amplification and sequencing with conserved primers. *Proc. Natl. Acad. Sci. USA* **1989**, *86*, 6196–6200. [CrossRef] [PubMed]

46. Hsieh, H.-M.; Chiang, H.-L.; Tsai, L.-C.; Lai, S.-Y.; Huang, N.-E.; Linacre, A.; Lee, J.C.-I. Cytochrome b gene for species identification of the conservation animals. *Forensic Sci. Int.* **2001**, *122*, 7–18. [CrossRef]

47. Lee, J.C.-I.; Tsai, L.-C.; Yang, C.-Y.; Liu, C.-L.; Huang, L.-H.; Linacre, A.; Hsieh, H.-M. DNA profiling of Shahtoosh. *Electrophoresis* **2006**, *27*, 3359–3362. [CrossRef] [PubMed]

48. Hebert, P.D.N.; Gregory, T.R. The Promise of DNA Barcoding for Taxonomy. *Syst. Biol.* **2005**, *54*, 852–859. [CrossRef]

49. Hebert, P.D.N.; Stoeckle, M.Y.; Zemlak, T.S.; Francis, C.M. Identification of Birds through DNA Barcodes. *PLoS Biol.* **2004**, *2*, e312. [CrossRef]

50. Ratnasingham, S.; Hebert, P.D.N. BARCODING: Bold: The Barcode of Life Data System (http://www.barcodinglife.org). *Mol. Ecol. Notes* **2007**, *7*, 355–364. [CrossRef]

51. Ball, S.L.; Hebert, P.D.N.; Burian, S.K.; Webb, J.M. Biological identifications of mayflies (Ephemeroptera) using DNA barcodes. *J. North Am. Benthol. Soc.* **2005**, *24*, 508. [CrossRef]

52. Hajibabaei, M.; Janzen, D.H.; Burns, J.M.; Hallwachs, W.; Hebert, P.D.N. DNA barcodes distinguish species of tropical Lepidoptera. *Proc. Natl. Acad. Sci. USA* **2006**, *103*, 968–971. [CrossRef]

53. Nelson, K.; Melton, T. Forensic Mitochondrial DNA Analysis of 116 Casework Skeletal Samples. *J. Forensic Sci.* **2007**, *52*, 557–561. [CrossRef]

54. Tobe, S.S.; Kitchener, A.C.; Linacre, A.M.T. Reconstructing Mammalian Phylogenies: A Detailed Comparison of the Cytochrome b and Cytochrome Oxidase Subunit I Mitochondrial Genes. *PLoS ONE* **2010**, *5*, e14156. [CrossRef]

55. Ahlers, N.; Creecy, J.; Frankham, G.; Johnson, R.N.; Kotze, A.; Linacre, A.; McEwing, R.; Mwale, M.; Rovie-Ryan, J.J.; Sitam, F.; et al. 'ForCyt' DNA database of wildlife species. *Forensic Sci. Int. Genet. Suppl. Series* **2017**, *6*, e466–e468. [CrossRef]

56. Pentinsaari, M.; Ratnasingham, S.; Miller, S.E.; Hebert, P.D.N. BOLD and GenBank revisited—Do identification errors arise in the lab or in the sequence libraries? *PLoS ONE* **2020**, *15*, e0231814. [CrossRef]

57. Kitpipit, T.; Tobe, S.S.; Kitchener, A.C.; Gill, P.; Linacre, A. The development and validation of a single SNaPshot multiplex for tiger species and subspecies identification—Implications for forensic purposes. *Forensic Sci. Int. Genet.* **2012**, *6*, 250–257. [CrossRef]

58. Santos, C.; Fondevila, M.; Ballard, D.; Banemann, R.; Bento, A.; Børsting, C.; Branicki, W.; Brisighelli, F.; Burrington, M.; Capal, T.; et al. Forensic ancestry analysis with two capillary electrophoresis ancestry informative marker (AIM) panels: Results of a collaborative EDNAP exercise. *Forensic Sci. Int. Genet.* **2015**, *19*, 56–67. [CrossRef]

59. Gettings, K.B.; Lai, R.; Johnson, J.L.; Peck, M.A.; Hart, J.A.; Gordish-Dressman, H.; Schanfield, M.S.; Podini, D.S. A 50-SNP assay for biogeographic ancestry and phenotype prediction in the U.S. population. *Forensic Sci. Int. Genet.* **2014**, *8*, 101–108. [CrossRef]

60. De La Puente, M.; Santos, C.; Fondevila, M.; Manzo, L.; Carracedo, Á.; Lareu, M.; Phillips, C. The Global AIMs Nano set: A 31-plex SNaPshot assay of ancestry-informative SNPs. *Forensic Sci. Int. Genet.* **2016**, *22*, 81–88. [CrossRef]

61. Kitpipit, T.; Thongjued, K.; Penchart, K.; Ouithavon, K.; Chotigeat, W. Mini-SNaPshot multiplex assays authenticate elephant ivory and simultaneously identify the species origin. *Forensic Sci Int Genet.* **2017**, *27*, 106–115. [CrossRef]

62. Tobe, S.S.; Linacre, A.M.T. A multiplex assay to identify 18 European mammal species from mixtures using the mitochondrial cytochrome b gene. *Electrophoresis* **2008**, *29*, 340–347. [CrossRef]

63. Zhang, J.; Wang, M.; Qi, X.; Shi, L.; Zhang, J.; Zhang, X.; Yang, T.; Ren, J.; Liu, F.; Zhang, G.; et al. Predicting the postmortem interval of burial cadavers based on microbial community succession. *Forensic Sci. Int. Genet.* **2021**, *52*, 8. [CrossRef]

64. Forger, L.V.; Woolf, M.S.; Simmons, T.L.; Swall, J.L.; Singh, B. A eukaryotic community succession based method for postmortem interval (PMI) estimation of decomposing porcine remains. *Forensic Sci. Int.* **2019**, *302*, 109838. [CrossRef] [PubMed]

65. López, C.D.; González, D.M.; Haas, C.; Vidaki, A.; Kayser, M. Microbiome-based body site of origin classification of forensically relevant blood traces. *Forensic Sci. Int. Genet.* **2020**, *47*, 102280. [CrossRef] [PubMed]

66. Williams, D.W.; Gibson, G. Classification of individuals and the potential to detect sexual contact using the microbiome of the pubic region. *Forensic Sci. Int. Genet.* **2019**, *41*, 177–187. [CrossRef] [PubMed]

67. Young, J.; Linacre, A. Massively parallel sequencing is unlocking the potential of environmental trace evidence. *Forensic Sci. Int. Genet.* **2021**, *50*, 102393. [CrossRef]

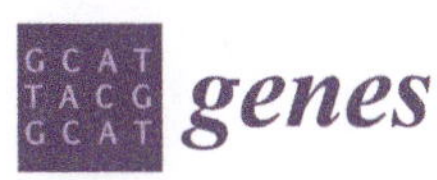

Review

DNA Transfer in Forensic Science: Recent Progress towards Meeting Challenges

Roland A. H. van Oorschot [1,2,*], Georgina E. Meakin [3,4], Bas Kokshoorn [5,6], Mariya Goray [7] and Bianca Szkuta [8]

[1] Office of the Chief Forensic Scientist, Victoria Police Forensic Services Department, Macleod, VIC 3085, Australia
[2] School of Molecular Sciences, La Trobe University, Bundoora, VIC 3086, Australia
[3] Centre for Forensic Science, University of Technology Sydney, Ultimo, NSW 2007, Australia; georgina.meakin@uts.edu.au
[4] Centre for the Forensic Sciences, Department of Security and Crime Science, University College London, London WC1H 9EZ, UK
[5] Netherlands Forensic Institute, 2497 GB The Hague, The Netherlands; b.kokshoorn@nfi.nl
[6] Faculty of Technology, Amsterdam University of Applied Sciences, 1097 DZ Amsterdam, The Netherlands
[7] College of Science and Engineering, Flinders University, Adelaide, SA 5042, Australia; mariya.goray@flinders.edu.au
[8] School of Life and Environmental Sciences, Deakin University, Geelong, VIC 3220, Australia; b.szkuta@deakin.edu.au
* Correspondence: roland.vanoorschot@police.vic.gov.au

Abstract: Understanding the factors that may impact the transfer, persistence, prevalence and recovery of DNA (DNA-TPPR), and the availability of data to assign probabilities to DNA quantities and profile types being obtained given particular scenarios and circumstances, is paramount when performing, and giving guidance on, evaluations of DNA findings given activity level propositions (activity level evaluations). In late 2018 and early 2019, three major reviews were published on aspects of DNA-TPPR, with each advocating the need for further research and other actions to support the conduct of DNA-related activity level evaluations. Here, we look at how challenges are being met, primarily by providing a synopsis of DNA-TPPR-related articles published since the conduct of these reviews and briefly exploring some of the actions taken by industry stakeholders towards addressing identified gaps. Much has been carried out in recent years, and efforts continue, to meet the challenges to continually improve the capacity of forensic experts to provide the guidance sought by the judiciary with respect to the transfer of DNA.

Keywords: DNA transfer; DNA persistence; DNA prevalence; DNA recovery; activity level evaluation; forensic science

Citation: van Oorschot, R.A.H.; Meakin, G.E.; Kokshoorn, B.; Goray, M.; Szkuta, B. DNA Transfer in Forensic Science: Recent Progress towards Meeting Challenges. *Genes* **2021**, *12*, 1766. https://doi.org/10.3390/genes12111766

Academic Editor: Antonio Amorim

Received: 12 October 2021
Accepted: 4 November 2021
Published: 7 November 2021

Publisher's Note: MDPI stays neutral with regard to jurisdictional claims in published maps and institutional affiliations.

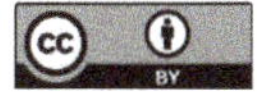

1. Introduction

Awareness and understanding of the transfer, persistence, prevalence and recovery of DNA (DNA-TPPR), as well as access to relevant data on these issues to support probability assignments, have become increasingly relevant to forensic scientists to assist with investigations of alleged criminal activities and to provide guidance to the triers of fact [1,2]. The desire to utilise DNA profiling methodologies is due to the high discrimination power of the profiles they are able to generate, and thus, their ability to exculpate or inculpate an individual [3–5]. Further, the sensitivity of these methods allows profiles to be generated from minute quantities of biological material [6–8]. Knowing that profiles can be readily collected from objects that have been touched by hands [9,10] or worn [11–14] significantly broadened the scope of objects and surfaces that are targeted for DNA sampling to assist investigations [15]. Such items may include weapons, tools, containers, bags, bottles, personal items, appliances, computers, phones, tie-wraps, ropes and cords, clothing items, glasses, tape, documents, handles, steering wheels, chairs, tables and benches, windows, cartridge cases, circuit boards, stones, etc., that may be associated with any type of criminal activity including robberies, sex offences, assaults, homicides, drug manufacturing and trafficking, and a range of other indictable offences as well as items associated with missing persons cases [6,15–23]. Within many jurisdictions, samples collected from these types of items form a substantial portion of the samples collected for profiling and are heavily relied on to assist investigations [16,20,24].

However, two elements have meant that increasingly, the question of relevance to the trier of fact has shifted from who the DNA is from, to how and when it got to the area from which it was collected [2,25–27]. The first is the knowledge that DNA can not only be deposited by a person contacting an object but can also be readily transferred by various other modes, including (a) from person to person to object; (b) from person to object to person to object; (c) from person to object to object [1,9]. The second is that many of the samples collected from touched objects and worn clothing [13,28–30], as well as samples of small stains of various biological materials such as blood, saliva and semen collected from various surfaces with pre-existing levels of background DNA [31–34], provide mixed profiles. Figure 1 depicts a general overview of the many potential sources (including who, what, when and how) that may contribute to a recovered sample and the DNA profile generated from it, as well as the many factors that could potentially impact the levels of transfer, persistence, prevalence and recovery of these contributions.

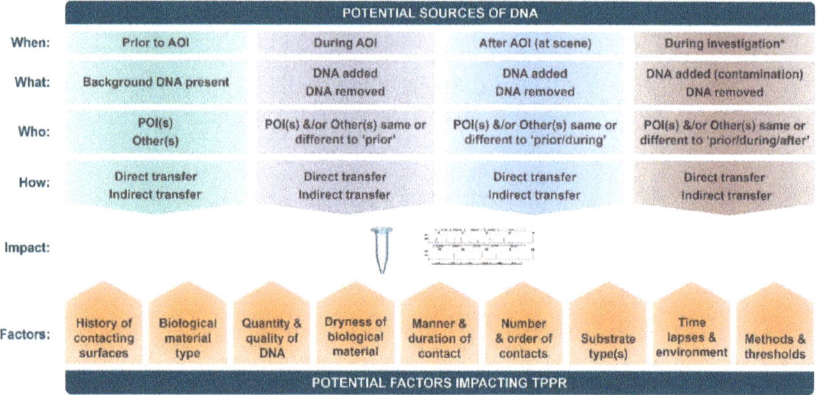

Figure 1. Potential sources contributing to, and factors impacting, the sample recovered and the DNA profile generated from it. The variable shading within each box represents that each source and factor can vary in relative contribution and impact. AOI = Action of Interest. POI = Person of Interest. * Apart from contamination of evidence by DNA from investigators and their associates during the investigation process, detection of AOI-related DNA could be due to cross contamination with another area of the same item or other item of the same case due to direct transfer events (for example, within packaging) or indirect transfer events (for example, via reused, uncleaned, or inadequately cleaned, tools, bench and/or gloves).

To provide guidance on the likelihood of DNA findings given competing propositions of interest with respect to the activities performed requires a thorough understanding of the factors and variables impacting DNA-TPPR, the availability of data in order to generate probabilities of particular types of profiles given specific sets of circumstances, and the knowledge of potential impact of the methodologies, processes and thresholds applied to generate the available data. In late 2018 and early 2019, three major reviews were published on elements of these, with each advocating the need for further research and other actions to support the conduct of DNA-related activity level evaluations. Firstly, van Oorschot et al. [1] conducted a review of the state of play with respect to DNA transfer in forensic science and highlighted areas requiring further attention. This was soon followed by two additional major reviews relating to DNA-TPPR: Burrill et al. [35] and Gosch and Courts [36].

In their review, van Oorschot et al. [1] provided a brief history of aspects relating to the transfer of DNA, indicated why understanding aspects of DNA-TPPR and availability of related data are important to the forensic and legal fraternity, plus gave a detailed summary of the many aspects pertaining to the transfer of DNA within the forensic science context. These included:

- What was known about DNA-TPPR at the time, including in relation to:
  - Potential means and complexities of transfer.
  - Core factors impacting transfer.
  - Prevalence and origins of non-self DNA on various surfaces.
  - Persistence of deposited DNA in various circumstances.
  - Potential relevance of activities performed between activities of interest.
  - Impact of using different recovery and processing methodologies on quantities of DNA retrieved and the profile types generated.

- Consideration of associated elements, including in relation to:
  - Contamination risks.
  - Type of sources of information, and tools, to utilise when addressing activity level questions.
  - Readiness of those addressing transfer-related questions, and the adequacies of training, competency/proficiency testing and accreditation programs.
  - Means of creating, gathering, sharing and using data.

The authors also highlighted several areas that could benefit from more attention/investment, including:

- Research to better understand the effect of the many variables impacting DNA-TPPR, and build the data necessary to facilitate more accurate probability assignments of generating particular types of profiles in a wide range of relevant casework situations. Specific areas of research include:
  - Impacts of physical and chemical differences of contacting surfaces, including those relating to their topography, chemical compositions, fibre type, weave, thickness, electrical charge, etc.
  - Assessment of transfer of primary touch deposits after long time periods.
  - Drying patterns and transfer rates of various relevant biological materials, such as semen, and the impact different substrates may have.
  - Effect of duration and/or frequency of use on the accumulation of DNA, and subsequent changes to profiles, for objects of different types and substrates.
  - Awareness of general levels of background DNA (including quantity, origin and quality), and the impact of factors such as a person's shedder status and frequency of item use.
  - Understanding of the influence of any background DNA on the interpretation of mixed profiles.
  - Acquisition of more accurate probabilities of finding non-self DNA, and of the different relative mixture proportions within a deposit made by a hand, by collecting more samples from random individuals in a wide range of situations.
  - Prevalence of non-self DNA on the bodies of both children and adults.
  - The quantity and quality of DNA from donors and other individuals in fingernail samples after various known contact activities; acquisition of non-self DNA during regular social interaction; indirect transfer by occupying another person's space for a certain amount of time; the effects of personal habits; and an individual's shedder status, on detection of donor and foreign DNA.
  - Awareness of contributors to the non-self component of DNA retrieved from personal objects and occupied spaces.

  ○ Persistence of the temporary user of an item after use by the original owner has resumed.

  ○ Probabilities of detection, and relative contribution, of individuals to profiles retrieved from a wider array of shared objects and surfaces within confined shared spaces (e.g., homes, offices, cars) and public spaces, given known histories.

  ○ Impact of handwashing on the amount and quality of DNA deposited from hands, including factors such as: different methods of washing hands, the natural accumulation of DNA on hands post-handwashing, and the different personal habits of individuals, and their effect on the accumulation of self and non-self DNA on hands.

  ○ Impacts of genetic factors and various non-genetic factors (e.g., behavioural traits, health situation, and/or environmental conditions), and their potential interactions, on shedder status, as well as identifying and understanding their underlying properties.

  ○ Understanding the impact of the absence/presence of the types of information one relies on that may be gathered by the crime scene attending officer, and to consider means of improving the gathering of relevant information in an efficient and consistent manner.

  ○ Studies to help establish more accurate probability distributions for relevant factors impacting transfer.

  ○ Determining the accuracy of 'experiential' assessment (i.e., based on experiences) relative to 'experimental' assessment (i.e., based on data from experiments).

- Enhancement of access to relevant data, including specific areas such as:

  ○ Availability of a quality controlled open access depository of relevant DNA-TPPR information that can be easily mined for various purposes.

  ○ Inclusion of relevant details of the methods, protocols and thresholds applied to generate the DNA-TPPR data presented.

- Recognition of DNA activity-associated expertise to be distinct and supported by dedicated training, competency testing, authorisation and ongoing proficiency testing.

In the review by Gosch and Courts [36], an excellent summary of the existing literature as of October 2018 was also provided with respect to our knowledge of the core variables influencing DNA-TPPR. They highlighted the limitations of much of the DNA transfer-related research studies conducted to date in terms of:

- Underestimating the complexities and multitude of factors needing to be considered.
- Recording relevant information to allow comparisons and appropriate use.
- Identifying the relative weight of different impacting variables.

Regarding the latter, they pointed out that factors such as casework-relevant persistence scenarios or the impact of inter-individual differences in handling an item are among those receiving limited attention. The authors further highlighted deficiencies in overall research study designs and documentation, lamented on the lack of agreement on the DNA analysis output parameters most appropriate to be utilised when comparing studies and addressing activity level questions and standardisation of recording these, and indicated a disequilibrium in the degree of studies relating to pertinent factors. Furthermore, they described and launched a new database ('DNA-TrAC') [37] to assist the accessibility of relevant DNA-TPPR information to aid addressing of activity level questions.

Around the same period, Burrill et al. [35] also provided a review of published research on aspects of transfer and persistence relating to 'touch DNA', including on:

- How much DNA can be recovered from handled items.
- Whether trace DNA can be detected under certain scenarios including varying degrees of indirect transfer.
- Factors which may influence these results.

Whilst the authors pointed to similar issues raised by the two above mentioned reviews, they also explored deeper the current knowledge in relation to the composition of touch deposits. They concluded that "Further exploration of relative contributions of hand-endogenous and -exogenous DNA contributions to touch deposits is warranted, along with more specific localization of DNA sources inside and outside a cellular infrastructure", and that "A more comprehensive picture of where the DNA in 'touch DNA' comes from will provide valuable information to practitioners seeking to utilize touch DNA typing results in a courtroom context, and will contribute to the ongoing effort to understand and predict the circumstances of DNA transfer in a forensic context more reliably".

A year prior to the three reviews mentioned above, in their Appendix B, Taylor et al. [38] identified 17 study areas that, if acted on, would improve our knowledge base and assist evaluations of evidence in light of propositions that suggest differing DNA transfer mechanisms. These specific studies related to areas including: efficiencies of different extraction methods, substrate considerations, environmental conditions, persistence of DNA in various situations, shedder consistency and shedder propensity determination, duration and manner of handling/contact, objects used habitually, accumulation of DNA from multiple contacts, levels of primary user's DNA on regularly used items, levels of background DNA, and value of profile degradation information.

Collectively, the aforementioned three reviews [1,35,36] and the research paper by Taylor et al. [38] acknowledged the importance of DNA-TPPR in investigations of criminal activity, highlighted the many limitations in our current knowledge and availability of required data, and provided some guidance on improvement opportunities. In this paper, we assess the extent to which we are meeting these challenges. This is achieved primarily by providing a synopsis of publications relevant to DNA-TPPR that have been published since these reviews. We then reflect on this and some of the actions taken by industry stakeholders in support of addressing identified gaps. Finally, we provide a general conclusion in relation to progress towards improving the guidance that experts are able to provide the courts in relation to the transfer of DNA.

2. Identification and Reporting of Recent DNA-TPPR Publications

Identification of recent relevant publications was achieved through the conduct of a systematic review. The search was conducted on 30 March 2021 for the period 2018 to the present within Scopus and Web of Science. Applying the Preferred Reporting Items for Systematic Reviews and Meta-Analyses (PRISMA) guidelines [39]. The search commenced by applying the following:

> TITLE-ABS-KEY ((DNA OR "deoxyribonucleic acid") AND (transfer* OR deposit* OR contact* OR persist* OR prevalen* OR background OR shedder) AND (human OR participant OR donor OR volunteer) AND (forensic* OR crim*)) AND (LIMIT-TO (PUBYEAR, 2021) OR LIMIT-TO (PUBYEAR, 2020) OR LIMIT-TO (PUBYEAR, 2019) OR LIMIT-TO (PUBYEAR, 2018)).

One hundred and forty-four papers were identified for inclusion in the synopsis of relevant publications within the given period presented in Section 3 (Figure 2). As we may not have captured some relevant publications, or inadvertently excluded some from further consideration, we advise those seeking publications relating to specific core topics to conduct additional searches relating to their narrower area of focus.

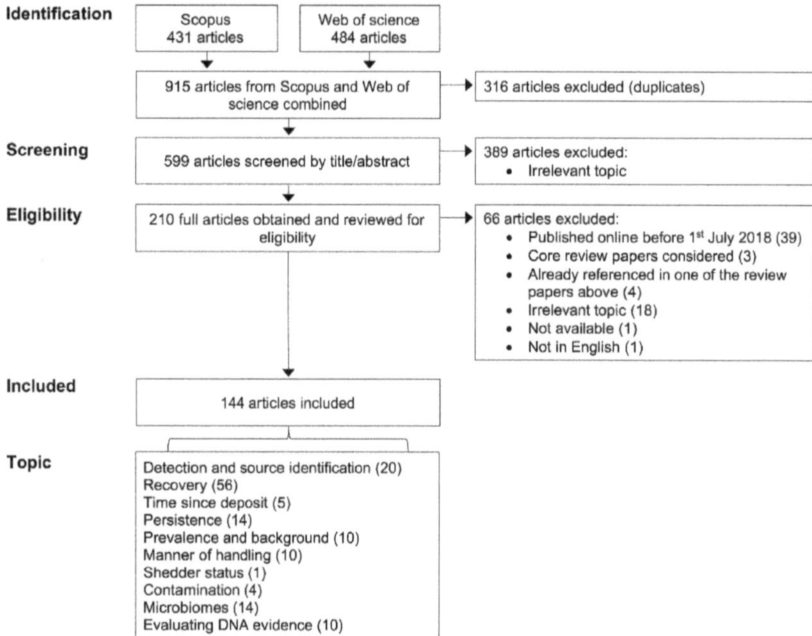

Figure 2. Process and outcome of review to identify articles to be included in synopsis. Topic categorisation of articles was based on their primary area of DNA-TPPR-related focus. Numbers of articles included/excluded are indicated in parentheses after each topic/exclusion criterion.

Based on the primary DNA-TPPR-related focus and content of the 144 included articles, each was assigned to one of the following topic categories: detection and source identification, recovery, time since deposit, persistence, prevalence and background, manner of handling, shedder status, contamination, microbiomes, evaluating DNA evidence. Where a paper was deemed to also contain information of relevance to an additional topic area, this information was also conveyed within the other topic subsection.

A synopsis is provided that gives a general overview of the focus areas and some general findings of the articles reviewed. The articles included in the synopsis were from many different journals, with *Forensic Science International: Genetics* (54) and *Forensic Science International* (23) providing the most articles. The majority of papers focused primarily on various aspects of DNA detection and recovery, with fewer concentrating on various elements of transfer, prevalence and persistence (Figure 2). The degrees of relevance of the publications identified vary, yet each is incorporated and referred to in the synopsis. The scope and depth of some of the presented publications are very limited. Further, some of the experimental designs within the studies conducted have limitations and while some acknowledge this, others do not. However, we have refrained from drawing attention to these and, instead, urge readers to delve fuller into the papers of interest to make their own assessment of such matters.

The reported findings of conducted research are those determined by the authors of the research and not our extrapolations. While in general we concur and/or are supportive of the vast majority of findings, conclusions and recommendations reported in the publications listed, their inclusion does not necessarily imply that we concur, and we do not make systematic comparisons of studies to inform a further judgement. For more details of the experimental designs, methodologies utilised, analyses employed, results obtained, and associated interpretations and discussion of the studies referred to, we recommend that the relevant specified references are consulted.

Several of the reported findings are new and broaden our understanding and/or improve the availability of relevant data and some produce findings verifying existing understandings/knowledge with or without making reference to relevant prior studies. We have chosen not to point out connections to prior studies here, but urge interested parties to consult the details of the publication of interest as well as any others on the relevant topic that were published prior to the period of publications bookending in this review to gain a fuller appreciation of the available knowledge and data. References within the papers of interest listed here and those listed within the aforementioned review articles can be a good start in such situations. Further, we are aware of some interesting and relevant papers that have been published since the cut-off date for inclusion within this review, and thus, are not included here. A selection of these more recent articles will be highlighted in the discussion section.

3. Synopsis of Recent DNA-TPPR-Related Publications

3.1. Detection and Source Identification

Twenty papers were identified that primarily addressed detection of biological sources and/or their identification (Figure 2), plus one additional study that also addressed this issue but was primarily focussed on another topic. Several studies investigated the visualisation and detection of biological materials. In addition to readily visualising biological stains, Yano et al. [40] demonstrated the ability of an acid-free *p*-dimethylaminocinnamaldehyde solution sprayed on glass slides and clothing and irradiated with blue-light-emitting diode light to visualise relatively fresh deposited finger and palm prints on clothing. This study also demonstrated that this technique does not adversely affect STR analyses, thus providing potentially useful methodology to localise areas on items of interest to assist better targeting for sampling. A number of other studies also demonstrated the ability of various treatments to potentially enhance detection of biological materials, including the use of:

- Trypan blue to improve visibility of shed skin flakes collected by adhesive film [41].
- Diamond™ Nucleic Acid Dye (DD) (Promega, Madison, WI, USA) to detect cellular material in lip-prints [42].
- DD to detect DNA on used swabs to potentially assess if further processing for DNA profiling is warranted [43].
- Ethidium Bromide to detect small amounts of DNA on swabs to possibly provide similar pre-screening benefits [44].
- Immunohistochemical staining of skin-expressed proteins to identify exfoliated epidermal cells to screen samples taken from handled/touched objects [45].
- NIR hyperspectral imaging to localise invisible traces of blood, urine and semen on various substrates [46].
- A test based on the click reaction between serum albumin and tetraphenylethene maleimide (TPE-MI) to visualise invisible blood stains (and showing that it may perform better than luminol) [47].
- Fluorescence spectroscopy to localise the presence of saliva stains [48] or detection of saliva on swab samples of human skin that had been licked [49].

Furthermore, Butler et al. [50] compared four methods that have been previously used as presumptive tests for the detection of traces of blood on dark materials, finding that luminol was, overall, the most effective method.

To explore source differences and gain insight into associations with DNA content, Burrill et al. [51] used flow cytometry and microscopic examination to generate granularity, size and nucleic acid fluorescence data of washed and unwashed hands, as well as saliva, nasal and eye wash that could be sources of transferred DNA onto hands. They found that hand rinses consisted mainly of anucleate corneocytes, many of which also stained positive for nucleic acids, and suggested the need for further research on the recovery and analysis of corneocyte DNA, which they report was previously assumed to be negligible.

The potential of a software tool for the automated detection and characterisation of epithelial cells from fingerprints based on fluorescence intensity across the cell surface and size/morphology was demonstrated by Olsen et al. [52]. This study also observed that trace cell populations from certain individuals may have distinct morphological and/or structural properties. The authors pointed out that this technique can, therefore, facilitate investigations into the deposit, transfer, and persistence of both cellular material and DNA in trace biological samples.

Tests for the detection of human PSA and human α-amylase for the identification of seminal fluid and saliva, respectively, in forensic samples are commonly used as presumptive tests in sexual assault-related cases to aid decisions on further testing procedures. It is relevant to know how frequent PSA and amylase are detectable by these tests in vaginal swabs that are void of seminal fluid and saliva. A study by Kishbaugh et al. [53] of 50 vaginal swabs from unique donors over the age of 18 years and relevant history, and a study by Sari et al. [54] of 20 pre-pubescent (3–9 years), 20 post-pubescent (16–45 years) and 20 post-menopausal (50–75 years) females, help fill this knowledge gap, and thus, assist the accuracy of interpretation of immunochromatographic testing results. In addition, a review of current methods of sperm detection, factors affecting sperm detection, and recent advances in sperm detection utilising alternative methodologies is provided by Suttipasit [55].

Traditional identification methods for the nature of the body fluids or tissues present in a sample collectively cater for a narrow range of biological materials tend to require one test per target fluid or tissue and may consume material compromising attaining a DNA profile. New methodologies, especially those utilising mRNA and proteomics approaches, have shown opportunities to identify a wider range of biological materials that may enhance forensic examination capacities. Molecular biology techniques continue to be explored to enhance the capacity to improve source identification. Abbas et al. [56] reported on the development of a protein microarray chip with enhanced fluorescence for sensitive identification of semen and vaginal fluid and pointed to the value of further development of highly sensitive chips for the identification of other biological body fluids. O'Leary and Glynn [57] highlighted the potential of a selection of miRNAs to identify forensically relevant body fluids. Hanson et al. [58], using cSNPs in body fluid-specific mRNA transcripts, demonstrated the ability to identify forensically relevant body fluids and skin, as well as differentiate blood, semen and saliva transcripts from different individuals. Those authors also indicated that, with further development, one may in the future be able to assign body fluids to DNA donors, which, in many instances, may provide additional probative value. Kamanna et al. [59] demonstrated the potential of proteomic analysis, using mass spectrometry-based approaches, MALDI-ToF MS/MS and n-LC-ESI-qToF MS/MS, to identify vaginal fluid and blood from only a few fibres plucked from a microswab used to collect a sample from underneath fingernails. In addition, Watanabe et al. [60] explored the simultaneous analyses of semen-specific methylated (or unmethylated) CpG markers and adjacent single nucleotide polymorphisms. By combining methylation-specific polymerase chain reaction and pyrosequencing technology, the authors developed a method to detect three semen-specific methylated/unmethylated regions that was able to identify semen-derived alleles from mixed stains. The authors suggested that this type of methodology may be a useful approach for genotyping from a mixture of body fluids.

3.2. Recovery

This section includes studies that investigated various aspects of DNA recovery, specifically sampling, storage, extraction, preferential recovery from mixed samples, profiling, and differences in the methodologies employed. Fifty-six papers are reported (Figure 2), along with some others that were primarily included in other topics.

3.2.1. Sampling

Several studies continue to elucidate the ability to generate DNA profiles from samples taken from touched objects [61–64]. Additional studies evaluated means of generating human DNA profiles from traces of biological material left on various items, including hair [65], bricks [66], dogs [67], bite marks in food [68], paper documents [69], eye wear [70], superabsorbent polymer-containing products (commonly found in nappies and sanitary towels) [71], improvised explosive devices [72], rifle magazines [73] and bullet cartridges [74–78]. Further, Gray et al. [79] demonstrated that STR DNA profiles can be generated from human blood found in *Anopheles* mosquitoes, from one or multiple individuals, and that the quality of the profiles declined as the duration between mosquito blood meal and sample collection increased.

The performance of different swabs on the collection and profiling of DNA continues to be explored. When considering touch DNA recovery, two studies compared the performance of different swabs, with each finding that a specific type of swab performed better than others [80,81]. A further study indicated that the use of pieces of absorbing paper moistened with 70% ethanol recovered epithelial cells/touch DNA from various surface types better than a cotton swab moistened with water [82]. In addition, Sherier et al. [83] illustrated the potential benefits of using the microFLOQ® Direct Swab (Copan, Brescia, Italy) for collecting DNA from minute stains, and possibly using it as a pre-screening methodology (i.e., sampling a small portion of a stain for initial screening and testing for expeditious processing) while saving the remainder of the stain for later testing. They also demonstrated that swabbing the centre of stains of blood, semen and saliva provided more DNA and complete profiles than swabbing the edge of stains.

Investigation also continues into the use of adhesives, such as tapes and gels, for DNA sampling. Kanokwongnuwut et al. [84] compared the efficiencies of different types of tape on collecting DNA from fingermarks and the effect of different numbers of applications, illustrating that particular tapes performed better than others and the benefits of ten applications compared to just one or two applications. Damsteeg-van Berkel et al. [85] showed that collection efficiency from textile substrates increased with increasing stubbing force in a concave down increasing function to a threshold depending on the substrate material. Zorbo and Jeuniaux [86] illustrated that DNA profiles can also be generated from cells, particularly those deposited by skin contact, collected using 1:1 tapings that are conventionally used to obtain microtraces of fibres and hairs prior to sampling for DNA from a body or clothing. However, the authors recommended taking additional samples from an area of interest post 1:1 taping using other techniques such as swabbing. Dierig et al. [41] compared DNA yields and profiles of single skin cells recovered from adhesive tape versus processing of 1×1 cm areas of adhesive tape after the adhesive tape had been applied to external areas of T-shirts after a period of wearing and where they had been vigorously grappled for 10 sec to mimic a physical assault. They found the approach of sampling 1×1 cm areas to be superior in regard to DNA yield, profile completeness and identification of the offender profile. Finally, gels have also been shown to be efficient methods for the recovery of DNA from fingermarks [87–90].

A few studies point to the potential benefits of applying different collection methods depending on the type of substrate [91], especially with respect to metal surfaces [80,92]. In addition, Sessa et al. [93] compared three sampling techniques (adhesive tape, cutting out, dry swab) for the detection of touch DNA from wearers and handlers of brassieres, and found no difference in the recovery of the handler's DNA among the three techniques, even though the cutting out technique showed the greatest recovery. However, recovery of the wearer's DNA was best achieved using adhesive tape. Overall, for their sets of samples, use of the dry swab collection method performed worst. However, for the subset of samples where in the experimental design the period of contact was shortest, out of the three techniques, samples collected using the dry swab technique yielded the highest number of handler profiles. The authors also demonstrated that when targeting for foreign DNA, the sample area should be narrowed as much as practicable to the smallest area possible to maximise target DNA recovery.

In addition to its use in visualising areas of cellular deposits, DD has also been used to determine how many cells are required to generate an informative DNA profile, either by direct PCR or conventional DNA profiling methodologies [94]. This study found that, when using direct PCR, ≥ 40 buccal cells collected from a saliva sample by either a swab or tapelift were required, whereas, from a touch sample, ≥ 800 corneocytes collected by swabbing or ≥ 4000 corneocytes collected by tapelift were required. However, more cells were required for the same DNA profile result when samples were processed through a DNA extraction workflow: ≥ 80 buccal cells from a swab and tapelift, ≥ 4000 corneocytes collected by a swab, ≥ 8000 corneocytes collected by a tapelift, illustrating that the use of direct PCR can be more efficient. The authors also concluded that cell-free DNA forms a major component of the DNA collected from touched deposits, and that tapelifting is not as efficient as swabbing in co-collecting this component of the total DNA deposited. Miller et al. [95] and Burrill et al. [96] also provided evidence that extracellular DNA can represent a substantial proportion of total DNA recovered from handled substrates. Additionally, Burrill et al. [96] determined a suitable technique to separate cellular and cell-free fractions of hand deposits (i.e., one that maintains the representative fraction of cell-free DNA at the time of collection) and the best of three methods tested to purify the cell-free DNA for DNA profiling. A separate study by Burrill et al. [97] demonstrated that enhanced lysis methods using a reducing agent and longer incubation may be valuable for the extraction of DNA from corneocytes, which make up the majority of the cellular material left in touch deposits by hands. The authors also showed that the corneocyte DNA is fragmented. The authors suggested that use of methods that extract the DNA from corneocytes more efficiently than standard methodologies, and application of profiling techniques more suitable to fragmented DNA, could enhance the ability to obtain useful profiles from touch DNA samples.

3.2.2. Storage

Three studies investigated the impact of storage conditions on the preservation of DNA in biological materials. Kaur et al. [98] looked at the degradation (using UV–visible spectroscopic profiles) of various types of forensic blood-related casework samples preserved under various conditions and different durations. They found that the preservation techniques had a greater impact on the quality of DNA than the aging of the sample, but not to the degree that STR profiles could not be generated. Badu-Boateng et al. [99] examined various storage conditions to determine the most appropriate means of storing crime scene soil–blood mixed samples prior to analysis at the laboratory, based on DNA quantification, DNA degradation and DNA profile parameters. They found that storage at $-20\ ^{\circ}\text{C}$ was the best for this sample type, followed by room temperature and $4\ ^{\circ}\text{C}$, respectively. Corradini et al. [100] showed that buccal cells collected directly on to FTA mini cards (GE Healthcare) and stored for 11 years still provided good quantities of DNA and good-quality DNA profiles. In addition to these studies, Suttipasit [55] emphasised the need for appropriate long-term specimen preservation in order to be able to take advantage of potential future methodological advances to interrogate samples beyond current abilities.

3.2.3. Extraction

Several studies reported the benefits of using direct PCR methods over processes that include a magnetic bead extraction step for the generation of DNA profiles from touched objects, including Kanokwongnuwut et al. [94]. Dierig et al. [41], comparing different DNA extraction methods, found that direct lysis methods (a Chelex solution method, Casework Direct Kit (Promega, Mannheim, Germany), Investigator Casework GO! Kit (Qiagen, Hilden, Germany)) were more suitable than a magnetic bead-based method (Maxwell RSC Blood DNA Kit (Promega)) for low template traces due to the limited loss of DNA. Meanwhile, de Oliveira Francisco et al. [101] found that the Casework Direct Kit (Promega) was much more efficient for processing touch DNA samples than the DNA IQ™ System (Promega), another magnetic bead-based DNA extraction method.

A couple of studies looked toward the future, considering how we might better understand and improve extraction efficiencies. LeSassier et al. [102] described means of developing artificial fingerprint samples and advocated their use to assist future studies on the efficiencies of various methods of collection and extraction of DNA from fingerprints. Liu et al. [103] summarised the recent development of magnetic solid-phase extraction in forensic science applications, including DNA extraction, and pointed out that modifications of functional materials on the surface of magnetic particles that could lead to potential improvements (e.g., to better cope with negative impacts of some pre-processing tools, such as fingerprint powder and tapes) and broadening of their application (e.g., detection of biomarkers, such as amino acids, peptides, hormones, etc.).

Two studies considered the extraction of non-DNA elements of biological samples for forensic applications. O'Leary and Glynn [57] identified the best of three methods investigated for the extraction of miRNAs from body fluids for the purpose of using miRNAs for body fluid identification. A study to support the potential future application of genetically variable peptide analysis of touched samples for forensic identification [104] considered a workflow for the collection, enrichment and fractionation of DNA and protein in latent fingerprint samples. The authors demonstrated that the workflow provided sufficient DNA and protein from touch samples for further analysis. Further, the authors observed that the quantity and quality of protein remained robust, regardless of fingerprint age, and that the proteomic content of the touch samples was consistent across donors and fingerprint age.

3.2.4. Preferential Recovery from Mixed Samples

Some studies considered the impact of different sampling and pre-sampling methods on preferential recovery of DNA from particular donor(s) in mixed samples. Hayden and Wallin [105], investigating the effectiveness of different methods of sampling from fingernails to minimise the collected amount of endogenous (female) DNA and maximise the amount of exogenous (male) DNA, concluded that their swabbing method did this better than two alternative methods tested. One study compared an automated procedure to a manual procedure for standard differential extraction of sperm-cell fractions, and found that similar levels of semen separation efficiency were achieved for sperm-cell fractions using both automated and manual procedures [106]. Three studies continue to look at novel means of separating sperm cells from other cells to assist the interpretation of DNA profiles generated downstream. These include the application of optical tweezers [107], acoustic differential extraction technologies [108], and capillary zone electrophoresis [109]. Furthermore, using DEPArray™ technology (Menarini Silicon Biosystems, Bologna, Italy), Anslinger et al. [110] demonstrated the ability to obtain complete DNA profiles from isolated single white cells from each of the two or three known contributors to mixed stains. They concluded that this technology opens up new possibilities with respect to mixture deconvolution, especially for mixtures composed of cells of the same type. However, as touch samples can contain a substantial proportion of extracellular DNA, Miller et al. [95] pointed out potential challenges for front-end cell sorting approaches to recovering DNA from touch samples, which necessitate the presence of cells with sufficient amounts of intracellular DNA.

3.2.5. Profiling

Two studies demonstrated improvements in the abilities to generate Y-STR profiles from non-semen sexual assault samples. Henry and Scandrett [111] showed that the Yfiler® Plus kit (Thermo Fisher Scientific, Melbourne, Australia) significantly outperformed AmpFlSTR Yfiler® (Thermo Fisher Scientific) in the ability to generate useful profiles from semen negative sexual assault samples, i.e., swabs that gave negative results to a screening test for acid phosphatase or ABAcard® p30 antigen test (Abacus Diagnostics, West Hills, CA, USA) in combination with the absence of spermatozoa by microscopy, and excluding samples that tested positive for the presence of human salivary amylase using the RSID™ Saliva test (Independent Forensics, Lombard, IL, USA). In contrast, Owers et al. [112] showed that Powerplex® Y23 (Promega, Madison, WI, USA) significantly outperformed

Yfiler (Thermo Fisher Scientific, Waltham, MA, USA) in the quality of profiles generated from vaginal swabs of alleged penetration where no semen was detected.

Two studies also investigated the use of non-traditional DNA profiling systems, specifically field-based systems and Massive Parallel Sequencing (MPS). While rapid field-based DNA identification systems have their benefits, Dawnay et al. [113] illustrated the limitations of the ParaDNA Field Instrument and Intelligence Test Chemistry (LGC) to collect viable DNA samples and produce profiles from the surfaces of the skin, exposed tissue or carrion larvae. The use of MPS in comparison to traditional Capillary Electrophoresis (CE) techniques to generate DNA profiles from real casework samples obtained from semen, saliva, blood, and epithelial material on various surfaces, as well as reference oral swabs, was evaluated by Avila et al. [114]. They found that the biological nature of the samples impacted various relevant MPS sequencing, and base-calling quality metrics associated with producing a DNA profile, not apparent when generating DNA profiles using CE; this was especially so for epithelial samples. The authors advocated for further research on MPS genotyping of forensic casework samples, including evaluation of DNA transfer effects, impact of the substrate or deposition surface for each sample and other aspects of the nature of individual samples.

Interpretation of DNA profiles and mixture deconvolution requires use of software and laboratory-specific interpretation methods. Mortera [115] reviewed the different methods and software available to assist in determining whether or not the DNA of a given individual is present in a sample. The author provided details on a quantitative method that used Bayesian Networks as a computational device for efficiently computing likelihoods. This method also allowed the combination of evidence from multiple samples to make inferences about relationships from DNA mixtures and other more complex scenarios [115]. Furthermore, Buckleton et al. [116] revisited a previously conducted interlaboratory exercise (comprising five mock cases, with each case consisting of an electropherogram file and typed reference profiles from individuals described as victims, consensual partners, or suspects) (NIST MIX13) to re-evaluate DNA mixture interpretation using currently available methods, especially several modern probabilistic genotyping systems. Their analyses demonstrated the benefits of utilising 'probabilistic genotyping' over 'combined probability of inclusion' methodology.

3.2.6. Methodology Differences

In the studies by Szkuta et al. [117] and Szkuta et al. [118] of DNA quantities and profiles generated from samples collected from clothing, and by Goray et al. [119] of DNA quantities and profiles generated from samples collected from items/surfaces within office spaces, similar sets of samples were processed by different laboratories using different suites of processing, from sample collection through to the generation and analyses of DNA. These studies showed that differences in methodologies applied between the laboratories appeared to impact the quantity of DNA recovered and the composition of the profiles produced. When determining probabilities using data from various studies, Gill et al. [120] stressed the need to consider the differences in methodologies used by different studies to generate the available data.

3.3. Time since Deposition

Five studies were identified that considered how one might determine time since deposition (TSD) of biological materials (Figure 2), specifically blood, semen and saliva. Weber and Lednev [121] provided an overview of what is known about the biochemical mechanisms of blood aging, how these are used to determine the age of a bloodstain, the current techniques for bloodstain age determination, emerging spectroscopic techniques and technology, and the limitations of all these methodologies. Stotesbury et al. [122] and Cossette et al. [123] presented further research on using visible absorbance spectroscopy and DNA degradation to explore their use in determining TSD of blood, with the latter publication focusing on the impact of temperature. Bird et al. [124] considered degradation patterns of semen-specific mRNA genes to assist with determining TSD of semen. Meanwhile, Asaghiar and Williams [125] evaluated the use of changes in the expression of a hypoxia-sensitive marker for determining the age of deposited samples of blood, semen and saliva. Each of these studies demonstrated scope for potential use of the methodologies they investigated in TSD determination. They also noted the limitations in the scope of sample types analysed and the accuracy of TSD analyses, and recommended further research. Additionally, Weber and Ladnev [121] pointed out the need of any methodology being considered for use in forensic casework to be validated and that this would require further research into the impacts of environmental and substrate effects.

3.4. Persistence

This section summarises the fourteen papers identified that investigated the persistence of DNA from various biological materials (Figure 2), plus one additional study that also provided comment on persistence but was primarily categorised in another topic. Whilst it is possible to generate DNA STR profiles from a 100 year old semen stain [126] and from fingerprints archived for several years [127], when considering persistence of DNA in fingermarks left at room temperature for up to just one week, Alketbi and Goodwin [128] indicated that the quantity of DNA recovered was not influenced by the duration that the fingermarks were left before sampling, but was influenced by the environmental conditions (temperature and humidity) and type of substrate on which they were deposited.

When investigating the persistence of DNA from blood and keratinocytes deposited on a variety of porous and non-porous substrates, as well as a range of mock exhibits with natural deposits of touch DNA and saliva, under various environmental conditions (indoor temperature controlled, indoors ambient temperature, outdoors forest area in Singapore where rainfall is abundant and relative humidity is high) for a duration up to 85 weeks, Lee et al. [129] found that degradation and persistence of DNA are highly dependent on the environment. DNA on articles left outdoors degraded rapidly, but most samples collected from the items kept within indoor environments were less affected and provided good profiles for long periods after deposition, similar to trends observed in studies performed in temperate countries.

Several studies investigated the persistence of DNA on surfaces of the body (skin, beneath fingernails and hands) when immersed or washed in water under varying conditions. Meixner et al. [130] found that DNA profiles can still be generated from blood stains and 'touch' deposits on skin specimens after several days of being immersed in water (cold, room-temperature or warm water as well as in a stream and a pond). The duration of persistence was dependent on the temperature and aquatic environment and was longest when immersed in cold water. Hayden and Wallin [105] demonstrated that DNA can remain under fingernails (female fingernail donor's consensual partner) and on the skin (male sweat donor's consensual partner) after showering. While Romero-García et al. [131] noted that samples taken from towels used once to dry hands immediately after having washed them with neutral pH soap only provided partial profiles of the person drying their hands. This was the case both after the individual's hand performed various daily activities and in separate tests where individuals had held hands with someone else for 5 min prior to washing their hands.

Other studies looked at the persistence of DNA and biological fluids on various non-porous and porous items after cleaning or washing. Helmus et al. [132] investigated whether DNA traces (blood, saliva, epithelial cells) on different objects (knives, plates, glasses, and plastic lids) can persist on the surface despite cleaning by different methods (such as washing by hand or use of a dishwasher). They found that small deposits of biological material often still provided sufficient DNA to generate full profiles after the item they were on was rinsed or washed by hand, while profiles were not able to be generated after cleaning in a dishwasher. Further studies showed that sufficient DNA for STR profiling could be recovered from cuttings of semen stains on polyester and/or cotton fabric after washing, with the amount of DNA dependent on the type of washing applied [133–135]. Noël et al. [133] showed that this was possible even after multiple washings, and that more DNA was recovered from cuttings than swabbing of stained cotton bedsheets. Both Noël et al. [133] and Karadayi et al. [134] also showed that the washed stains were able to be visually detected using a light source and provided positive prostate-specific antigen test results. Similarly, Hofmann et al. [136] showed that washed blood stains can generally also be detected using luminol, but the quality of the bloodstains is dependent on a number of factors including the type of washing machine, the washing temperature, the filling degree of the washing machine, and the drying conditions of the blood stain (temperature, duration).

To provide a dataset that may help guide sample targeting and prioritisation, as well as manage expectations of stakeholders regarding observing positive or negative results, Fonneløp et al. [137] performed a retrospective study on the transfer, persistence and recovery of sperm (from internal vaginal swabs, external vaginal swabs, rectal swabs, oral swabs and skin surfaces) and epithelial cells (from external genital swabs, hand swabs, skin swabs, penile swabs, internal vaginal swabs, rectal swabs and oral swabs) collected in sexual assault casework. The samples collected from different areas of the skin to assess the presence of the person of interest (POI)-derived epithelial DNA included face, lips and around the mouth, neck/throat, breast/chest, arm, leg, seat, thigh, rest of body. The authors found that sperm cells had the highest persistence rate in internal vaginal swabs, and were detected up to 72 h post assault, but the majority of the positive samples (i.e., case specific POI DNA profile detected) were collected within 48 h. Analysis of skin and penile swabs demonstrated the persistence of case-specific POI DNA from epithelial cells up to 48 h, and the majority of positive samples were within 24 h. The authors also found that POI-derived epithelial cells were not detected in external genital swabs when collected beyond 12 h post assault.

In addition to DNA, the persistence of mRNA and miRNA in laundered or cleaned biological fluid stains has also been investigated. Mayes et al. [138] showed that mRNA and miRNA markers were able to detect blood and semen from stains exposed to various laundering conditions. They also tested blood and semen stains exposed to various environmental conditions relating to temperature, humidity and light for six months, and found that mRNA targets were observed through six months for some conditions but undetectable after 30 days for other conditions, whereas their miRNA targets persisted under all test conditions for the duration of the study. Furthermore, when investigating the level of blood-derived DNA and miRNA inside firearm barrels after cleaning with DNA-ExitusPlus™ (AppliChem GmbH, Darmstadt, Germany), Schyma et al. [139] found that while the DNA had been removed, the blood-specific miRNA was still detectable.

3.5. Prevalence and Background

This section summarises the ten papers identified that investigated the prevalence of DNA and presence of background DNA (Figure 2), plus one additional study that also provided comment on this subject matter but was primarily categorised in another topic. The prevalence of DNA from drivers, passengers and other individuals on a wide range of locations within vehicles driven regularly by one individual has been explored in three studies [140–142]. These studies found that DNA was able to be collected from all targeted sites, and yields and profile compositions varied between sites, with relatively higher yields retrieved from steering wheels and seats. The authors found that the driver was always observed as a contributor in DNA profiles from sites on the driver's side, in most instances being the sole or a major contributor, and the driver was also observed as a sole or a major contributor at several sites on the passenger side. They also found that DNA profiles of known recent passengers, close associates of the driver, and unknown individuals were observed on many of the sites on both the passenger and driver sides.

The prevalence of DNA from users in an office space was considered by Goray et al. [119]. They investigated the extent to which DNA, left by a temporary user of the office space that had been occupied by a regular user for an extended period, is detectable when the duration of their temporary occupancy and their general activities are known, as well as how readily the DNA of the regular user is still detectable after a known period of occupancy by another person. From samples collected from several items/surfaces within single use office spaces that had been used temporarily by another occupant for 2.5–7 h, the authors found that sufficient DNA for profiling was recovered from nearly all areas sampled. They found that the regular user of the office space was the major or majority contributor (as defined by the authors) to profiles from most items within the space, even after temporary use by another person. It was reported that detectability of the temporary occupier varied among offices and items tested, and whilst the temporary occupier was not observed on all items they touched, in most instances when detected, it was known that they had touched the surface at some stage. The authors also observed profiles from other individuals, including colleagues, family members and unknowns, that were present on several items, mostly as minor contributors.

The study by Szkuta et al. [143] considered background levels of DNA on common entry points to homes (rarely contacted external and internal windowsills and edges, and frequently contacted entrance door handles) occupied by known individuals with some general knowledge on the history of use. They found that interpretable DNA profiles were able to be generated from nearly all door handles (all mixed profiles) and internal windowsills and edges (mostly mixed profiles), but the majority of external windowsills and edges yielded limited to no DNA profile information. The authors reported that the individuals living in the house tended to be main contributors to the profiles, and that the last person to make contact with a door handle was observed as a contributor in most but not all profiles. The authors also observed unknown contributors in the profiles of many of the door handle, internal windowsill and edge samples, and in most situations, but not all, they were a minor contributor.

The study by Albani et al. [144] investigated the extent of male-derived DNA presence on unused feminine sanitary products (tampons, pads, liners). The authors postulated, but did not test, that if such DNA was present, it could possibly be transferred onto the wearer and subsequently be detected in samples taken from intimate areas during a medical examination. However, the authors found no to very little background DNA present, with only 4 of the 52 items (1 tampon and 3 liners) exhibiting one or two Y-STR alleles and 1 additional item (pad) exhibiting two alleles using an autosomal STR kit, with all alleles appearing with low RFU signals.

To elucidate the level and origins of background DNA on worn upper garments, Szkuta et al. [117] and Szkuta et al. [118] collected samples from several areas (two internal and six external) of two garments (both owned and previously worn by the participant) each worn on separate occasions, for 6 to 15 h on a work day and a non-work day, after being washed. They also recorded details of the history of the garment, and the interactions and activities during wearing, and collected samples for reference DNA profiles from participants and their close associates. They found variation in the DNA quantity, profile composition and inclusion/exclusion of the wearer and their associates, among participants, garments worn on different occasions and the garment areas sampled. The authors reported that DNA from the wearer of a garment was found on all internal and external areas sampled, with the best quality profiles corresponding to the wearer obtained from internal collars followed by internal cuffs. They also found that DNA from individuals living or sharing a space with the wearer was frequently detected in samples from external areas of the garment. In such samples, the contribution of the wearer to the DNA profile was occasionally absent or minor relative to the presence of the close associate; this was most frequently observed in samples taken from the external back of the garment.

A further study by Murphy et al. [145] examined the background levels of male DNA on the inside front of clean, but not new, pairs of underpants worn for a day by a female who was asked to abstain from sexual intercourse for 48 h prior to taking part in the study. The authors reported that, of the 103 samples taken after a day of wearing, 83 showed the presence of male DNA to varying quantities (as detected by the Quantifiler

Trio DNA quantification kit (Thermo Fisher Scientific, Warrington, UK)) and 24 contained sufficient DNA to proceed to profiling. Of those 24 profiled samples, 12 samples showed the detection of the Y chromosome and varying numbers of minor alleles (not from the female wearer) using the autosomal NGM SElect kit (Thermo Fisher Scientific, Warrington, UK), 5 gave a complete Y-STR profile, and 18 gave incomplete Y-STR profiles. Each of the samples that gave a complete Y-STR profile was from a female who cohabited with a male partner and the profile matched that of the partner where a reference profile was available (four of five). Based on the results of their study, the authors concluded that the finding of a Y-filer profile on the inside front of underpants worn by a female is not expected in the absence of sexual contact. Further, in the absence of sexual contact, a Y-STR profile, if present, is more likely to be obtained from a cohabitating male rather than from a non-cohabitating male in social contact with a female.

Two studies included investigation of the impact of cleaning on levels and composition of background DNA on various surfaces. Reither et al. [146] found that domestic cleaning methods (e.g., vacuuming, mopping with cleaning agents that did not contain cholic acid) had limited impact on the quantity of DNA recovered from various types of flooring (e.g., carpet, tiles), but often altered the DNA profile composition of the samples collected when comparing the profile from the post-cleaned area with the profile from the corresponding pre-cleaned area. Similarly, in experiments to determine the impact of a range of cleaning agents and cleaning actions using DNA-free towel pieces and sponges on small blood stains, saliva stains and fingermarks on plastic table tops and fabric surfaces, Helmus et al. [147] found that the DNA was redistributed to other areas of the item by the cleaning action. They also found that the cleaning agent had little impact on the ability to generate DNA profiles of the sample collected, with the exception of chloric agents, which the authors asserted rendered almost everything DNA-free.

3.6. Manner of Handling

This section reports ten studies that investigated manner of handling (Figure 2). We have broken down this section into further subtopics to categorise the studies into elements of handling, including time, pressure, and testing of various scenarios. We have also included studies on non-contact DNA transfer in this section.

3.6.1. Handling Time

In their study of the impact of handling time by a non-wearer of a worn brassiere, Sessa et al. [93] found that the contact duration does not appear to have an effect on the amount of DNA deposited and when a major contributor is detected on a garment. Outcomes of their experiments (which included small specific target areas of known contact by the 'handler') also showed that the person handling the garment last contributed the most to the recovered DNA, even though they may have touched the garment for only a few seconds.

3.6.2. Pressure

Examining the effect of deposition pressure (using weights from 0.1 to 10 kg) applied by fingers on the quality of latent fingermarks and DNA STR profiles, Hefetz et al. [148] found that as deposition pressure increased, so did the length and width of fingermarks and the efficiency of DNA profiling from the fingermarks. The latter was based on increases in the amount of DNA recovered, number of amplified loci, and number of forensically useful DNA profiles, which were observed for each of the substrates tested (glass, polythene, paper).

3.6.3. Scenario Testing

The transfer of DNA to clothing under a number of case-relevant scenarios was investigated by Szkuta et al. [118] and De Wolff et al. [149]. Szkuta et al. [118] examined whether an 'activity partner' was discernible on clothing worn by another individual after specific interactions: 'contact' where the final action during the wearing of the garment was an embrace with a known other individual; 'close proximity' where the final action during the wearing of the garment was to travel to and from a nearby café to have a meal with a known other individual; 'physical absence' where the wearer of the garment spent most of a working day in an office of a known other individual, in the absence of the other individual. The study did not find any DNA from the activity partner on the garments after the wearer had gone on an outing, even though they had been in close proximity with each other for a while. However, the study did observe DNA from the activity partner on several areas of the garments following the embrace and after temporarily occupying another person's office. It was reported that particular areas of the garment were more prone to acquiring DNA from the hugging partner or the office owner than others, and their detection as a major or minor component was deemed activity dependent. When investigating DNA transfer to clothing within vehicles, De Wolff et al. [149] found that in many instances, DNA from a regular driver of a vehicle could be recovered from samples collected from the external back of the upper garment, and from the seat of the trousers pants, worn by an incidental driver (30 min) of that vehicle soon after departing the vehicle. This highlighted a potential avenue of indirect transfer that may be relevant during investigations of particular types of offences.

DNA transfer within specific scenarios that can occur during sexual assaults was investigated by Ramos et al. [150]. Their study recorded where underwear was contacted and how much DNA was transferred by volunteer 'offenders' during six types of mock sexual assault scenarios: removing underwear; removing brassiere; digital penetration of the vagina from the front; grabbing breasts over the top of the brassiere; digital penetration of the vagina from the rear; grabbing the breasts under the brassiere from the rear. The authors found that the pattern of contact varied for different activities and identified the areas of underwear most commonly contacted from various sexual assault activities. They demonstrated that some areas corresponded to areas typically sampled during casework and others less so, thus providing information to help improve sample targeting. They too observed several instances of a colleague or cohabitating partner of mock offenders being detected within a DNA sample.

A study by Gosch et al. [151] considered trace DNA characteristics (including DNA yield, number of contributors, relative profile contribution for known and unknown contributors, LRs) of samples recovered from various surfaces of two types of firearms handled in four realistic casework-relevant scenarios. In each scenario, the firearm had background DNA deposited over four days by the mock owner. The four different activities then undertaken with the firearms included: the mock owner performed a shooting scenario; a second individual performed the same shooting scenario as the mock owner; a second individual imitated a longer and more intensive contact with the firearm; a second individual performed the same shooting scenario as the mock owner, then wiped the firearm using a dry cotton towel for 15 s simulating fingerprint removal. The authors observed a large variability of trace characteristics that was partly attributable to the way the firearms were handled, the firearm surface types sampled, and factors of inter- as well as intra-individual variability.

When considering DNA transfer to knife handles, particularly within opportunistic crimes, Butcher et al. [152] conducted experiments to generate data to help address consideration of questions relating to whether the DNA obtained comes from the regular user, the last user (ostensibly, the user at the time of the crime) or from indirect transfer events. The authors found that regularly used knives that were then used for just 2–60 s by a second person, performing a stabbing action, resulted for three of the four participant pairings in a decrease in contribution from the regular user's DNA with simultaneous increase in contribution from the second user's DNA. They reported that the trend appeared to be due to a decrease in regular user DNA via transfer to the second user's hands, rather than an increase in DNA deposited from the second user, but a deviation from this general trend was observed for the fourth participant pairing. While they found a low level contribution of the non-handler's DNA on most knife handles, one volunteer deposited a similar amount of DNA through regular use as the amount of indirectly transferred unknown DNA deposited by another volunteer's hands, leading the authors to indicate that caution should be taken when relying solely on absolute quantities of DNA to inform evaluative interpretations and that other parameters, such as profile quality and relative contributions to mixed profiles, should also be taken into account. However, when also considering DNA transfer within stabbing scenarios, Samie et al. [153] observed that the quantity of DNA generally reduced when moving from hand (the quantity collected when sampling directly from a hand) to primary transfer (the quantity collected from a surface handled by a hand) and, subsequently, to secondary transfer.

To assist activity level evaluation, Euteneuer et al. [154] investigated the correlation between shooting distance and the amount of blood backspatter in/on a used firearm. The authors could not establish any meaningful correlation between backspatter distribution and DNA yields, the shooting distance and the condition of the wound channel.

3.6.4. Non-Contact Transfer

The first study to consider non-contact transfer with dried biological materials was published by Thornbury et al. [155]. They investigated the possibility of indirect DNA transfer without contact from various substrates (two different non-porous hard substrates and two different porous, soft substrates) after various biological materials (blood, saliva, semen, vaginal fluid, touch DNA) deposited on them had dried and after applying two types of agitation (tapping—all substrates; stretching—all fabric substrates). The authors found that detectable levels of indirect transfer of DNA without contact were possible. They also demonstrated that the type of biological material and substrate affected the drying time and characteristics of deposits, and that the rate and percentage transfer appeared to be dependent on the type of agitation, substrate, biological material and its drying properties.

3.7. Shedder Status

This section summarises the one paper where shedder status was deemed the most relevant DNA-TPPR aspect (Figure 2), plus seven additional studies that also provided comment on this subject matter but were primarily categorised in other topics. When investigating shedder status as a possible factor influencing the extent of secondary DNA transfer to a crime scene when the offender wears working gloves, Otten et al. [156] initially determined the shedder status of a group of individuals, finding that good shedders deposited higher amounts and quality of DNA onto objects compared to bad shedders. The authors then conducted experiments where participants were paired into groups of various combinations of good and bad shedders, with the first participant of each pair wearing working gloves to pack and carry boxes, and then, two days later, the same gloves were worn by the second participant to break-in using a screwdriver. The study reported that good shedders, overall, deposited more DNA than bad shedders, both onto the outside and inside of the gloves regardless of being the first or second wearer and user of the gloves. The authors also found that a DNA profile of the first wearer was found on the screwdriver in several instances, and in each of the situations where this was observed, the first user had been a designated good shedder, confirming the possibility of a person's DNA profile being found on an object they never handled.

Several other papers demonstrated or alluded to observing differences in the quantities of DNA deposited, which was attributed to differences in shedder status, for example [51, 78,150,152]. However, Miller et al. [95] found that individuals who deposited extremely large amounts of DNA by touch one day may deposit no detectable DNA on another day despite a restriction on handwashing close in time to deposition, leading the authors to question the concept that there are consistently good shedders, at least through the palms of hands. Similarly, Samie et al. [153] noted that while a person could be judged as a good shedder overall, when considering a single experiment, that same person could be a very poor shedder. They suggest that when assessing the probability of observing a given quantity of DNA, for a given donor, the whole distribution should be accounted for and not only its mean value. The authors also showed that the 'transfer proportion' (quantity of DNA transferred onto a surface over the initial quantity on the hand) may vary between participants and will depend on the type of transfer (primary versus secondary), indicating that the quantification of DNA on one hand cannot be used to infer the shedder status and asses what will be transferred onto a surface.

Like shedder status determination from finger/hand marks, a study by Kanok-wongnuwut et al. [42] found that the amounts of cellular material deposited by lip-prints is consistent for individuals, but different among individuals. The authors were able to categorise lip shedder status from heavy to light, but they did not observe a correlation between lip-print shedder status and the shedder status of the individual determined from thumb prints.

3.8. Contamination

The potential unwanted transfer of DNA during a forensic examination (or contamination) can also be relevant and has been considered in four of the studies identified (Figure 2). Three of these studies looked at the potential of DNA contamination via items used during an examination in the laboratory, specifically gloves and fingerprint brushes [157–159]. In the study by Goray et al. [157], a number of laboratory-based evidence recovery personnel were videoed performing a range of examinations and several factors were assessed to evaluate the risks of DNA loss, addition and redistribution via gloves. The factors included: what each glove touched and in what sequence; the number, duration and type of contact made by each glove with the item under examination, tools used and other surfaces; when gloves were replaced; DNA profiles of samples taken from worn gloves at the time of replacement against those relating to the item under investigation, the examiner, and other staff members. The authors observed that many different surface areas are touched by gloves during examinations, and differences exist among examiners in what they touch and when they change gloves. They reported that, in many instances, the case-associated person of interest was observed within the profile generated from DNA retrieved from outer surfaces of most gloves sampled at time of replacement. They also observed DNA profiles of the examiner, or other staff members, predominantly in samples taken from the first and last gloves used during the examination, which were associated with removing the exhibit from the packaging and repackaging it. Their evaluation deemed that several of the observed contacts made by the gloves were a high contamination risk event. Furthermore, Van den Berge et al. [158] performed tests showing that DNA from hands transferred to various parts of the external side of laboratory gloves while being donned. With respect to used fingerprint brushes, the study by Nontiapirom et al. [159] produced results verifying findings that human DNA can persist on fingerprint brushes after use, such that fingerprint brushes can be a potential contamination risk when reused.

Two of the identified studies also considered the effectiveness of contamination-minimisation procedures within the laboratory [158,160]. In the above study by Van den Berge et al. [158], they also performed tests providing outcomes supporting the use of 0.3% sodium hypochlorite solution or commercially available RNase AWAY™ (Thermo Fisher Scientific, Waltham, MA, USA) as decontamination reagents to clean and subsequently dry the exterior of donned gloves prior to entering the laboratory and/or handling items of evidence. The authors reported that the results precipitated an update to their laboratory's contamination risk reduction strategy. The study by Basset and Castella [160] compared the number of DNA contamination events by laboratory staff before and after the implementation of additional contamination minimisation procedures (that included: physical separation between living environments (e.g., offices, cafeteria) and laboratory zones; personal objects prohibited from laboratory zones; double gloving; use of different disposable lab coats within different laboratory rooms; lab coats changed daily; stain collection split among different operators so that the person in contact with the swab does not touch other surfaces; automation of DNA extraction for standard traces) and found that the number of such contamination events declined by more than 70% after implementation of the procedures.

3.9. Microbiomes

Fourteen studies (Figure 2) delve into the opportunities to identify individuals, or associate them with a location or an activity, that may be offered from analysing microbiomes in the absence of and/or in addition to traditional DNA evidence. These include investigations into:

- Classification of individuals and the potential to detect sexual contact using the microbiome of the pubic region [161].
- Bacterial communities associated with cell phones and shoes of the same person [162].
- Microbial communities of a wide range of known body sites and the detection of the source of different microbial contributions in mixtures of different body sites or with soil [163].
- Distinguishing microbiome communities of saliva, skin and mixtures of both as a potential tool for identifying samples of single and mixed biological materials [164].
- Correlations between the presence of certain bacterial species on a donor's hands and personal characteristics [165].
- The direct and indirect transfer of microbiomes between individuals [166].
- The ability of several commercial kits to recover sufficient bacterial DNA from fingerprints to generate a microbiome profile [167].
- Generating both STR profiles and microbial population profiles from the same DNA extract of each sample to evaluate the sub-source and source questions, respectively in two forensic cases [168].
- The usefulness of the likelihood ratio approach for the evaluation of source attribution in microbial forensic cases to facilitate the interpretation of evidence in legal proceedings [169].

In addition, Young and Linacre [170] provided a review of studies on the potential and limitations of utilising microbiome analyses in forensic science, especially in relation to skin microbiome. Meanwhile, Jurkevitch and Pasternal [171] provided a review on the use of soil bacterial community comparisons to assist investigation of alleged crimes. Each of these studies and reviews, as well as a review by Neckovic et al. [172], indicated some positive results and potential useful applications, but also highlighted a range of limitations of their applicability and the challenges of microbial profiling for forensic science casework applications. These challenges are further illustrated by investigations of the presence of microbiomes within forensic evidence recovery laboratories, and the potential for microbiomes to transfer during examinations [173,174].

3.10. Evaluating DNA Evidence

This final section of the synopsis reports papers that consider the evaluation of DNA evidence given propositions at different levels within the Hierarchy of Propositions. Ten papers with a primary focus on this subject matter are included (Figure 2), along with one other that was primarily included in another topic, and are reported within two subsections: setting propositions and use of Bayesian Networks, and other activity level assessment-related matters.

3.10.1. Setting Propositions and Use of Bayesian Networks

When evaluating the value of biological evidence, it is important that the propositions are formulated appropriately. Gill et al. [120] presented guidelines from the DNA Commission of the International Society for Forensic Genetics (ISFG) on determining and formulating the propositions for the evaluation of biological traces, given activity level propositions. This paper included eleven specific recommendations and provided examples to illustrate the principles espoused. The authors also noted that suitable propositions are ideally set before knowledge of the trace DNA evidence, that data relevant to the case in question be gathered to assign probabilities, and that Bayesian Networks (BNs) are useful to help consider all relevant possibilities. Taylor et al. [175] also stressed the importance of properly constructing the propositions. The authors indicated the need for a clear summary of propositions representing the views of the prosecution and defence, accompanied with details on the agreed and contested information and assumptions by the scientist, to assist in carrying out an evaluation and in understanding by the courts. Furthermore, Buckleton et al. [176] showed an example where considerations of DNA-TPPR are required to inform sub-source level proposition setting, specifically to condition the calculation on the presence of DNA of an assumed contributor. The authors showed this in relation to the number of contributors, as this is likely to impact on the LR at the sub-source level.

Several studies focussed on the use of BNs to evaluate DNA results given competing propositions, including Taylor et al. [177], Gill et al. [120], Volgin [178], De March and Tarino [179], and Samie et al. [180]. Examples of the use of BNs to evaluate biological traces given activity level propositions are provided in: the supplementary material within the article of Gill et al. [120] (that is accessible in the online version); and by Volgin [178] involving the use of a T-shirt as a balaclava. Further, De March and Tarino [179] provided an insight into the application of BNs to real criminal cases through the assessment of the probative value of different analyses related to some biological material retrieved from an object of interest.

Two studies went further to consider the applicability of BNs to the complexities of issues of DNA transfer. Taylor et al. [177] showed the value of an Object-Oriented Bayesian Network (OOBN) to tackle cases involving repeating elements of complex and various DNA transfer mechanisms and indicated that, as new data on DNA-TPPR factors become available, these can be readily accommodated by the general overall OOBN architecture. Further, Samie et al. [180] showed that BNs can handle the complexity of variables associated with DNA-TPPR to inform activity level assessments. Their study demonstrated the uses of BNs and simulation methods to identify the variables impacting the value of evidence assessed under activity level propositions. The authors did so by focussing on trace DNA evidence recovered from knife handles allegedly involved in stabbing instances, showing that some variables had greater bearing on the variation of the LR than others. In the situation they investigated, the authors reported that the identified key variables were associated with the sampling, the extraction efficiency, the background and the quantity of DNA on hands, and they asserted that data acquisition should focus mainly on those variables with the greatest impact.

3.10.2. Other Activity Level Assessment-Related Matters

In his commentary, Gill [181] pointed out that the increased sensitivity of modern DNA profiling techniques means that DNA may be recovered that is irrelevant to the crime and stressed the importance of scientists, lawyers and judges to be aware of the limitations of DNA profiling evidence. This was echoed by Sessa et al. [93], who also pointed out the need for everyone in the medico-legal community to know the power of touch DNA and understand the potential limitations associated with it. Gill [181] went on to note that the presence of DNA does not tell us when or how it got there, so additional context is needed from other non-DNA evidence, which if ignored could result in miscarriages of justice. He provided several real case examples to highlight how ignorance of key aspects, such as background DNA, secondary transfer, and laboratory contamination, can influence case outcomes. Similarly, Perepechina [182] referred to a retrospective analysis of a case where consideration of transfer issues was pertinent. Given these issues, he [181] also pointed out the need to educate stakeholders, including all parties engaged in the criminal justice system, with respect to the various facets relating to activity level assessments.

An additional concern highlighted by Gill [181] is the occurrence of carryover of the strength of evidence associated with a DNA 'match' to weight of evidence associated with activity level propositions. He reported that this cannot be done; activity level assessments are to be undertaken separately using different information and generating a different statistic. This point is also made by the DNA Commission of the ISFG [120].

Apart from the few calls for specific further research noted above, many of the other publications incorporated in this synopsis, in their discussion sections, also incorporate suggestions/recommendations/advocacy for further research to enlighten our understandings and advance the acquisition of relevant data to improve our abilities to provide activity level assessments. From challenges encountered in their study, Dunhill and Chapman [183] encouraged authors to publish results of studies on indirect transfer of DNA in a more streamlined fashion to allow for systematic analysis of data across studies. Further, De March and Tarino [179] indicated that while the data available to inform probabilities are limited and extrapolation from published data for practical use in a case analysis can be troublesome, this should not prevent the forensic scientist from providing a statement at the activity level when the circumstances of a case require it.

4. Reflections on the Research Efforts to Meet the Challenges

Based on the focus, scope and depth of the research activities published over the last few years, we reflect that overall, some progress has been made to meet the many challenges, but much of the challenges noted in the introduction remain and require more effort to address them. While several of the recent studies have provided means of improving the detection and recovery of DNA and DNA profiles of relevance from crime-related items, more effort will be required to determine the best practices given the specific circumstances encountered. Of the 144 articles included in the synopsis, relatively few (35) primarily focus on aspects of persistence, DNA prevalence and background DNA, manner of handling and shedder status (Figure 2). Of these, few provide the highly desired data to help assign probabilities of obtaining profile types given particular sets of circumstances, especially those that are relatively commonly encountered. The latter is partly due to the relatively recent and increasing need for such data, and the requirement for sufficient repeats to be conducted to generate robust frequency data, which may place this type of research beyond the scope of some research groups. The multitude of situations and associated variables for which probabilities are desired provides scope for conducting many future research projects to provide welcomed outputs.

Some additional research efforts have been directed at determining and mitigating risks of contamination of evidence (see Section 3.8). Further research may highlight additional risk factors and means of mitigating these, thus providing opportunities to enhance the integrity of the evidence throughout the forensic process and the interpretation thereof.

Some research has been conducted on other elements of information that may be gleaned from deposits of biological materials to facilitate activity level evaluations (see Section 3.1, Section 3.3, Section 3.9). Further studies towards improving abilities to accurately determine the TSD of various types of biological material in various circumstances (preferably even of different components within mixed samples), and into microbiome profiles that inform on the environment that a sample is associated with, and/or its source, and/or provide an avenue for identity determination in the absence of human DNA, may assist future activity level evaluations.

To assist with activity level evaluations, BNs are starting to be utilised more (see Section 3.10.1), such that any developments towards making BN-related software packages even more user friendly for forensic practitioners may further facilitate their utilisation and the standard of the guidance provided to the court. However, there appears to be little recent human factors-related research effort directed towards facilitating the development of competencies of those tasked with providing activity level-related guidance and how to best convey this guidance to other stakeholders. Such research, as well as human factors research relating to individuals and processes associated with the collection of evidence and maintaining its integrity, would be welcomed as they may identify improvement opportunities in the means of training experts and the quality of tasks undertaken and the services provided.

Encouragingly, very recent publications (i.e., articles published after conducting the systematic search, or during the search period but not captured) demonstrate the realisation of the need for, and the efforts supporting, ongoing research activity towards meeting the broad range of outstanding challenges. Examples of such publications of studies addressing identified knowledge and data gaps include:

- DNA profile success of samples from casework-related items [24].
- Impacts of surface roughness and physicochemical interactions on deposits of biological materials [184].
- Impacts of chewing gum on drying properties of saliva [185].
- Prevalence and persistence of saliva in vehicles [186].
- Exploring means of determining an individual's shedder status.
- Consideration of distance and time with respect to accumulation of DNA within offices on surfaces that are not touched [187].
- Evaluation of profiles retrieved from the outside of gloves after simulating transfer scenarios related to breaking and entering [188].
- Findings indicating that cities around the globe have distinct microbial taxonomic signatures [189].
- Development of an LR framework incorporating sensitivity analysis to model multiple direct and secondary transfer events on skin surfaces [190].
- Highlighting the importance/value of considering common sources of unknown DNA [191].
- Assigning weight of cell type testing results [192] when evaluating findings given activity level propositions.

These studies demonstrate the realisation of the need for, and the efforts supporting, ongoing research activity towards meeting the broad range of outstanding challenges.

5. Industry Actions towards Addressing Challenges

5.1. Research

Many of the reviews and research papers referenced in the previous sections note the need for more research to better inform our understanding of variables affecting DNA-TPPR and supplying relevant data to determine probabilities given a set of circumstances. Meakin et al. [193], apart from also advocating this, urged for better designed research studies to cater for this need. In particular, they expanded on the recommendation of Gosch and Courts [36] for different experimental designs to be employed when generating probabilities for activity level evaluations as opposed to investigating DNA transfer mechanisms. They recommended that the former requires iterations of realistic experiments (e.g., a casework-relevant scenario performed once by multiple participants), whereas the latter require repetitions of highly controlled and potentially unrealistic experiments (e.g., a single participant performing the same action multiple times). Meakin et al. [193] also directed readers to the ISFG recommendations [120], which provide further advice for designing experiments to generate activity level probabilities.

Evident from the authorships and their affiliations, forensic laboratories, alone or in collaboration with other forensic laboratories and/or academic institutions, are major contributors to much of the published DNA-TPPR-related research. Much of this is being funded by internal resources. Major research funding bodies are also increasingly supporting DNA-TPPR-related research. For example, the National Institute of Justice (NIJ) in the United States of America has funded over 60 DNA-related projects to the value in excess of USD 42 million during 2018–2020 [194,195], which include a wide range of DNA-TPPR-related research projects, and the European Network of Forensic Institutes (ENSFI) has recently funded a large multi-institutional collaborative project to generate accessible DNA transfer rate data [196].

5.2. Education and Training

Apart from the need for research to improve our understanding and generate data to allow the assignment of probabilities given a set of circumstances, there are other challenges to be met by relevant industry stakeholders. These include aspects relating to the education and training of those tasked with providing expert evidence on DNA-TPPR-related matters, building of awareness of aspects associated with DNA-TPPR among crime scene attendees and those within the legal fraternity, availability and utility of published data, and setting of standards associated with DNA-related activity level evaluative reporting. Steps are being taken to address these challenges.

DNA-TPPR-related research findings, including unpublished findings, are being presented and discussed within dedicated sessions and workshops at international forensic conferences attended by forensic, policing and legal practitioners as well as academia. For example, Congresses of the International Society of Forensic Genetics [197]; Gordon Research Conferences: Forensic Analysis of Human DNA [198]; American Academy of Forensic Sciences (AAFS) conferences [199]; the International Symposium on Human Identification ((ISHI) [200]; and the symposium on Recent Progress on Forensic Sciences and DNA Transfer organised by Laboratoire d'Hématologie Médico-Légale [201].

Further education/upskilling of stakeholders on the topic of DNA-TPPR and the associated activity level evaluative reporting is also being made possible through the development and availability of dedicated programs such as summer schools on various aspects of forensic genetics organised by the International Society of Forensic Genetics [202] and university-based courses such as the Certificate of Advanced Studies on 'Statistics and the evaluation of forensic evidence' run by the University of Lausanne [203]. Freely accessible courses and webinars have also been produced, such as that on 'Challenging Forensic Science: How Science Should Speak to Court' made available by the University of Lausanne [204] and the series of webinars on DNA mixture interpretation and probabilistic genotyping organised by the Federal Bureau of Investigation (FBI) Laboratory and NIJ's Forensic Technology Center of Excellence [205].

The skill set required to become expert at the provision of guidance on DNA-TPPR at the activity level is distinct from those required to provide guidance at the DNA sub-source level, biological material source level or non-DNA activity level. Recognition of this can be an important first step for laboratories to help define the necessary enrichments and changes to a suite of methodologies, protocols, training units and authorisations. Introduction of these is then to be managed, such that the increasing demands for such services can be met at the expected standards. Most forensic DNA experts trained over the last twenty years have been trained to provide statements at the sub-source level. A forensic expert solely trained and competent at providing DNA evidence at the sub-source level should not provide opinion at the activity level without also being trained and authorised to do so.

An example of a jurisdiction with a competency testing program specific to evaluation of forensic biology findings given activity level propositions can be found in the Netherlands [206]. Experts can submit an application for registration as an expert in the field to the Netherlands Register of Court Experts (www.nrgd.nl). They are subsequently assessed by a committee of both scientific experts and legal professionals against a standard that has been developed by a group of international experts in the field. The standards demarcate the field of 'DNA activity' from 'DNA source' and 'DNA kinship' and list the minimum requirements for experts in these fields. These requirements cover training, experience, methodology, reporting, and knowledge of the Dutch legal system [207]. Registered individuals must demonstrate their ongoing competency to the Board on a regular (five year) basis.

5.3. Availability and Sharing of Data

Kokshoorn et al. [208] and Gosch and Courts [36] advocated the need for sharing of research data associated with DNA-TPPR. They also indicated the type of information that is relevant when interpreting the generated data and should be made available when publishing DNA-TPPR-related research (or making it available on sharing platforms). These included information on: item (type of item, construction and surface composition, etc.); item history (handling, packaging, etc.); sampling (surface area targeted, sampling method, etc.); analysis (DNA extraction, amplification, CE, etc.); and interpretation (allele calling, statistical model, parameter settings, proposition setting, NoC determination, etc.). Kokshoorn et al. [208] also advocated for harmonisation and standardisation in how some of this information should be recorded, to further assist utilisation of the data. Gosch and Courts [36] constructed a database for entry and accessibility of such data, added the data from relevant publications and requested researchers to submit the relevant data to DNA-TrAC [37]. DNA-TrAC contains 311 entries of relevant research articles published in the period 1993–2017. Detailed information is provided per publication covering a wide range of aspects relevant to understanding DNA-TPPR and utilising data for activity level evaluations. It also provides the ability to sort information based on various parameters including general details of the publications, questions being addressed by the studies, transfer scenarios in the context of a specific type of activity, categories of study object (e.g., primary deposit, further transfer, background DNA, persistence, recovery), and variables affecting DNA-TPPR. The website also includes a list of 17 review articles published in the period 2002–2020 with a summary of the topics addressed by each as well as a file listing 33 articles relevant to DNA-TPPR published during the period 2018–2020 for which the details have not yet been entered into the DNA-TrAC database. The last version fully and actively curated by the Gosch and Courts was uploaded in December 2019 and a request is issued for others to assist with the maintenance of the database. DNA-TrAC is a useful portal to source DNA-TPPR information and data that may be relevant to a range of stakeholders. Maintenance and upkeep of this database, or the creation of something similar, would be an asset to the forensic community and thus desirable.

A separate relevant database ('BDATT-TTADB'), constructed with funding support from research grants from the Social Sciences and Humanities Research Council of Canada, has recently become available [209,210]. The database was built with the aim of being relevant for practitioners to interpret transfer traces at activity level, integrating transfer experiments in an operational situation [209]. It provides information for a wide range of trace types, including DNA and biological fluids. It allows for easy searching according to type of trace, type of study (including transfer, persistence, recovery, background, contamination), key words (as determined by the database custodians, not the ones listed in the associated publication) as well as aspects such as authors. Apart from the general information regarding the publication (i.e., title, authors, journal), it provides a copy of the published abstract, a summary statement regarding the studies' experimental conditions and results, a summary statement regarding the relevancy of the study for the Canadian environment, and a link to the publication. The database includes several hundred papers relating to DNA-TPPR and is updated regularly [209,210]. This database resource provides an excellent means for any interested parties to identify potentially relevant studies. However, those seeking some of the finer details often required when conducting activity level evaluations, as described above, will need to examine the identified literature more closely. An additional source of relevant data will also be made available in early 2022, when the UK Body Fluid Forum launches a digital collection of casework-informed research and case reports to facilitate sharing of experiences and data specifically relevant to informing evaluation of biological findings given activity level propositions. When available, these articles will be accessible here: https://www.sciencedirect.com/journal/science-and-justice/special-issues. Further development and maintenance of databases containing all the relevant information that allow easy mining of desired finer details, and further efforts towards harmonisation and standardisation of the data generated and shared as suggested by Kokshoorn et al. [208], would be welcomed.

5.4. Standards and Guidance

Many standards and guidance on how to conduct DNA-related activity level evaluative reporting are being provided by governing bodies. For example, the Forensic Science Regulator in England and Wales [211] and the DNA Commission of the ISFG [120,212]; there is also an ISO standard relating to forensic science reporting currently under development [213]. Additionally, some of the fallacies associated with the reporting of DNA-TPPR matters, that forensic practitioners need be cognisant of and avoid when providing guidance to the triers of fact, are highlighted by Meakin et al. [193].

Forensic laboratories are also investing in developing in-house methods, procedures and training modules to facilitate the conduct of DNA-related activity level evaluations and the training of their staff to do so. However, unlike many other forensic disciplines, independent ongoing proficiency testing in all the relevant elements associated with DNA-related activity level evaluations for those authorised to provide expert opinion to assist triers of fact is not readily available. Creation of a good fit for purpose internationally available proficiency testing program would facilitate the provision of high-quality guidance by forensic practitioners.

The National Institute of Standards and Technology (NIST) in the USA has very recently (June 2021) published a draft of a scientific foundation review in relation to the interpretation of DNA mixtures [214]. It also contemplates several of the points we raised earlier. It is a wide ranging comprehensive in-depth review that provides an overview of the past, present and future of DNA mixture interpretation and identifies challenges and pathways to deal with them. It includes a general introduction; principles and practices relating to DNA mixture interpretation; sources of data and information; delving into the issues pertaining to the reliability of DNA mixture measurements and interpretation as well as the context and relevance of DNA mixture interpretation (with details on various factors associated with DNA transfer); consideration of the potential and limitations of new technologies to provide solutions to existing problems. The chapters and appendices are accompanied with highlighted key takeaways, principal points and/or future considerations. Takeaways that directly relate to DNA transfer and activity level reporting, presented in chapter 5 of the review [214], include:

- #5.1: DNA can be transferred from one surface or person to another, and this can potentially happen multiple times. Therefore, the DNA present on an evidence item may be unrelated (irrelevant) to the crime being investigated.
- #5.2: Highly sensitive DNA methods increase the likelihood of detecting irrelevant DNA. When assessing evidence that involves very small quantities of DNA, it is especially important to consider relevance.
- #5.3: Highly sensitive methods increase the likelihood of detecting contaminating DNA that might affect an investigation. Contamination avoidance procedures should be robust both at the crime scene and in the laboratory.
- #5.4: DNA statistical results such as a sub-source likelihood ratio do not provide information about how or when DNA was transferred, or whether it is relevant to a case. Therefore, using the likelihood ratio as a standalone number without context can be misleading.
- #5.5: The fact that DNA transfers easily between objects does not negate the value of DNA evidence. However, the value of DNA evidence depends on the circumstances of the case.
- #5.6: There is a growing body of knowledge about DNA transfer and persistence, but significant knowledge gaps remain.

5.5. Cooperation with Other Scientific Disciplines, the Legal Community, and Police

The compartmentalised nature of the scientific disciplines in many modern forensic laboratories hampers the proper evaluation of forensic findings [215]. Interdisciplinary assessments of traces increase the impact of the forensic sciences on the criminal justice system (CJS), both improving efficiency by reducing unnecessary examinations and improving understanding of the combined weight of the findings given case-relevant propositions at the activity level [216].

Case-relevant information is structured in propositions, assumptions, and other, undisputed case information [175]. For any evaluation of findings given activity level propositions that a scientist is asked to perform, it is crucial that all parties in the CJS are in a position to share task-relevant information with the scientist.

Education and training of stakeholders in the CJS is a crucial step to reduce common misconceptions of what evaluations given propositions at the activity level are, as well as to achieve the desired communication and collaboration between the scientist and the other actors in the CJS. Efforts are being made in several jurisdictions, for instance, by providing guidance documents for legal professionals [217–220].

6. Concluding Remarks

Much progress has been made recently towards addressing identified challenges concerning the provision of expert guidance in relation to DNA-TPPR-associated activity level evaluations sought to facilitate just outcomes during legal proceedings. However, many challenges remain. These include in relation to:

- Quantity and quality of research directed at informing our understanding of DNA-TPPR and building the data needed to assign probabilities to DNA quantities and profile types being obtained given a vast range of circumstances.
- Harmonisation, standardisation, and accessibility of available data.
- Development of validated standardised methodologies and protocols to perform DNA-related activity level evaluations.
- Training and authorisation of experts to perform such evaluations and provide the guidance when needed as well as recognition of this expertise as a separate discipline.
- Education and cooperation of stakeholders within the legal fraternity.

Continued investment in addressing these challenges will improve the value and understanding of the data and the guidance given to the triers of fact.

Author Contributions: Conceptualisation, R.A.H.v.O.; investigation, R.A.H.v.O., B.S.; writing—original draft preparation, R.A.H.v.O., G.E.M., B.K., M.G., B.S.; writing—review and editing, R.A.H.v.O., G.E.M., B.K., M.G., B.S.; visualisation, R.A.H.v.O. and B.S.; project administration, R.A.H.v.O. All authors have read and agreed to the published version of the manuscript.

Funding: This research received no external funding.

Conflicts of Interest: The authors declare no conflict of interest.

References

1. Van Oorschot, R.A.H.; Szkuta, B.; Meakin, G.E.; Kokshoorn, B.; Goray, M. DNA transfer in forensic science: A review. *Forensic Sci. Int. Genet.* **2019**, *38*, 140–166. [CrossRef] [PubMed]
2. Taylor, D.; Kokshoorn, B.; Biedermann, A. Evaluation of forensic genetics findings given activity level propositions: A review. *Forensic Sci. Int. Genet.* **2018**, *36*, 34–49. [CrossRef] [PubMed]
3. Gill, P.; Haned, H.; Bleka, O.; Hansson, O.; Dørum, G.; Egeland, T. Genotyping and interpretation of STR-DNA: Low-template, mixtures and database matches—Twenty years of research and development. *Forensic Sci. Int. Genet.* **2015**, *18*, 100–117. [CrossRef] [PubMed]
4. Børsting, C.; Morling, N. Next generation sequencing and its applications in forensic genetics. *Forensic Sci. Int. Genet.* **2015**, *18*, 78–89. [CrossRef] [PubMed]
5. Butler, J.M. *Advanced Topics in Forensic DNA Typing: Methodology*; Academic Press: San Diego, CA, USA, 2012.
6. Van Oorschot, R.A.H.; Ballantyne, K.N.; Mitchell, J.R. Forensic trace DNA: A review. *Investig. Genet.* **2010**, *1*, 1–17. [CrossRef] [PubMed]
7. Ballantyne, K.N.; Poy, A.L.; van Oorschot, R.A.H. Environmental DNA monitoring: Beware of the transition to more sensitive typing methodologies. *Aust. J. Forensic Sci.* **2013**, *45*, 323–340. [CrossRef]
8. Farash, K.; Hanson, E.K.; Ballantyne, J. Single source DNA profile recovery from single cells isolated from skin and fabric from touch DNA mixtures in mock physical assaults. *Sci. Justice* **2018**, *58*, 191–199. [CrossRef] [PubMed]
9. Van Oorschot, R.A.H.; Jones, M.K. DNA fingerprints from fingerprints. *Nature* **1997**, *387*, 767. [CrossRef]
10. Lowe, A.; Murray, C.; Whitaker, J.; Tully, G.; Gill, P. The propensity of individuals to deposit DNA and secondary transfer of low level DNA from individuals to inert surfaces. *Forensic Sci. Int.* **2002**, *129*, 25–34. [CrossRef]
11. Van Oorschot, R.A.H.; Glavich, G.; Mitchell, R.J. Persistence of DNA deposited by the original user on objects after subsequent use by a second person. *Forensic Sci. Int. Genet.* **2014**, *8*, 219–225. [CrossRef] [PubMed]

12. Breathnach, M.; Williams, L.; McKenna, L.; Moore, E. Probability of detection of DNA deposited by habitual wearer and/or the second individual who touched the garment. *Forensic Sci. Int. Genet.* **2016**, *20*, 53–60. [CrossRef] [PubMed]

13. Magee, A.M.; Breathnach, M.; Doak, S.; Thornton, F.; Noone, C.; McKenna, L.G. Wearer and non-wearer DNA on the collars and cuffs of upper garments of worn clothing. *Forensic Sci. Int. Genet.* **2018**, *34*, 152–161. [CrossRef] [PubMed]

14. Poetsch, M.; Pfeifer, M.; Konrad, H.; Bajanowski, T.; Helmus, J. Impact of several wearers on the persistence of DNA on clothes—A study with experimental scenarios. *Int. J. Legal Med.* **2018**, *132*, 117–123. [CrossRef] [PubMed]

15. Wickenheiser, R.A. Trace DNA: A review, discussion of theory, and application of the transfer of trace quantities of DNA through skin contact. *J. Forensic Sci.* **2002**, *47*, 442–450. [CrossRef]

16. Harbison, S.-A.; Fallow, M.; Bushell, D. An analysis of the success rate of 908 trace DNA samples submitted to the Crime Sample Database Unit in New Zealand. *Aust. J. Forensic Sci.* **2008**, *40*, 49–53. [CrossRef]

17. Castella, V.; Mangin, P. DNA profiling success and relevance of 1739 contact stains from caseworks. *Forensic Sci. Int. Genet. Suppl. Ser.* **2008**, *1*, 405–407. [CrossRef]

18. Raymond, J.J.; van Oorschot, R.A.H.; Walsh, S.J.; Roux, C.; Gunn, P.R. Trace DNA and street robbery: A criminalistic approach to DNA evidence. *Forensic Sci. Int. Genet. Suppl. Ser.* **2009**, *2*, 544–546. [CrossRef]

19. Mapes, A.A.; Kloosterman, A.D.; de Poot, C.J.; van Marion, V. Objective data on DNA success rates can aid the selection process of crime samples for analysis by rapid mobile DNA technologies. *Forensic Sci. Int.* **2016**, *264*, 28–33. [CrossRef] [PubMed]

20. Mapes, A.A.; Kloosterman, A.D.; van Marion, V.; de Poot, C.J. Knowledge on DNA success rates to optimize the DNA analysis process: From crime scene to laboratory. *J. Forensic Sci.* **2016**, *61*, 1055–1061. [CrossRef] [PubMed]

21. Dziak, R.; Peneder, A.; Buetter, A.; Hageman, C. Trace DNA sampling success from evidence items commonly encountered in forensic casework. *J. Forensic Sci.* **2018**, *63*, 835–841. [CrossRef]

22. Martin, B.; Blackie, R.; Taylor, D.; Linacre, A. DNA profiles generated from a range of touched sample types. *Forensic Sci. Int. Genet.* **2018**, *36*, 13–19. [CrossRef] [PubMed]

23. Van Oorschot, R.A.H.; Szkuta, B.; Verdon, T.J.; Mitchell, R.J.; Ballantyne, K.N. Trace DNA profiling in missing persons investigations. In *Handbook of Missing Persons*; Morewitz, S.J., Sturdy Colls, C., Eds.; Springer: Cham, Switzerland, 2016; pp. 353–363.

24. Krosch, M.N. Variation in forensic DNA profiling success among sampled items and collection methods: A Queensland perspective. *Aust. J. Forensic Sci.* **2020**, *53*, 612–625. [CrossRef]

25. Taroni, F.; Biedermann, A.; Vuille, J.; Morling, N. Whose DNA is this? How relevant a question? (A note for forensic scientists). *Forensic Sci. Int. Genet.* **2013**, *7*, 467–470. [CrossRef] [PubMed]

26. Meakin, G.; Jamieson, A. DNA transfer: Review and implications for casework. *Forensic Sci. Int. Genet.* **2013**, *7*, 434–443. [CrossRef] [PubMed]

27. Gill, P. Analysis and implications of the miscarriages of justice of Amanda Knox and Raffaele Sollecito. *Forensic Sci. Int. Genet.* **2016**, *23*, 9–18. [CrossRef]

28. Blackie, R.; Taylor, D.; Linacre, A. DNA profiles from clothing fibers using direct PCR. *Forensic Sci. Med. Pathol.* **2016**, *12*, 331–335. [CrossRef]

29. Ruan, T.; Barash, M.; Gunn, P.; Bruce, D. Investigation of DNA transfer onto clothing during regular daily activities. *Int. J. Leg. Med.* **2018**, *132*, 1035–1042. [CrossRef]

30. Hess, S.; Haas, C. Recovery of trace DNA on clothing: A comparison of mini-tape lifting and three other forensic evidence collection techniques. *J. Forensic Sci.* **2017**, *62*, 187–191. [CrossRef]

31. Van den Berge, M.; Ozcanhan, G.; Zijlstra, S.; Lindenbergh, A.; Sijen, T. Prevalence of human cell material: DNA and RNA profiling of public and private objects and after activity scenarios. *Forensic Sci. Int. Genet.* **2016**, *21*, 81–89. [CrossRef]

32. Van den Berge, M.; van de Merwe, L.; Sijen, T. DNA transfer and cell type inference to assist activity level reporting: Post-activity background samples as a control in dragging scenario. *Forensic Sci. Int. Genet. Suppl. Ser.* **2017**, *6*, e591–e592. [CrossRef]

33. Fonneløp, A.E.; Ramse, M.; Egeland, T.; Gill, P. The implications of shedder status and background DNA on direct and secondary transfer in an attack scenario. *Forensic Sci. Int. Genet.* **2017**, *29*, 48–60. [CrossRef] [PubMed]

34. Noël, S.; Lagacé, K.; Rogic, A.; Granger, D.; Bourgoin, S.; Jolicoeur, C.; Séguin, D. DNA transfer during laundering may yield complete genetic profiles. *Forensic Sci. Int. Genet.* **2016**, *23*, 240–247. [CrossRef]

35. Burrill, J.; Daniel, B.; Frascione, N. A review of trace "Touch DNA" deposits: Variability factors and an exploration of cellular composition. *Forensic Sci. Int. Genet.* **2019**, *39*, 8–18. [CrossRef] [PubMed]

36. Gosch, A.; Courts, C. On DNA transfer: The lack and difficulty of systematic research and how to do it better. *Forensic Sci. Int. Genet.* **2019**, *40*, 24–36. [CrossRef]

37. DNA-TrAC Database. Available online: https://bit.ly/2R4bFgL (accessed on 15 August 2021).

38. Taylor, D.; Biedermann, A.; Samie, L.; Pun, K.M.; Hicks, T.; Champod, C. Helping to distinguish primary from secondary transfer events for trace DNA. *Forensic Sci. Int. Genet.* **2017**, *28*, 155–177. [CrossRef] [PubMed]

39. Moher, D.; Liberati, A.; Tetzlaff, J.; Altman, D.G. Preferred reporting items for systematic reviews and meta-analyses: The PRISMA statement. *BMJ* **2009**, *339*, b2535. [CrossRef] [PubMed]

40. Yano, R.; Shimoda, O.; Okitsu, T.; Sakurada, M.; Ueno, Y. Development of a modified p-dimethylaminocinnamaldehyde solution for touch DNA analysis and its application to STR analysis. *Forensic Sci. Int. Genet.* **2019**, *38*, 86–92. [CrossRef] [PubMed]

41. Dierig, L.; Schmidt, M.; Wiegand, P. Looking for the pinpoint: Optimizing identification, recovery and DNA extraction of micro traces in forensic casework. *Forensic Sci. Int. Genet.* **2020**, *44*, 102191. [CrossRef]

42. Kanokwongnuwut, P.; Kirkbride, K.P.; Linacre, A. Detection of cellular material in lip-prints. *Forensic Sci. Med. Pathol.* **2019**, *15*, 362–368. [CrossRef]
43. Kanokwongnuwut, P.; Kirkbride, P.; Linacre, A. Visualising latent DNA on swabs. *Forensic Sci. Int.* **2018**, *291*, 115–123. [CrossRef]
44. Kitchner, E.; Chavez, J.; Ceresa, L.; Bus, M.M.; Budowle, B.; Gryczynski, Z. A novel approach for visualization and localization of small amounts of DNA on swabs to improve DNA collection and recovery process. *Analyst* **2021**, *146*, 1198–1206. [CrossRef] [PubMed]
45. Akutsu, T.; Ikegaya, H.; Watanabe, K.; Miyasaka, S. Immunohistochemical staining of skin-expressed proteins to identify exfoliated epidermal cells for forensic purposes. *Forensic Sci. Int.* **2019**, *303*, 109940. [CrossRef]
46. Malegori, C.; Alladio, E.; Oliveri, P.; Manis, C.; Vincenti, M.; Garofano, P.; Barni, F.; Berti, A. Identification of invisible biological traces in forensic evidences by hyperspectral NIR imaging combined with chemometrics. *Talanta* **2020**, *215*, 120911. [CrossRef]
47. Wang, Z.; Zhang, P.; Liu, H.; Zhao, Z.; Xiong, L.; He, W.; Kwok, R.T.K.; Lam, J.W.Y.; Ye, R.; Tang, B.Z. Robust Serum Albumin-Responsive AIEgen Enables Latent Bloodstain Visualization in High Resolution and Reliability for Crime Scene Investigation. *ACS Appl. Mater. Interfaces* **2019**, *11*, 17306–17312. [CrossRef] [PubMed]
48. Denny, S.E.; Nazeer, S.S.; Sivakumar, T.T.; Nair, B.J.; Jayasree, R.S. Forensic application of fluorescence spectroscopy: An efficient technique to predict the presence of human saliva. *J. Lumin.* **2018**, *203*, 696–701. [CrossRef]
49. Raj, C.K.; Garlapati, K.; Karunakar, P.; Badam, R.; Soni, P.; Lavanya, R. Saliva as Forensic Evidence using Fluorescent Spectroscopy: A Pilot Study. *J. Clin. Diagn. Res.* **2018**, *12*, ZC27–ZC29. [CrossRef]
50. Butler, J.; Chaseling, J.; Wright, K. A Comparison of Four Presumptive Tests for the Detection of Blood on Dark Materials. *J. Forensic Sci.* **2019**, *64*, 1838–1843. [CrossRef]
51. Burrill, J.; Daniel, B.; Frascione, N. Illuminating touch deposits through cellular characterization of hand rinses and body fluids with nucleic acid fluorescence. *Forensic Sci. Int. Genet.* **2020**, *46*, 102269. [CrossRef] [PubMed]
52. Olsen, A.; Miller, M.; Yadavalli, V.K.; Ehrhardt, C.J. Open source software tool for the automated detection and characterization of epithelial cells from trace biological samples. *Forensic Sci. Int.* **2020**, *312*, 110300. [CrossRef] [PubMed]
53. Kishbaugh, J.M.; Cielski, S.; Fotusky, A.; Lighthart, S.; Maguire, K.; Quarino, L.; Conte, J. Detection of prostate specific antigen and salivary amylase in vaginal swabs using SERATEC® immunochromatographic assays. *Forensic Sci. Int.* **2019**, *304*, 109899. [CrossRef]
54. Sari, D.; Hitchcock, C.; Collins, S.; Cochrane, C.; Bruce, D. Amylase testing on intimate samples from pre-pubescent, post-pubescent and post-menopausal females: Implications for forensic casework in sexual assault allegations. *Aust. J. Forensic Sci.* **2020**, *52*, 618–625. [CrossRef]
55. Suttipasit, P. Forensic Spermatozoa Detection. *Am. J. Forensic Med. Pathol.* **2019**, *40*, 304–311. [CrossRef]
56. Abbas, N.; Lu, X.; Badshah, M.A.; In, J.B.; Heo, W.I.; Park, K.Y.; Lee, M.-K.; Kim, C.H.; Kang, P.; Chang, W.-J.; et al. Development of a protein microarray chip with enhanced fluorescence for identification of semen and vaginal fluid. *Sensors* **2018**, *18*, 3874. [CrossRef] [PubMed]
57. O'Leary, K.R.; Glynn, C.L. Investigating the Isolation and Amplification of microRNAs for Forensic Body Fluid Identification. *MicroRNA* **2018**, *7*, 187–194. [CrossRef] [PubMed]
58. Hanson, E.; Ingold, S.; Dorum, G.; Haas, C.; Lagace, R.; Ballantyne, J. Assigning forensic body fluids to DNA donors in mixed samples by targeted RNA/DNA deep seqeuncing of coding region SNPs using ion torrent technology. *Forensic Sci. Int. Genet. Suppl. Ser.* **2019**, *7*, 23–24. [CrossRef]
59. Kamanna, S.; Henry, J.; Voelcker, N.; Linacre, A.; Kirkbride, K.P. A complementary forensic 'proteo-genomic' approach for the direct identification of biological fluid traces under fingernails. *Anal. Bioanal. Chem.* **2018**, *410*, 6165–6175. [CrossRef] [PubMed]
60. Watanabe, K.; Taniguchi, K.; Akutsu, T. Development of a DNA methylation-based semen-specific SNP typing method: A new approach for genotyping from a mixture of body fluids. *Forensic Sci. Int. Genet.* **2018**, *37*, 227–234. [CrossRef]
61. Mishra, I.K.; Singh, B.; Mishra, A.; Mohapatra, B.K.; Kaushik, R.; Behera, C. Touch DNA as forensic aid: A review. *Indian J. Forensic Med. Toxicol.* **2020**, *14*, 58–62.
62. Yudianto, A.; Indah Nuraini, M.; Furqoni, A.H.; Manyanza Nzilibili, S.M.; Harjanto, P. The use of touch DNA analysis in forensic identification focusing on Short Tandem Repeat-Combined DNA Index System loci THO1, CSF1PO and TPOX. *Infect. Dis. Rep.* **2020**, *12*, 8716. [CrossRef] [PubMed]
63. Wong, H.Y.; Tan, J.; Lim, Z.G.; Kwok, R.; Lim, W.; Syn, C.K.C. DNA profiling success rates of commonly submitted crime scene items. *Forensic Sci. Int. Genet. Suppl. Ser.* **2019**, *7*, 597–599. [CrossRef]
64. Ferrara, M.; Sessa, F.; Rendine, M.; Spagnolo, L.; De Simone, S.; Riezzo, I.; Ricci, P.; Pascale, N.; Salerno, M.; Bertozzi, G.; et al. A multidisciplinary approach is mandatory to solve complex crimes: A case report. *Egypt. J. Forensic Sci.* **2019**, *9*, 11. [CrossRef]
65. Naue, J.; Sänger, T.; Lutz-Bonengel, S. Get it off, but keep it: Efficient cleaning of hair shafts with parallel DNA extraction of the surface stain. *Forensic Sci. Int. Genet.* **2020**, *45*, 102210. [CrossRef] [PubMed]
66. Cahill, M.J.; Chapman, B. The novel use of a spray-on rubber coating to recover cellular material from the surface of bricks. *Forensic Sci. Int. Genet.* **2020**, *49*, 102404. [CrossRef] [PubMed]
67. Brower, A.; Akridge, B.; Siemens-Bradley, N. Human DNA collection from police dogs: Technique and application. *Forensic Sci. Med. Pathol.* **2021**, *17*, 230–234. [CrossRef]

68. Musse, J.O.; Marques, J.A.M.; Remualdo, V.; Pitlovanciv, A.K.; da Silva, C.A.L.; Corte-Real, F.; Vieira, D.N.; Vieira, W.A.; Paranhos, L.R.; Corte-Real, A.T. Deoxyribonucleic acid extraction and quantification from human saliva deposited on foods with bitemarks. *J. Contemp. Dent. Pract.* **2019**, *20*, 548–551. [PubMed]

69. Thakar, M.K.; Sahajpal, V.; Bhambara, A.K.; Bhandari, D.; Sharma, A. DNA profiling of saliva traces habitually deposited on various documents: A pilot study. *Egypt. J. Forensic Sci.* **2020**, *10*, 14. [CrossRef]

70. Aparna, R.; Shanti Iyer, R. Tears and Eyewear in Forensic Investigation—A Review. *Forensic Sci. Int.* **2020**, *306*, 110055. [CrossRef] [PubMed]

71. O'Connor, A.M.; Watts, J.E.M. The development of a rapid and reliable method (SAPSWash): For the extraction and recovery of spermatozoa from superabsorbent polymer containing products. *Forensic Sci. Int.* **2020**, *316*, 110501. [CrossRef]

72. Vanderheyden, N.; Verhoeven, E.; Vermeulen, S.; Bekaert, B. Survival of forensic trace evidence on improvised explosive devices: Perspectives on individualisation. *Sci. Rep.* **2020**, *10*, 12813. [CrossRef] [PubMed]

73. Tasker, E.; Roman, M.G.; Akosile, M.; Mayes, C.; Hughes, S.; LaRue, B. Efficacy of "touch" DNA recovery and room-temperature storage from assault rifle magazines. *Leg. Med.* **2020**, *43*, 101658. [CrossRef] [PubMed]

74. Booth, N.; Chapman, B. DNA recovery from fired hollow point ammunition. *Aust. J. Forensic Sci.* **2019**, *51*, S107–S110. [CrossRef]

75. Sterling, S.A.; Mason, K.E.; Anex, D.S.; Parker, G.J.; Hart, B.; Prinz, M. Combined DNA Typing and Protein Identification from Unfired Brass Cartridges. *J. Forensic Sci.* **2019**, *64*, 1475–1481. [CrossRef] [PubMed]

76. Thanakiatkrai, P.; Rerkamnuaychoke, B. Direct STR typing from fired and unfired bullet casings. *Forensic Sci. Int.* **2019**, *301*, 182–189. [CrossRef] [PubMed]

77. Holland, M.M.; Bonds, R.M.; Holland, C.A.; McElhoe, J.A. Recovery of mtDNA from unfired metallic ammunition components with an assessment of sequence profile quality and DNA damage through MPS analysis. *Forensic Sci. Int. Genet.* **2019**, *39*, 86–96. [CrossRef]

78. Jansson, L.; Forsberg, C.; Akel, Y.; Dufva, C.; Ansell, C.; Ansell, R.; Hedman, J. Factors affecting DNA recovery from cartridge cases. *Forensic Sci. Int. Genet.* **2020**, *48*, 102343. [CrossRef] [PubMed]

79. Gray, S.L.; Tiedge, T.M.; Butkus, J.M.; Earp, T.J.; Lindner, S.E.; Roy, R. Determination of human identity from Anopheles stephensi mosquito blood meals using direct amplification and massively parallel sequencing. *Forensic Sci. Int. Genet.* **2020**, *48*, 102347. [CrossRef] [PubMed]

80. Bonsu, D.O.M.; Higgins, D.; Austin, J.J. Forensic touch DNA recovery from metal surfaces—A review. *Sci. Justice* **2020**, *60*, 206–215. [CrossRef]

81. Comte, J.; Baechler, S.; Gervaix, J.; Lock, E.; Milon, M.-P.; Delémont, O.; Castella, V. Touch DNA collection—Performance of four different swabs. *Forensic Sci. Int. Genet.* **2019**, *43*, 102113. [CrossRef]

82. Janssen, K.; Aune, M.; Olsen, M.; Olsen, G.H.; Berg, T. Biological stain collection—Absorbing paper is superior to cotton swabs. *Forensic Sci. Int. Genet. Suppl. Ser.* **2019**, *7*, 468–469. [CrossRef]

83. Sherier, A.J.; Kieser, R.E.; Novroski, N.M.M.; Wendt, F.R.; King, J.L.; Woerner, A.E.; Ambers, A.; Garofano, P.; Budowle, B. Copan microFLOQ® Direct Swab collection of bloodstains, saliva, and semen on cotton cloth. *Int. J. Legal Med.* **2020**, *134*, 45–54. [CrossRef]

84. Kanokwongnuwut, P.; Kirkbride, K.P.; Linacre, A. An assessment of tape-lifts. *Forensic Sci. Int. Genet.* **2020**, *47*, 102292. [CrossRef] [PubMed]

85. Damsteeg-van Berkel, S.; Beemster, F.; Dankelman, J.; Loeve, A.J. The influence of contact force on forensic trace collection efficiency when sampling textiles with adhesive tape. *Forensic Sci. Int.* **2019**, *298*, 278–283. [CrossRef] [PubMed]

86. Zorbo, S.; Jeuniaux, P.P.J.M.H. DNA Recovery From Tape-Lifting Kits: Methodology and Practice. *J. Forensic Sci.* **2020**, *65*, 641–648. [CrossRef] [PubMed]

87. Zieger, M.; Schneider, C.; Utz, S. DNA recovery from gelatin fingerprint lifters by direct proteolytic digestion. *Forensic Sci. Int.* **2019**, *295*, 145–149. [CrossRef] [PubMed]

88. Fieldhouse, S.; Parsons, R.; Bleay, S.; Walton-Williams, L. The effect of DNA recovery on the subsequent quality of latent fingermarks: A pseudo-operational trial. *Forensic Sci. Int.* **2020**, *307*, 110076. [CrossRef] [PubMed]

89. Harush-Brosh, Y.; Hefetz, I.; Hauzer, M.; Mayuoni-Kirshenbaum, L.; Mashiach, Y.; Faerman, M.; Levin-Elad, M. Clean and clear (out): A neat method for the recovery of latent fingermarks from crime-scenes. *Forensic Sci. Int.* **2020**, *306*, 110049. [CrossRef]

90. Harush-Brosh, Y.; Mayuoni-Kirshenbaum, L.; Mashiach, Y.; Hauzer, M.; Hefetz, I.; Bengiat, R.; Levin-Elad, M.; Faerman, M. An efficient and eco-friendly workflow for dual fingermark processing and STR profiling. *Forensic Sci. Int. Genet.* **2020**, *47*, 102310. [CrossRef]

91. Hartless, S.; Walton-Williams, L.; Williams, G. Critical evaluation of touch DNA recovery methods for forensic purposes. *Forensic Sci. Int. Genet. Suppl. Ser.* **2019**, *7*, 379–380. [CrossRef]

92. Bonsu, D.O.M.; Higgins, D.; Henry, J.; Austin, J.J. Evaluation of the efficiency of Isohelix™ and Rayon swabs for recovery of DNA from metal surfaces. *Forensic Sci. Med. Pathol.* **2021**, *17*, 199–207. [CrossRef]

93. Sessa, F.; Salerno, M.; Bertozzi, G.; Messina, G.; Ricci, P.; Ledda, C.; Rapisarda, V.; Cantatore, S.; Turillazzi, E.; Pomara, C. Touch DNA: Impact of handling time on touch deposit and evaluation of different recovery techniques: An experimental study. *Sci. Rep.* **2019**, *9*, 9542. [CrossRef]

94. Kanokwongnuwut, P.; Martin, B.; Taylor, D.; Kirkbride, K.P.; Linacre, A. How many cells are required for successful DNA profiling? *Forensic Sci. Int. Genet.* **2021**, *51*, 102453. [CrossRef] [PubMed]

95. Miller, M.; Philpott, M.K.; Olsen, A.; Tootham, M.; Yadavalli, V.K.; Ehrhardt, C.J. Technical note: Survey of extracellular and cell-pellet-associated DNA from 'touch'/trace samples. *Forensic Sci. Int.* **2021**, *318*, 110557. [CrossRef] [PubMed]

96. Burrill, J.; Kombara, A.; Daniel, B.; Frascione, N. Exploration of cell-free DNA (cfDNA) recovery for touch deposits. *Forensic Sci. Int. Genet.* **2021**, *51*, 102431. [CrossRef] [PubMed]

97. Burrill, J.; Rammenou, E.; Alawar, F.; Daniel, B.; Frascione, N. Corneocyte lysis and fragmented DNA considerations for the cellular component of forensic touch DNA. *Forensic Sci. Int. Genet.* **2021**, *51*, 102428. [CrossRef]

98. Kaur, S.; Saini, V.; Dalal, R. UV-Visible spectroscopic effect on Haemoglobin & DNA degradation: A forensic approach. *Forensic Sci. Int.* **2020**, *307*, 110078. [PubMed]

99. Badu-Boateng, A.; Twumasi, P.; Salifu, S.P.; Afrifah, K.A. A comparative study of different laboratory storage conditions for enhanced DNA analysis of crime scene soil-blood mixed sample. *Forensic Sci. Int.* **2018**, *292*, 97–109. [CrossRef]

100. Corradini, B.; Alù, M.; Magnanini, E.; Galinier, M.E.; Silingardi, E. The importance of forensic storage support: DNA quality from 11-year-old saliva on FTA cards. *Int. J. Legal Med.* **2019**, *133*, 1743–1750. [CrossRef] [PubMed]

101. Francisco, D.D.O.; Lopez, L.F.; Gonçalves, F.D.T.; Fridman, C. Casework direct kit as an alternative extraction method to enhance touch DNA samples analysis. *Forensic Sci. Int. Genet.* **2020**, *47*, 102307. [CrossRef]

102. LeSassier, D.S.; Schulte, K.Q.; Manley, T.E.; Smith, A.R.; Powals, M.L.; Albright, N.C.; Ludolph, B.C.; Weber, K.L.; Woerner, A.E.; Gardner, M.W.; et al. Artificial fingerprints for cross-comparison of forensic DNA and protein recovery methods. *PLoS ONE* **2019**, *14*, e0223170. [CrossRef] [PubMed]

103. Liu, C.; Wu, S.; Yan, Y.; Dong, Y.; Shen, X.; Huang, C. Application of magnetic particles in forensic science. *TrAC Trends Anal. Chem.* **2019**, *121*, 115674. [CrossRef]

104. Schulte, K.Q.; Hewitt, F.C.; Manley, T.E.; Reed, A.J.; Baniasad, M.; Albright, N.C.; Powals, M.E.; LeSassier, D.S.; Smith, A.R.; Zhang, L.; et al. Fractionation of DNA and protein from individual latent fingerprints for forensic analysis. *Forensic Sci. Int. Genet.* **2021**, *50*, 102405. [CrossRef] [PubMed]

105. Hayden, D.D.; Wallin, J.M. A comparative study for the isolation of exogenous trace DNA from fingernails. *Forensic Sci. Int. Genet.* **2019**, *39*, 119–128. [CrossRef] [PubMed]

106. Timken, M.D.; Klein, S.B.; Kubala, S.; Scharnhorst, G.; Buoncristiani, M.R.; Miller, K.W.P. Automation of the standard DNA differential extraction on the Hamilton AutoLys STAR system: A proof-of-concept study. *Forensic Sci. Int. Genet.* **2019**, *40*, 96–104. [CrossRef] [PubMed]

107. Auka, N.; Valle, M.; Cox, B.D.; Wilkerson, P.D.; Cruz, T.D.; Reiner, J.E.; Seashols-Williams, S.J. Optical tweezers as an effective tool for spermatozoa isolation from mixed forensic samples. *PLoS ONE* **2019**, *14*, e0211810. [CrossRef]

108. Clark, C.P.; Xu, K.; Scott, O.; Hickey, J.; Tsuei, A.C.; Jackson, K.; Landers, J.P. Acoustic trapping of sperm cells from mock sexual assault samples. *Forensic Sci. Int. Genet.* **2019**, *41*, 42–49. [CrossRef]

109. Wright, S.N.; Huge, B.J.; Dovichi, N.J. Capillary zone electrophoresis separation and collection of spermatozoa for the forensic analysis of sexual assault evidence. *Electrophoresis* **2020**, *41*, 1344–1353. [CrossRef] [PubMed]

110. Anslinger, K.; Graw, M.; Bayer, B. Deconvolution of blood-blood mixtures using DEPArray TM separated single cell STR profiling. *Rechtsmedizin* **2019**, *29*, 30–40. [CrossRef]

111. Henry, J.; Scandrett, L. Assessment of the Yfiler® Plus PCR amplification kit for the detection of male DNA in semen-negative sexual assault cases. *Sci. Justice* **2019**, *59*, 480–485. [CrossRef]

112. Owers, R.; McDonald, A.; Montgomerie, H.; Morse, C. A casework study comparing success rates and expectations of detecting male DNA using two different Y-STR multiplexes on vaginal swabs in sexual assault investigations where no semen has been detected. *Forensic Sci. Int. Genet.* **2018**, *37*, 1–5. [CrossRef]

113. Dawnay, N.; Flamson, R.; Hall, M.J.R.; Steadman, D.W. Impact of sample degradation and inhibition on field-based DNA identification of human remains. *Forensic Sci. Int. Genet.* **2018**, *37*, 46–53. [CrossRef]

114. Avila, E.; Cavalheiro, C.P.; Felkl, A.B.; Graebin, P.; Kahmann, A.; Alho, C.S. Brazilian forensic casework analysis through MPS applications: Statistical weight-of-evidence and biological nature of criminal samples as an influence factor in quality metrics. *Forensic Sci. Int.* **2019**, *303*, 109938. [CrossRef] [PubMed]

115. Mortera, J. DNA Mixtures in Forensic Investigations: The Statistical State of the Art. *Annu. Rev. Stat. Appl* **2020**, *7*, 111–142. [CrossRef]

116. Buckleton, J.S.; Bright, J.A.; Cheng, K.; Budowle, B.; Coble, M.D. NIST interlaboratory studies involving DNA mixtures (MIX13): A modern analysis. *Forensic Sci. Int. Genet.* **2018**, *37*, 172–179. [CrossRef] [PubMed]

117. Szkuta, B.; Ansell, R.; Boiso, L.; Connolly, E.; Kloosterman, A.D.; Kokshoorn, B.; McKenna, L.G.; Steensma, K.; van Oorschot, R.A.H. Assessment of the transfer, persistence, prevalence and recovery of DNA traces from clothing: An inter-laboratory study on worn upper garments. *Forensic Sci. Int. Genet.* **2019**, *42*, 56–68. [CrossRef] [PubMed]

118. Szkuta, B.; Ansell, R.; Boiso, L.; Connolly, E.; Kloosterman, A.D.; Kokshoorn, B.; McKenna, L.G.; Steensma, K.; van Oorschot, R.A.H. DNA transfer to worn upper garments during different activities and contacts: An inter-laboratory study. *Forensic Sci. Int. Genet.* **2020**, *46*, 102268. [CrossRef] [PubMed]

119. Goray, M.; Kokshoorn, B.; Steensma, K.; Szkuta, B.; van Oorschot, R.A.H. DNA detection of a temporary and original user of an office space. *Forensic Sci. Int. Genet.* **2020**, *44*, 102203. [CrossRef] [PubMed]

120. Gill, P.; Hicks, T.; Butler, J.M.; Connolly, E.; Gusmão, L.; Kokshoorn, B.; Morling, N.; van Oorschot, R.A.H.; Parson, W.; Prinz, M.; et al. DNA commission of the International society for forensic genetics: Assessing the value of forensic biological evidence—Guidelines highlighting the importance of propositions. Part II: Evaluation of biological traces considering activity level propositions. *Forensic Sci. Int. Genet.* **2020**, *44*, 102186. [CrossRef] [PubMed]

121. Weber, A.R.; Lednev, I.K. Crime clock—Analytical studies for approximating time since deposition of bloodstains. *Forensic Chem.* **2020**, *19*, 100248. [CrossRef]

122. Stotesbury, T.; Cossette, M.L.; Newell-Bell, T.; Shafer, A.B.A. An Exploratory Time Since Deposition Analysis of Whole Blood Using Metrics of DNA Degradation and Visible Absorbance Spectroscopy. *Pure Appl. Geophys.* **2021**, *178*, 735–743. [CrossRef]

123. Cossette, M.L.; Stotesbury, T.; Shafer, A.B.A. Quantifying visible absorbance changes and DNA degradation in aging bloodstains under extreme temperatures. *Forensic Sci. Int.* **2021**, *318*, 110627. [CrossRef]

124. Bird, T.A.G.; Walton-Williams, L.; Williams, G. Time since deposition of biological fluids using RNA degradation. *Forensic Sci. Int. Genet. Suppl. Ser.* **2019**, *7*, 401–402. [CrossRef]

125. Asaghiar, F.; Williams, G.A. Evaluating the use of hypoxia sensitive markers for body fluid stain age prediction. *Sci. Justice* **2020**, *60*, 547–554. [CrossRef] [PubMed]

126. Mameli, A.; Scudiero, C.M.; Delogu, G.; Ghiani, M.E. Successful analysis of a 100 years old semen stain generating a complete DNA STR profile. *J. Forensic Leg. Med.* **2019**, *61*, 78–81. [CrossRef] [PubMed]

127. Romano, C.G.; Mangiaracina, R.; Donato, L.; D'Angelo, R.; Scimone, C.; Sidoti, A. Aged fingerprints for DNA profile: First report of successful typing. *Forensic Sci. Int.* **2019**, *302*, 109905. [CrossRef] [PubMed]

128. Alketbi, S.K.; Goodwin, W. The effect of time and environmental conditions on Touch DNA. *Forensic Sci. Int. Genet. Suppl. Ser.* **2019**, *7*, 701–703. [CrossRef]

129. Lee, L.Y.C.; Wong, H.Y.; Lee, J.Y.; Waffa, Z.B.M.; Aw, Z.Q.; Fauzi, S.N.A.B.M.; Hoe, S.Y.; Lim, M.-L.; Syn, C.K.-C. Persistence of DNA in the Singapore context. *Int. J. Legal Med.* **2019**, *133*, 1341–1349. [CrossRef]

130. Meixner, E.; Kallupurackal, V.; Kratzer, A.; Voegeli, P.; Thali, M.J.; Bolliger, S.A. Persistence and detection of touch DNA and blood stain DNA on pig skin exposed to water. *Forensic Sci. Med. Pathol.* **2020**, *16*, 243–251. [CrossRef]

131. Romero-García, C.; Rosell-Herrera, R.; Revilla, C.J.; Baeza-Richer, C.; Gomes, C.; Palomo-Díez, S.; Arroyo-Pardo, E.; López-Parra, A.M. Effect of the activity in secondary transfer of DNA profiles. *Forensic Sci. Int. Genet. Suppl. Ser.* **2019**, *7*, 578–579. [CrossRef]

132. Helmus, J.; Poetsch, J.; Pfeifer, M.; Bajanowski, T.; Poetsch, M. Cleaning a crime scene 2.0—What to do with the bloody knife after the crime? *Int. J. Legal Med.* **2020**, *134*, 171–175. [CrossRef]

133. Noël, S.; Lagacé, K.; Raymond, S.; Granger, D.; Loyer, M.; Bourgoin, S.; Jolicoeur, C.; Séguin, D. Repeatedly washed semen stains: Optimal screening and sampling strategies for DNA analysis. *Forensic Sci. Int. Genet.* **2019**, *38*, 9–14. [CrossRef]

134. Karadayi, S.; Moshfeghi, E.; Arasoglu, T.; Karadayi, B. Evaluating the persistence of laundered semen stains on fabric using a forensic light source system, prostate-specific antigen Semiquant test and DNA recovery-profiling. *Med. Sci. Law* **2020**, *60*, 122–130. [CrossRef] [PubMed]

135. Basyoni, H.A.; Mohamed, K.M.; El-Barrany, U.M.; Rashed, L.A.; Aboubakr, H.M.; Razik, H.A.A. How possible is it to recover semen DNA from laundered cotton and polyester fabrics? *Indian J. Forensic Med. Toxicol.* **2020**, *14*, 2941–2948.

136. Hofmann, M.; Adamec, J.; Anslinger, K.; Bayer, B.; Graw, M.; Peschel, O.; Schulz, M.M. Detectability of bloodstains after machine washing. *Int. J. Legal Med.* **2019**, *133*, 3–16. [CrossRef] [PubMed]

137. Fonneløp, A.E.; Johannessen, H.; Heen, G.; Molland, K.; Gill, P. A retrospective study on the transfer, persistence and recovery of sperm and epithelial cells in samples collected in sexual assault casework. *Forensic Sci. Int. Genet.* **2019**, *43*, 102153. [CrossRef]

138. Mayes, C.; Houston, R.; Seashols-Williams, S.; LaRue, B.; Hughes-Stamm, S. The stability and persistence of blood and semen mRNA and miRNA targets for body fluid identification in environmentally challenged and laundered samples. *Leg. Med.* **2019**, *38*, 45–50. [CrossRef] [PubMed]

139. Schyma, C.; Madea, B.; Müller, R.; Zieger, M.; Utz, S.; Grabmüller, M. DNA-free does not mean RNA-free—The unwanted persistence of RNA. *Forensic Sci. Int.* **2021**, *318*, 110632. [CrossRef]

140. Boyko, T.; Mitchell, R.J.; van Oorschot, R.A.H. DNA within cars: Prevalence of DNA from driver, passenger and others on steering wheels. *Aust. J. Forensic Sci.* **2019**, *51*, S91–S94. [CrossRef]

141. Boyko, T.; Szkuta, B.; Mitchell, R.J.; van Oorschot, R.A.H. Prevalence of DNA from the driver, passengers and others within a car of an exclusive driver. *Forensic Sci. Int.* **2020**, *307*, 110139. [CrossRef]

142. De Wolff, T.R.; Aarts, L.H.J.; van den Berge, M.; Boyko, T.; van Oorschot, R.A.H.; Zuidberg, M.; Kokshoorn, B. Prevalence of DNA of regular occupants in vehicles. *Forensic Sci. Int.* **2021**, *320*, 110713. [CrossRef]

143. Szkuta, B.; Reither, J.B.; Conlan, X.A.; van Oorschot, R.A.H. The presence of background DNA on common entry points to homes. *Forensic Sci. Int. Genet. Suppl. Ser.* **2019**, *7*, 784–786. [CrossRef]

144. Albani, P.P.; Patel, J.; Fleming, R.I. DNA on feminine sanitary products. *Forensic Sci. Int.* **2018**, *293*, 24–26. [CrossRef] [PubMed]

145. Murphy, C.; Kenna, J.; Flanagan, L.; Lee Gorman, M.; Boland, C.; Ryan, J. A Study of the Background Levels of Male DNA on Underpants Worn by Females. *J. Forensic Sci.* **2020**, *65*, 399–405. [CrossRef] [PubMed]

146. Reither, J.B.; Gray, E.; Durdle, A.; Conlan, X.A.; van Oorschot, R.A.H.; Szkuta, B. Background DNA on flooring: The effect of cleaning. *Forensic Sci. Int. Genet. Suppl. Ser.* **2019**, *7*, 787–790. [CrossRef]

147. Helmus, J.; Pfeifer, M.; Feiner, L.-K.; Krause, L.J.; Bajanowski, T.; Poetsch, M. Unintentional effects of cleaning a crime scene—When the sponge becomes an accomplice in DNA transfer. *Int. J. Legal Med.* **2019**, *133*, 759–765. [CrossRef] [PubMed]

148. Hefetz, I.; Einot, N.; Faerman, M.; Horowitz, M.; Almog, J. Touch DNA: The effect of the deposition pressure on the quality of latent fingermarks and STR profiles. *Forensic Sci. Int. Genet.* **2019**, *38*, 105–112. [CrossRef] [PubMed]

149. De Wolff, T.; Aarts, L.H.J.; van den Berge, M.; Boyko, T.; van Oorschot, R.A.H.; Zuidberg, M.; Kokshoorn, B. Prevalence of DNA in vehicles: Linking clothing of a suspect to car occupancy. *Aust. J. Forensic Sci.* **2019**, *51*, S103–S106. [CrossRef]

150. Ramos, P.; Handt, O.; Taylor, D. Investigating the position and level of DNA transfer to undergarments during digital sexual assault. *Forensic Sci. Int. Genet.* **2020**, *47*, 102316. [CrossRef]

151. Gosch, A.; Euteneuer, J.; Preuß-Wössner, J.; Courts, C. DNA transfer to firearms in alternative realistic handling scenarios. *Forensic Sci. Int. Genet.* **2020**, *48*, 102355. [CrossRef]

152. Butcher, E.V.; van Oorschot, R.A.H.; Morgan, R.M.; Meakin, G.E. Opportunistic crimes: Evaluation of DNA from regularly-used knives after a brief use by a different person. *Forensic Sci. Int. Genet.* **2019**, *42*, 135–140. [CrossRef]

153. Samie, L.; Taroni, F.; Champod, C. Estimating the quantity of transferred DNA in primary and secondary transfers. *Sci. Justice* **2020**, *60*, 128–135. [CrossRef]

154. Euteneuer, J.; Gosch, A.; Cachée, P.; Courts, C. A distant relationship?—Investigation of correlations between DNA isolated from backspatter traces recovered from firearms, wound profile characteristics, and shooting distance. *Int. J. Legal Med.* **2020**, *134*, 1619–1628. [CrossRef] [PubMed]

155. Thornbury, D.; Goray, M.; van Oorschot, R.A.H. Indirect DNA transfer without contact from dried biological materials on various surfaces. *Forensic Sci. Int. Genet.* **2021**, *51*, 102457. [CrossRef] [PubMed]

156. Otten, L.; Banken, S.; Schürenkamp, M.; Schulze-Johann, K.; Sibbing, U.; Pfeiffer, H.; Vennemann, M. Secondary DNA transfer by working gloves. *Forensic Sci. Int. Genet.* **2019**, *43*, 102126. [CrossRef]

157. Goray, M.; Pirie, E.; van Oorschot, R.A.H. DNA transfer: DNA acquired by gloves during casework examinations. *Forensic Sci. Int. Genet.* **2019**, *38*, 167–174. [CrossRef]

158. Van den Berge, M.; Wagner, S.; Meijers, E.; Kokshoorn, B.; Kloosterman, A.; van der Scheer, M.; Sijen, T. Minimizing hand-to-glove DNA contamination. *Forensic Sci. Int. Genet. Suppl. Ser.* **2019**, *7*, 19–20. [CrossRef]

159. Nontiapirom, K.; Bunakkharasawat, W.; Sojikul, P.; Panvisavas, N. Assessment and prevention of forensic DNA contamination in DNA profiling from latent fingerprint. *Forensic Sci. Int. Genet. Suppl. Ser.* **2019**, *7*, 546–548. [CrossRef]

160. Basset, P.; Castella, V. Positive impact of DNA contamination minimization procedures taken within the laboratory. *Forensic Sci. Int. Genet.* **2019**, *38*, 232–235. [CrossRef]

161. Williams, D.W.; Gibson, G. Classification of individuals and the potential to detect sexual contact using the microbiome of the pubic region. *Forensic Sci. Int. Genet.* **2019**, *41*, 177–187. [CrossRef] [PubMed]

162. Coil, D.A.; Neches, R.Y.; Lang, J.M.; Jospin, G.; Brown, W.E.; Cavalier, D.; Hampton-Marcell, J.; Gilbert, J.A.; Eisen, J.A. Bacterial communities associated with cell phones and shoes. *PeerJ* **2020**, *8*, e9235. [CrossRef] [PubMed]

163. Tackmann, J.; Arora, N.; Schmidt, T.S.B.; Rodrigues, J.F.M.; Von Mering, C. Ecologically informed microbial biomarkers and accurate classification of mixed and unmixed samples in an extensive cross-study of human body sites. *Microbiome* **2018**, *6*, 192. [CrossRef]

164. Yao, T.; Han, X.; Guan, T.; Zhai, C.; Liu, C.; Liu, C.; Zhu, B.; Chen, L. Exploration of the microbiome community for saliva, skin, and a mixture of both from a population living in Guangdong. *Int. J. Legal Med.* **2021**, *135*, 53–62. [CrossRef]

165. Phan, K.; Barash, M.; Spindler, X.; Gunn, P.; Roux, C. Retrieving forensic information about the donor through bacterial profiling. *Int. J. Legal Med.* **2020**, *134*, 21–29. [CrossRef]

166. Neckovic, A.; van Oorschot, R.A.H.; Szkuta, B.; Durdle, A. Investigation of direct and indirect transfer of microbiomes between individuals. *Forensic Sci. Int. Genet.* **2020**, *45*, 102212. [CrossRef]

167. Assenmacher, D.M.; Fields, S.D.; Crupper, S.S. Comparison of Commercial Kits for Recovery and Analysis of Bacterial DNA From Fingerprints. *J. Forensic Sci.* **2020**, *65*, 1310–1314. [CrossRef] [PubMed]

168. Quaak, F.C.A.; van de Wal, Y.; Maaskant-van Wijk, P.A.; Kuiper, I. Combining human STR and microbial population profiling: Two case reports. *Forensic Sci. Int. Genet.* **2018**, *37*, 196–199. [CrossRef]

169. Lindgren, P.; Myrtennäs, K.; Forsman, M.; Johansson, A.; Stenberg, P.; Nordgaard, A.; Ahlinder, J. A likelihood ratio-based approach for improved source attribution in microbiological forensic investigations. *Forensic Sci. Int.* **2019**, *302*, 109869. [CrossRef]

170. Young, J.M.; Linacre, A. Massively parallel sequencing is unlocking the potential of environmental trace evidence. *Forensic Sci. Int. Genet.* **2021**, *50*, 102393. [CrossRef]

171. Jurkevitch, E.; Pasternak, Z. A walk on the dirt: Soil microbial forensics from ecological theory to the crime lab. *FEMS Microbiol. Rev.* **2021**, *45*, fuaa053. [CrossRef] [PubMed]

172. Neckovic, A.; van Oorschot, R.A.H.; Szkuta, B.; Durdle, A. Challenges in Human Skin Microbial Profiling for Forensic Science: A Review. *Genes* **2020**, *11*, 1015. [CrossRef]

173. Neckovic, A.; van Oorschot, R.A.H.; Szkuta, B.; Durdle, A. Investigation into the presence and transfer of microbiomes within a forensic laboratory setting. *Forensic Sci. Int. Genet.* **2021**, *52*, 102492. [CrossRef] [PubMed]

174. Neckovic, A.; van Oorschot, R.A.H.; Szkuta, B.; Durdle, A. Identifying background microbiomes in an evidence recovery laboratory: A preliminary study. *Sci. Justice* **2021**, *61*, 280–290. [CrossRef]

175. Taylor, D.; Kokshoorn, B.; Hicks, T. Structuring cases into propositions, assumptions, and undisputed case information. *Forensic Sci. Int. Genet.* **2020**, *44*, 102199. [CrossRef]

176. Buckleton, J.; Taylor, D.; Bright, J.-A.; Hicks, T.; Curran, J. When evaluating DNA evidence within a likelihood ratio framework, should the propositions be exhaustive? *Forensic Sci. Int. Genet.* **2021**, *50*, 102406. [CrossRef]

177. Taylor, D.; Samie, L.; Champod, C. Using Bayesian networks to track DNA movement through complex transfer scenarios. *Forensic Sci. Int. Genet.* **2019**, *42*, 69–80. [CrossRef]

178. Volgin, L. The importance of evaluating findings given activity level propositions in order to avoid misleading evidence. *Aust. J. Forensic Sci.* **2019**, *51*, S10–S13. [CrossRef]

179. De March, I.; Taroni, F. Bayesian networks and dissonant items of evidence: A case study. *Forensic Sci. Int. Genet.* **2020**, *44*, 102172. [CrossRef] [PubMed]

180. Samie, L.; Champod, C.; Taylor, D.; Taroni, F. The use of Bayesian Networks and simulation methods to identify the variables impacting the value of evidence assessed under activity level propositions in stabbing cases. *Forensic Sci. Int. Genet.* **2020**, *48*, 102334. [CrossRef] [PubMed]

181. Gill, P. DNA evidence and miscarriages of justice. *Forensic Sci. Int.* **2019**, *294*, e1–e3. [CrossRef]

182. Perepechina, I.O. Considering DNA transfer issues in a retrospective analysis of forensic examinations. *Forensic Sci. Int. Genet. Suppl. Ser.* **2019**, *7*, 853–855. [CrossRef]

183. Dunhill, T.; Chapman, B. Meta-analysis of the secondary transfer of DNA. *Aust. J. Forensic Sci.* **2019**, *51*, S44–S47. [CrossRef]

184. Hughes, D.A.; Szkuta, B.; van Oorschot, R.A.H.; Yang, W.; Conlan, X.A. Impact of surface roughness on the deposition of saliva and fingerprint residue on non-porous substrates. *Forensic Chem.* **2021**, *23*, 100318. [CrossRef]

185. Thornbury, D.; Goray, M.; van Oorschot, R.A.H. Drying properties and DNA content of saliva samples taken before, during and after chewing gum. *Aust. J. Forensic Sci.* **2021**, 1–10. [CrossRef]

186. Kelly, P.; Connolly, E. The prevalence and persistence of saliva in vehicles. *Forensic Sci. Int. Genet.* **2021**, *53*, 102530. [CrossRef]

187. Puliatti, L.; Handt, O.; Taylor, D. The level of DNA an individual transfers to untouched items in their immediate surroundings. *Forensic Sci. Int. Genet.* **2021**, *54*, 102561. [CrossRef] [PubMed]

188. Tanzhaus, K.; Reiß, M.-T.; Zaspel, T. "I've never been at the crime scene!"—Gloves as carriers for secondary DNA transfer. *Int. J. Legal Med.* **2021**, *135*, 1385–1393. [CrossRef] [PubMed]

189. Danko, D.; Bezdan, D.; Afshin, E.E.; Ahsanuddin, S.; Bhattacharya, C.; Butler, D.J.; Chng, K.R.; Donnellan, D.; Hecht, J.; Jackson, K.; et al. A global metagenomic map of urban microbiomes and antimicrobial resistance. *Cell* **2021**, *184*, 3376–3393.e3317. [CrossRef]

190. Gill, P.; Bleka, Ø.; Roseth, A.; Fonneløp, A.E. An LR framework incorporating sensitivity analysis to model multiple direct and secondary transfer events on skin surface. *Forensic Sci. Int. Genet.* **2021**, *53*, 102509. [CrossRef]

191. Taylor, D.; Volgin, L.; Kokshoorn, B.; Champod, C. The importance of considering common sources of unknown DNA when evaluating findings given activity level propositions. *Forensic Sci. Int. Genet.* **2021**, *53*, 102518. [CrossRef] [PubMed]

192. Ypma, R.J.F.; Maaskant van Wijk, P.A.; Gill, R.; Sjerps, M.; van den Berge, M. Calculating LRs for presence of body fluids from mRNA assay data in mixtures. *Forensic Sci. Int. Genet.* **2021**, *52*, 102455. [CrossRef]

193. Meakin, G.E.; Kokshoorn, B.; van Oorschot, R.A.H.; Szkuta, B. Evaluating forensic DNA evidence: Connecting the dots. *WIREs Forensic Sci.* **2020**, *3*, e1404.

194. Jones, N.S.; Fornaro, E. *National Institute of Justice Forensic Science Research and Development Symposium*; RTI Press: Research Triangle, NC, USA, 2021. [CrossRef]

195. National Institute of Justice. Available online: https://nij.ojp.gov (accessed on 15 August 2021).

196. European Network of Forensic Science Institutes (ENFSI). Monopoly Programmes. Available online: https://enfsi.eu/projects (accessed on 15 August 2021).

197. International Society of Forensic Genetics (ISFG). Conferences. Available online: https://www.isfg.org/Meeting (accessed on 15 August 2021).

198. Gordon Research Conferences (GRC). Forensic Analysis of Human DNA. Available online: https://www.grc.org/forensic-analysis-of-human-dna-conference/ (accessed on 15 August 2021).

199. American Academy of Forensic Sciences (AAFS). Conference Proceedings. Available online: https://aafs.org/aafs/Resources/Proceedings/AAFS/Resources/Proceedings.aspx?hkey=b8e1fc6b-2c69--411a-a386--7d38929ca963 (accessed on 10 October 2021).

200. Promega. International Symposium on Human Identification (ISHI). Available online: https://www.ishinews.com (accessed on 15 August 2021).

201. Budowle, B.; van Oorschot, R.A.H.; Morling, N.; Martinez de Pancorbo, M.; Doutremepuich, C.; Piters, A.; Esponda, A.; Monique, G. *Les Progrès Récents en Empreintes Génétiques et en ADN de Transfert (Recent Progress on Forensic Sciences and DNA Transfer)*; Librairie Mollat: Bordeaux, France, 2020. Available online: https://www.expertise-adn.fr/actualites-adn/les-progres-recents-en-empreintes-genetiques-et-en-adn-de-transfert (accessed on 15 August 2021).

202. International Society of Forensic Genetics (ISFG). Summer School. Available online: https://isfgsummerschool.events.idloom.com/virtual-edition-2021 (accessed on 15 August 2021).

203. University of Lausanne. Statistics and the Evaluation of Forensic Evidence. Available online: https://www.formation-continue-unil-epfl.ch/formation/statistics-evaluation-forensic-evidence-cas/ (accessed on 15 August 2021).

204. University of Lausanne. Challenging Forensic Science: How Science Should Speak to Court. Available online: https://www.coursera.org/learn/challenging-forensic-science (accessed on 15 August 2021).

205. Forensic Technology Center of Excellence; National Institute of Justice. Probabilistic Genotyping of Evidentiary DNA Typing Results: Online Workshop Series. Available online: https://forensiccoe.org/online-workshop-series-probabilistic-genotyping-of-evidentiary-dna-typing-results (accessed on 15 August 2021).
206. Netherlands Register of Court Experts (NRGD). Register Open for Applications DNA Activity Level. 2021. Available online: https://english.nrgd.nl/news/register-open-for-applications-dna-activity-level.aspx (accessed on 8 October 2021).
207. Netherlands Register of Court Experts (NRGD). Standards: Human DNA Analysis and Interpretation (001.1–001.3). 2021. Available online: https://english.nrgd.nl/binaries/10321%20-%20Standards%20Human%20DNA%20Analysis%20and%20Interpretation%20v4.1_tcm40--493992.pdf (accessed on 10 October 2021).
208. Kokshoorn, B.; Aarts, L.H.J.; Ansell, R.; Connolly, E.; Drotz, W.; Kloosterman, A.D.; McKenna, L.G.; Szkuta, B.; van Oorschot, R.A.H. Sharing data on DNA transfer, persistence, prevalence and recovery: Arguments for harmonization and standardization. *Forensic Sci. Int. Genet.* **2018**, *37*, 260–269. [CrossRef]
209. Université Du Québec À Trois-Rivières. BDATT-TTADB (Transfer Traces Activity DataBase). Available online: http://www.uqtr.ca/LRC/BDATT-TTADB (accessed on 15 August 2021).
210. Cadola, L.; Charest, M.; Lavallée, C.; Crispino, F. The occurrence and genesis of transfer traces in forensic science: A structured knowledge database. *J. Can. Soc. Forensic Sci* **2021**, *54*, 86–100. [CrossRef]
211. GOV.UK. Forensic Science Providers: Codes of Practice and Conduct. Available online: https://www.gov.uk/government/collections/forensic-science-providers-codes-of-practice-and-conduct (accessed on 15 August 2021).
212. Gill, P.; Hicks, T.; Butler, J.M.; Connolly, E.; Gusmão, L.; Kokshoorn, B.; Morling, N.; van Oorschot, R.A.H.; Parson, W.; Prinz, M.; et al. DNA Commission of the International Society for Forensic Genetics: Assessing the value of forensic biological evidence—Guidelines highlighting the importance of propositions: Part I: Evaluation of DNA profiling comparisons given (sub-) source propositions. *Forensic Sci. Int. Genet.* **2018**, *36*, 189–202. [CrossRef] [PubMed]
213. International Organization for Standardization. Forensic Sciences—Part 5: Reporting. ISO/CD 21043–5. 2021. Available online: https://www.iso.org/standard/73896.html?browse=tc (accessed on 16 August 2021).
214. Butler, J.M.; Iyer, H.; Press, R.; Taylor, M.K.; Vallone, P.M.; Willis, S. National Institute of Standards and Technology. DNA Mixture Interpretation: A NIST Scientific Foundation Review. 2021. Available online: https://nvlpubs.nist.gov/nistpubs/ir/2021/NIST.IR.8351-draft.pdf (accessed on 10 October 2021).
215. Roux, C.; Willis, S.; Weyermann, C. Shifting forensic science focus from means to purpose: A path forward for the discipline? *Sci. Justice* **2021**, *61*, 678–686. [CrossRef]
216. De Koeijer, J.A.; Sjerps, M.J.; Vergeer, P.; Berger, C.E.H. Combining evidence in complex cases—A practical approach to interdisciplinary casework. *Sci. Justice* **2020**, *60*, 20–29. [CrossRef] [PubMed]
217. National Institute of Forensic Science Australia New Zealand. An Introductory Guide to Evaluative Reporting. 2017. Available online: http://www.anzpaa.org.au/forensic-science/our-work/projects/evaluative-reporting (accessed on 10 October 2021).
218. Willis, S.M.; McKenna, L.; McDermott, S.D.; O'Donnell, G.; Barrett, A.; Rasmusson, B.; Höglund, T.; Berger, C.E.H.; Sierps, M.J.; Lucena-Molina, J.J.; et al. ENFSI Guideline for Evaluative Reporting in Forensic Science. 2015. Available online: http://enfsi.eu/wp-content/uploads/2016/09/m1_guideline.pdf (accessed on 10 October 2021).
219. Kokshoorn, B.; Aarts, B.; De Blaeij, T.; Maaskant-van Wijk, P.; Blankers, B. Bewijskracht van onderzoek naar biologische sporen en DNA. Deel 3: Activiteitniveau. *Expert. en Recht* **2014**, *6*, 213–219.
220. Robertson, P.; Aitken, C.; Royal Statistical Society. The Logic of Forensic Proof: Inferential Reasoning in Criminal Evidence and Forensic Science. 2014. Available online: https://rss.org.uk/RSS/media/File-library/Publications/rss-inferential-reasoning-criminal-evidence-forensic-science.pdf (accessed on 10 October 2021).

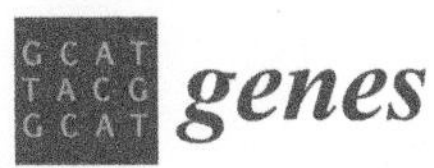

Review

Predicting Physical Appearance from DNA Data—Towards Genomic Solutions

Ewelina Pośpiech [1], Paweł Teisseyre [2,3], Jan Mielniczuk [2,3] and Wojciech Branicki [1,4,*]

1   Malopolska Centre of Biotechnology, Jagiellonian University, 30-387 Kraków, Poland; ewelina.pospiech@uj.edu.pl
2   Institute of Computer Science, Polish Academy of Sciences, 01-248 Warsaw, Poland; Pawel.Teisseyre@ipipan.waw.pl (P.T.); jan.mielniczuk@ipipan.waw.pl (J.M.)
3   Faculty of Mathematics and Information Science, Warsaw University of Technology, 00-662 Warsaw, Poland
4   Central Forensic Laboratory of the Police, 00-583 Warsaw, Poland
*   Correspondence: wojciech.branicki@uj.edu.pl; Tel.: +48-126-645-024

Abstract: The idea of forensic DNA intelligence is to extract from genomic data any information that can help guide the investigation. The clues to the externally visible phenotype are of particular practical importance. The high heritability of the physical phenotype suggests that genetic data can be easily predicted, but this has only become possible with less polygenic traits. The forensic community has developed DNA-based predictive tools by employing a limited number of the most important markers analysed with targeted massive parallel sequencing. The complexity of the genetics of many other appearance phenotypes requires big data coupled with sophisticated machine learning methods to develop accurate genomic predictors. A significant challenge in developing universal genomic predictive methods will be the collection of sufficiently large data sets. These should be created using whole-genome sequencing technology to enable the identification of rare DNA variants implicated in phenotype determination. It is worth noting that the correctness of the forensic sketch generated from the DNA data depends on the inclusion of an age factor. This, however, can be predicted by analysing epigenetic data. An important limitation preventing whole-genome approaches from being commonly used in forensics is the slow progress in the development and implementation of high-throughput, low DNA input sequencing technologies. The example of palaeoanthropology suggests that such methods may possibly be developed in forensics.

Keywords: physical appearance; human genome variation; DNA-based prediction; investigative leads; forensic DNA intelligence; forensic genomics

Citation: Pośpiech, E.; Teisseyre, P.; Mielniczuk, J.; Branicki, W. Predicting Physical Appearance from DNA Data—Towards Genomic Solutions. *Genes* **2022**, *13*, 121. https://doi.org/10.3390/genes13010121

Academic Editor: Fulvio Cruciani

Received: 10 December 2021
Accepted: 4 January 2022
Published: 10 January 2022

Publisher's Note: MDPI stays neutral with regard to jurisdictional claims in published maps and institutional affiliations.

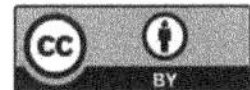

1. Introduction

The information included in genomic data can be used to generate investigative leads that, when properly used, can speed up the process of human identification in forensic investigations. Such forensic DNA intelligence can use a variety of methods, including relatedness testing, the inference of ancestry, the prediction of physical phenotype, and age estimation [1–4]. As an inherently interdisciplinary science, forensic science today can benefit from the rapidly developing methods in the areas of genomics and machine learning, which is particularly beneficial for the further development of forensic DNA intelligence. Studies of human genome variation conducted today on an unprecedented scale are revealing how genes control phenotypes. This knowledge has fundamental meaning for understanding the genome–phenome relationship. Importantly, the growing knowledge of human genome variation allows for the development of algorithms that can more accurately predict phenotypes, providing more reliable investigative leads to help identify an unnamed perpetrator or victim and solve a case. It is worth noting that the DNA-based predictive tools developed in the forensic field are also useful in evolutionary anthropology. In this review paper, we will summarise how the advances in understanding the genetic architectures of various human physical characteristics, and the progress in high-throughput genotyping technologies in combination with machine-learning methods, allow the prediction of physical appearance traits. We will also highlight the evolution of the approach to the genetic prediction of physical traits, which has moved from building predictive models based on variables that show genetic association to building models based on variables that improve predictive performance (Figure 1).

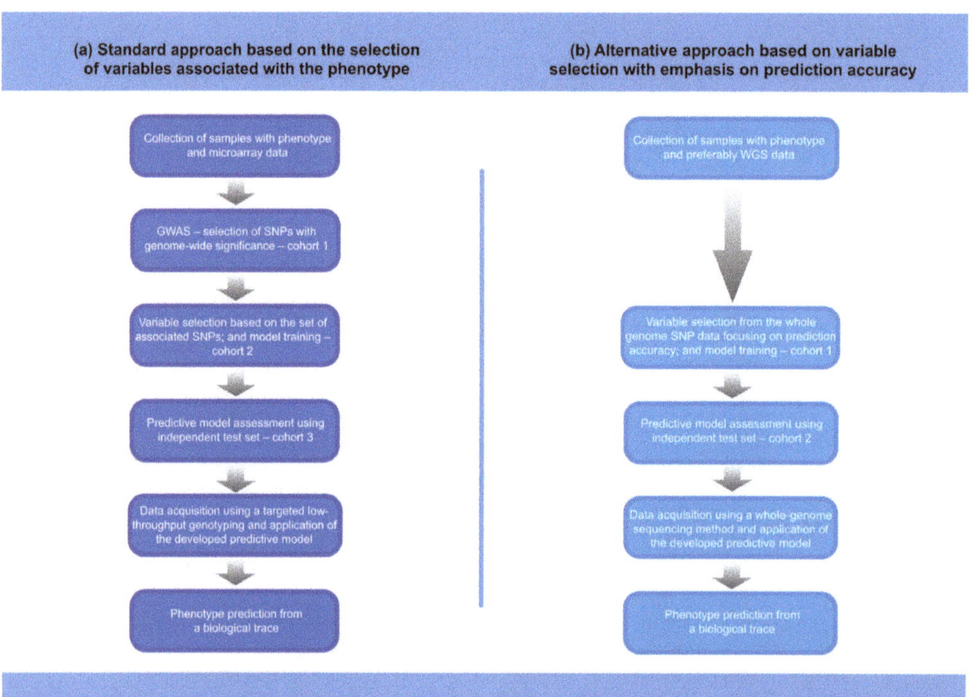

Figure 1. Procedure for the development and application of a phenotype prediction tool. The main differences in the procedures for developing a predictive model using the standard or alternative approach concern the selection of variables and the number of variables in the model. Consequently, the method of acquiring genetic data in the practical forensic applications of the next-generation predictive models may require whole-genome sequencing methods. Thus: (**a**) only phenotype-associated SNPs are included in prediction modelling, the models are not very extensive, and the methods of data acquisition can be less complex (SNaPshot, targeted MPS); (**b**) the selection of relevant variables (SNPs) is targeted towards improving the prediction accuracy of the model, and much more advanced variable selection methods are required. Some complex models may involve many thousands of SNPs, which, in biological traces, must be analysed using whole-genome sequencing methods that are effective for low DNA input samples.

2. Explaining the Heritability of Appearance Traits

A large meta-analysis of twin studies has confirmed that all human traits are heritable and showed that most of the traits can be explained by an additive genetic variation [5]. The extreme similarity of physical appearance of monozygotic twins clearly indicates the role of genes, but their identification is not simple due to the complex nature of appearance traits. Linkage mapping, which relies on the co-segregation of causal DNA variants with marker variants (SNP or STR) within pedigrees, has been very successful at identifying the gene variants affecting simple mendelian traits [6], but mostly failed to identify the DNA variants involved in the determination of complex traits [7]. The breakthrough in explaining the heritability of complex phenotypes has come with the advent of genome-wide association studies (GWAS), which are effective at discovering common variants with small effect sizes on traits [7]. GWAS is used to identify associations between genotypes and phenotypes by testing for differences in the allele frequency of DNA variants between individuals who differ phenotypically. Technically, the analysis of hundreds of thousands of DNA variants in the genomes of these individuals enables finding those statistically associated with a specific phenotype [8].

2.1. Pigmentation Phenotype

GWAS data have been very effective at explaining the heritability of physical appearance traits. The heritability of human pigmentation traits has been assessed to be above 80% and, thus, provides a good starting point for DNA-based prediction, because it means that 80% of the variation in pigmentation in a population is due to genetic variation between individuals and that the influence of the environment is relatively small [9–11].

Many candidate genes for human pigmentation were identified before the GWAS era through animal models and the linkage to diseases with mendelian inheritance modes, such as oculocutaneous albinism. Genome-wide association scans confirmed the importance of these genes and identified many of the novel gene variants influencing the variability of normal human pigmentation. The collected data confirmed a very promising perspective for the genetic prediction of pigmentation traits. The less complex nature of some pigmentation phenotypes, such as blue and brown eye colours and red hair colour, and the availability of DNA variants with relatively large effect sizes, similar to the genetic effects observed for mendelian traits, were particularly encouraging. The region on chromosome 15, including the *OCA2* gene, was implicated in eye colour via linkage and subsequent fine-mapping analyses [12,13]. The evidence of a relationship between *OCA2* genotypes and eye colour became stronger with additional reports [14–16]. This was an Icelandic GWAS that implicated the involvement of neighbouring *HERC2* in the determination of eye colour and suggested that this genomic region was responsible for the regulation of *OCA2* gene expression [17]. This speculation was soon confirmed by other studies that showed that the DNA variant rs12913832 was responsible for brown and blue eye colour in humans [18,19]. The postulated interaction between these two genes in determining eye colour was also confirmed [20]. Most of the SNP heritability of red hair colour is explained by the single *MC1R* gene, which was also discovered long before the genome-wide association scans and confirmed in various population samples across the globe [21,22]. The effect of this gene was extended to skin colour and freckling [23,24]. These early genome-wide association scans for pigmentation also clearly demonstrated their agnostic power to detect novel, sometimes unexpected genotype–phenotype relationships, as in the case of the *IRF4* gene, which is now an important predictor of pigmentation phenotypes [17,25]. The success of GWAS was clear, but a significant proportion of heritability remained missing, which could be attributed mainly to the insufficiently large sample sizes used in genome-wide association scans, insufficient phenotyping regimes generating heterogeneity, the insufficient density of the GWA arrays and the significance of non-additive variation [26,27]. Indeed, the improved statistical power to detect small effect-size variants more effectively in the next series of genome-wide association scans enabled the identification of multiple new DNA variants involved in the heritability of hair and eye colour. For example, a large study of 192,986 European individuals from 10 populations identified 50 new loci for eye colour [28]. The study revealed signals with genome-wide significance for 12,192 SNPs from 52 genomic regions in the discovery set of 157,485 individuals. By combining discovery and replication sets, the study finally identified 124 independent associations from 61 genomic regions and concluded that the known variants explain 53.2% of eye colour variation. Notably, the study also investigated Asian cohorts and found consistency in the genetic architecture of eye colour in populations from Europe and Asia [28].

Human skin colour is highly variable at continental and intercontinental levels, complicating research on the genetic architecture and heritability of this trait [29]. The rs1426654 in *SLC24A5*, discovered thanks to a Zebrafish study, plays an important role in skin colour differences at the continental level, explaining more than 30% of skin colour differences between African and European populations [30]. GWAS on skin colour conducted on various population samples discovered multiple genes and gene variants involved in skin colour variation at the intercontinental level [25,31–34]. Notably, the studies of African populations showed large differences in skin colour, revealing the high complexity of the genetic architecture of skin colour in Africa and the significance of genes unknown to European studies [35,36].

A meta-analysis that involved almost 300,000 genomes from individuals of European ancestry included in two different cohorts (23andMe, UK Biobank) discovered 124 loci relevant to human hair colour, mostly novel associations, including genes with strong effect, such as *SLC45A1*, *DSTYK*, *FOSL2*, *LHX2*, *EDNRB*, *SHC4*, *KRT31*, and *BCAS1*. The study was highly successful at explaining up to 34.6% (red hair) of the heritability of human hair colour, despite an imperfect phenotyping regime involving self-reported hair colour in adulthood [37]. Another study based on UK Biobank resources examined 343,234 genomes from participants reporting British descent and these were, thus, more homogeneous. This study assessed that all identified variants explain 90% of the SNP heritability of red hair colour but, surprisingly, it found that a DNA variant located 97 kb from the 5′ end of the *MC1R* gene may be more important for explaining red hair colour than the polymorphism within the *MC1R* exon, and it identified an additional eight loci that contribute to the genetics of red hair colour. This research also revealed 213 variants important to the determination of blond hair colour, accounting for 73% of SNP heritability. In addition, a set of 56 DNA variants was found to be important for brown hair colour and was assessed to account for 47% of SNP heritability of this hair category [38].

2.2. Hair Features

Along with hair colour, other features describing the properties of human hair can be useful to define the physical appearance of an individual. Research shows that genetics plays a key role in the determination of hair features. However, the level of heritability may differ for various hair traits. Very high heritability (85–95%) was estimated for hair shape [39]. Heritability of around 70% was reported for monobrow and beard thickness [40]. Studies are contradictory in terms of the heritability level of hair loss (~40–80%) [40–43] and hair greying (~30–90%) [40,44], but the accuracy of the heritability measurement may be affected by the definition of heritability, the study design and the method of analysis used [45]. It is worth noting that heritability values calculated from the entire SNPs analysed in GWA studies tend to be underestimated compared to estimates of pedigree heritability, because the former do not include phenotypic variation due to rare variants that are not correctly determined by the SNPs genotyped on microarrays or common variants with small effect sizes that are not correctly identified if the sample size is not large enough. In turn, pedigree heritability may be biased by the common environmental factors to which families are typically exposed [43,45]. Notably, heritability estimates may vary due to changes in allele frequencies in populations caused by different evolutionary mechanisms and environmental contributions that change with the age of individuals [46]. The genetic basis of hair loss and hair shape are the most investigated so far. Androgenetic alopecia, known in men as male pattern baldness (MPB), is the most common type of progressive loss of hair from the scalp and is particularly frequent among men in Europe. Over the last >10 years, several GWA studies on hair loss have been carried out, with the vast majority of research conducted on Europeans [43,47–53]. These studies revealed multiple genes that are associated with the risk of MPB, with two loci showing the strongest effect of association, Xq12 (*AR/EDA2R*) and 20p11 (*PAX1/FOXA2*). Of these two loci, only 20p11 is known to act in Asians, indicating the significance of population heterogeneity [54,55]. A long list of additional loci, representing smaller effect sizes, identified through GWAS and/or candidate gene approaches, is available in the literature (e.g., *HDAC9*, *WNT10*, *TARDBP*, *EBF1*, *SUCNR1*, *AUTS2*, *FGF5*, *IRF4*, *C1orf127*, *RUNX1*, and *TWIST2*). Studies published in

2017–2018 led to significant advances in research on the genetics of hair loss. Four large GWA scans have been conducted on individuals of European descent. The first three of those studies, which investigated 20,000–50,000 genomes each, detected altogether more than 300 GWA signals, including 253 novel MPB associations [42,52,53]. The largest study, which investigated 200,000 genomes, allowed the identification of >600 genome-wide associations, explaining altogether 25% of the phenotypic variation observed in alopecia [43]. These large-scale studies not only discovered many new loci involved in alopecia, but also highlighted the implicated molecular pathways and discovered the genetic links of alopecia with different traits/conditions, including bone mineral density, puberty, metabolic traits, and Parkinson's disease. However, a significant part of MPB heritability remains missing. Recent studies showed that the use of advanced statistical methods and the incorporation of functional genomics data prior to association tests may improve the efficiency of SNP detection in GWAS and these approaches were proved to be successful in MPB research by increasing the number of SNP hits by an additional ~4% [56,57].

For hair morphology (shape), four GWA studies have been published so far, two of which were carried out on Europeans, with one study on Latin Americans and one on East Asians [40,58–60]. Hair shape, usually defined as straight vs. wavy vs. curly, is a highly distinctive feature of human appearance. As with hair loss, genetic heterogeneity between populations is observed with different mechanisms and genes underlying straight hair formation in Europeans and East Asians. The *TCHH* gene is known to act only in Europeans, while *EDAR* is the main contributor to straight hair in East Asians [58,59,61]. However, the proportion of known heritability attributed to both genes in respective populations was found to be small (<10%). The *TCHH* gene was discovered in the first GWA study published in 2009, which was conducted on three cohorts with a total of more than 4800 individuals of European descent [58]. *TCHH* was the only gene in this study that reached genome-wide significance, but suggestive associations were also disclosed for several additional loci, including the *FRAS1* and *WNT10* genes. The role of the *EDAR* gene in hair straightness and thickness in Asians was discovered through candidate gene analyses [61,62] and confirmed in a later GWA study conducted in 2016 on ~2900 Chinese people, with no additional genes reaching GWA significance in this study [59]. A GWA study conducted on >6000 Latin Americans discovered a novel association for *PRSS53* [40]. The latest meta-analysis of European GWA studies, exploring a total of more than 16,000 samples, allowed the identification of 12 hair shape genes, including eight novel association signals (*ERRFI1/SLC45A1, PEX14, PADI3, TGFA, LGR4, HOXC13, KRTAP,* and *PTK6*) [60]. The study showed that a model consisting of 14 SNPs across novel and literature loci, together with sex, explains 10% of the total hair shape variability. Further research pointed to the role of gene–gene interactions in hair shape determination as one of the factors underlying missing heritability [63]. The *RPTN* gene has been implicated in straight hair formation in Europeans and East Asians, but throughout interactions with different previously known head hair shape genes.

Only a few studies have addressed the genetic basis of other hair traits. In recent years, the first genes responsible for the thickness of the eyebrows, e.g., *EDAR, FOXL2, LIMS1, TMEM174,* SOX2, and *FOXD1* [40,64,65], monobrows, e.g., *PAX3* and 5q13.2 [40,51], beard thickness, e.g., *EDAR, LNX1, PREP,* and *FOXP2* [40], and hair greying, e.g., *IRF4,* and *KIF1A* [40,66], have been identified through whole-genome or whole-exome analyses.

2.3. Human Height

Human height is heritable in approximately 80%, but only the single genes associated with this trait were known before the era of GWA studies. The study of human height genetics is a good example of the effectiveness of explaining the heritability of complex traits through the GWAS approach. An important advantage of stature studies is undoubtedly the ease of measuring this phenotype and thus the homogeneity of the phenotypic data. The genome-wide association scans for human stature identified gene variants with a small effect size, clearly confirming the high polygenicity of this trait. The first three GWA studies of human height, which collectively included more than 50,000 samples, detected only 54 loci with a statistically significant association with stature [67–69]. Most of these loci have not been previously linked to human height and, in many cases, the known biological function did not make them candidates for the regulation of human stature. The genes discovered explained only about 5% of the variation in height, which was very discouraging, especially for predicting this distinctive feature. A huge meta-analysis that considered GWAS data for more than 180,000 genomes made only a small advance in explaining the heritability of human growth, enabling the discovery of 180 loci. The work demonstrated the importance of allelic heterogeneity in explaining the complex genetic architecture of human stature [70]. At the same time, it has been argued that testing each SNP individually for an association with a trait, which is typical for GWAS investigations, leads to missing many real associations, especially when the effect sizes of individual SNPs on a trait are small. By fitting all SNPs simultaneously, Yang et al. provided an unbiased estimate of the variance explained by the SNPs in total, and showed that common genetic variants are able to explain as much as 45% of the variance in human height [71]. However, consistently increasing the number of genomes analysed with high-density DNA microarrays has proven to be an effective method for elucidating the still-missing genetic variation responsible for human height. The large meta-analysis that included 700,000 European genomes (250,000 previously investigated [72] and 450,000 from the UK Biobank) identified 3290 near-independent SNPs associated with human stature which were found to explain 24.6% of variance of this trait [73]. Still, unpublished data suggest that the large proportion of missing heritability may be hiding in rare genetic variants (≤ 0.01) that can be detected via the whole genome sequencing of a sufficient number of genomes [74]. Notably, Zoledziewska et al. showed that human height can be under pressure from natural selection, presenting data showing that known height-decreasing alleles were found at higher frequency in Sardinians than would be expected to be caused by genetic drift [75]. Research on the genetic architecture of human stature, on a smaller scale, is also being conducted in populations in Asia and Africa. A meta-analysis of 93,926 individuals from East Asia identified 98 loci, including 17 novel for human height [76]. A GWA study based on 191,787 Japanese genomes disclosed 573 height-associated variants and assessed that 64 rare (<0.01) and low-frequency (<0.05) variants explain 1.7% of the height variance. The study revealed genes not previously associated with stature [77]. Eighty-three low-frequency variants affecting human height have also been reported in [78].

2.4. Facial Morphology

The human face represents a set of correlated complex phenotypes that are highly variable at inter- and intra-population levels and define what is apparently the most differentiating human trait [79]. The high similarity of the faces of monozygotic twins clearly indicates that most of this variability is genetically determined. Despite this, research into the heritability of facial features has caused quite a few problems, probably due to the three-dimensional nature of human faces. Only a recent face heritability study performed on 952 British twins using an advanced phenotyping and landmarking system confirmed the high heritability (>65%) of many facial traits [80]. Indeed, contrary to some physical phenotype traits, collecting phenotypic data for faces can be challenging. A self-reported categorisation is less useful, and measurement ideally requires the involvement of methods that are able to capture the three-dimensionality of faces. The approaches used to collect facial appearance data for studying the genetics of craniofacial variation that can be found in the literature are standard 2D photographs, magnetic resonance imaging (MRI) and 3D scanning. The latter has quickly gained a dominant position in craniofacial genetics research. It should be noted that the phenotypic assessment of facial variability from 3D images is not an easy task and makes large-scale studies and comparisons between different studies difficult. Initially, the process relied on a labour-intensive process of the manual determination of landmarks, and later, several automated landmarking methods applicable to 3D images have facilitated research on the association of facial phenotype with genotype [80–83]. In one of the first works on the genetics of natural craniofacial variation, 11 DNA variants previously associated with cleft-lip phenotypes were tested in two European cohorts with the phenotypes captured using 2D photos or magnetic resonance images [84]. A DNA variant near the *GREM1* gene was associated with nose width, and another near the *CCDC26* gene was associated with bizygomatic distance. The first GWAS scan that was aimed at investigating normal facial variation identified only a single intronic DNA variant in the *PAX3* gene, which showed association with nasion position. This first study was conducted on a relatively small group of 2185 adolescents. The study used a 3D laser scanning method to collect phenotypic data. The 22 identified landmarks were then used to generate 54 3D and 2D distances featuring different facial characteristics. Additionally, following a previous method, a principal component analysis enabled the identification of 14 independent groups of correlated coordinates [85]. These parameters were used in association testing, which identified four associations, but only *PAX3* was replicated in an independent cohort of 1622 participants [86]. A larger GWAS analysis of almost 10,000 individuals of European origin from several cohorts used 3D MRI scans and 2D photos, and identified five genes involved in facial variation. *PAX3*, *PRDM16*, and *TP63* have previously been linked to craniofacial development, while *C5orf50* and *COL17A1* were new findings [87]. The strongest signal was again obtained for *PAX3*, which soon gained further confirmation in an independent study of about 6000 Latin Americans investigated in the large CANDELA project [40]. It is worth noting that rare variants in *PAX3*, the most replicated gene for natural variation in facial appearance, cause Waardenburg syndrome, which involves some facial dysmorphism, including a broad nasal bridge. The phenotyping regime in Adhikari's study involved a simple approach based on standard 2D photographs, and the study also implicated *DCHS2*, *RUNX2*, *GLI3*, and *PAX1* in nose morphology and *EDAR* in chin protrusion [40]. Another GWAS study, which included 3D images of 3118 individuals of European ancestry that were used to derive 20 facial distance measurements, identified several genomic regions and implicated *MAFB*, *PAX9*, *MIPOL1*, *ALX3*, *HDAC8*, and *PAX1* in normal facial variation, including the measures of eye, nose, and facial breadth. The study also provided additional evidence for the association between *PRDM16* and *C5orf50* and facial features [88]. Crouch et al. investigated the hypothesis that the DNA variants responsible for large effects on facial morphology exist in the human genome, and focused on individuals displaying extreme facial characteristics to find them. The study included 3D images of 1832 individuals from the general population as a discovery set and 1567 3D scans of twins from the TwinsUK databank, plus 33 of East Asians for replication. The original 3D scans were used to manually mark each face with 14 well-defined landmarks, allowing a mesh of 50,000–150,000 surface points in 3D space to be transformed into a set of 29,658 surface points for each face. This approach enabled the identification of three SNPs in *PCDH15*, *MBTPS1*, and *TMEM163*, genes that have previously been associated with various pathological phenotypes involving craniofacial dysmorphias [89]. The study by Claes et al. (2018) involved 2329 individuals at the discovery stage and an additional 1719 at the replication stage, and found associations for 15 loci with facial features, including four new genes, nine consistently confirmed, and two linked with pleiotropic facial phenotypic features. The study used an innovative, data-driven facial phenotyping approach based on structural correlations between about 10,000 3D quasi-landmarks, which enabled the hierarchical (global-to-local) clustering of the human face into segments [90]. This approach also yielded good results for a meta-analysis, which included 8246 European individuals and enabled the identification of 203 loci associated with normal facial variation [91] and for a study of facial features in East Africans, which investigated 2595 3D facial images collected on Tanzanian children [92]. The latter cohort was previously investigated, with two genes, *SCHIP1* and *PDE8A*, identified that were associated with measures of human facial size [83]. GWA studies investigating human facial morphology in non-European cohorts are rare. Worth noting is a GWAS conducted on an exploratory panel of Uyghurs that identified six loci important for the genetic architecture of the human face, four of which were replicated in independent cohorts of Uyghur or southern Han Chinese [93].

3. DNA-Based Predictive Tools for Forensic Applications

Several factors determine the accuracy of DNA-based predictive methods, including high heritability of a trait, the identification of appropriate predictors, and the selection of the best mathematical approach to model development. The forensic community very early recognised the investigative potential of extracting phenotypes from DNA data. The practical importance of a simple amelogenin genetic sex test [94], and also of the inference of biogeographical ancestry [95,96], made it clear that a description of the phenotypic characteristics of a person of undetermined identity can provide important investigative leads. The variation of the *MC1R* gene was soon proposed as an indicator of red hair colour [97], while the predictive potential of the *OCA2* variation was proposed for the inference of eye colour [14]. The availability of GWAS data has made it possible to develop tools for predicting human appearance traits more effectively. The research carried out has made it possible to develop predictive tools with varying performances and practicalities of application for different physical characteristics (Table 1).

Table 1. Examples of various approaches proposed for genetic prediction of physical traits.

Physical Trait	Statistical Model	Number of Predictors in the Model	Prediction Accuracy Parameters	Ref.
Eye colour	Multinomial logistic regression (IrisPlex) [1]	6 SNPs	$AUC_{brown} = 0.93$ [2] $AUC_{intermediate} = 0.72$ $AUC_{blue} = 0.91$	[98]
	Likelihood ratio	4 SNPs	$LR_{light\text{-}dark}$ depends on genotypes	[99]
	Multiple linear regression	3 SNPs	$R^2 = 0.764$	[100]
	No statistical model, classification based on genotypes	6 SNPs	Overall classification success rate (blue–green–brown): 98.94%	[101]
	Likelihood ratio	6 SNPs	$LR_{light\text{-}dark}$ depends on genotypes $AUC_{light\text{-}dark} = 0.925$	[102]
	Bayesian naïve classifier (Snipper)	23 SNPs	Classification success rate: blue = 98.27%, green-hazel = 97.81% brown = 96.67%.	[103]
	Multiple response classification tree	4 SNPs	Classification success rate: blue = 89% intermediate = 46% brown = 94%	[104]
	No statistical model, prediction based on genotypes	5 SNPs	Overall classification success rate (blue–green–brown): 97.64%	[105]
Hair colour	Multinomial logistic regression + prediction guide (HIrisPlex) [1]	22 SNPs	Classification success rate: $AUC_{blond} = 0.81$ $AUC_{brown} = 0.82$ $AUC_{black} = 0.87$ $AUC_{red} = 0.93$	[106]

Table 1. *Cont.*

Physical Trait	Statistical Model	Number of Predictors in the Model	Prediction Accuracy Parameters	Ref.
Hair colour	Bayesian naïve classifier (Snipper)	12 SNPs	Classification success rate: blond = 92.3% brown = 76.7% black = 74.6% red = 85% Sex-related prediction accuracy differences noted	[107]
	Multinomial logistic regression	270 SNPs	$AUC_{blond} = 0.74$ $AUC_{brown} = 0.68$ $AUC_{black} = 0.86$ $AUC_{red} = 0.86$	[37]
Skin colour	Multiple linear regression, including interaction	3 SNPs	$R^2 = 0.496$	[100]
	No statistical model, classification based on genotypes	5 SNPs	Overall classification success rate (dark–medium–light): 62% 38% of results inconclusive	[105]
	Bayesian naïve classifier (Snipper)	10 SNPs	$AUC_{white} = 0.999$ $AUC_{intermediate} = 0.803$ $AUC_{black} = 0.966$	[108]
	Multinomial logistic regression (HIrisPlex-S) [1]	36 SNPs	$AUC_{light} = 0.97$ $AUC_{dark} = 0.83$ $AUC_{dark\text{-}black} = 0.96$ or $AUC_{very\text{-}pale} = 0.74$ $AUC_{pale} = 0.72$ $AUC_{intermediate} = 0.73$ $AUC_{dark} = 0.87$ $AUC_{dark\text{-}black} = 0.97$	[109]
	Multiple linear regression	9 SNPs	$R^2 = 0.65$	[110]
Freckles	Binomial logistic regression	34 SNPs + sex	$AUC_{freckled} = 0.809$	[111]
	Multinomial logistic regression	20 SNPs + sex	$AUC_{non\text{-}freckled} = 0.754$ $AUC_{freckled} = 0.657$ $AUC_{heavily\text{-}freckled} = 0.792$	[112]
Hair loss	Binomial logistic regression	20 SNPs	$AUC_{bald} = 0.66$ $AUC_{bald} = 0.76$ in men ≥ 50 years old	[113]
	Binomial logistic regression	14 SNPs	$AUC_{early\text{-}onset\ baldness} = 0.74$	[114]
	Polygenic scores (weighted allele sums)	261 autosomal SNPs; 70 X chromosomal SNPs	$AUC_{severe\ baldness} = 0.748$ (autosomal SNPs) $AUC_{severe\ baldness} = 0.621$ (X chromosome SNPs) With autosomal and X SNPs + age included in the model: $AUC_{severe\ baldness} = 0.79$; $AUC_{moderate\ baldness} = 0.70$; $AUC_{slight\ baldness} = 0.61$	[52]

Table 1. *Cont.*

Physical Trait	Statistical Model	Number of Predictors in the Model	Prediction Accuracy Parameters	Ref.
	Binomial logistic regression	3 SNPs	$AUC_{straight} = 0.62$	[115]
Hair shape	Binomial and multinomial logistic regression	32 SNPs in binomial modelor33 SNPs in multinomial model	$AUC_{straight} = 0.66$ in Europeans $AUC_{straight} = 0.79$ in non-Europeans or $AUC_{straight} = 0.67$ in Europeans $AUC_{wavy} = 0.60$ in Europeans $AUC_{curly} = 0.60$ in Europeans $AUC_{straight} = 0.80$ in non-Europeans $AUC_{wavy} = 0.61$ in non-Europeans $AUC_{curly} = 0.74$ in non-Europeans	[116]
Hair greying	Binary and multi-class neural network	10 SNPs + age and sex in binary model or 12 SNPs + age and sex in multi-class model	$AUC_{greying} = 0.87$ (mostly based on age) or $AUC_{no\ greying} = 0.86$ $AUC_{mild\ greying} = 0.79$ $AUC_{severe\ greying} = 0.86$	[66]
Height	Polygenic scores (weighted allele sums)	54 SNPs	$AUC_{tall\ stature} = 0.65$	[117]
	Polygenic scores (weighted allele sums)	180 SNPs	$AUC_{tall\ stature} = 0.75$	[118]
	Polygenic scores (weighted allele sums)	689 SNPs	$AUC_{tall\ stature} = 0.79$	[119]
	L_1-penalized regression (LASSO)	>20,000 SNPs	$r = 0.64$	[120]
Face	Partial least squares regression	Genomic ancestry (68 DNA variants) + sex + 24 SNPs	Genomic ancestry explains 9.6% of the total facial variation; sex independently from ancestry explains 12.9%; SNPs make a small contribution to improving facial distinctiveness	[82]
	Ridge regression	Genomic ancestry (1000 genomic Principal Components) + sex, BMI and age	Genomic ancestry and sex explain large proportion of the predictive accuracy of the model; age and BMI improve the accuracy of the model	[121]
	Simple quantitative method (principal component analysis and partial least square analysis used to extract new face traits)	277 SNPs	SSA statistic [3]: no difference between SNP-based prediction and random predictions in females; SNP-based predictions significantly better than random predictions in males	[93]

[1] SNaPshot and MPS forensically validated genetic tests for data collection available; [2] AUC—area under the ROC (receiver operating characteristic) curve, describes the general performance of the model, 1 means perfect prediction and 0.5 means random assignment; [3] SSA—a shape similarity statistic (shape space angle) developed to measure the angle between two shapes in the 3D face modelling data space.

3.1. Pigmentation Traits

In particular, the discovery of eye colour markers with large phenotypic effects has made it easy to develop pretty accurate genetic predictors of this trait. The best-known tool commonly used in the forensic field today is the IrisPlex predictive system, which includes both a genetic test for data acquisition and a mathematical algorithm for predicting the three categories of eye colour [98]. The algorithm was developed based on the systematic selection of markers made by Liu et al., who reported 24 variants from eight genes, enabling the prediction of blue and brown eye colour with a prediction accuracy expressed by an AUC of 0.91 and 0.93, respectively [122]. AUC, which stands for area under the ROC (receiver operating characteristic) curve, describes the general performance of the model in such a way that 1 means perfect classification and 0.5 means random assignment to the phenotype categories. For forensic purposes, the number of markers from the originally identified 24 was restricted to the six with the largest effect [98,122]. The six crucial predictors included *HERC2* rs12913832, *OCA2* rs1800407, *SLC24A4* rs12896399, *SLC45A2* rs16891982, *TYR* rs1393350, and *IRF4* rs12203592. The original IrisPlex method implements a multinomial logistic regression algorithm and a simple single base extension method based on SNaPshot minisequencing, which allows the PCR amplification and genotyping of several SNPs in a multiplex reaction. Importantly, the products of primer extension are analysed using capillary electrophoresis platforms, which are commonly used in human identification testing laboratories. Other tools based on other mathematical solutions were soon developed but, essentially, each of these algorithms relied on exploiting information in the *HERC2-OCA2* gene complex. In general, these works were limited to the development of predictive algorithms using various sets of samples and mathematical approaches, but did not present specific tools for the collection of genetic data [99–104]. Notably, IrisPlex and other forensic methods of eye colour prediction can accurately predict blue and brown iris colours, but have difficulty with the prediction of intermediate eye colours [3]. Moreover, in some populations, the effect of sex was noted on prediction results [123–125]. The IrisPlex tool for the genotyping and prediction of eye colour evolved to HIrisPlex [106] and finally to the HIrisPlex-S tool [109], which were developed based on the same strategy as IrisPlex. The algorithm for hair colour prediction implemented in HIrisPlex was developed based on the investigation of a Polish population sample, which enabled the selection of 22 crucial SNPs from 11 genes for hair colour. The study showed a high level of accuracy for red and black hair colour prediction (AUC ~ 0.9) and a lower prediction accuracy for blond and brown hair colour (AUC ~ 0.8) [126]. The skin colour predictor was proposed by Walsh et al. after a systematic study of skin colour candidate variants in a sample of 2025 individuals from 31 worldwide populations. The algorithm predicted skin colour with very high accuracy, with an AUC = 0.97 for light skin colour, 0.83 dark, and 0.96 for dark-black skin colour [127]. Notably, it has been demonstrated that the original SNaPshot protocol can be replaced by the targeted massive parallel sequencing (MPS) method [128], and the HIrisPlex-S method was also adopted in a tool combining pigmentation prediction capability with ancestry inference developed by the VISAGE consortium [129]. Other studies also investigated the possibility of hair and skin colour prediction in the forensic field [100,105,107,108,110]. The Snipper Application suite deserves more attention because it provides an online tool that allows the performance of predictive calculations based on data generated by any genotyping method. The tool was originally developed for the statistical interpretation of data in ancestry inference studies, but a number of new functionalities have subsequently been added to enable the prediction of pigmentation and even age [130]. A more complete prediction of pigmentation will be provided by the developed algorithms for freckle prediction [111,112]. It is worth noting that the use of extended DNA variant sets for prediction has begun to be explored, which may lead to the development of next-generation prediction tools. For example, the previously described association work of Hysi et al. was extended to predictive modelling. Hair colour prediction was compared in two independent cohorts using prediction models based on the 258 associated SNPs and the original HIrisPlex method, and these new models outperformed the previous HIrisPlex model [37]. Further development of pigmentation predictors may also require the use of sex information, and age will naturally be needed for the final interpretation of the data [37,123]. This issue is also addressed later in the article, as sex in particular can be important for predicting other appearance traits.

3.2. Hair Loss

Numerous association studies conducted for MPB raised questions about the predictive ability of the discovered genetic variants. In 2015, a compact regression model was developed based on analysis of five SNPs from five genomic regions (Xq12, 20p11,

EBF1, *TARDBP*, and *HDAC9*), trained and validated on >600 samples from six European populations [113]. The model was shown to enable the prediction of hair loss in Europeans at an acceptable level, but only in two extreme phenotype categories, i.e., young men with significant alopecia vs. older men without symptoms of alopecia with AUC of 0.76. In the same study, Marcińska et al. also pointed to the potential role of allelic heterogeneity in determining scalp hair loss. Expanding the number of DNA variants in both crucial regions, i.e., Xq12 and 20p11, improved the accuracy of prediction, suggesting that there might be more functional variants in these loci. The extended 20-SNP regression model predicted hair loss with an AUC of 0.66 in all samples of all age categories and had the highest AUC value for the age category of $\geq$50 years old (AUC = 0.76; sensitivity = 67.7%; specificity = 90%), where the sensitivity refers to the ability of the model to correctly classify individuals with the particular phenotype (here baldness), while the specificity refers to the ability of the model to correctly classify individuals without this phenotype [113].

Liu et al. conducted a parallel study on the prediction of MPB in >2700 Europeans and developed a 14-SNP model that was found to predict early-onset MPB cases with a cross-validated AUC of 0.74 [114]. The accuracy of hair loss prediction status in elderly and middle-aged individuals was lower, with an AUC of 0.69–0.71. In 2017, Hagenaars and colleagues developed a polygenic predictor based on the genome-wide data generated for a large cohort of 40,000 individuals and showed that it can discriminate individuals with no signs of hair loss from those with severe baldness, with an AUC = 0.78, sensitivity = 0.74, and specificity = 0.69 [52].

3.3. Hair Shape and Other Hair Features

The first preliminary model for head hair shape was developed as a follow-up to the first GWA study conducted on hair characteristics [58], and included an analysis of three SNPs in three genes (*TCHH*, *WNT10A*, *FRAS1*), and was trained on data generated for 528 samples from Polish individuals [115]. The model was reported to predict straight hair with high accuracy but low specificity (cross-validated AUC = 0.622, sensitivity = 93.2%, specificity = 15.4%). The application of the model on an independent test set consisting of samples from six European populations and using a 65% probability threshold allowed for higher sensitivity (81.4%) and improved specificity (50.0%) of prediction, but at the same time with a very high rate of inconclusive results (66.9%). In 2018, a large-scale prediction study for hair shape prediction was conducted with more than 9600 samples used for predictor selection and model development and more than 2400 samples used for prediction model validation, collected from both European and non-European populations [116]. The binomial logistic regression model was developed to predict hair shape, defined as straight vs. non-straight, based on 32 informative SNPs from 26 loci. The model was reported to explain ~12% of hair shape variation and can predict straight vs. non-straight hair in European populations with an accuracy of AUC of 0.66, a sensitivity of 84.1% and a specificity of 34.2%. It was shown that the same set of SNP markers can predict hair shape with significantly different accuracies in Europeans and non-Europeans. For non-European samples, the AUC value was 0.79, sensitivity = 82.9%, and specificity = 49.8%. The higher prediction accuracy obtained for non-European populations compared to Europeans is due to the effect of the *EDAR* gene, which has a significant effect on the determination of straight hair in non-European populations, primarily East Asian. In addition to the binomial model, a multinomial logistic regression model was developed to allow for a higher resolution of hair shape prediction, considering three categories—straight, wavy and curly—based on an analysis of 33 SNP positions. There are few or no prediction studies of the remaining hair features. In 2016, Adhikari et al. predicted different hair traits using the GWAS data generated for Latin Americans and reported the highest accuracy of prediction for beard thickness and the lowest for hair greying, with ~18% and ~7% of the phenotypic variation explained by the associated SNPs, respectively [40]. Interestingly, for both of these traits, a large effect of age and sex on prediction was observed, explaining the additional ~11% and ~20% of the phenotypic variation, respectively, for beard thickness and greying. Age was found to be a main predictor of hair greying in a study conducted in 2020, explaining around 48% of the variation observed in hair greying in a cohort of 849 people from Poland [66]. A binary neural network model for greying vs. no greying prediction was developed in this study based on information relating to age, sex, and 10 SNPs selected using whole-exome sequencing data analysis (e.g., *KIF1A* rs59733750, *SEMA4D* rs45483393) and literature resources (*IRF4* rs12203592, *FGF5* rs7680591). The model achieved a high accuracy of prediction with a cross-validated AUC = 0.87 (sensitivity = 0.73; specificity = 0.85) but most of the prediction information was driven by age itself, while SNPs were found to explain merely ~7% of the variation in hair greying. As mentioned earlier, age is a very important factor in predicting hair loss. Sex and age were also shown to slightly improve the accuracy of prediction of hair shape [116].

This implies that there is a need to determine the sex and age of an individual from the analysed biological sample. Information on a person's sex is usually available in criminal investigations due to the inclusion of marker for the amelogenin gene located on the X and Y chromosome in standard STR DNA profiling, as previously mentioned, whereas age can be estimated via epigenetic analysis [131].

3.4. Human Stature

Attempts at forensic human height prediction have not been particularly numerous and have been limited to the development of predictive algorithms that are not equipped with data collection tools. The reasons are related to the limitations of DNA analysis technology and stem from the need to analyse too many DNA variants. While the 5% heritability explained by the 54 DNA variants identified by the initial GWAS scans for human height was unlikely to predict the full range of human height, Aulchenko et al. tested whether it would allow the reliable prediction of extreme height. However, this turned out to be possible with only limited accuracy. Tall stature prediction was possible at AUC of 0.65, thus only moderately improving the accuracy resulting from a random hit (AUC = 0.5) [117]. Using the 180 height markers identified in the Lango Allen et al. paper improved the prediction of tall stature to AUC of 0.75 [118]. The study suggested the importance of allelic heterogeneity for the prediction of human stature. Further increasing the number of predictors to 697 reported in the paper by [72] enabled the prediction of tall stature with an AUC of 0.79 [119]. The possibilities of human height prediction have also been explored outside the forensic mainstream using a non-standard approach that has nevertheless yielded very promising results, enabling the prediction of the full range of human height at a good level of accuracy [120]. Based on the results obtained, the authors suggested changing the approach to phenotype prediction, pointing out the benefits of also including as predictors polymorphisms that do not show an association with a given trait, but only on the basis of the improved prediction accuracy obtained after their inclusion in the prediction model [132].

3.5. The Human Face

Drawing a forensic sketch based on the instructions of a witness in a criminal case is a tool that has been used for years to identify the perpetrator of a crime. People recognise each other through the high variability of facial features. Therefore, having a good understanding of the genetics of human facial variation and being able to predict this complex phenotype is a very exciting prospect for forensic DNA intelligence. The small amount of explained heritability for craniofacial traits does not bring good prospects for the prediction of human facial phenotypes. Nevertheless, attempts have been made to develop models that would allow the prediction of facial appearance. The proposed methods are based on the indirect prediction of facial phenotypes, with ancestry and sex prediction DNA data playing a key role in this regard. The method by Claes et al. implements a bootstrapped response-based imputation modelling that makes use of information on genomic ancestry and sex first to create a sketch called a base-face. At the second stage, the information in 24 SNPs associated with facial variation is used to improve the prediction outcome [82]. A similar strategy was proposed by Lippert et al., who used the whole genome sequencing data to gain information about the sex and ancestry proportions of the individual [121]. The data on genetic face predictors did not improve facial appearance predictions, but the study showed a positive effect on the prediction of age and body mass index. The genetic prediction of facial features was also explored by Qiao at el., who developed a quantitative model based on multiple SNP loci and tried to simulate 3D face models. The study suggests that epistasis is part of the genetic architecture of facial features and concludes that the model developed should be treated as an exploratory basis for future, more advanced predictive models [93].

4. Appearance Prediction in the Era of Big Data

4.1. Appearance Trait Predicition as a Supervised Learning Task

The prediction of human externally visible characteristics using DNA markers can be treated as a supervised learning problem in which the considered appearance trait corresponds to a response (target) variable, whereas genetic markers correspond to explanatory variables (also known as features or predictors). The supervised learning models are fitted using training data, which consist of observations for which the value of the target variable is known. Depending on the type of the target variable, three tasks can be distinguished: regression (for a quantitative trait, e.g., human height), binary classification (for a binary trait, e.g., the presence of freckles), and multi-class classification (for a categorical trait, e.g., eye colour).

The specificity of the problem and the greatest challenge lies in the large number of potential features (genetic markers), which may significantly exceed the number of observations in the training data. Due to this, the use of traditional models and estimation methods (such as the maximum likelihood method in logistic regression) is not feasible. The simplest solution is to use some initial filtering method to reduce the total number of markers. However, simple filters only assess the marginal dependence between the variable and the trait; they may exclude variables that are potentially useful for the model, for example, variables that contribute by interacting with already selected ones. Therefore, there is a need to apply the estimation methods as well as feature selection approaches specially tailored to high-dimensional settings. This is one of the greatest challenges in designing learning models for appearance trait prediction.

Finally, it is important to note that traditional genome-wide association studies focus on detecting the genetic variants associated with the trait with high statistical confidence, which, in particular, includes controlling the probability of at least one rejection via multiple-testing procedures. When the prediction is the main task, the paradigm shift is needed, because focusing on the accuracy of the model becomes the main objective [133]. This approach requires the careful selection of variables. On one hand, unlike in GWAS, it is allowed to include a certain number of non-significant variables in the model, since the excessive pruning of SNPs, which may result in the discarding of some significant variables, can negatively affect prediction accuracy [132]. On the other hand, including too many spurious variables may cause the overfitting of the model and decrease its accuracy [134].

4.2. Linear Easily Interpretable Models

Despite its simplicity, the linear model and its generalisations are powerful tools for appearance trait prediction. The theory [135] and empirical evidence [136,137] suggest that in many cases the dependence between the trait and genetic markers can be captured using linear models. Several studies indicate that they frequently work on par or even better than more complex models, such as ensemble methods or neural networks [120,132,135–137], as they are not liable to overfitting. A distinct advantage of the linear models is their interpretability; the parameter value indicates how the given variable influences the dependent variable for fixed values of the remaining variables. Within the linear models, there are many methods of parameter estimation, among which the regularised (also known as penalised) maximum likelihood methods play the most prominent role in modern genetic data analysis. First, for the regularisation methods, there are theoretical guarantees that the solution of the related optimisation problem exists and is unique, even for a high-dimensional setting. Second, some forms of the regularisation, such as lasso, ensure the sparsity of the vector of estimated coefficients, meaning that a majority of coefficients will be zero. Under some unfortunately stringent conditions, this majority will correspond to non-significant variables in the model. Thus, the selected regularisation techniques can be seen as methods of simultaneous parameter estimation and feature selection. Below, we discuss the three most important generalised linear models (linear regression, logistic regression, and multinomial regression) and the methods of parameter estimation within them.

In the case of the quantitative trait, it is natural to consider the *linear regression model*, which assumes that for an i-th observation, we have $y_i = \beta_0 + x_i^T \beta + \epsilon_i$, where y_i is the value of the target variable, β_0 is an intercept, $\beta = (\beta_1, \ldots, \beta_p)^T$ is the coefficients vector, ϵ_i is noise, and $x_i = (x_{i,1}, \ldots, x_{i,p})^T$ is a vector of features. Coordinates $x_{i,1}, \ldots, x_{i,p}$ denote the genetic markers for the i-th observation. They can be coded numerically as 0, 1, or 2, where 0 indicates the homozygosity of the major allele, 1 the heterozygosity and 2 the homozygosity of the minor allele. In the penalised least squares method, we solve:

$$\hat{\beta}_0, \hat{\beta} = \arg\min_{b_0 \in R, b \in R^p} \sum_{i=1}^{n} (y_i - b_0 - x_i^T b)^2 + \lambda \mathrm{pen}(b),$$

where $\lambda > 0$ is the regularisation parameter that controls the penalty strength and $\mathrm{pen}(b)$ is the penalty. For example, in the lasso method, $\mathrm{pen}(b) = ||b||_1 = \sum_{j=1}^{p} |b_j|$, we discuss other choices below. In the case of a binary trait, the logistic regression model is usually used in which the posterior probability is modelled as:

$$P(y_i = 1 | x_i) = \frac{\exp(\beta_0 + x_i^T \beta)}{1 + \exp(\beta_0 + x_i^T \beta)}$$

and parameters are estimated using the penalised maximum likelihood method:

$$\hat{\beta}_0, \hat{\beta} = \arg\max_{b_0 \in R, b \in R^p} \sum_{i=1}^{n} [y_i \log(\sigma(b_0 + x_i^T b)) + (1 - y_i) \log(1 - \sigma(b_0 + x_i^T b))] + \lambda \mathrm{pen}(b),$$

where $\sigma(s) = \exp(s)/(1 + \exp(s))$ is the sigmoid logistic function. The multinomial logistic regression (MLR) extends the logistic model when the number of categories of the dependent variable $K > 2$. This is the most commonly used model, as usually the considered trait has multiple categories (eye colour, skin colour, hair type, etc.). The posterior probability for the k-th category is:

$$P(y_i = k | x_i) = \frac{\exp(\beta_{0k} + x_i^T \beta_k)}{1 + \sum_{k=1}^{K-1} \exp(\beta_{0k} + x_i^T \beta_k)},$$

for $k = 1, \ldots, K - 1$, where β_k is a coefficients vector corresponding to the k-th category and $P(y_i = K | x_i) = 1 - \sum_{k=1}^{K-1} P(y_i = k | x_i)$. In this model, we have $K \times p$ parameters, which are estimated using the penalised maximum likelihood method. The interaction terms $x_{i,j} \times x_{i,k}$ can be included in the above models, at the cost of a significant increase in the number of parameters. In addition to linear models, additive models are an important class of models in which, instead of the linear combination $\beta_0 + x_i^T \beta$, the combination of M non-linear base functions $\beta_0 + \sum_{m=1}^{M} \beta_m h_m(x_i)$ is used. In this group, the notable approach is the MARS method (multivariate adaptive regression splines; see Section 9 in [134]) in which the functions h_m are constructed as products of so-called hinge functions in a forward stage-wise manner. Importantly, the functions h_m in MARS can capture non-linear dependencies as well as interactions between variables. Note that the considered model is linear in predictors $h_m(x_i)$ and is an important example of the transformation of predictors method.

Regarding regularisation in the above models, the lasso penalty $\text{pen}(b) = ||b||_1$ is the most popular choice, which was successfully used in appearance trait prediction, e.g., in prediction of human height [120] or eye colour [137]. The lasso method selects features with non-zero estimated coefficients, and the number selected depends on parameter $\lambda > 0$. A small value of λ will result in a larger number of features included in the model, whereas for a larger λ, we obtain a more parsimonious model. The optimal value of λ is chosen using cross-validation or by minimising the prediction error with a validation set. An alternative to the lasso is ridge penalty $\text{pen}(b) = ||b||_2$ which, instead of performing feature selection, only shrinks the estimated parameters towards zero. The ridge penalty facilitates a reduction in the variance of the estimators, especially when the variables are highly correlated, and thus may yield an even higher accuracy for the prediction than the lasso method.

Although the lasso method has many excellent properties and high predictive power, in recent years, several modifications have been proposed in statistical and machine learning literature. For example, it has been noticed that the lasso method produces biased estimators for truly significant variables with large coefficients, and this bias does not necessarily disappear for a large sample size. To overcome this drawback, non-convex penalties, such as SCAD (smoothly clipped absolute deviation) [138] or MCP (minimax concave penalty) [139] have been proposed and effective algorithms for solving the related optimisation problems have been developed [140]. Another important line of research is focused on controlling the false discovery rate (FDR) (the expected fraction of non-significant variables that are selected for the model) instead of the much stronger control of probability that at least one non-significant variable is selected (familywise error rate). Unfortunately, the standard lasso does not control the FDR, which means that, among the selected variables, we can expect a significant portion of spurious variables. The problem is exacerbated by the fact that there is no known way of testing the significance of a specific feature based on its estimated lasso coefficient that would allow the application of one of multiple testing approaches, such as the Benjamini-Hochberg procedure [141], to control the FDR.

A notable alternative approach is the knockoff filter method [142]. It can be seen as a refinement of randomisation methods [143,144] that, by permuting the values of a studied predictor (which renders the resulting artificial predictor non-significant), creates a benchmark situation in which its usefulness can be checked. The basic idea in [142] is to construct extra variables called 'knockoff' variables, which are noisy copies of original ones but which have a certain similar correlation structure, as they allow for FDR control when standard variable selection methods (such as lasso) are applied. Namely, the lasso method is run using both the original variables and knockoff variables (thus there are $2 \times p$ variables in total). The original variable is deemed useful when its pertaining estimated coefficient is significantly larger than that of the corresponding knockoff.

The nonconvex penalties, as well as the randomisation methods, seem to be worthwhile alternatives to the lasso method for predicting human traits. The above methods are implemented, e.g., in R software, see packages glmnet (lasso and ridge), ncvreg (MCP, SCAD), knockoff (knockoff filter), and earth (MARS method).

4.3. Complex Black-Box Models

The black-box model is a class of predictive models that are able to recover complex dependencies between explanatory variables and the dependent variable, including interaction terms, and which can potentially achieve higher accuracy then linear models. The main limitations are the high computational complexity, the difficulty in interpreting the model, and the necessity of parameter tuning. In this group, ensemble methods and neural networks play the leading role. The former are usually based on decision trees [145] and overcome two limitations of single trees: their instability and tendency to overfitting. The simplest approach is bagging (bootstrap aggregating) [146] in which each tree in the ensemble is trained using a bootstrap sample, i.e., a sample drawn with replacements from the original training data. In order to classify a new instance, each decision tree provides the classification for the input data. The majority vote classification is then chosen as the final prediction. In the case of regression, the predictions from individual tress are averaged. Another important class of models are random subspace methods (RSM), in which each base classifier is learnt using the randomly selected subset of variables [147,148]. One of the most successful and commonly used methods is random forest (RF), which can be seen as a combination of bagging and RSM. The RF uses a modified tree learning algorithm that selects, at each candidate split in the learning process, a random subset of the features of size m, where m is a hyper-parameter. Making m smaller helps to avoid the danger of overfitting. Nowadays, the most powerful class of ensemble methods are gradient boosting (GB) algorithms (Section 10 in [134]). In GB, the subsequent models $F_1(x), \ldots, F_M(x)$ are learned sequentially, and the last model $F_M(x)$ serves as a final model. The main advantage of GB algorithms is that they are able to optimise different loss functions, depending on the considered task. The classifier in step $m + 1$ (usually a decision tree) is learnt using current training data, in which the residuals from the previous model are treated as the current target variable (where the squared loss is considered, and the residuals are $y_i - F_m(x_i)$). The residuals are related to the so-called functional gradient of the loss function and, therefore, GB methods can be seen as gradient descent algorithms, which take steps in the direction of the steepest descent and converge to the minimum of the loss function. The common property of all boosting algorithms is that the current model zooms in on samples where its predecessor failed. Usually, some regularisation techniques are used in boosting algorithms to prevent overfitting. There are many versions of gradient boosting algorithms, among which XGB (extreme gradient boosting) is considered to be one of the most powerful variants [149]. The ensemble methods are controlled by different parameters, whose optimal choice may significantly improve the performance: the number of trees, the size of the random subspace (in RF and RSM), as well as the regularisation and pruning parameters.

The ensemble methods described above (RF and XGB) are often used to assess the importance of the features. The simplest approach is based on a permutation scheme and is very similar to the randomisation feature selection described above. The first method (called mean decrease accuracy) involves fitting two ensemble models (e.g., RF or XGB): the first is based on the original training data and the second is based on training data in which the values of the j-th variable are randomly permuted. The variable importance measure for the j-th variable is defined as the difference in accuracies corresponding to these two models. A large value of the difference indicates the significance of the variable. The second measure (called mean decrease impurity) is based on observing how well the given variable separates the classes. The Boruta algorithm [150], based on the above two measures, contains a testing procedure that allows the rejecting of the noisy variables. Other more sophisticated variable importance measures are also advocated for, e.g., the MCFS method [151], in which one of its major advantages is that the predictive power of each tree in the ensemble is taken into account in the measure definition.

The second important group of black-box models is artificial neural networks (ANN) [152]. The latest advances in computational and optimisation methods have made it possible to train networks with very complex architectures corresponding to large families of functions, such as convolution networks (in image recognition) and recurrent networks (in text analysis). The deep networks used today may consist of hundreds of hidden layers and can model very complex dependencies [153]. In appearance trait prediction, the feed-forward neural network is usually used. In such networks, the input signal (the vector of features for the i-th observation) is transmitted from the input layer to the output layer, which yields the prediction of the response. The hidden layers consist of artificial neurons in which the linear combination of the signals from the previous layers is computed and the signal is passed through the activation function as the input for the following layers. The models are trained using gradient algorithms (the ADAM algorithm [154] is now the state-of-the-art method) and the back-propagation algorithm is used to effectively compute the gradient of the considered risk function [153]. A number of parameters need to be tuned in ANN, such as the number of layers, the number of neurons in each layer, and the value of the learning rate. Other spectacular advances with ANN, such as variational autoencoders (VAE), which enable latent feature analysis (see [155]), are of potential interest in appearance trait prediction. For the methods described here, see R packages randomForest, xgboost, rmcfs, Boruta, and tensorflow.

4.4. Feature Selection

Feature selection is an essential element when building predictive models, as it prevents overfitting and allows discovering the dependency structure between variables and, in particular, recovering the features that affect the target variable. In the models described above, feature selection is usually embedded in learning algorithms. For example, in linear models as well as neural networks, selection is performed via regularisation, whereas in tree-based methods, the relevant features are selected when building the tree. However, including too many potential features may significantly increase the computational cost of fitting the model. Thus, very often in practice, there is a need to apply some fast preliminary filtering method. In the machine learning community, methods based on information theory have gained the most popularity in recent years [156]. They are fast, model free, and are able to detect non-linear dependencies and interactions between variables, as well as take into account redundancies. The basic quantity used in such methods is mutual information (MI):

$$I(Y, X_k) = \sum_{x,y} P(X_k = x, Y = y) \log \frac{P(X_k = x, Y = y)}{P(X_k = x)P(Y = y)}$$

which is a non-parametric measure of dependence between some feature X_k and target variable Y. Moreover, analogously defined, the conditional mutual information $I(Y, X_k|Z)$ quantifies the dependence strength between X_k and Y given the possibly multivariate variable Z. It is commonly used in feature selection of a new predictor X_k when Z consists of predictors already chosen. Another important quantity used in genome-wise interaction studies (GWIS) is interaction information (*II*):

$$II(Y, X_j, X_k) = I((X_k, X_j), Y) - I(Y, X_k) - I(Y, X_j)$$

which measures the interaction strength between X_k and X_j for the prediction of Y. The positive value of *II* indicates a synergistic interaction, whereas a negative value indicates redundancy. *II* has been successfully used in many genetic studies to detect epistasis [157,158], and also in the context of appearance trait prediction, such as human pigmentation [159]. It has been shown that the methods based on *II* are able to detect interactions that remain undetected by the logistic regression model [160].

The existing filters based on MI are forward sequential procedures that, in each step, add a candidate feature X_k to the set of already selected features S. The quality of a candidate feature can be assessed using various criteria, and the representative one is CIFE (conditional infomax feature extraction) [156,161]. It adds candidate X_k, being the maximizer of $I(Y, X_k) + \sum_{j \in S} II(Y, X_k, X_j)$. The CIFE takes into account the marginal dependence between a candidate feature and the target variable, as well as interactions between the candidate feature and the previously selected features. Methods taking into account higher order interactions are also considered [162]. In practice, it is important to decide at which step to stop the procedure of adding new candidate variables, with the possible solution based on the approximate distribution of the criterion function when a candidate feature is not significant, as proposed in [163].

5. The Need for a High-Throughput, Low-Input DNA Sequencing Method in Forensic Science

The limitations of DNA sequencing technologies used in the forensic field are increasingly problematic because they are hindering the implementation of new methods that can improve law enforcement and justice, and which are therefore important for the safety of society. The lack of a suitable method for generating large amounts of SNP data from degraded DNA, validated for use in forensics, was considered to be a barrier to the forensic implementation of investigative genetic genealogy, an approach that was very successful at solving a number of criminal cases [1,164]. Such a method also seems to be essential for developing next-generation tools for the DNA-based prediction of appearance traits, which requires information derived from hundreds or even thousands of SNPs. It may be argued that the optimal method for all the applications developed for forensic DNA intelligence would be whole-genome sequencing (WGS). Notably, WGS that uses high-throughput methods (massively parallel sequencing) has revolutionised the studies of ancient DNA and enabled a better understanding of human evolutionary history. Similarities between forensic genetics and palaeogenetics, especially in terms of the specificity of research material with a high content of inhibitors and small amounts of highly fragmented DNA, and the enormous success of palaeogenetics in the analysis of such samples, prompts a closer look at the methods developed in this field. Several technological advancements were crucial for the effective analysis of ancient DNA, including the very efficient extraction of short ancient DNA fragments, the implementation of the uracil-DNA glycosylase (UDG) protocol for the selective removal of damaged sections of ancient DNA, improved protocols for library preparation, and, finally, progress has also been made in high-throughput DNA sequencing [165,166]. The major advantage for ancient DNA research brought about by high-throughput sequencing technology is the ability to sequence very short DNA fragments. Research material analysed in forensic DNA laboratories is not as degraded as ancient samples, and current DNA extraction methods are efficient and effective at removing inhibitors. Therefore, the transfer of DNA analysis protocols from palaeogenomics to forensic genomics should perhaps primarily focus on library preparation methods that work well with low-input DNA. Standard library preparation protocols are optimised for large amounts of DNA and perform poorly in the case of samples containing degraded DNA. However, a number of modified protocols have been proposed to reduce the requirement for DNA inputs to be at subnanogram quantities.

One category of protocols involves library construction based on double-stranded DNA. A first protocol was described by Meyer and Kircher in 2010, and this was laborious and had limitations that resulted in the losses of ancient DNA sequences due to incompatible adapter combinations and three purification steps prior to amplification [167]. Double-stranded library preparation protocols involve the blunt-end repair of the degraded DNA fragments, the non-directional blunt-end ligation of two adapters and the fill-in of the nicks formatted between adapters and the DNA fragment [168]. A more advanced alternative of double stranded library preparation method is the protocol proposed by Carøe et al., named blunt-end-single-tube. As the name suggests, the protocol is carried out in a single tube and relies on heat denaturation instead of purification between the subsequent steps of end-repair, the ligation of double-stranded adapters to the 5′ ends, and adapter fill-in [169].

The second approach for library preparation from samples containing low amounts of degraded DNA is particularly interesting, as it implies a process of library construction based on single-stranded DNA, allowing the use of DNA that was preserved in a single-stranded state and which is considered to be more efficient compared to double-stranded approaches. The original protocol for single-stranded library preparation, although it recovered more endogenous DNA, was very expensive and laborious [170]. However, the protocol evolved to a simplified version proposed in Gansauge et al., 2017 [171]. This is a method that involves the dephosphorylation of the template DNA, the splinted ligation of a biotinylated adapter to the 3′ end, bonding to streptavidin beads, annealing an extension primer to allow the synthesis of a second strand, and the ligation of the 5′ end of a double-stranded adapter to the 3′ end of the newly synthesized strand. The authors also proposed an automated version of this protocol [172]. An interesting modification of the single-strand library preparation method was recently proposed by Kapp et al. (2021). The advantage of the method, named the Santa Cruz Reaction, relies on simplicity and cost effectiveness. The method converts single-stranded DNA into sequencing libraries using a single enzymatic reaction, enabling the simultaneous directional splinted ligation of Illumina's P5 and P7 adapters [173]. Technological improvements in ancient DNA analysis have resulted in significant progress in sequencing efficiency. Whole-genome data from ancient hominin material were generated with an average sequence coverage of only 1.3-fold in 2010 [174] and 30-fold in 2012 [175]. The usefulness of these protocols was also confirmed in clinical research of problematic biological material, including formalin-fixed paraffin embedded tissues [176]. The future will show whether the protocols developed in palaeogenomics can be easily transferred to forensic genomics. This would undoubtedly be extremely helpful for the further development of forensic DNA intelligence methods.

6. Concluding Remarks

Research on the genetic architecture of natural variation in the human physical phenotype is growing in scale and involves different human populations. The genetic prediction of physical appearance traits occupies an important place in forensic research, although the available tools are limited to the least complex traits, mainly pigmentation. Notably, there are examples of using predictive methods that have been developed by the forensic community in ancient DNA research, and which have been carried out in the field of molecular anthropology [177–179] and in the identification of historical figures [180–182], which is further evidence that molecular anthropology and forensic genetics have a lot in common. Some DNA-based predictive tools developed by the forensic community have been implemented in commercial kits. The most famous ForenSeq kit allows the analysis of HIrisPlex SNPs and therefore the prediction of eye and hair colour [183]. The HIrisPlex-S variants are also available in the Ion AmpliSeq™ PhenoTrivium Panel [184]. Predicting reliable sketches in forensic science is highly desirable at the investigation stage. For this reason, there are reports of police using private companies offering services in this regard, particularly for facial appearance prediction. For example, the Snapshot Forensic DNA Phenotyping System offered by Parabon NanoLabs claims to facilitate the accurate prediction of genetic ancestry, eye colour, hair colour, skin colour, freckling, and face shape [185]. Further research offers the opportunity to better understand the evolutionary and genetic basis of human appearance traits. The prospect of future studies on the heritability of complex traits and the exploration of the importance of rare DNA variants, as well as epistatic interactions of the second and higher orders, seems interesting. The explanation of heritability will consequently enable a more reliable prediction of physical phenotype. Undoubtedly, however, the application of next-generation predictive methods, which must rely on much larger sets of predictors and more sophisticated statistical and machine learning algorithms, will require improvements in the technology of DNA polymorphism analysis used in the forensic field. Proper interpretation of the data requires knowledge of age, which is best determined via DNA methylation analysis. However, DNA methylation analysis requires the largest amounts of DNA, so in studying biological traces for intelligence purposes, it would be beneficial to develop more sensitive age prediction methods. The application of novel predictive approaches will also require answers to important ethical questions arising from the use of high-throughput DNA analysis methods.

Funding: This research received no external funding.

Conflicts of Interest: The authors declare no conflict of interest.

References

1. Kling, D.; Phillips, C.; Kennett, D.; Tillmar, A. Investigative genetic genealogy: Current methods, knowledge and practice. *Forensic Sci. Int. Genet.* **2021**, *52*, 102474. [CrossRef]
2. Phillips, C. Forensic genetic analysis of bio-geographical ancestry. *Forensic Sci. Int. Genet.* **2015**, *18*, 49–65. [CrossRef] [PubMed]
3. Kayser, M. Forensic DNA Phenotyping: Predicting human appearance from crime scene material for investigative purposes. *Forensic Sci. Int. Genet.* **2015**, *18*, 33–48. [CrossRef]
4. Lee, H.Y.; Lee, S.D.; Shin, K.J. Forensic DNA methylation profiling from evidence material for investigative leads. *BMB Rep.* **2016**, *49*, 359–369. [CrossRef] [PubMed]
5. Polderman, T.J.; Benyamin, B.; de Leeuw, C.A.; Sullivan, P.F.; van Bochoven, A.; Visscher, P.M.; Posthuma, D. Meta-analysis of the heritability of human traits based on fifty years of twin studies. *Nat. Genet.* **2015**, *47*, 702–709. [CrossRef]
6. Botstein, D.; Risch, N. Discovering genotypes underlying human phenotypes: Past successes for mendelian disease, future approaches for complex disease. *Nat. Genet.* **2003**, *33*, 228–237. [CrossRef]
7. Visscher, P.M.; Brown, M.A.; McCarthy, M.I.; Yang, J. Five years of GWAS discovery. *Am. J. Hum. Genet.* **2012**, *90*, 7–24. [CrossRef] [PubMed]
8. Uffelmann, E.; Huang, Q.Q.; Munung, N.S.; DeVries, J.; Okada, Y.; Martin, A.R.; Martin, H.C.; Lappalainen, T.; Posthuma, D. Genome-wide association studies. *Nat. Rev. Methods Primers* **2021**, *1*, 59. [CrossRef]
9. Clark, P.; Stark, A.E.; Walsh, R.J.; Jardine, R.; Martin, N.G. A twin study of skin reflectance. *Ann. Hum. Biol.* **1981**, *8*, 529–541. [CrossRef] [PubMed]
10. Lin, B.D.; Mbarek, H.; Willemsen, G.; Dolan, C.V.; Fedko, I.O.; Abdellaoui, A.; De Geus, E.J.; Boomsma, D.I.; Hottenga, J.-J. Heritability and Genome-Wide Association Studies for Hair Color in a Dutch Twin Family Based Sample. *Genes* **2015**, *6*, 559–576. [CrossRef]
11. Bito, L.Z.; Matheny, A.; Cruickshanks, K.J.; Nondahl, D.M.; Carino, O.B. Eye Color Changes Past Early Childhood: The Louisville Twin Study. *Arch. Ophthalmol.* **1997**, *115*, 659–663. [CrossRef]
12. Eiberg, H.; Mohr, J. Assignment of genes coding for brown eye colour (BEY2) and brown hair colour (HCL3) on chromosome 15q. *Eur. J. Hum. Genet.* **1996**, *4*, 237–241. [CrossRef] [PubMed]
13. Rebbeck, T.R.; Kanetsky, P.A.; Walker, A.H.; Holmes, R.; Halpern, A.C.; Schuchter, L.M.; Elder, D.E.; Guerry, D. P gene as an inherited biomarker of human eye color. *Cancer Epidemiol. Biomark. Prev.* **2002**, *11*, 782–784.
14. Frudakis, T.; Thomas, M.; Gaskin, Z.; Venkateswarlu, K.; Chandra, K.S.; Ginjupalli, S.; Gunturi, S.; Natrajan, S.; Ponnuswamy, V.K.; Ponnuswamy, K.N. Sequences associated with human iris pigmentation. *Genetics* **2003**, *165*, 2071–2083. [CrossRef] [PubMed]
15. Duffy, D.L.; Montgomery, G.W.; Chen, W.; Zhao, Z.Z.; Le, L.; James, M.R.; Hayward, N.K.; Martin, N.G.; Sturm, R.A. A three-single-nucleotide polymorphism haplotype in intron 1 of OCA2 explains most human eye-color variation. *Am. J. Hum. Genet.* **2007**, *80*, 241–252. [CrossRef] [PubMed]
16. Branicki, W.; Brudnik, U.; Kupiec, T.; Wolańska-Nowak, P.; Szczerbińska, A.; Wojas-Pelc, A. Association of polymorphic sites in the OCA2 gene with eye colour using the tree scanning method. *Ann. Hum. Genet.* **2008**, *72*, 184–192. [CrossRef]
17. Sulem, P.; Gudbjartsson, D.F.; Stacey, S.N.; Helgason, A.; Rafnar, T.; Magnusson, K.P.; Manolescu, A.; Karason, A.; Palsson, A.; Thorleifsson, G.; et al. Genetic determinants of hair, eye and skin pigmentation in Europeans. *Nat. Genet.* **2007**, *39*, 1443–1452. [CrossRef]
18. Sturm, R.A.; Duffy, D.L.; Zhao, Z.Z.; Leite, F.P.; Stark, M.S.; Hayward, N.K.; Martin, N.G.; Montgomery, G.W. A single SNP in an evolutionary conserved region within intron 86 of the HERC2 gene determines human blue-brown eye color. *Am. J. Hum. Genet.* **2008**, *82*, 424–431. [CrossRef]
19. Eiberg, H.; Troelsen, J.; Nielsen, M.; Mikkelsen, A.; Mengel-From, J.; Kjaer, K.W.; Hansen, L. Blue eye color in humans may be caused by a perfectly associated founder mutation in a regulatory element located within the HERC2 gene inhibiting OCA2 expression. *Hum. Genet.* **2008**, *123*, 177–187. [CrossRef]
20. Visser, M.; Kayser, M.; Grosveld, F.; Palstra, R.J. Genetic variation in regulatory DNA elements: The case of OCA2 transcriptional regulation. *Pigment Cell Melanoma Res.* **2014**, *27*, 169–177. [CrossRef] [PubMed]
21. Valverde, P.; Healy, E.; Jackson, I.; Rees, J.L.; Thody, A.J. Variants of the melanocyte-stimulating hormone receptor gene are associated with red hair and fair skin in humans. *Nat. Genet.* **1995**, *11*, 328–330. [CrossRef] [PubMed]
22. Rees, J.L. Genetics of hair and skin color. *Annu. Rev. Genet.* **2003**, *37*, 67–90. [CrossRef] [PubMed]
23. Flanagan, N.; Healy, E.; Ray, A.; Philips, S.; Todd, C.; Jackson, I.J.; Birch-Machin, M.A.; Rees, J.L. Pleiotropic effects of the melanocortin 1 receptor (MC1R) gene on human pigmentation. *Hum. Mol. Genet.* **2000**, *9*, 2531–2537. [CrossRef] [PubMed]
24. Bastiaens, M.; ter Huurne, J.; Gruis, N.; Bergman, W.; Westendorp, R.; Vermeer, B.J.; Bouwes Bavinck, J.N. The melanocortin-1-receptor gene is the major freckle gene. *Hum. Mol. Genet.* **2001**, *10*, 1701–1708. [CrossRef]
25. Han, J.; Kraft, P.; Nan, H.; Guo, Q.; Chen, C.; Qureshi, A.; Hankinson, S.E.; Hu, F.B.; Duffy, D.L.; Zhao, Z.Z.; et al. A genome-wide association study identifies novel alleles associated with hair color and skin pigmentation. *PLoS Genet.* **2008**, *4*, e1000074. [CrossRef]
26. Manolio, T.A.; Collins, F.S.; Cox, N.J.; Goldstein, D.B.; Hindorff, L.A.; Hunter, D.J.; McCarthy, M.I.; Ramos, E.M.; Cardon, L.R.; Chakravarti, A.; et al. Finding the missing heritability of complex diseases. *Nature* **2009**, *461*, 747–753. [CrossRef] [PubMed]
27. Nelson, R.M.; Pettersson, M.E.; Carlborg, Ö. A century after Fisher: Time for a new paradigm in quantitative genetics. *Trends Genet.* **2013**, *29*, 669–676. [CrossRef]

28. Simcoe, M.; Valdes, A.; Liu, F.; Furlotte, N.A.; Evans, D.M.; Hemani, G.; Ring, S.M.; Smith, G.D.; Duffy, D.L.; Zhu, G.; et al. Genome-wide association study in almost 195,000 individuals identifies 50 previously unidentified genetic loci for eye color. *Sci. Adv.* **2021**, *7*, eabd1239. [CrossRef] [PubMed]

29. Norton, H.L. The color of normal: How a Eurocentric focus erases pigmentation complexity. *Am. J. Hum. Biol.* **2021**, *33*, e23554. [CrossRef]

30. Lamason, R.L.; Mohideen, M.A.; Mest, J.R.; Wong, A.C.; Norton, H.L.; Aros, M.C.; Jurynec, M.J.; Mao, X.; Humphreville, V.R.; Humbert, J.E.; et al. SLC24A5, a putative cation exchanger, affects pigmentation in zebrafish and humans. *Science* **2005**, *310*, 1782–1786. [CrossRef]

31. Liu, F.; Visser, M.; Duffy, D.L.; Hysi, P.G.; Jacobs, L.C.; Lao, O.; Zhong, K.; Walsh, S.; Chaitanya, L.; Wollstein, A.; et al. Genetics of skin color variation in Europeans: Genome-wide association studies with functional follow-up. *Hum. Genet.* **2015**, *134*, 823–835. [CrossRef]

32. Sulem, P.; Gudbjartsson, D.F.; Stacey, S.N.; Helgason, A.; Rafnar, T.; Jakobsdottir, M.; Steinberg, S.; Gudjonsson, S.A.; Palsson, A.; Thorleifsson, G.; et al. Two newly identified genetic determinants of pigmentation in Europeans. *Nat. Genet.* **2008**, *40*, 835–837. [CrossRef] [PubMed]

33. Edwards, M.; Bigham, A.; Tan, J.; Li, S.; Gozdzik, A.; Ross, K.; Jin, L.; Parra, E.J. Association of the OCA2 polymorphism His615Arg with melanin content in east Asian populations: Further evidence of convergent evolution of skin pigmentation. *PLoS Genet.* **2010**, *6*, e1000867. [CrossRef]

34. Stokowski, R.P.; Pant, P.V.; Dadd, T.; Fereday, A.; Hinds, D.A.; Jarman, C.; Filsell, W.; Ginger, R.S.; Green, M.R.; van der Ouderaa, F.J.; et al. A genomewide association study of skin pigmentation in a South Asian population. *Am. J. Hum. Genet.* **2007**, *81*, 1119–1132. [CrossRef]

35. Crawford, N.G.; Kelly, D.E.; Hansen, M.E.B.; Beltrame, M.H.; Fan, S.; Bowman, S.L.; Jewett, E.; Ranciaro, A.; Thompson, S.; Lo, Y.; et al. Loci associated with skin pigmentation identified in African populations. *Science* **2017**, *358*, eaan8433. [CrossRef] [PubMed]

36. Martin, A.R.; Lin, M.; Granka, J.M.; Myrick, J.W.; Liu, X.; Sockell, A.; Atkinson, E.G.; Werely, C.J.; Möller, M.; Sandhu, M.S.; et al. An Unexpectedly Complex Architecture for Skin Pigmentation in Africans. *Cell* **2017**, *171*, 1340–1353. [CrossRef]

37. Hysi, P.G.; Valdes, A.M.; Liu, F.; Furlotte, N.A.; Evans, D.M.; Bataille, V.; Visconti, A.; Hemani, G.; McMahon, G.; Ring, S.M.; et al. Genome-wide association meta-analysis of individuals of European ancestry identifies new loci explaining a substantial fraction of hair color variation and heritability. *Nat. Genet.* **2018**, *50*, 652–656. [CrossRef]

38. Morgan, M.D.; Pairo-Castineira, E.; Rawlik, K.; Canela-Xandri, O.; Rees, J.; Sims, D.; Tenesa, A.; Jackson, I.J. Genome-wide study of hair colour in UK Biobank explains most of the SNP heritability. *Nat. Commun.* **2018**, *9*, 5271. [CrossRef] [PubMed]

39. Medland, S.E.; Zhu, G.; Martin, N.G. Estimating the heritability of hair curliness in twins of European ancestry. *Twin Res. Hum. Genet.* **2009**, *12*, 514–518. [CrossRef] [PubMed]

40. Adhikari, K.; Fontanil, T.; Cal, S.; Mendoza-Revilla, J.; Fuentes-Guajardo, M.; Chacón-Duque, J.C.; Al-Saadi, F.; Johansson, J.A.; Quinto-Sanchez, M.; Acuña-Alonzo, V.; et al. A genome-wide association scan in admixed Latin Americans identifies loci influencing facial and scalp hair features. *Nat. Commun.* **2016**, *7*, 10815. [CrossRef]

41. Nyholt, D.R.; Gillespie, N.A.; Heath, A.C.; Martin, N.G. Genetic basis of male pattern baldness. *J. Investig. Dermatol.* **2003**, *121*, 1561–1564. [CrossRef] [PubMed]

42. Pirastu, N.; Joshi, P.K.; de Vries, P.S.; Cornelis, M.C.; McKeigue, P.M.; Keum, N.; Franceschini, N.; Colombo, M.; Giovannucci, E.L.; Spiliopoulou, A.; et al. GWAS for male-pattern baldness identifies 71 susceptibility loci explaining 38% of the risk. *Nat. Commun.* **2017**, *8*, 1584, Erratum in: *Nat Commun.* **2018**, *9*, 2536. [CrossRef] [PubMed]

43. Yap, C.X.; Sidorenko, J.; Wu, Y.; Kemper, K.E.; Yang, J.; Wray, N.R.; Robinson, M.R.; Visscher, P.M. Dissection of genetic variation and evidence for pleiotropy in male pattern baldness. *Nat. Commun.* **2018**, *9*, 5407. [CrossRef] [PubMed]

44. Gunn, D.A.; Rexbye, H.; Griffiths, C.E.; Murray, P.G.; Fereday, A.; Catt, S.D.; Tomlin, C.C.; Strongitharm, B.H.; Perrett, D.I.; Catt, M. Why some women look young for their age. *PLoS ONE* **2009**, *4*, e8021. [CrossRef]

45. Weissbrod, O.; Flint, J.; Rosset, S. Estimating SNP-Based Heritability and Genetic Correlation in Case-Control Studies Directly and with Summary Statistics. *Am. J. Hum. Genet.* **2018**, *103*, 89–99. [CrossRef] [PubMed]

46. Visscher, P.M.; Hill, W.G.; Wray, N.R. Heritability in the genomics era—concepts and misconceptions. *Nat. Rev. Genet.* **2008**, *9*, 255–266. [CrossRef] [PubMed]

47. Richards, J.B.; Yuan, X.; Geller, F.; Waterworth, D.; Bataille, V.; Glass, D.; Song, K.; Waeber, G.; Vollenweider, P.; Aben, K.K.; et al. Male-pattern baldness susceptibility locus at 20p11. *Nat. Genet.* **2008**, *40*, 1282–1284. [CrossRef]

48. Hillmer, A.M.; Brockschmidt, F.F.; Hanneken, S.; Eigelshoven, S.; Steffens, M.; Flaquer, A.; Herms, S.; Becker, T.; Kortüm, A.K.; Nyholt, D.R.; et al. Susceptibility variants for male-pattern baldness on chromosome 20p11. *Nat. Genet.* **2008**, *40*, 1279–1281. [CrossRef] [PubMed]

49. Brockschmidt, F.F.; Heilmann, S.; Ellis, J.A.; Eigelshoven, S.; Hanneken, S.; Herold, C.; Moebus, S.; Alblas, M.A.; Lippke, B.; Kluck, N.; et al. Susceptibility variants on chromosome 7p21.1 suggest HDAC9 as a new candidate gene for male-pattern baldness. *Br. J. Dermatol.* **2011**, *165*, 1293–1302. [CrossRef]

50. Li, R.; Brockschmidt, F.F.; Kiefer, A.K.; Stefansson, H.; Nyholt, D.R.; Song, K.; Vermeulen, S.H.; Kanoni, S.; Glass, D.; Medland, S.E.; et al. Six novel susceptibility Loci for early-onset androgenetic alopecia and their unexpected association with common diseases. *PLoS Genet.* **2012**, *8*, e1002746. [CrossRef]

51. Pickrell, J.K.; Berisa, T.; Liu, J.Z.; Ségurel, L.; Tung, J.Y.; Hinds, D.A. Detection and interpretation of shared genetic influences on 42 human traits. *Nat. Genet.* **2016**, *48*, 709–717. [CrossRef]

52. Hagenaars, S.P.; Hill, W.D.; Harris, S.E.; Ritchie, S.J.; Davies, G.; Liewald, D.C.; Gale, C.R.; Porteous, D.J.; Deary, I.J.; Marioni, R.E. Genetic prediction of male pattern baldness. *PLoS Genet.* **2017**, *13*, e1006594. [CrossRef] [PubMed]

53. Heilmann-Heimbach, S.; Herold, C.; Hochfeld, L.M.; Hillmer, A.M.; Nyholt, D.R.; Hecker, J.; Javed, A.; Chew, E.G.; Pechlivanis, S.; Drichel, D.; et al. Meta-analysis identifies novel risk loci and yields systematic insights into the biology of male-pattern baldness. *Nat. Commun.* **2017**, *8*, 14694. [CrossRef]

54. Liang, B.; Yang, C.; Zuo, X.; Li, Y.; Ding, Y.; Sheng, Y.; Zhou, F.; Cheng, H.; Zheng, X.; Chen, G.; et al. Genetic variants at 20p11 confer risk to androgenetic alopecia in the Chinese Han population. *PLoS ONE* **2013**, *8*, e71771. [CrossRef]

55. Zhuo, F.L.; Xu, W.; Wang, L.; Wu, Y.; Xu, Z.L.; Zhao, J.Y. Androgen receptor gene polymorphisms and risk for androgenetic alopecia: A meta-analysis. *Clin. Exp. Dermatol.* **2012**, *37*, 104–111. [CrossRef]

56. Loh, P.R.; Kichaev, G.; Gazal, S.; Schoech, A.P.; Price, A.L. Mixed-model association for biobank-scale datasets. *Nat. Genet.* **2018**, *50*, 906–908. [CrossRef]

57. Kichaev, G.; Bhatia, G.; Loh, P.R.; Gazal, S.; Burch, K.; Freund, M.K.; Schoech, A.; Pasaniuc, B.; Price, A.L. Leveraging Polygenic Functional Enrichment to Improve GWAS Power. *Am. J. Hum. Genet.* **2019**, *104*, 65–75. [CrossRef] [PubMed]

58. Medland, S.E.; Nyholt, D.R.; Painter, J.N.; McEvoy, B.P.; McRae, A.F.; Zhu, G.; Gordon, S.D.; Ferreira, M.A.; Wright, M.J.; Henders, A.K.; et al. Common variants in the trichohyalin gene are associated with straight hair in Europeans. *Am. J. Hum. Genet.* **2009**, *85*, 750–755. [CrossRef] [PubMed]

59. Wu, S.; Tan, J.; Yang, Y.; Peng, Q.; Zhang, M.; Li, J.; Lu, D.; Liu, Y.; Lou, H.; Feng, Q.; et al. Genome-wide scans reveal variants at EDAR predominantly affecting hair straightness in Han Chinese and Uyghur populations. *Hum. Genet.* **2016**, *135*, 1279–1286. [CrossRef]

60. Liu, F.; Chen, Y.; Zhu, G.; Hysi, P.G.; Wu, S.; Adhikari, K.; Breslin, K.; Pospiech, E.; Hamer, M.A.; Peng, F.; et al. Meta-analysis of genome-wide association studies identifies 8 novel loci involved in shape variation of human head hair. *Hum. Mol. Genet.* **2018**, *27*, 559–575. [CrossRef]

61. Fujimoto, A.; Kimura, R.; Ohashi, J.; Omi, K.; Yuliwulandari, R.; Batubara, L.; Mustofa, M.S.; Samakkarn, U.; Settheetham-Ishida, W.; Ishida, T.; et al. A scan for genetic determinants of human hair morphology: EDAR is associated with Asian hair thickness. *Hum. Mol. Genet.* **2008**, *17*, 835–843. [CrossRef]

62. Tan, J.; Yang, Y.; Tang, K.; Sabeti, P.C.; Jin, L.; Wang, S. The adaptive variant EDARV370A is associated with straight hair in East Asians. *Hum. Genet.* **2013**, *132*, 1187–1191. [CrossRef]

63. Pospiech, E.; Lee, S.D.; Kukla-Bartoszek, M.; Karłowska-Pik, J.; Woźniak, A.; Boroń, M.; Zubańska, M.; Bronikowska, A.; Hong, S.R.; Lee, J.H.; et al. Variation in the RPTN gene may facilitate straight hair formation in Europeans and East Asians. *J. Dermatol. Sci.* **2018**, *91*, 331–334. [CrossRef]

64. Endo, C.; Johnson, T.A.; Morino, R.; Nakazono, K.; Kamitsuji, S.; Akita, M.; Kawajiri, M.; Yamasaki, T.; Kami, A.; Hoshi, Y.; et al. Genome-wide association study in Japanese females identifies fifteen novel skin-related trait associations. *Sci. Rep.* **2018**, *8*, 8974. [CrossRef] [PubMed]

65. Wu, S.; Zhang, M.; Yang, X.; Peng, F.; Zhang, J.; Tan, J.; Yang, Y.; Wang, L.; Hu, Y.; Peng, Q.; et al. Genome-wide association studies and CRISPR/Cas9-mediated gene editing identify regulatory variants influencing eyebrow thickness in humans. *PLoS Genet.* **2018**, *14*, e1007640. [CrossRef] [PubMed]

66. Pospiech, E.; Kukla-Bartoszek, M.; Karłowska-Pik, J.; Zieliński, P.; Woźniak, A.; Boroń, M.; Dąbrowski, M.; Zubańska, M.; Jarosz, A.; Grzybowski, T.; et al. Exploring the possibility of predicting human head hair greying from DNA using whole-exome and targeted NGS data. *BMC Genom.* **2020**, *21*, 538. [CrossRef]

67. Gudbjartsson, D.F.; Walters, G.B.; Thorleifsson, G.; Stefansson, H.; Halldorsson, B.V.; Zusmanovich, P.; Sulem, P.; Thorlacius, S.; Gylfason, A.; Steinberg, S.; et al. Many sequence variants affecting diversity of adult human height. *Nat. Genet.* **2008**, *40*, 609–615. [CrossRef]

68. Lettre, G.; Jackson, A.U.; Gieger, C.; Schumacher, F.R.; Berndt, S.I.; Sanna, S.; Eyheramendy, S.; Voight, B.F.; Butler, J.L.; Guiducci, C.; et al. Identification of ten loci associated with height highlights new biological pathways in human growth. *Nat. Genet.* **2008**, *40*, 584–591. [CrossRef] [PubMed]

69. Weedon, M.N.; Lango, H.; Lindgren, C.M.; Wallace, C.; Evans, D.M.; Mangino, M.; Freathy, R.M.; Perry, J.R.; Stevens, S.; Hall, A.S.; et al. Genome-wide association analysis identifies 20 loci that influence adult height. *Nat. Genet.* **2008**, *40*, 575–583. [CrossRef]

70. Lango Allen, H.; Estrada, K.; Lettre, G.; Berndt, S.I.; Weedon, M.N.; Rivadeneira, F.; Willer, C.J.; Jackson, A.U.; Vedantam, S.; Raychaudhuri, S.; et al. Hundreds of variants clustered in genomic loci and biological pathways affect human height. *Nature* **2010**, *467*, 832–838. [CrossRef]

71. Yang, J.; Benyamin, B.; McEvoy, B.P.; Gordon, S.; Henders, A.K.; Nyholt, D.R.; Madden, P.A.; Heath, A.C.; Martin, N.G.; Montgomery, G.W.; et al. Common SNPs explain a large proportion of the heritability for human height. *Nat. Genet.* **2010**, *42*, 565–569. [CrossRef]

72. Wood, A.R.; Esko, T.; Yang, J.; Vedantam, S.; Pers, T.H.; Gustafsson, S.; Chu, A.Y.; Estrada, K.; Luan, J.; Kutalik, Z.; et al. Defining the role of common variation in the genomic and biological architecture of adult human height. *Nat. Genet.* **2014**, *46*, 1173–1186. [CrossRef]

73. Yengo, L.; Sidorenko, J.; Kemper, K.E.; Zheng, Z.; Wood, A.R.; Weedon, M.N.; Frayling, T.M.; Hirschhorn, J.; Yang, J.; Visscher, P.M. Meta-analysis of genome-wide association studies for height and body mass index in ~700,000 individuals of European ancestry. *Hum. Mol. Genet.* **2018**, *27*, 3641–3649. [CrossRef] [PubMed]

74. Kaiser, J. Growth spurt for height genetics. *Science* **2020**, *370*, 645. [CrossRef] [PubMed]

75. Zoledziewska, M.; Sidore, C.; Chiang, C.W.K.; Sanna, S.; Mulas, A.; Steri, M.; Busonero, F.; Marcus, J.H.; Marongiu, M.; Maschio, A.; et al. Height-reducing variants and selection for short stature in Sardinia. *Nat. Genet.* **2015**, *47*, 1352–1356. [CrossRef] [PubMed]

76. He, M.; Xu, M.; Zhang, B.; Liang, J.; Chen, P.; Lee, J.Y.; Johnson, T.A.; Li, H.; Yang, X.; Dai, J.; et al. Meta-analysis of genome-wide association studies of adult height in East Asians identifies 17 novel loci. *Hum. Mol. Genet.* **2015**, *24*, 1791–1800. [CrossRef]

77. Akiyama, M.; Ishigaki, K.; Sakaue, S.; Momozawa, Y.; Horikoshi, M.; Hirata, M.; Matsuda, K.; Ikegawa, S.; Takahashi, A.; Kanai, M.; et al. Characterizing rare and low-frequency height-associated variants in the Japanese population. *Nat. Commun.* **2019**, *10*, 4393. [CrossRef]

78. Marouli, E.; Graff, M.; Medina-Gomez, C.; Lo, K.S.; Wood, A.R.; Kjaer, T.R.; Fine, R.S.; Lu, Y.; Schurmann, C.; Highland, H.M.; et al. Rare and low-frequency coding variants alter human adult height. *Nature* **2017**, *542*, 186–190. [CrossRef]

79. Roosenboom, J.; Hens, G.; Mattern, B.C.; Shriver, M.D.; Claes, P. Exploring the Underlying Genetics of Craniofacial Morphology through Various Sources of Knowledge. *Biomed. Res. Int.* **2016**, *2016*, 3054578. [CrossRef] [PubMed]

80. Tsagkrasoulis, D.; Hysi, P.; Spector, T.; Montana, G. Heritability maps of human face morphology through large-scale automated three-dimensional phenotyping. *Sci. Rep.* **2017**, *7*, 45885. [CrossRef]

81. Guo, J.; Mei, X.; Tang, K. Automatic landmark annotation and dense correspondence registration for 3D human facial images. *BMC Bioinform.* **2013**, *14*, 232. [CrossRef]

82. Claes, P.; Liberton, D.K.; Daniels, K.; Rosana, K.M.; Quillen, E.E.; Pearson, L.N.; McEvoy, B.; Bauchet, M.; Zaidi, A.A.; Yao, W.; et al. Modeling 3D facial shape from DNA. *PLoS Genet.* **2014**, *10*, e1004224. [CrossRef] [PubMed]

83. Cole, J.B.; Manyama, M.; Kimwaga, E.; Mathayo, J.; Larson, J.R.; Liberton, D.K.; Lukowiak, K.; Ferrara, T.M.; Riccardi, S.L.; Li, M.; et al. Genomewide Association Study of African Children Identifies Association of SCHIP1 and PDE8A with Facial Size and Shape. *PLoS Genet.* **2016**, *12*, e1006174. [CrossRef]

84. Boehringer, S.; van der Lijn, F.; Liu, F.; Günther, M.; Sinigerova, S.; Nowak, S.; Ludwig, K.U.; Herberz, R.; Klein, S.; Hofman, A.; et al. Genetic determination of human facial morphology: Links between cleft-lips and normal variation. *Eur. J. Hum. Genet.* **2011**, *19*, 1192–1197. [CrossRef] [PubMed]

85. Toma, A.M.; Zhurov, A.I.; Playle, R.; Marshall, D.; Rosin, P.L.; Richmond, S. The assessment of facial variation in 4747 British school children. *Eur. J. Orthod.* **2012**, *34*, 655–664. [CrossRef] [PubMed]

86. Paternoster, L.; Zhurov, A.I.; Toma, A.M.; Kemp, J.P.; St Pourcain, B.; Timpson, N.J.; McMahon, G.; McArdle, W.; Ring, S.M.; Smith, G.D.; et al. Genome-wide association study of three-dimensional facial morphology identifies a variant in PAX3 associated with nasion position. *Am. J. Hum. Genet.* **2012**, *90*, 478–485. [CrossRef]

87. Liu, F.; van der Lijn, F.; Schurmann, C.; Zhu, G.; Chakravarty, M.M.; Hysi, P.G.; Wollstein, A.; Lao, O.; de Bruijne, M.; Ikram, M.A.; et al. A genome-wide association study identifies five loci influencing facial morphology in Europeans. *PLoS Genet.* **2012**, *8*, e1002932. [CrossRef] [PubMed]

88. Shaffer, J.R.; Orlova, E.; Lee, M.K.; Leslie, E.J.; Raffensperger, Z.D.; Heike, C.L.; Cunningham, M.L.; Hecht, J.T.; Kau, C.H.; Nidey, N.L.; et al. Genome-Wide Association Study Reveals Multiple Loci Influencing Normal Human Facial Morphology. *PLoS Genet.* **2016**, *12*, e1006149. [CrossRef] [PubMed]

89. Crouch, D.J.M.; Winney, B.; Koppen, W.P.; Christmas, W.J.; Hutnik, K.; Day, T.; Meena, D.; Boumertit, A.; Hysi, P.; Nessa, A.; et al. Genetics of the human face: Identification of large-effect single gene variants. *Proc. Natl. Acad. Sci. USA* **2018**, *115*, E676–E685. [CrossRef]

90. Claes, P.; Roosenboom, J.; White, J.D.; Swigut, T.; Sero, D.; Li, J.; Lee, M.K.; Zaidi, A.; Mattern, B.C.; Liebowitz, C.; et al. Genome-wide mapping of global-to-local genetic effects on human facial shape. *Nat. Genet.* **2018**, *50*, 414–423. [CrossRef] [PubMed]

91. White, J.D.; Indencleef, K.; Naqvi, S.; Eller, R.J.; Hoskens, H.; Roosenboom, J.; Lee, M.K.; Li, J.; Mohammed, J.; Richmond, S.; et al. Insights into the genetic architecture of the human face. *Nat. Genet.* **2021**, *53*, 45–53. [CrossRef] [PubMed]

92. Liu, C.; Lee, M.K.; Naqvi, S.; Hoskens, H.; Liu, D.; White, J.D.; Indencleef, K.; Matthews, H.; Eller, R.J.; Li, J.; et al. Genome scans of facial features in East Africans and cross-population comparisons reveal novel associations. *PLoS Genet.* **2021**, *17*, e1009695. [CrossRef]

93. Qiao, L.; Yang, Y.; Fu, P.; Hu, S.; Zhou, H.; Peng, S.; Tan, J.; Lu, Y.; Lou, H.; Lu, D.; et al. Genome-wide variants of Eurasian facial shape differentiation and a prospective model of DNA based face prediction. *J. Genet. Genom.* **2018**, *45*, 419–432. [CrossRef]

94. Sullivan, K.M.; Mannucci, A.; Kimpton, C.P.; Gill, P. A rapid and quantitative DNA sex test: Fluorescence-based PCR analysis of X-Y homologous gene amelogenin. *Biotechniques* **1993**, *15*, 636–638, 640–641. [PubMed]

95. Evett, I.W.; Pinchin, R.; Buffery, C. An investigation of the feasibility of inferring ethnic origin from DNA profiles. *J. Forensic Sci. Soc.* **1992**, *32*, 301–306. [CrossRef]

96. Shriver, M.D.; Smith, M.W.; Jin, L.; Marcini, A.; Akey, J.M.; Deka, R.; Ferrell, R.E. Ethnic-affiliation estimation by use of population-specific DNA markers. *Am. J. Hum. Genet.* **1997**, *60*, 957–964.

97. Grimes, E.A.; Noake, P.J.; Dixon, L.; Urquhart, A. Sequence polymorphism in the human melanocortin 1 receptor gene as an indicator of the red hair phenotype. *Forensic Sci. Int.* **2001**, *122*, 124–129. [CrossRef]

98. Walsh, S.; Liu, F.; Ballantyne, K.N.; van Oven, M.; Lao, O.; Kayser, M. IrisPlex: A sensitive DNA tool for accurate prediction of blue and brown eye colour in the absence of ancestry information. *Forensic Sci. Int. Genet.* **2011**, *5*, 170–180. [CrossRef]

99. Mengel-From, J.; Børsting, C.; Sanchez, J.J.; Eiberg, H.; Morling, N. Human eye colour and HERC2, OCA2 and MATP. *Forensic Sci. Int. Genet.* **2010**, *4*, 323–328. [CrossRef]

100. Valenzuela, R.K.; Henderson, M.S.; Walsh, M.H.; Garrison, N.A.; Kelch, J.T.; Cohen-Barak, O.; Erickson, D.T.; John Meaney, F.; Bruce Walsh, J.; Cheng, K.C.; et al. Predicting phenotype from genotype: Normal pigmentation. *J. Forensic Sci.* **2010**, *55*, 315–322. [CrossRef] [PubMed]

101. Spichenok, O.; Budimlija, Z.M.; Mitchell, A.A.; Jenny, A.; Kovacevic, L.; Marjanovic, D.; Caragine, T.; Prinz, M.; Wurmbach, E. Prediction of eye and skin color in diverse populations using seven SNPs. *Forensic Sci. Int. Genet.* **2011**, *5*, 472–478. [CrossRef] [PubMed]

102. Pośpiech, E.; Draus-Barini, J.; Kupiec, T.; Wojas-Pelc, A.; Branicki, W. Prediction of eye color from genetic data using Bayesian approach. *J. Forensic Sci.* **2012**, *57*, 880–886. [CrossRef]

103. Ruiz, Y.; Phillips, C.; Gomez-Tato, A.; Alvarez-Dios, J.; de Cal, M.C.; Cruz, R.; Maroñas, O.; Söchtig, J.; Fondevila, M.; Rodriguez-Cid, M.J.; et al. Further development of forensic eye color predictive tests. *Forensic Sci. Int. Genet.* **2013**, *7*, 28–40. [CrossRef]

104. Allwood, J.S.; Harbison, S. SNP model development for the prediction of eye colour in New Zealand. *Forensic Sci. Int. Genet.* **2013**, *7*, 444–452. [CrossRef] [PubMed]

105. Hart, K.L.; Kimura, S.L.; Mushailov, V.; Budimlija, Z.M.; Prinz, M.; Wurmbach, E. Improved eye- and skin-color prediction based on 8 SNPs. *Croat. Med. J.* **2013**, *54*, 248–256. [CrossRef]

106. Walsh, S.; Liu, F.; Wollstein, A.; Kovatsi, L.; Ralf, A.; Kosiniak-Kamysz, A.; Branicki, W.; Kayser, M. The HIrisPlex system for simultaneous prediction of hair and eye colour from DNA. *Forensic Sci. Int. Genet.* **2013**, *7*, 98–115. [CrossRef]

107. Söchtig, J.; Phillips, C.; Maroñas, O.; Gómez-Tato, A.; Cruz, R.; Alvarez-Dios, J.; de Cal, M.Á.; Ruiz, Y.; Reich, K.; Fondevila, M.; et al. Exploration of SNP variants affecting hair colour prediction in Europeans. *Int. J. Legal Med.* **2015**, *129*, 963–975. [CrossRef] [PubMed]

108. Maroñas, O.; Phillips, C.; Söchtig, J.; Gomez-Tato, A.; Cruz, R.; Alvarez-Dios, J.; de Cal, M.C.; Ruiz, Y.; Fondevila, M.; Carracedo, Á.; et al. Development of a forensic skin colour predictive test. *Forensic Sci. Int. Genet.* **2014**, *13*, 34–44. [CrossRef]

109. Chaitanya, L.; Breslin, K.; Zuñiga, S.; Wirken, L.; Pośpiech, E.; Kukla-Bartoszek, M.; Sijen, T.; Knijff, P.; Liu, F.; Branicki, W.; et al. The HIrisPlex-S system for eye, hair and skin colour prediction from DNA: Introduction and forensic developmental validation. *Forensic Sci. Int. Genet.* **2018**, *35*, 123–135. [CrossRef]

110. Andersen, J.D.; Meyer, O.S.; Simão, F.; Jannuzzi, J.; Carvalho, E.; Andersen, M.M.; Pereira, V.; Børsting, C.; Morling, N.; Gusmão, L. Skin pigmentation and genetic variants in an admixed Brazilian population of primarily European ancestry. *Int. J. Legal Med.* **2020**, *134*, 1569–1579. [CrossRef]

111. Hernando, B.; Ibañez, M.V.; Deserio-Cuesta, J.A.; Soria-Navarro, R.; Vilar-Sastre, I.; Martinez-Cadenas, C. Genetic determinants of freckle occurrence in the Spanish population: Towards ephelides prediction from human DNA samples. *Forensic Sci. Int. Genet.* **2018**, *33*, 38–47. [CrossRef]

112. Kukla-Bartoszek, M.; Pośpiech, E.; Woźniak, A.; Boroń, M.; Karłowska-Pik, J.; Teisseyre, P.; Zubańska, M.; Bronikowska, A.; Grzybowski, T.; Płoski, R.; et al. DNA-based predictive models for the presence of freckles. *Forensic Sci. Int. Genet.* **2019**, *42*, 252–259. [CrossRef]

113. Marcińska, M.; Pośpiech, E.; Abidi, S.; Andersen, J.D.; van den Berge, M.; Carracedo, Á.; Eduardoff, M.; Marczakiewicz-Lustig, A.; Morling, N.; Sijen, T.; et al. Evaluation of DNA variants associated with androgenetic alopecia and their potential to predict male pattern baldness. *PLoS ONE* **2015**, *10*, e0127852. [CrossRef] [PubMed]

114. Liu, F.; Hamer, M.A.; Heilmann, S.; Herold, C.; Moebus, S.; Hofman, A.; Uitterlinden, A.G.; Nöthen, M.M.; van Duijn, C.M.; Nijsten, T.E.; et al. Prediction of male-pattern baldness from genotypes. *Eur. J. Hum. Genet.* **2016**, *24*, 895–902. [CrossRef] [PubMed]

115. Pośpiech, E.; Karłowska-Pik, J.; Marcińska, M.; Abidi, S.; Andersen, J.D.; Berge, M.V.D.; Carracedo, Á.; Eduardoff, M.; Freire-Aradas, A.; Morling, N.; et al. Evaluation of the predictive capacity of DNA variants associated with straight hair in Europeans. *Forensic Sci. Int. Genet.* **2015**, *19*, 280–288. [CrossRef] [PubMed]

116. Pośpiech, E.; Chen, Y.; Kukla-Bartoszek, M.; Breslin, K.; Aliferi, A.; Andersen, J.D.; Ballard, D.; Chaitanya, L.; Freire-Aradas, A.; van der Gaag, K.J.; et al. Towards broadening Forensic DNA Phenotyping beyond pigmentation: Improving the prediction of head hair shape from DNA. *Forensic Sci. Int. Genet.* **2018**, *37*, 241–251. [CrossRef]

117. Aulchenko, Y.S.; Struchalin, M.V.; Belonogova, N.M.; Axenovich, T.I.; Weedon, M.N.; Hofman, A.; Uitterlinden, A.G.; Kayser, M.; Oostra, B.A.; van Duijn, C.M.; et al. Predicting human height by Victorian and genomic methods. *Eur. J. Hum. Genet.* **2009**, *17*, 1070–1075. [CrossRef] [PubMed]

118. Liu, F.; Hendriks, A.E.; Ralf, A.; Boot, A.M.; Benyi, E.; Sävendahl, L.; Oostra, B.A.; van Duijn, C.; Hofman, A.; Rivadeneira, F.; et al. Common DNA variants predict tall stature in Europeans. *Hum. Genet.* **2014**, *133*, 587–597. [CrossRef]

119. Liu, F.; Zhong, K.; Jing, X.; Uitterlinden, A.G.; Hendriks, A.E.J.; Drop, S.L.S.; Kayser, M. Update on the predictability of tall stature from DNA markers in Europeans. *Forensic Sci. Int. Genet.* **2019**, *42*, 8–13. [CrossRef]

120. Lello, L.; Avery, S.G.; Tellier, L.; Vazquez, A.I.; de Los Campos, G.; Hsu, S.D.H. Accurate Genomic Prediction of Human Height. *Genetics* **2018**, *210*, 477–497. [CrossRef]

121. Lippert, C.; Sabatini, R.; Maher, M.C.; Kang, E.Y.; Lee, S.; Arikan, O.; Harley, A.; Bernal, A.; Garst, P.; Lavrenko, V.; et al. Identification of individuals by trait prediction using whole-genome sequencing data. *Proc. Natl. Acad. Sci. USA* **2017**, *114*, 10166–10171. [CrossRef]

122. Liu, F.; van Duijn, K.; Vingerling, J.R.; Hofman, A.; Uitterlinden, A.G.; Janssens, A.C.; Kayser, M. Eye color and the prediction of complex phenotypes from genotypes. *Curr. Biol.* **2009**, *19*, R192–R193. [CrossRef] [PubMed]

123. Martinez-Cadenas, C.; Peña-Chilet, M.; Ibarrola-Villava, M.; Ribas, G. Gender is a major factor explaining discrepancies in eye colour prediction based on HERC2/OCA2 genotype and the IrisPlex model. *Forensic Sci. Int. Genet.* **2013**, *7*, 453–460. [CrossRef]

124. Pietroni, C.; Andersen, J.D.; Johansen, P.; Andersen, M.M.; Harder, S.; Paulsen, R.; Børsting, C.; Morling, N. The effect of gender on eye colour variation in European populations and an evaluation of the IrisPlex prediction model. *Forensic Sci. Int. Genet.* **2014**, *1*, 1–6. [CrossRef] [PubMed]

125. Pośpiech, E.; Karłowska-Pik, J.; Ziemkiewicz, B.; Kukla, M.; Skowron, M.; Wojas-Pelc, A.; Branicki, W. Further evidence for population specific differences in the effect of DNA markers and gender on eye colour prediction in forensics. *Int. J. Legal. Med.* **2016**, *130*, 923–934. [CrossRef]

126. Branicki, W.; Liu, F.; van Duijn, K.; Draus-Barini, J.; Pośpiech, E.; Walsh, S.; Kupiec, T.; Wojas-Pelc, A.; Kayser, M. Model-based prediction of human hair color using DNA variants. *Hum. Genet.* **2011**, *129*, 443–454. [CrossRef] [PubMed]

127. Walsh, S.; Chaitanya, L.; Breslin, K.; Muralidharan, C.; Bronikowska, A.; Pospiech, E.; Koller, J.; Kovatsi, L.; Wollstein, A.; Branicki, W.; et al. Global skin colour prediction from DNA. *Hum. Genet.* **2017**, *136*, 847–863. [CrossRef]

128. Breslin, K.; Wills, B.; Ralf, A.; Ventayol Garcia, M.; Kukla-Bartoszek, M.; Pospiech, E.; Freire-Aradas, A.; Xavier, C.; Ingold, S.; de La Puente, M.; et al. HIrisPlex-S system for eye, hair, and skin color prediction from DNA: Massively parallel sequencing solutions for two common forensically used platforms. *Forensic Sci. Int. Genet.* **2019**, *43*, 102152. [CrossRef] [PubMed]

129. Xavier, C.; de la Puente, M.; Mosquera-Miguel, A.; Freire-Aradas, A.; Kalamara, V.; Vidaki, A.; Gross, T.; Revoir, A.; Pośpiech, E.; Kartasińska, E.; et al. Development and validation of the VISAGE AmpliSeq basic tool to predict appearance and ancestry from DNA. *Forensic Sci. Int. Genet.* **2020**, *48*, 102336. [CrossRef]

130. Phillips, C.; Salas, A.; Sánchez, J.J.; Fondevila, M.; Gómez-Tato, A.; Alvarez-Dios, J.; Calaza, M.; de Cal, M.C.; Ballard, D.; Lareu, M.V.; et al. Inferring ancestral origin using a single multiplex assay of ancestry-informative marker SNPs. *Forensic Sci. Int. Genet.* **2007**, *1*, 273–280. [CrossRef] [PubMed]

131. Noroozi, R.; Ghafouri-Fard, S.; Pisarek, A.; Rudnicka, J.; Spólnicka, M.; Branicki, W.; Taheri, M.; Pośpiech, E. DNA methylation-based age clocks: From age prediction to age reversion. *Ageing Res. Rev.* **2021**, *68*, 101314. [CrossRef]

132. De Los Campos, G.; Vazquez, A.I.; Hsu, S.; Lello, L. Complex-Trait Prediction in the Era of Big Data. *Trends Genet.* **2018**, *34*, 746–754. [CrossRef]

133. Shmueli, G. To Explain or to Predict? *Stat. Sci.* **2010**, *25*, 289–310. [CrossRef]

134. Hastie, T.; Tibshirani, R.; Friedman, J. *The Elements of Statistical Learning*, 2nd ed.; Springer: New York, NY, USA, 2009.

135. Hill, G.H.; Goddard, M.E.; Vissher, P.M. Data and Theory Point to Mainly Additive Genetic Variance for Complex Traits. *PLoS Genet.* **2008**, *4*, 1–10. [CrossRef]

136. Katsara, M.A.; Branicki, W.; Walsh, S.; Kayser, M.; Nothnagel, M. Evaluation of supervised machine-learning methods for predicting appearance traits from DNA. *Forensic Sci. Int. Genet.* **2021**, *53*, 1–9. [CrossRef] [PubMed]

137. Kukla-Bartoszek, M.; Teisseyre, P.; Pośpiech, E.; Karłowska-Pik, J.; Zieliński, P.; Woźniak, A.; Boroń, M.; Dąbrowski, M.; Zubańska, M.; Jarosz, A.; et al. Searching for improvements in predicting human eye colour from DNA. *Int. J. Legal Med.* **2021**, *135*, 2175–2187. [CrossRef] [PubMed]

138. Fan, J.; Li, R. Variable selection via nonconcave penalized likelihood and its oracle properties. *J. Amer. Stat. Assoc.* **2001**, *96*, 1348–1361. [CrossRef]

139. Zhang, C.H. Nearly unbiased variable selection under minimax concave penalty. *Ann. Stat.* **2001**, *38*, 894–942. [CrossRef]

140. Breheny, P.; Huang, J. Coordinate descent algorithms for nonconvex penalized regression, with applications to biological feature selection. *Ann. Appl. Stat.* **2011**, *5*, 232–253. [CrossRef]

141. Benjamini, Y.; Hochberg, Y. Controlling the false discovery rate: A practical and multiple approach to multiple testing. *J. R. Stat. Soc. Ser. B* **1995**, *57*, 289–300.

142. Barber, R.F.; Candes, E.J. Controlling the False Discovery Rate by knockoffs. *Ann. Stat.* **2015**, *43*, 2055–2085. [CrossRef]

143. Tsamardinos, I.; Borboudakis, G. Permutation testing improves Bayesian Network learning. In Proceedings of the Joint European Conference on Machine Learning and Knowledge Discovery in Databases, Barcelona, Spain, 19–23 September 2010; pp. 322–337.

144. Tansey, W.; Veitch, V.; Zhang, H.; Rabadan, R.; Blei, D. The Holdout Randomisation Test for Feature Selection in Black Box Models. *J. Comput. Graph. Stat.* **2021**, 1–37. Available online: https://arxiv.org/abs/1811.00645 (accessed on 8 December 2021).

145. Bishop, C. *Pattern Recognition and Machine Learning*, 1st ed.; Springer: New York, NY, USA, 2006.

146. Breiman, L. Bagging Predictors. *Mach. Learn.* **1996**, *24*, 123–140. [CrossRef]

147. Ho, T.K. The Random Subspace Method for Constructing Decision Forests. *IEEE Trans. Pattern Anal. Mach. Intell.* **1998**, *20*, 832–844.

148. Mielniczuk, J.; Teisseyre, P. Using Random Subspace Method for Prediction and Variable Importance Assessment in Regression. *Comput. Stat. Data Anal.* **2014**, *71*, 725–742. [CrossRef]

149. Chen, T.; Guestrin, C. XGBoost: A Scalable Tree Boosting System. In Proceedings of the 22nd ACM SIGKDD International Conference on Knowledge Discovery and Data Mining, San Francisco, CA, USA, 13–17 August 2016; pp. 785–794.

150. Kursa, M.; Rudnicki, W. Feature Selection with the Boruta Package. *J. Stat. Softw.* **2010**, *36*, 1–13. [CrossRef]

151. Dramiński, M.; Rada-Iglesias, A.; Enroth, S.; Wadelius, C.; Koronacki, J.; Komorowski, J. Monte Carlo feature selection for supervised classification. *Bioinformatics* **2008**, *24*, 110–117. [CrossRef] [PubMed]

152. Rosenblatt, F. The Perceptron—A Perceiving and Recognizing Automaton, Report. 1957. Available online: https://blogs.umass.edu/brain-wars/files/2016/03/rosenblatt-1957.pdf (accessed on 8 December 2021).

153. Goodfellow, J.; Bengio, Y.; Courville, A. *Deep Learning*, 1st ed.; MIT Press: Cambridge, MA, USA, 2016.

154. Kingma, D.; Ba, J. Adam: A Method for Stochastic Optimization. In Proceedings of the International Conference on Learning Representations, San Diego, CA, USA, 7–9 May 2015; pp. 1–13.

155. Kingsma, D.; Welling, M. Autoencoding variational Bayes. In Proceedings of the 2nd Conference on Learning Representations, Banff, AB, Canada, 14–16 April 2014; pp. 1–14.

156. Brown, G.; Pocock, A.; Zhao, M.-J.; Luján, M. Conditional Likelihood Maximisation: A Unifying Framework for Information Theoretic Feature Selection. *J. Mach. Learn. Res.* **2012**, *13*, 27–66.

157. Moore, J.H.; Hu, T. Epistatic analysis using information theory. *Methods Mol. Biol.* **2015**, *1253*, 257–268. [PubMed]

158. Cordell, H.J. Epistasis: What it means, what it doesn't mean, and statistical methods to detect it in humans. *Hum. Mol. Genet.* **2002**, *11*, 2463–2468. [CrossRef]

159. Pośpiech, E.; Wojas-Pelc, A.; Walsh, S.; Liu, F.; Maeda, H.; Ishikawa, T.; Skowron, M.; Kayser, M.; Branicki, W. The common occurrence of epistasis in the determination of human pigmentation and its impact on DNA-based pigmentation phenotype prediction. *Forensic Sci. Int. Genet.* **2014**, *11*, 64–72. [CrossRef] [PubMed]

160. Mielniczuk, J.; Teisseyre, P. Deeper Look at Two Concepts of Measuring Gene-Gene Interactions: Logistic Regression and Interaction Information Revisited. *Genet. Epidemiol.* **2018**, *42*, 187–200. [CrossRef] [PubMed]

161. Lin, D.; Tang, X. Conditional infomax learning: An integrated framework for feature extraction and fusion. In Proceedings of the European Conference on Computer Vision, Graz, Austria, 7–13 May 2006; pp. 68–82.

162. Vinh, N.X.; Zhou, S.; Chan, J.; Bailey, J. Can high-order dependencies improve mutual information based feature selection? *Pattern Recognit.* **2016**, *53*, 46–58. [CrossRef]

163. Mielniczuk, J.; Teisseyre, P. Stopping rules for mutual information-based feature selection. *Neurocomputing* **2019**, *358*, 255–274. [CrossRef]

164. Tillmar, A.; Sjölund, P.; Lundqvist, B.; Klippmark, T.; Älgenäs, C.; Green, H. Whole-genome sequencing of human remains to enable genealogy DNA database searches—A case report. *Forensic Sci. Int. Genet.* **2020**, *46*, 102233. [CrossRef] [PubMed]

165. Hofman, C.A.; Warinner, C. Ancient DNA 101: An introductory guide in the era of high-throughput sequencing. *SAA Rec.* **2019**, *19*, 18–25.

166. Hofreiter, M.; Sneberger, J.; Pospisek, M.; Vanek, D. Progress in forensic bone DNA analysis: Lessons learned from ancient DNA. *Forensic Sci. Int. Genet.* **2021**, *54*, 102538. [CrossRef]

167. Meyer, M.; Kircher, M. Illumina sequencing library preparation for highly multiplexed target capture and sequencing. *Cold Spring Harb. Protoc.* **2010**, *2010*, pdb.prot5448. [CrossRef]

168. Psonis, N.; Vassou, D.; Kafetzopoulos, D. Testing a series of modifications on genomic library preparation methods for ancient or degraded DNA. *Anal. Biochem.* **2021**, *623*, 114193. [CrossRef]

169. Carøe, C.; Gopalakrishnan, S.; Vinner, L.; Mak, S.S.T.; Sinding, M.-H.S.; Samaniego, J.A.; Wales, N.; Sicheritz-Pontén, T.; Gilbert, M.T.P. Single-tube library preparation for degraded DNA. *Methods Ecol. Evol.* **2018**, *9*, 410–419. [CrossRef]

170. Gansauge, M.T.; Meyer, M. Single-stranded DNA library preparation for the sequencing of ancient or damaged DNA. *Nat. Protoc.* **2013**, *8*, 737–748. [CrossRef]

171. Gansauge, M.T.; Gerber, T.; Glocke, I.; Korlevic, P.; Lippik, L.; Nagel, S.; Riehl, L.M.; Schmidt, A.; Meyer, M. Single-stranded DNA library preparation from highly degraded DNA using T4 DNA ligase. *Nucleic Acids Res.* **2017**, *45*, e79. [CrossRef]

172. Gansauge, M.T.; Aximu-Petri, A.; Nagel, S.; Meyer, M. Manual and automated preparation of single-stranded DNA libraries for the sequencing of DNA from ancient biological remains and other sources of highly degraded DNA. *Nat. Protoc.* **2020**, *15*, 2279–2300. [CrossRef] [PubMed]

173. Kapp, J.D.; Green, R.E.; Shapiro, B. A Fast and Efficient Single-stranded Genomic Library Preparation Method Optimized for Ancient DNA. *J. Hered.* **2021**, *112*, 241–249. [CrossRef] [PubMed]

174. Green, R.E.; Krause, J.; Briggs, A.W.; Maricic, T.; Stenzel, U.; Kircher, M.; Patterson, N.; Li, H.; Zhai, W.; Fritz, M.H.; et al. A draft sequence of the Neandertal genome. *Science* **2010**, *328*, 710–722. [CrossRef] [PubMed]

175. Meyer, M.; Kircher, M.; Gansauge, M.T.; Li, H.; Racimo, F.; Mallick, S.; Schraiber, J.G.; Jay, F.; Prüfer, K.; de Filippo, C.; et al. A high-coverage genome sequence from an archaic Denisovan individual. *Science* **2012**, *338*, 222–226. [CrossRef] [PubMed]

176. Stiller, M.; Sucker, A.; Griewank, K.; Aust, D.; Baretton, G.B.; Schadendorf, D.; Horn, S. Single-strand DNA library preparation improves sequencing of formalin-fixed and paraffin-embedded (FFPE) cancer DNA. *Oncotarget* **2016**, *7*, 59115–59128. [CrossRef]

177. Rasmussen, M.; Li, Y.; Lindgreen, S.; Pedersen, J.S.; Albrechtsen, A.; Moltke, I.; Metspalu, M.; Metspalu, E.; Kivisild, T.; Gupta, R.; et al. Ancient human genome sequence of an extinct Palaeo-Eskimo. *Nature* **2010**, *463*, 757–762. [CrossRef]

178. Keller, A.; Graefen, A.; Ball, M.; Matzas, M.; Boisguerin, V.; Maixner, F.; Leidinger, P.; Backes, C.; Khairat, R.; Forster, M.; et al. New insights into the Tyrolean Iceman's origin and phenotype as inferred by whole-genome sequencing. *Nat. Commun.* **2012**, *3*, 698. [CrossRef] [PubMed]

179. Olalde, I.; Allentoft, M.E.; Sánchez-Quinto, F.; Santpere, G.; Chiang, C.W.; DeGiorgio, M.; Prado-Martinez, J.; Rodríguez, J.A.; Rasmussen, S.; Quilez, J.; et al. Derived immune and ancestral pigmentation alleles in a 7000-year-old Mesolithic European. *Nature* **2014**, *507*, 225–228. [CrossRef]
180. Bogdanowicz, W.; Allen, M.; Branicki, W.; Lembring, M.; Gajewska, M.; Kupiec, T. Genetic identification of putative remains of the famous astronomer Nicolaus Copernicus. *Proc. Natl. Acad. Sci. USA* **2009**, *106*, 12279–12282. [CrossRef]
181. Kupiec, T.; Branicki, W. Genetic examination of the putative skull of Jan Kochanowski reveals its female sex. *Croat. Med. J.* **2011**, *52*, 403–409. [CrossRef] [PubMed]
182. King, T.E.; Fortes, G.G.; Balaresque, P.; Thomas, M.G.; Balding, D.; Maisano Delser, P.; Neumann, R.; Parson, W.; Knapp, M.; Walsh, S.; et al. Identification of the remains of King Richard III. *Nat. Commun.* **2014**, *5*, 5631. [CrossRef] [PubMed]
183. Salvo, N.M.; Janssen, K.; Kirsebom, M.K.; Meyer, O.S.; Berg, T.; Olsen, G.H. Predicting eye and hair colour in a Norwegian population using Verogen's ForenSeq™ DNA signature prep kit. *Forensic Sci. Int. Genet.* **2021**, *56*, 102620. [CrossRef]
184. Diepenbroek, M.; Bayer, B.; Schwender, K.; Schiller, R.; Lim, J.; Lagacé, R.; Anslinger, K. Evaluation of the Ion AmpliSeq™ PhenoTrivium Panel: MPS-Based Assay for Ancestry and Phenotype Predictions Challenged by Casework Samples. *Genes* **2020**, *11*, 1398. [CrossRef] [PubMed]
185. Parabon NanoLabs. Available online: https://snapshot.parabon-nanolabs.com (accessed on 8 December 2021).

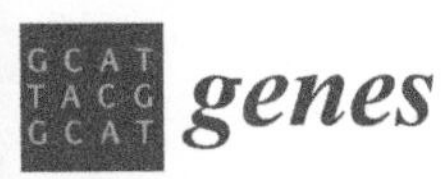

Article

Development and Evaluation of the Ancestry Informative Marker Panel of the VISAGE Basic Tool

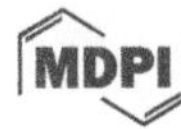

María de la Puente [1], Jorge Ruiz-Ramírez [1], Adrián Ambroa-Conde [1], Catarina Xavier [2], Jacobo Pardo-Seco [3], Jose Álvarez-Dios [4], Ana Freire-Aradas [1], Ana Mosquera-Miguel [1], Theresa E. Gross [5,6], Elaine Y. Y. Cheung [5], Wojciech Branicki [7], Michael Nothnagel [8,9], Walther Parson [2,10], Peter M. Schneider [5], Manfred Kayser [11], Ángel Carracedo [1,12], Maria Victoria Lareu [1], Christopher Phillips [1,*] and on behalf of the VISAGE Consortium [†]

1   Forensic Genetics Unit, Institute of Forensic Sciences, University of Santiago de Compostela, 15782 Santiago de Compostela, Spain; m.delapuente.vila@gmail.com (M.d.l.P.); ruizramirez.jorge@gmail.com (J.R.-R.); ambroa.adrian@gmail.com (A.A.-C.); ana.freire3@hotmail.com (A.F.-A.); ana.mosquera@usc.es (A.M.-M.); angel.carracedo@usc.es (Á.C.); mvictoria.lareu@usc.es (M.V.L.)
2   Institute of Legal Medicine, Medical University of Innsbruck, 6020 Innsbruck, Austria; catarinagaxavier@hotmail.com (C.X.); walther.parson@i-med.ac.at (W.P.)
3   Genetics, Vaccines, Infectious Diseases and Pediatrics Research Group (GENVIP Group), Instituto de Investigación Sanitaria de Santiago de Compostela, 15706 Santiago de Compostela, Spain; j.pardoseco@gmail.com
4   Faculty of Mathematics, University of Santiago de Compostela, 15705 Santiago de Compostela, Spain; joseantonio.alvarez.dios@usc.es
5   Institute of Legal Medicine, Faculty of Medicine and University Clinic, University of Cologne, 50823 Cologne, Germany; gross.theresa@gmail.com (T.E.G.); elaine.yy.cheung@outlook.com (E.Y.Y.C.); peter.schneider@uk-koeln.de (P.M.S.)
6   Hessisches Landeskriminalamt, 65187 Wiesbaden, Germany
7   Malopolska Centre of Biotechnology, Jagiellonian University, 30-387 Kraków, Poland; wojciech.branicki@uj.edu.pl
8   Cologne Center for Genomics, University of Cologne, 50823 Cologne, Germany; mnothnag@ini-koeln.de
9   University Hospital Cologne, 50937 Cologne, Germany
10   Forensic Science Program, The Pennsylvania State University, University Park, State College, PA 16802, USA
11   Department of Genetic Identification, Erasmus MC University Medical Center Rotterdam, 3015 CN Rotterdam, South Holland, The Netherlands; m.kayser@erasmusmc.nl
12   Fundación Pública Galega de Medicina Xenómica (FPGMX), 15706 Santiago de Compostela, Spain
*   Correspondence: c.phillips@mac.com
†   A complete list of the centers and investigators in the VISAGE GROUP is provided in Appendix A.

Citation: de la Puente, M.; Ruiz-Ramírez, J.; Ambroa-Conde, A.; Xavier, C.; Pardo-Seco, J.; Álvarez-Dios, J.; Freire-Aradas, A.; Mosquera-Miguel, A.; Gross, T.E.; Cheung, E.Y.Y.; et al. Development and Evaluation of the Ancestry Informative Marker Panel of the VISAGE Basic Tool. *Genes* **2021**, *12*, 1284. https://doi.org/10.3390/genes12081284

Academic Editor: Niels Morling

Received: 21 July 2021
Accepted: 18 August 2021
Published: 22 August 2021

Abstract: We detail the development of the ancestry informative single nucleotide polymorphisms (SNPs) panel forming part of the VISAGE Basic Tool (BT), which combines 41 appearance predictive SNPs and 112 ancestry predictive SNPs (three SNPs shared between sets) in one massively parallel sequencing (MPS) multiplex, whereas blood-based age analysis using methylation markers is run in a parallel MPS analysis pipeline. The selection of SNPs for the BT ancestry panel focused on established forensic markers that already have a proven track record of good sequencing performance in MPS, and the overall SNP multiplex scale closely matched that of existing forensic MPS assays. SNPs were chosen to differentiate individuals from the five main continental population groups of Africa, Europe, East Asia, America, and Oceania, extended to include differentiation of individuals from South Asia. From analysis of 1000 Genomes and HGDP-CEPH samples from these six population groups, the BT ancestry panel was shown to have no classification error using the Bayes likelihood calculators of the *Snipper* online analysis portal. The differentiation power of the component ancestry SNPs of BT was balanced as far as possible to avoid bias in the estimation of co-ancestry proportions in individuals with admixed backgrounds. The balancing process led to very similar cumulative population-specific divergence values for Africa, Europe, America, and Oceania, with East Asia being slightly below average, and South Asia an outlier from the other groups. Comparisons were made of the African, European, and Native American estimated co-ancestry proportions in the six admixed 1000 Genomes populations, using the BT ancestry panel SNPs and 572,000 Affymetrix Human Origins array SNPs. Very similar co-ancestry proportions were observed down to a minimum value of 10%, below which, low-level co-ancestry was not always reliably detected by BT SNPs. The *Snipper* analysis portal provides a comprehensive population dataset for the BT ancestry panel SNPs, comprising a 520-sample standardised reference dataset; 3445 additional samples from 1000 Genomes, HGDP-CEPH, Simons Foundation and Estonian Biocentre genome diversity projects; and 167 samples of six populations from in-house genotyping of individuals from Middle East, North and East African regions complementing those of the sampling regimes of the other diversity projects.

Keywords: bio-geographical ancestry; massively parallel sequencing; ancestry informative markers; SNPs; 1000 Genomes; Human Origins SNP array

1. Introduction

In the last ten years, forensic DNA analysis has been extended beyond identification tests that link a suspect to crime-scene evidence using STR profiling, into areas of genetic analysis designed to predict a range of physical characteristics of unidentified trace donors, mainly defined by single nucleotide polymorphisms (SNPs). Such SNP tests, applicable when no suspect has been identified by investigators, have been termed forensic DNA phenotyping (FDP), and until recently, consisted of tests to infer bio-geographical ancestry (BGA) [1], or to predict certain externally visible characteristics (EVCs) [2]. These SNP-based tests have now been supplemented with DNA analyses that measure the methylation status of carefully chosen CpG sites showing age-correlated methylation patterns in order to estimate a donor's chronological age from the same DNA samples used for BGA and EVC tests [3]. The array of FDP tests now being adopted can serve to progress a major criminal investigation lacking strong leads, resurrect cold cases by providing new genetic data about old crime-scene DNA samples, and aid in the identification of the missing or historical remains [4]. While FDP tests have been gaining traction as supplementary analysis regimes available to forensic laboratories, the emergence of massively parallel sequencing (MPS) now provides major enhancements for forensic DNA analysis, including improved sensitivity to analyse minimal amounts of evidential material, larger multiplexes that can combine conventional identification STRs with SNPs for FDP analysis, and greater detail about the detectable variation within a sequence. The VISible Attributes through GEnomics (VISAGE) Consortium was initiated in 2017 to develop new MPS-based tools for predicting the BGA, appearance based on common EVCs, and age of an unidentified crime-scene DNA donor.

VISAGE adopted a two-step program to create MPS tools for FDP: developing a Basic Tool as a pilot assay, followed by the development of an Enhanced Tool with more markers and extended capabilities. The VISAGE Basic Tool (herein BT) is the first forensic MPS test combining markers for predicting eye, hair, and skin colour with those for BGA inference in a single assay, along with a saliva-blood focused age estimation assay requiring a parallel assay and workflow due to the bisulphite conversion steps needed to measure methylation. The VISAGE BT was founded on marker panels which have been shown to be informative for the three pigmentation traits [5–7] and for continental-scale population differentiation [8–12]. The level of multiplexing necessary to accommodate sufficient SNPs to yield optimum predictions of both EVCs and continental BGA was in part dictated by experience of building multiplexes for forensic MPS analysis [8,12,13]. Therefore, for the BT assay, which acts as a pilot test, we decided to design a moderate PCR scale of 150 to 160 SNPs by combining the 41 well-established HIrisPlex-S markers, which have been successfully applied in previous SNaPshot and MPS assays [5–7,13], with up to 120 ancestry-informative marker (AIM) SNPs. A panel of 120 AIM SNPs represents a reduced multiplex size compared to the one commercially available forensic ancestry panel for MPS, i.e., the Thermo Fisher Precision ID Ancestry Panel, comprising 165 AIMs [14], although similar in scale to another panel of 127 AIMs [8]. For this reason, we selected markers with the maximum possible ancestry informativeness for any given population, and then balanced these to ensure the major population groups had broadly comparable levels of differentiation. In contrast to the previous development of the 127-SNP Global AIMs panel (gAIMs [8]), South Asians, i.e., individuals from the Indian subcontinent, were treated as a separate population group.

This paper describes the compilation of component SNPs into the ancestry informative marker set forming the major portion of the VISAGE Basic Tool for appearance-ancestry. The development of the AIMs set and its evaluation involved four stages: i. Selection of markers and balancing of their relative population informativeness proportions in the multiplex to ensure comparable levels of continental population group differentiation; ii. Generation of a large-scale reference dataset built on open-access, genome-wide variant datasets, plus our own MPS genotyping of in-house population samples from which to apply the statistical analysis pipelines accompanying the BT assay; iii. Genotype concordance studies and an audit of existing genome-wide variant datasets for the selected AIM SNPs by analysing whole-genome sequence data released by the 1000 Genomes Project in 2020 [15–17]; and iv. Evaluation of the panel's capacity to make efficient population differentiations using existing likelihood-based ancestry inference tests.

2. Materials and Methods

2.1. Selection and Balancing of Component Ancestry Informative SNPs

The BT assay design targeted an AIMs panel of approximately 120 SNPs, based on the fact that ~25% of the full multiplex would be occupied with the 41 markers of HIrisPlex-S, and shared use of key SNPs rs16891982 (in *SLC45A2* gene), rs1426654 (*SLC24A5*), rs12913832 (*HERC2*) for both ancestry and appearance predictive purposes. Because tri-allelic SNPs have been found to be useful for the detection of mixed DNA [18], but when carefully selected have also been informative for ancestry to comparable levels as binary SNPs [19], we expanded their number in the multiplex above those of the previous gAIMs panel (which had six tri-allelic SNPs of a total 127 loci [8]). Twenty tri-allelic SNPs showing the highest levels of population divergence were selected from a very large candidate pool created from a genome-wide compilation of this type of human variation [20].

Careful consideration was made to balance the differentiation of the five main continental population groups of sub-Saharan Africa, Europe, East Asia, Oceania and America (herein, AFR, EUR, EAS, OCE and AMR) with differentiation of the South Asian sub-group (SAS). We decided to target 60–70 SNPs for continental differentiation, plus 20 SNPs to distinguish South Asia from the neighbouring population groups of Europe and East Asia.

SNPs for continental differentiation were compiled from four well-established AIM sets: i. the 127-SNP gAIMs ancestry panel; ii. the 446-SNP LACE (Latin American Cancer Epidemiology) ancestry panel [21]; iii–iv. the 165-SNP Thermo Fisher Precision ID Ancestry Panel (PIAP) [14], which includes the widely used 56-SNP Kiddlab ancestry panel [22]. SNPs differentiating South Asian and European populations were compiled from the above panels and three dedicated AIM sets for such geographic distinctions: v. the best European differentiating SNPs from the EUROFORGEN NAME panel [23]; vi. the Shriver group's US admixture mapping panel, with many highly European-informative loci [24]; and vii. the *Eurasiaplex* South Asian informative panel [9].

The continental SNPs in BT were balanced in terms of their individual population differentiation power to equilibrate as far as possible the five continental groups, ensuring that no one population group had excessive numbers of indicative SNPs, which could potentially bias calculations of co-ancestry proportions in persons with admixed backgrounds (e.g., excessive numbers of African-informative SNPs in such a small panel could overestimate this co-ancestry compared to the others). For each SNP, this process records the population specific divergence ($I_{n\ AFR}$; $I_{n\ EUR}$; $I_{n\ E\ ASN}$; etc., the metric divergence is capitalised and measures the degree of differentiation per marker) to guide the removal or addition of SNPs for a specific population comparison in order to improve overall I_n balance. To reach this balance, the *Snipper* online ancestry analysis portal [25] was used to estimate cumulative I_n values, as previously described for the development of the gAIMs panel [8]. As BT had a smaller number of SNPs than gAIMs, we did not expect to reach a comparably narrow range of finely balanced I_n values.

2.2. Compilation of a 4132-Sample Population Dataset

A comprehensive population dataset for the BT ancestry SNPs was generated by compiling online whole-genome-sequencing variant data from 3965 samples and adding in-house genotyping of 167 samples from six populations, chosen to cover geographic gaps in data for several under-represented regions, i.e., 30 from Eritrea, 16 from Somalia, 32 from Morocco, 32 from Central Iraq, 28 from the Kurdistan region of Iraq and 29 from Turkey (Turkish resident in Germany). An additional 277 DNA samples from the HGDP-CEPH human diversity panel were genotyped with the BT assay with the goal of further extending the geographic coverage of Oceanian, Native American and Middle East (herein ME) population variation, i.e., regions not covered by 1000 Genomes Phase 3 populations. However, the 1000 Genomes Consortium completed whole-genome-sequencing of the full HGDP-CEPH panel in 2019 soon after our in-house genotyping had been completed, so we compiled the complete dataset from 1000 Genomes and used the overlapping sample data to measure the MPS genotyping concordance of BT. This was accomplished for the whole marker set of BT (i.e., including the 41 appearance markers) to gauge sequencing performance across the complete multiplex.

Of the total 4132 SNP genotype profiles compiled, 520 were used as a standardised six population group reference dataset for uploading as training sets to the *Snipper* ancestry analysis portal, with the aim of providing the closest possible equivalence of sample sizes amongst the continental and South Asian regions. The standardised reference dataset consisted of: sub-Saharan Africans represented by 108 1000 Genomes 30X sequence coverage (1KG-30) Yoruba from Nigeria (YRI); Europeans by 99 1KG-30 CEPH Europeans from Utah (CEU); East Asians by 103 1KG-30 Han Chinese from Beijing (CHB); South Asians by 103 1KG-30 Gujarati from Houston (GIH); Oceanians by 28 HGDP-CEPH Papuans from Bougainvillea and Papua New Guinea; Native Americans by 79 samples, comprising 61 HGDP-CEPH samples from Maya, Pima populations, Colombians and Amazonian Surui and Karitiana populations, supplemented by 18 1KG-30 Peruvians from Lima, Peru (PEL) which we had previously analysed and showed no detectable non-American co-ancestry (in-silico analysis of 572,743 Affymetrix Human Origins SNPs, see Table 10.5 of [26]).

Although we established the above standardised reference dataset, the additional populations compiled can be flexibly included in *Snipper* or can replace those in the reference set at the user's discretion by adjusting the Excel-based training set file uploaded to the 'multiple profiles' classifier portal (http://mathgene.usc.es/snipper/analysismultipleprofiles.html, accessed on 20 August 2021), which generates a Bayes likelihood ratio statistical test for ancestry and a matched 2D principal component analysis (PCA) plot. For maximum flexibility, the other population data was arranged into a series of worksheets in the same core Excel reference file, allowing the end-user to select alternative reference populations from 1000 Genomes or HGDP-CEPH (e.g., HGDP-CEPH Pakistani South Asian samples rather than 1KG-30 Gujarati, or other populations from the Indian sub-continent). The same user-driven options apply to the VISAGE in-house population samples provided in a separate worksheet. The admixed populations in 1000 Genomes, comprising 96 African Caribbean individuals in Barbados (ACB), 61 Americans of African Ancestry in SW USA (ASW), 64 individuals with Mexican Ancestry from Los Angeles USA (MXL,) 94 Colombians from Medellin, Colombia (CLM), 104 Puerto Ricans from Puerto Rico (PUR), 67 of 85 PEL (i.e., with detected co-ancestry) were also compiled in a separate worksheet but would not be expected to be useful as training set data from which representative allele frequency estimates could be obtained, given their high levels of individual admixture.

Genome-wide variant data from Simons Foundation human genome diversity project (herein SGDP) has been available for several years [27], and offers additional information on geographic areas outside of those covered by 1000 Genomes or the HGDP-CEPH sampling regimes, in particular, Northeast Asia (broadly, Eastern Siberia east towards the Bering

Straits); Southeast Island Asia; and Central South Asia (broadly, the Caucasus' east towards the central Asian Steppe immediately north of South Asia). There are 278 genome-wide SNP datasets, of which 22 overlap with 1000 Genomes and 126 overlap with the HGDP-CEPH panel samples, leaving 130 unique samples, from 67 populations. The small sample size of SGDP highlights the very limited number of 1, 2 or 3 samples per region. Nevertheless, we compiled the 130 SGDP-unique BT AIM profiles into a dedicated worksheet and completed population analyses using the standardised reference set.

Genome-wide variant data from the Estonian Biocentre genome diversity project (herein, EGDP) largely mirrors the sampling regimes of SGDP [28], with a maximum of 16 samples per region, but mainly 1, 2 or 3 per region. EGDP has 402 whole-genome datasets from the sampling of 126 populations that almost all complement those of SGDP and provides extensive coverage of regions in Siberia, Northeast Asia, Eastern Europe, and Central South Asia. As with SGDP, the 402 EGDP BT AIM profiles were compiled into a dedicated worksheet and population analyses made with the standardised reference set. Note that the tri-allelic SNPs forming part of the BT AIMs panel are not reported by EGDP and an additional four ancestry SNPs do not have genotypes, so data completeness is ~83.5% (96/115 SNPs).

2.3. Genotyping Concordance amongst MPS Sequence Data and Online Databases

Genotyping concordance for the BT SNPs was assessed in two ways. First, a direct comparison was made between the MPS genotypes generated during developmental runs genotyping 277 HGDP-CEPH DNA samples for all 153 SNPs in BT, and the SNP genotypes reported by 1000 Genomes for the same DNA samples [16], providing 42,381 comparisons. Second, the genotypes listed by 1000 Genomes Phase 3 database for 2504 worldwide population samples (and available in the Ensembl browser at: http://www.ensembl.org/Homo_sapiens/Info/Index, accessed on 20 August 2021) were compared to the high coverage re-sequencing dataset for the same samples, released in early 2020 by the New York Genome Centre [17]. The high sequence coverage genotypes correspond to an average 30X coverage, while the current Phase 3 genotypes were produced from an average 2-3X coverage. We considered the high coverage data to represent more reliable genotype calls for the SNPs of BT, so these were compiled as the major part of the reference population data we used for statistical analysis of ancestry, as described above.

The Coriell control DNA samples originally used as the genotyping concordance standards in the inter-laboratory evaluations of the BT assay [29] were also run as positive controls on each sequencing run performed for the in-house population studies.

2.4. Evaluation of Ancestry and Co-Ancestry Inference Efficiency of the BT AIMs

The efficiency of the BT AIMs to infer ancestry was assessed for a six-group differentiation of African, European, East Asian, South Asian, American and Oceanian ancestries. To measure classification error, one-out cross-validation of the standardised reference dataset of 520 samples was performed using the verbose cross validation option in *Snipper* (http://mathgene.usc.es/Snipper/analysispopfile2_new.html, accessed on 20 August 2021). For all other samples, STRUCTURE, PCA and neighbour joining tree (NJT) analyses were performed on each of the separate population sets, comprising admixed and unadmixed 1000 Genomes samples not used as reference data; HGDP-CEPH samples not used as reference data (i.e., no Oceanian, American population data); SGDP samples, with the six in-house populations included in the same analysis run; and EGDP samples (for 100 binary SNPs of 115 ancestry SNPs in BT). STRUCTURE v.2.3.4 [30] was used for runs consisting of five iterations per K (genetic cluster values K:2 to K:8 evaluated) consisting of 100,000 burnin steps and 100,000 MCMC steps, using correlated allele frequencies under the Admixture model. The optimum 'K' cluster number was inferred by plotting log probability of K and magnitude of ΔK, following the analyses of Evanno et al. [31]. Allele frequencies were updated only using individuals marked POPFLAG = 1 at the optimum genetic cluster number of K:6. Cluster membership proportion plots were constructed with CLUMPAK v.1.1 [32]. Multi-dimensional scaling (MDS) analysis and construction of neighbour-joining trees was implemented using R software v.3.5.0 [33] over an allele-distance matrix computed with the *pegas* R package [34].

The reliable identification of co-ancestry in DNA donors with admixed backgrounds can be considered important information that can be reported to investigators. Although there is likely to be some imprecision in the estimation of co-ancestry ratios when using relatively small-scale AIMs panels like BT, if the markers have been carefully balanced, they are more likely to be free of bias towards one particular co-ancestral population group and therefore match more closely the actual co-ancestry proportions in such individuals. To measure the reliability of co-ancestry estimation from identifying genetic clusters using the BT AIMs, we ran all 504 admixed 1000 Genomes samples described above (including all 85 PEL), together with the unadmixed populations from AFR, EUR, AMR and EAS, to keep the identified genetic clusters simple (K:4). The ACB and ASW samples represent typical African Caribbean and African American co-ancestry patterns of majority African co-ancestry and 0–30% European co-ancestry. The MXL, CLB, PUR and PEL samples represent more complex three-way co-ancestry patterns of major European co-ancestry, with Native American and African co-ancestries at varied ratios, with a few PEL individuals showing detectable East Asian co-ancestry [15]. We compared the BT data to the co-ancestry ratio estimates from the detailed genetic cluster analysis of the same 1000 Genomes-CEPH populations using 572,743 Affymetrix Human Origins SNPs (see Section 2.2. Although the parallel analyses with the Human Origins SNPs used the ADMIXTURE algorithm [35] to identify clusters, because data input for this algorithm uses only binary variant data, we applied STRUCTURE to ensure the tri-allelic SNP genotypes were assessed. Co-ancestry ratios were grouped into 10-percentiles (i.e., bins of one tenth of the samples from any one population) and the mean ratios of each of these 10-percentile groups in both analyses were assessed for goodness-of-fit using linear regression. Finally, we included a comparison with the genetic distance algorithm (GDA) co-ancestry estimator available in *Snipper*, developed from the work of Cheung et al. 2017 [36].

2.5. Evaluation of Ancestry and Co-Ancestry Inference Efficiency of the BT AIMs

The current gnomAD version 3.1 genome database compiles variation in almost 100,000 individuals from ten populations, so it provides a very efficient system for the detection of rare variation which could be potentially population informative. We screened the gnomAD 3.1 database to make a genomic audit of rare variations associated with the selected BT ancestry SNPs, comprising two types: i. rare, but potentially informative 'flanking' SNPs present on the same amplified fragment as the target SNP; and ii. additional polymorphic alleles in the binary ancestry SNPs, in the form of a third nucleotide substitution—creating a tri-allelic SNP where the allele-3 is either very rare or linked to a specific population group and hitherto undetected. Cataloguing rare third nucleotide substitutions is an important MPS quality control step, as it forewarns the user that the detected nucleotide at the target site is not a spurious sequencing result, but has been detected as a low frequency allele. We confined out searches for flanking SNPs within an arbitrary +/− 25 nucleotides of the target SNP position.

3. Results and Discussion

3.1. Ancestry Informative SNPs in BT

One hundred binary SNPs were compiled into the final BT ancestry panel, comprising 7 SNPs informative for sub-Saharan African populations, 15 European, 16 East Asian, 20 South Asian, 13 Oceanian and 17 American populations. The extra 12 ancestry SNPs of the total 100 loci were selected as they showed a high level of differentiation between European and other Eurasian population groups, namely East and South Asian and Middle Eastern populations. Table 1 outlines the source of each of these binary SNPs from the previous forensic AIMs panel studies described in Section 2.1 [8,9,21–24], with just one

OCE-informative SNP added from a separate study that developed the *Pacifiplex* panel [11]. Over a quarter of SNPs (28 of 100) have been selected as forensic AIMs in multiple panels.

Balancing population specific divergence (PSD) values (excluding the 12 Eurasian divergent SNPs) was successful to a large extent and the cumulative PSD values for each of the six population groups are shown in Figure 1 (individual values per SNP in Table S1). AFR, EUR, OCE and AMR were well balanced with cumulative PSD values of 13.54, 13.30, 11.99 and 11.8, respectively. EAS with a cumulative value of 9.43 did not have enough informative SNPs to reach these levels of divergence, while SAS, with much less differentiation from EUR and EAS, only reached a cumulative value of 2.7. It is noteworthy that two BT appearance SNPs, rs6437783 (in *MYH15* gene) and rs1800414 (*OCA2*), shown in Table 1, had been selected for previous forensic ancestry panels as an EAS-informative SNP in gAIMs and Kiddlab AIM sets, respectively. Given the lower cumulative PSD value for EAS compared to other population groups, these two markers would be worth considering as joint ancestry-appearance SNPs along with the three already used in this way.

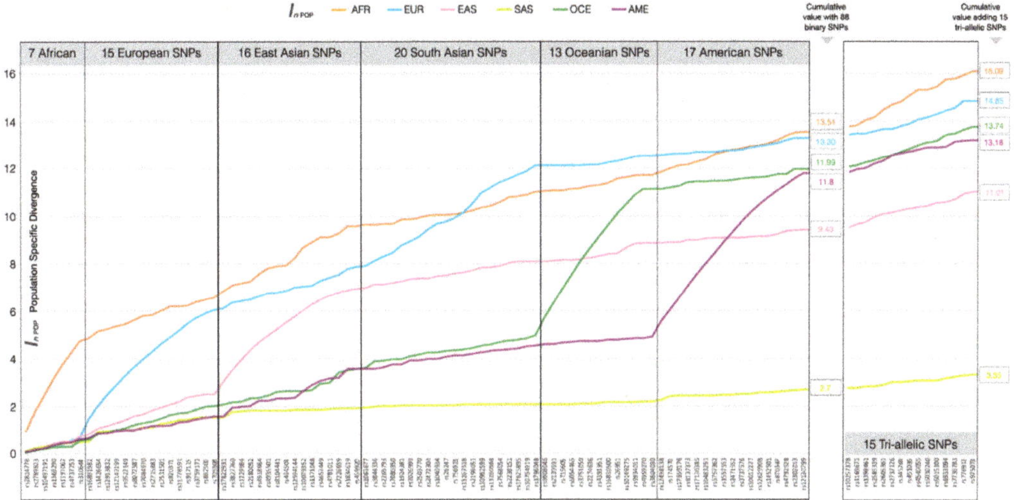

Figure 1. Accumulating population specific divergence values for each of the main population groups and the six sets of SNPs informative for their differentiation. The cumulative values are shown obtained from 88 binary SNPs (i.e., excluding 12 Eurasian-informative SNPs) and from the addition of the 15 tri-allelic SNPs in BT (VISAGE Basic Tool).

From a candidate list of 20 tri-allelic SNPs, rs11238577, rs11990024, rs9845503, rs7853487 and rs809540 were rejected from the assay design, bringing the total number of AIMs in BT to 115, including the three shared appearance SNPs. When the 15 tri-allelic SNPs were added to the cumulative PSD plot of Figure 1 the balance was marginally improved for EAS with a cumulative PSD value of 11.01 closer to the average value for the other population groups.

Table 1. Commonality between SNPs selected for the BT ancestry panel and established forensic ancestry panels: Kiddlab 56; Thermo Fisher Precision ID Ancestry Panel (PIAP); Euroforgen Global AIMs (gAIMs); the LACE panel; the NAME panel; Eurasiaplex; and Shriver et al. US admixture mapping panel [24]. The two markers lower right are BT appearance SNPs previously selected as AIMs.

No.	Pop.	SNP	KK/PIAP	gAIMs	LACE	Other
1	AFR	rs10497191	Kiddlab	-	LACE	
2	AFR	rs1197062	-	gAIMs	LACE	
3	AFR	rs1369290	-	gAIMs	-	
4	AFR	rs2789823	-	gAIMs	-	
5	AFR	rs2814778	Kiddlab	gAIMs	-	
6	AFR	rs310644	Kiddlab	gAIMs	-	
7	AFR	rs4737753	-	-	-	NAME
1	EUR	rs11778591	-	gAIMs	LACE	
2	EUR	rs12142199	-	gAIMs	-	
3	EUR	rs12913832	Kiddlab	gAIMs	-	
4	EUR	rs1426654	Kiddlab	gAIMs	-	
5	EUR	rs16891982	Kiddlab	gAIMs	-	
6	EUR	rs2715883	-	gAIMs	-	
7	EUR	rs3759171	-	gAIMs	LACE	
8	EUR	rs705308	PIAP	-	-	
9	EUR	rs7084970	-	gAIMs	-	
10	EUR	rs7531501	-	gAIMs	-	
11	EUR	rs8072587	-	gAIMs	-	
12	EUR	rs820371	-	gAIMs	LACE	
13	EUR	rs862500	-	gAIMs	LACE	
14	EUR	rs917115	Kiddlab	gAIMs	-	
15	EUR	rs9522149	Kiddlab	gAIMs	-	
1	OCE	rs10149275	-	gAIMs	-	
2	OCE	rs16830500	-	gAIMs	-	
3	OCE	rs2139931	-	gAIMs	-	
4	OCE	rs2274636	-	gAIMs	-	
5	OCE	rs26951	-	gAIMs	-	
6	OCE	rs3751050	-	gAIMs	-	
7	OCE	rs3804030	-	gAIMs	-	
8	OCE	rs4391951	-	gAIMs	-	
9	OCE	rs4959270	-	x	-	Pacifiplex *
10	OCE	rs6054465	-	gAIMs	-	
11	OCE	rs715605	-	gAIMs	-	
12	OCE	rs9908046	-	gAIMs	-	
13	OCE	rs9934011	-	gAIMs	-	

No.	Pop.	SNP	KK/PIAP	gAIMs	LACE	Other
1	AME	rs10012227	-	gAIMs	-	
2	AME	rs10483251	-	gAIMs	LACE	
3	AME	rs12130799	PIAP	-	-	
4	AME	rs12498138	Kiddlab	gAIMs	-	
5	AME	rs12629908	PIAP	-	-	
6	AME	rs1452501	-	gAIMs	LACE	
7	AME	rs1557553	-	gAIMs	LACE	
8	AME	rs17130385	-	gAIMs	LACE	
9	AME	rs17359176	-	gAIMs	LACE	
10	AME	rs174570	Kiddlab	gAIMs	LACE	
11	AME	rs2302013	-	gAIMs	-	
12	AME	rs2471552	-	gAIMs	-	
13	AME	rs3737576	Kiddlab	-	-	
14	AME	rs4792928	-	gAIMs	-	
15	AME	rs5757362	-	-	LACE	
16	AME	rs8137373	-	gAIMs	-	
17	AME	rs870347	Kiddlab	-	-	
1	EAS	rs10079352	-	gAIMs	LACE	
2	EAS	rs1229984	Kiddlab	gAIMs	-	
3	EAS	rs12594144	-	gAIMs	-	
4	EAS	rs1371048	-	gAIMs	-	
5	EAS	rs17822931	-	gAIMs	-	
6	EAS	rs1834619	Kiddlab	gAIMs	-	
7	EAS	rs2180052	-	gAIMs	-	
8	EAS	rs3827760	Kiddlab	gAIMs	-	
9	EAS	rs434504	-	gAIMs	-	
10	EAS	rs459920	Kiddlab	-	-	
11	EAS	rs4657449	-	gAIMs	-	
12	EAS	rs4781011	PIAP	-	-	
13	EAS	rs4918664	Kiddlab	gAIMs	-	
14	EAS	rs4935501	-	gAIMs	-	
15	EAS	rs7226659	Kiddlab	-	-	
16	EAS	rs8104441	-	gAIMs	-	

Other No.	Pop.	SNP	KK/PIAP	gAIMs	LACE	Other
1	Eurasia	rs1495085	-	-	-	NAME
2	Eurasia	rs1757928	-	-	-	NAME
3	Eurasia	rs2337024	-	-	-	NAME
4	Eurasia	rs6989963	-	-	-	NAME
5	Eurasia	rs6990312	Kiddlab	-	-	
6	Eurasia	rs7148809	-	-	-	NAME
7	Eurasia	rs12203115	-	-	-	NAME
8	Eurasia	rs2227203	-	-	-	NAME
9	Eurasia	rs39897	-	-	-	Eurasiaplex
10	Eurasia	rs4308478	-	-	-	NAME
11	Eurasia	rs7570971	-	-	-	NAME
12	Eurasia	rs984038	-	-	-	NAME
1	SAS	rs1040934	-	-	-	Shriver
2	SAS	rs1063677	-	-	-	Shriver
3	SAS	rs10764919	-	-	LACE	
4	SAS	rs10962599	-	-	-	Eurasiaplex
5	SAS	rs13267318	-	-	-	Shriver
6	SAS	rs13280988	-	-	LACE	
7	SAS	rs17625895	-	-	-	Eurasiaplex
8	SAS	rs1796048	-	-	-	Shriver
9	SAS	rs1924381	-	gAIMs	LACE	
10	SAS	rs2026999	-	-	-	Shriver
11	SAS	rs2196051	Kiddlab	-	-	
12	SAS	rs2238151	Kiddlab	-	-	
13	SAS	rs2269793	PIAP	-	-	
14	SAS	rs2472304	-	-	-	Eurasiaplex
15	SAS	rs2503770	-	gAIMs	LACE	
16	SAS	rs26247	-	-	-	Shriver
17	SAS	rs3844336	-	-	-	Shriver
18	SAS	rs7080350	-	-	LACE	
19	SAS	rs7568054	-	-	LACE	
20	SAS	rs756913	-	-	-	Eurasiaplex
MYH15°	EAS	rs6437783	-	gAIMs	-	-
OCA2°	EAS	rs1800414	Kiddlab	-	-	-

* A single SNP developed for the Pacifiplex panel was not incorporated into gAIMs. ° Gene locations of the two BT appearance SNPs previously selected for other ancestry panels.

Allele frequency estimates of the 115 BT AIMs based on the standardised reference grid outlined in Section 2.2 (YRI, CEU, CHB, GIH, plus HGDP-CEPH Americans and Oceanians) are given in File S1. Middle East allele frequency estimates are included based on 134 HGDP-CEPH samples from the Israeli Bedouin, Druze and Palestinian populations. Figure S1A–G summarise in simple bar charts the allelic variation in each binary AIM, arranged in sets of the AIMs informative for each population group and ranked by a simple delta allele frequency differential calculation comparing the informative-allele frequency in each target population against the average frequency in the other populations (except SAS-informative SNPs, ranked by SAS-EUR delta values). Figure S1G shows the allele frequencies of 12 Eurasian-informative SNPs in the relevant population groups. For comparison purposes we included North African (NAF) allele frequency estimates based on HGDP-CEPH Mozabite from Algeria, and delta values were estimated for EUR compared to a NAF-ME-SAS average).

3.2. Compilation of Reference and Test Population Datasets

File S2 contains all the Excel worksheets necessary for generating Bayes likelihood calculations and linked PCA analyses by uploading the BT ancestry SNP genotype data to *Snipper*. The active worksheet of reference and query SNP profiles uploaded to *Snipper* is in position 1 in Excel and has the label '1' applied to all reference population profiles in the rightmost column, and '0' to unknown profiles such as those compiled from a forensic sample. The values in cells A1, B1, C1 provide numbers of reference/query profiles, markers, and populations in the worksheet, respectively. All other SNP profiles compiled in the six supporting worksheets can be treated as test samples (i.e., marked with a '0'), or used as alternative or additional reference population datasets (e.g., the HGDP-CEPH or VISAGE in-house ME population genotypes can be added to the reference profiles as a seventh population group).

3.3. Genotyping Concordance

3.3.1. HGDP-CEPH in-House BT Genotypes vs. 1000 Genomes Whole-Genome-Sequence Data

File S3A lists all the pairwise genotype comparisons between in-house data for HGDP-CEPH samples and the data from 1000 Genomes published in 2020 [16]. This file examines all SNPs in BT except for one appearance marker, rs796296176, which did not have genotype data from the in-house analyses of HGDP-CEPH samples. Five HGDP-CEPH Middle East samples had excessive numbers of data gaps from in-house sequencing and were not included in genotype comparisons. Of the 153 total markers in BT, two ancestry SNPs had higher than average discordancy rates, indicating a problem with genotyping either from 1000 Genomes sequence analysis, or the BT MPS assay. First, tri-allelic SNP rs2737126 had 15/277 (5.4%) genotype discordancy, seemingly arising from failure to detect a G allele, when present as a GT or CG heterozygote, but not for all such genotypes. This phenomenon was not explained by detailed scrutiny of sequence data at this variant site. Second, the binary SNP rs3804030 had a disproportionately high genotype discordancy rate of 29/277 (10.47%), which appeared to be due to a failure to detect the rare, OCE-indicative C allele outside of Oceanian populations examined by 1000 Genomes. Interestingly, no discordances were seen for this SNP amongst pairwise comparisons of 27 HGDP-CEPH Oceanians.

File S3A shows that for the 151 SNPs of BT without apparent problems, the genotyping concordance was very high, reaching 99.96% concordance with 17 discordances largely appearing at random across the data grid, rather than systematically as detected in the above two SNPs. This high level of genotype concordance between the BT assay developed vs. 1000 Genomes whole genome sequence-based variant detection indicates the robustness of the MPS method and the BT multiplex developed by VISAGE. The no-call rate (unreported genotypes) was also low at 0.2% for 1000 Genomes, and 0.6% for our MPS genotyping.

3.3.2. 1000 Genomes Phase 3 Genotypes vs. 1000 Genomes High Sequence Coverage Genotypes

File S3B gives the pairwise comparisons for all BT SNPs between the current 1000 Genomes Phase 3 genotypes listed online by Ensembl, and the genotypes published following high coverage sequence analysis of the same samples by the New York Genome Centre [17]. As we have relied extensively on the online genotype data produced by 1000 Genomes Phase 3 for several years, the cross-checks of genotype calls comparing 30X and 2-3X sequence coverage that this concordance analysis provides are important. Amongst all 153 BT SNPs, 73 had zero genotype discordances and 66 showed largely inconsequential discordances numbering 1–5 genotype differences between each sequencing dataset (a locus-specific concordance of 99.96–99.8%). However, 14 SNPs had higher levels of six or more discordances, comprising 11 ancestry SNPs. Three ancestry SNPs: rs2789823, rs9522149 and rs2196051 had concordance rates $\leq$ 98.2% due to 25, 27 and 46 discordances, respectively. The BT ancestry SNPs genotype discordances of two or more in number are summarised in Figure 2. It can be assumed that higher sequence coverage provides more secure genotyping for a small, but significant proportion of SNPs in the 1000 Genomes variant database, of which 14 with higher-than-average levels of discordancy are part of BT. For this reason, all reference population data compiled from 1000 Genomes for VISAGE ancestry analyses with BT are based on the high coverage (30X) genotype datasets, which have yet to be made available in the Ensemble variant browser for 1000 Genomes.

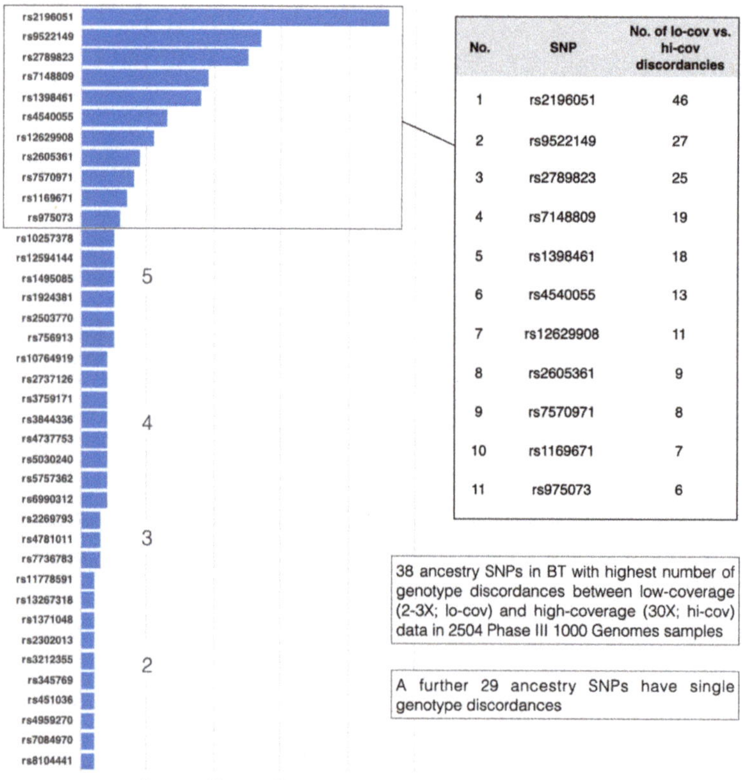

No.	SNP	No. of lo-cov vs. hi-cov discordancies
1	rs2196051	46
2	rs9522149	27
3	rs2789823	25
4	rs7148809	19
5	rs1398461	18
6	rs4540055	13
7	rs12629908	11
8	rs2605361	9
9	rs7570971	8
10	rs1169671	7
11	rs975073	6

38 ancestry SNPs in BT with highest number of genotype discordances between low-coverage (2-3X; lo-cov) and high-coverage (30X; hi-cov) data in 2504 Phase III 1000 Genomes samples

A further 29 ancestry SNPs have single genotype discordances

Figure 2. The 38 BT ancestry SNPs with the highest numbers of discordant genotypes between 1000 Genomes low coverage vs. high coverage sequence data. An additional 29 had only one discordant genotype. The full set of genotype comparisons for all BT SNPs and all 1000 Genomes samples are given in File S3B.

3.4. Ancestry Inference Efficiency of the BT Ancestry SNPs

One-out cross validation of the reference dataset gave 100% correct classification in all cases, i.e., all 520 reference profiles were successfully assigned to their true population of origin. The likelihood ratio values produced by cross validation were consistently high and most samples gave likelihoods greater than 'The profile is more than 1 billion times more likely to be from the true population of origin than another population' (data not shown).

Figure 3A shows the STRUCTURE analysis K:6 cluster plots for the reference populations (1–6) in worksheet 1 of File S1. Figure 3B shows the accompanying probability of data and Delta K statistical analyses indicating an optimum cluster number of 6 for these analyses. Figure 3C shows colour-matched MDS plots for the same samples for coordinate 1 vs. 2 (left plot), 1 vs. 3 (mid) and 2 vs. 3. Only a small degree of overlap between the OCE and EAS MDS clusters-of-points remains when comparing all three coordinate plots. Figure 3D shows the Neighbour Joining Tree (NJT) distance matrix results, which indicate a clear arrangement of branch lengths and spatial separation, apart from two SAS outliers close to the OCE set. The summary of cross-validation classification results in Figure 3E completes the ancestry analysis of these sample sets.

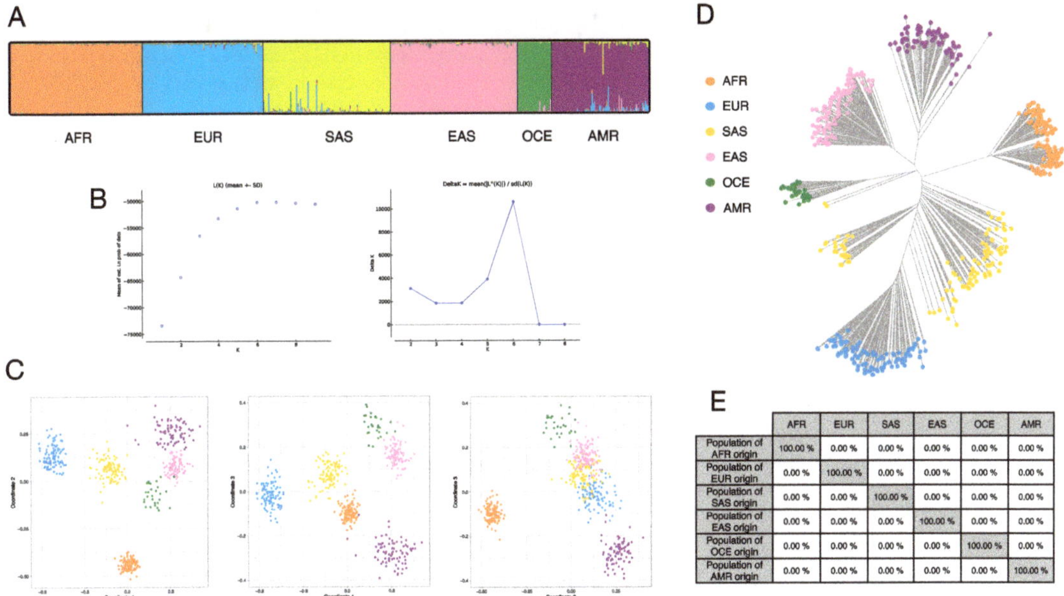

Figure 3. Ancestry analysis with 115 BT ancestry SNPs of the six populations of the standardised reference dataset (AFR: brown; EUR: blue; SAS: yellow; EAS: pink; OCE: green; AMR: purple), with consistent colours across three statistical analyses of A, C and D. (**A**) STRUCTURE cluster membership proportions at K = 6, indicated to be the optimum K number of genetic clusters by: (**B**) the mean L(K) (log probability of data) and ΔK plots from STRUCTURE runs, following the analyses of Evanno et al. [31]. (**C**) Multi-dimensional scaling (MDS) analysis showing principal component (PC) 1 vs. PC2 coordinates, PC1 vs. PC3 and PC2 vs. PC3 two-dimensional plots. (**D**) Neighbour joining tree (NJT) analysis. (**E**) Summary classification success table of cross validation of the standardised reference set.

Figure S2.1 summarises the same type of population analyses as Figure 3 applied to unadmixed (8–11, 14–25) and admixed (12–13, 26–29) 1000 Genomes samples (30X coverage genotypes) analysed against the reference population set. In nearly all cases, unadmixed samples show low levels of joint cluster membership. The admixed African populations give similar patterns to those found in other studies (but see Section 3.5) with European co-ancestry ranging from 5–30% K2 cluster membership. The admixed

American samples from 1000 Genomes also show the expected proportions from K:2 and K:6 in the STRUCTURE analysis, with K:1 cluster membership forming the third African co-ancestry component, most evident in Puerto Ricans. The carefully curated Peruvian reference Native American samples are clearly discernible on the left of the columns of the K6 cluster. Equally consistently, admixed samples occupy the middle ground between the MDS clusters-of-points formed by the unadmixed samples, depending on the degree of their separation in coordinates 1 vs. 3 or 1 vs. 2 MDS plots, particularly the admixed Africans in 1 vs. 2.

Figure S2.2–S2.4 show identical analysis output and using the same reference populations for HGDP-CEPH samples, SGDP-VISAGE in-house samples and EGDP samples, respectively. The HGDP-CEPH samples show a degree of joint cluster membership proportions in regions whose populations occupy continental margins, e.g., Mozabite show African-European co-ancestry patterns (joint membership proportions) and Pakistani populations show some European co-ancestry. The SGDP and EGDP sample analyses are the most varied, reflecting the more widespread sampling locations and emphasis on continental margin regions such as Central South Asia. The SGDP-EGDP Oceanian and American samples give clear, unequivocal cluster memberships, underlining the careful choice of informative SNPs for these population groups. However, it should be noted that BT and all other equivalent MPS ancestry panels show Oceanian ancestry to be only a small proportion of the STRUCTURE cluster patterns in the single SGDP Maori and Hawaiian samples, indicating that AIMs selected from analysis of Melanesians (i.e., HGDP-CEPH Papuans) are not sufficiently informative to infer Polynesian ancestry.

3.5. Co-Ancestry Analysis of Known Admixed Individuals in 1000 Genomes with BT Ancestry SNPs
3.5.1. Comparison of Co-Ancestry Patterns Obtained with the Human Origins Panel and BT

Figure 4 shows a direct pairwise comparison of the co-ancestry patterns (cluster membership proportions) of 504 admixed samples from 1000 Genomes (see File S1C), analysed in combination with the standardised reference set with the >572,000 Human Origins array SNPs (using ADMIXTURE due to SNP data density) and the 115 ancestry SNPs of BT (using STRUCTURE). File S4 gives the genetic cluster proportions from both analyses on which the Figure 4 cluster plots are based. These plots show a very good match of co-ancestry patterns in the two African admixed ACB and ASW populations. The correlation analysis and r^2 values aligned below the cluster plots in Figure 4 indicate high levels of correlation between Origins and BT co-ancestry proportion estimates for ACB and ASW, notably for the AFR proportions (although they are combined with AMR co-ancestry in these assessments). The EUR co-ancestry proportions tend to be slightly underestimated by BT SNPs or go undetected when very small. The four admixed populations with AMR co-ancestry are arranged in descending overall proportions of this co-ancestry and all show the same tendency for BT SNPs to underestimate the EUR proportions, but the PEL, MXL and CLM patterns still show a good match and relatively high r^2 values for both main EUR and AMR co-ancestries. When three co-ancestries are detected, the BT SNPs have less precision to detect AMR and AFR co-ancestry at levels below 25%, particularly evident in the PUR non-EUR co-ancestry proportion estimates. Overall, the patterns match very well for simple two-way co-ancestry across most ratios, with BT only failing to detect very minor co-ancestry when it falls below 5%. The match of patterns only tends to reduce when 3-way co-ancestry is more prevalent, notably when the two minor co-ancestries are both below 10%. BT SNPs can detect two-way co-ancestry using STRUCTURE with sufficient accuracy for proportions to be reliably reported down to about 10% minor co-ancestry, although when three-way co-ancestry is detected, more caution would be required in reporting minor ratios below this 10% threshold and the lack of accuracy in such cases should be highlighted in the report.

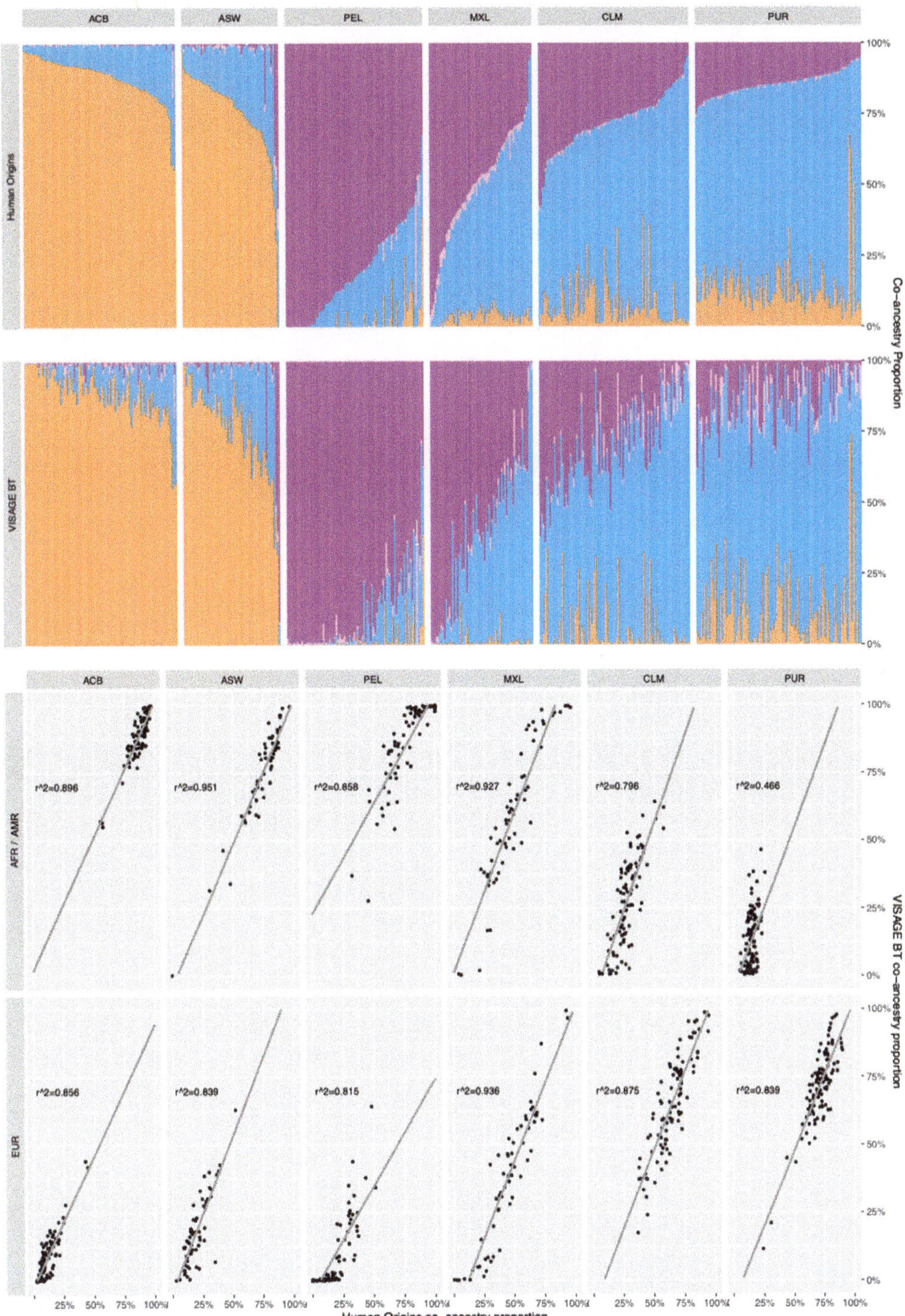

Figure 4. Pairwise comparison of individual co-ancestry proportions (cluster membership proportions) in 504 admixed samples from 1000 Genomes, analysed using the standardised reference set with Human Origins array, comprising

>572,000 SNPs (using ADMIXTURE) and 115 VISAGE BT ancestry SNPs (using STRUCTURE). Co-ancestry proportions in four genetic clusters representing, African, European, Native American and East Asian, ancestries are given in File S4. The r^2 correlation analysis plots of each admixed population group are shown below the corresponding cluster patterns.

3.5.2. Using GDA as a Simple Snipper-Based Evaluation of Admixture

From the STRUCTURE analysis of the BT SNPs, co-ancestry proportion estimates were compared to equivalent proportions provided by GDA in *Snipper*. This intended to test the efficiency of GDA to detect admixture and alert the user to the need to perform STRUCTURE analysis, if this initial analysis of the sample data does not suggest straight-forward unadmixed ancestry. Figure S3A shows cluster plots for the STRUCTURE run and for the co-ancestry proportions based on GDA values, with r^2 plots below arranged as in Figure 4. The r^2 values indicate a good match between each approach, but GDA underestimates the EUR co-ancestry to a significant degree in ACB and ASW, to the point where GDA did not detect this co-ancestry in a large proportion of individuals, and it was underestimated by more than 50% of the true value (from Human Origins SNP array data) in most of the others. The trend of GDA underestimating European co-ancestry continues across all the PEL, MXL, CLM and PUR samples, where additionally, AFR co-ancestry is consistently overestimated in each population. The EUR underestimation is partly explained by detection of significant proportions of EAS co-ancestry by GDA, likely to be falsely created by a close relationship between AMR and EAS population groups, which STRUCTURE differentiates more efficiently as distinct genetic clusters compared to GDA's measure of distance between EUR and both AMR and EAS.

3.5.3. Comparisons of 10-Percentile Co-Ancestry Ratio Patterns

A final visual comparison of co-ancestry patterns was made by plotting the mean co-ancestry ratios per 10-percentile group of individuals to smooth the data and allow easier assessment of trends in both the use of the small-scale BT ancestry panel to detect co-ancestry and GDA as an initial measure of the presence of admixture. Mean STRUCTURE co-ancestry proportions obtained with Origins SNPs and BT SNPs, plus GDA proportions, are plotted in Figure S3B. When admixture patterns are summarised into percentile groups, it is much easier to see the very close match in estimated co-ancestry ratios between Origins and BT SNP-based STRUCTURE runs. This is particularly evident in the 10th ASW percentile with a three-way co-ancestry pattern, and the 10th PEL percentile with a fourth EAS co-ancestry. However, co-ancestry proportions below 10% regularly fail to be detected by BT (1st ACB percentile, 3rd–5th PEL, 1st–2nd MXL, 9th–10th CLM percentiles). Therefore, it remains prudent to recognise that BT will not consistently detect co-ancestry ratios $\leq 10\%$. The presence of EAS co-ancestry at very small proportions in many of the MXL-CLM-PUR BT percentile groups indicates this component should be ignored when it is less than 10% and AMR co-ancestry is present above this ratio at the same time. The percentile group patterns in GDA emphasise that it is not an efficient technique for detecting admixture accurately when co-ancestral ratios are below 20%, so it does not provide an accurate measure of individuals with these proportions and STRUCTURE would be required in all cases, particularly as the bulk of the PEL-MXL-CLM percentile groups show spurious EAS co-ancestry ratios above this threshold value).

3.6. Audit of Additional Variation in BT SNPs from the GnomAD 3.1 Database

File S5 lists the co-amplified flanking SNPs and extra third-substitution alleles amongst both ancestry and appearance binary BT SNPs detected in the gnomAD 3.1 database. Twelve ancestry SNPs and three appearance SNPs had a third substitution allele, which reached the highest allele frequency of only 0.0002 in rs2302013 and rs917115 (both in East Asians). Ancestry SNP rs1063677 and appearance SNP rs12821256 showed all four substitution alleles, with the highest frequency for allele T of 0.0005 in Europeans in the GC SNP rs1063677.

The power of gnomAD to detect low frequency variants across the genome enabled sequence screens that indicated a large number of flanking SNPs within 25 nucleotides of the target site of many BT SNPs. Amongst the 115 ancestry SNPs, 49 had flanking SNPs, while in the 41 appearance (EVC) SNPs, there were 23, notably markers targeted in the SNP-rich MC1R gene. Four ancestry SNPs showed informative combinations of alleles in close proximity which show unlinked allele frequencies between the two loci—in other words, forming population-informative 2-SNP microhaplotypes (i.e., diplotypes). These four are detailed in Figure S4. The Chr-3 pair rs1169671-rs76444263 (target SNP in bold), Chr-8 pair rs75064826-rs13280988 and Chr-19 pair rs2337025-rs2337024 all show SAS-informative diplotypes, while the Chr-20 pair rs4809578-rs310644 has a range of diplotypes, which are most differentiating for AFR and EAS population groups. Microhaplotype rs1169671-rs76444263 combines a tri-allelic and binary SNP, but the latter has low levels of polymorphism so is less informative than the other binary SNP pairs. Diplotype SNP allele combinations can be analysed in *Snipper* by assigning A, C, G, T allele nomenclature to the alphabetic arrangement of diplotypes, which, for the above binary SNP pairs, would be A=AA, C=AG, G=CA, T=CG combinations; A=AA, C=AG, G=GA, T=GG combinations; and A=AC, C=AT, G=TC, T=TT combinations, respectively. While the phase of each SNP pair's alleles needs to be detected from the sequence data to do this, it indicates the potential extra variant information, which is accessible from MPS analysis of forensic SNPs.

4. Concluding Remarks

The primary aim of the VISAGE Consortium of creating an all-in-one forensic intelligence tool based on MPS technology requires the development of a full analytical pipeline. This should include population reference data and predictive algorithms for the inference of age, ancestry and appearance characteristics associated with the genotyped SNPs, plus an optimum sequencing protocol which is applicable to the two main forensic MPS platforms in current use. The strategy of starting with a prototype tool of simple age predictors in one multiplex, and established pigmentation phenotype and continental ancestry predictors in the second, allowed us to build a strong foundation on which to develop the more ambitious VISAGE Enhanced Tool (ET). ET represents substantial expansion of all three 'AAA' predictive systems in the same parallel MPS multiplex setup as BT (i.e., separate DNA workflows dedicated to methylation analysis and SNP genotyping). The ancestry panel of BT therefore took the best ancestry informative SNPs from several well-established forensic ancestry panels, with particular regard to known MPS sequence reliability as well as optimum ancestry informativeness. For this reason, BT has provided very good sequencing performance with forensic DNA [29,37], and enables ancestry inferences to be made for populations of continental and South Asian origin with the highest levels of statistical likelihood.

Although we dedicated considerable resources to genotyping BT SNPs in populations addressing several geographic gaps in coverage left by large-scale genomic sequencing projects, many global regions remain to be characterised with new studies. The dynamic system in *Snipper*, i.e., compiling the largest possible array of population data and allowing the end-user to select which samples extend or modify the standardised reference set, provides flexibility for statistical analyses of BT SNP data. It also allows new population data to be uploaded to the webpages holding reference sets (http://mathgene.usc.es/snipper/forensic_mps_aims.html, accessed on 20 August 2021) and the additional populations shown in File S1. Although genetic cluster analyses using STRUCTURE can be challenging for forensic practitioners analysing population data for the first time, in our view, it is the best way to detect and analyse individual co-ancestry in persons with admixed backgrounds. The comparisons of GDA and STRUCTURE made in this study indicate that GDA is not accurate enough to evaluate low level co-ancestry when admixture patterns are complex and an individual has more than two co-ancestries. However, when the BT ancestry SNPs are compared to the much larger panel of Human Origins SNPs, the level of detail obtained using STRUCTURE is well matched and indicates

BT SNPs are informative enough to accurately detect co-ancestral components present above 10% proportions.

Lastly, the care taken in selecting the BT ancestry SNPs based on their recorded reliability and sensitivity in previous MPS-based forensic ancestry panels [8,12,18,20,23] has helped to ensure predictable performance going forward with evaluation of both forensic MPS platforms. This extends to the sequencing chemistry, library preparation and sequence read balance (between strands, between alleles, within loci, between loci) observed so far in the forensic validations the VISAGE Consortium has made following SWGDAM guidelines for newly developed forensic DNA techniques (AmpliSeq chemistry [29], PowerSeq chemistry [37], and ForenSeq chemistry with a manuscript in submission). These same principals have been applied to the development of the ET ancestry panel, providing the means to increase the overall multiplex size of the tool and extending the range of populations among which ET ancestry SNPs can differentiate.

Supplementary Materials: The following are available online at https://www.mdpi.com/article/10.3390/genes12081284/s1, Files S1: Allele frequency estimates in seven population groups for the 115 ancestry SNPs of BT; S2A: Snipper Reference Grid; S2B: 1KG Unadmixed Populations; S2C: 1KG Admixed Populations; S2D: HGDP-CEPH Populations; S2E: VISAGE In-house Populations; S2F: SGDP Test Samples; S2G: EGDP Test Samples, S3A: Genotype comparisons of 1000 Genomes HGDP-CEPH data (red) vs VISAGE in-house HGDP-CEPH data (black); S3B: Genotype comparisons of 1000 Genomes Phase III low-coverage data based on 2-3X sequence coverage (black) vs. 1000 Genomes high coverage data based on New York Genome Centre's 30X resequencing of the same samples (blue); S4: Genetic cluster membership proportions from the four major contributing populations to American admixture with 572K SNPs of Human Origins array analyses using ADMIXTURE vs 115 BT SNPs using STRUCTURE, for 1511 unadmixed and 504 admixed 1000 Genomes samples; S5: Screen of all 153 BT SNPs of gnomAD genome database information for current GRCh37-38 positions, gene identifiers, third alleles and high frequency flanking SNPs (present on the same sequence strand as the target site within +/− 25 nucleotides). Figures S1A: 7 African-informative SNPs; S1B: 15 European-informative SNPs; S1C: 16 East Asian-informative SNPs; S1D: 20 South Asian-informative SNPs; S1E: 13 Oceanian-informative SNPs; S1F: 17 American-informative SNPs; S1G: 12 Eurasian divergent SNPs, S2.1: Bio-geographical ancestry analysis based on the six reference populations (1–6, summarised in Figure 1) plus unadmixed (8–11, 14–25) and admixed (12–13, 26–29) populations available from 1000 Genomes 30X high coverage data (1KG-30); S2.2: Bio-geographical ancestry analysis based on the six reference populations presented in Figure 1, plus populations available from HGDP-CEPH Whole Genome Sequencing Data; S2.3: Bio-geographical ancestry analysis based on the six reference populations presented in Figure 1, plus populations available from in-house genotyping with the VISAGE BT tool and SGDP data; S2.4: Bio-geographical ancestry analysis based on the six reference populations presented in Figure 1, plus populations available from EGDP data, with ~85% (95/115 SNPs) profile completeness. S3.1: (A) Co-ancestry proportions sample-by-sample in 504 1000 Genomes admixed individuals based on STRUCTURE and GDA analyses. (B) Correlation analyses and r2 values comparing the combined African-American and European co-ancestry proportion estimates with both techniques. S3.2: Mean co-ancestry proportions summarised as 10-percentile columns (10 bins of 10% of each set of individuals), of varyingnumbers per bin: ACB: 10, ACB: 10, ASW: 6, PEL: 8, ACB: 10, MXL: 6, CLM: 9, PUR: 10. S4: Four BT ancestry SNP target sites and population informative flanking SNPs within 25 nucleotides (nt) on the 5' or 3' side. Table S1: Individual and cumulative population specific Divergence (PSD) values for the 115 ancestry SNPs arranged in descending order of PSD value per population.

Author Contributions: Conceptualization, C.P., M.d.l.P., M.K., M.N., W.B., W.P., P.M.S., M.V.L. and J.Á.-D.; Methodology, C.P., J.R-R., A.A.-C., M.d.l.P., J.P.-S., A.M.-M., A.F.-A., C.X., E.Y.Y.C. and T.E.G.; Data Curation, C.P., A.A.-C., J.R.-R., M.d.l.P., A.F.-A., J.Á.-D., J.P.-S., E.Y.Y.C., P.M.S., T.E.G. and A.M.-M.; Writing and Editing Manuscript; C.P., M.d.l.P., M.V.L. and Á.C. All authors have read and agreed to the published version of the manuscript.

Funding: The study was supported by the European Union's Horizon 2020 Research and Innovation Programme under grant agreement No. 740580 within the framework of the VISible Attributes through GEnomics (VISAGE) Project and Consortium. MdlP is supported by a post-doctorate grant funded by the Consellería de Cultura, Educación e Ordenación Universitaria e da Consellería de

Economía, Emprego e Industria from Xunta de Galicia, Spain (ED481D-2021-008). J.R. is supported by the "Programa de axudas á etapa predoutoral" funded by the Consellería de Cultura, Educación e Ordenación Universitaria e da Consellería de Economía, Emprego e Industria from Xunta de Galicia, Spain (ED481A-2020/039).

Institutional Review Board Statement: In-house population samples were previously obtained from: i. Moroccan volunteers resident in Madrid for analysis at the University of Santiago de Compostela, Spain in 2008, originally collected by the Comisaría General de Policía Científica, Madrid, with Institutional Review Board approval for their use in population studies from University of Santiago de Compostela, Spain, reference no. 08-00844 (dated 1.5.2008); ii. Eritrean, Somali, Central Iraqi, Kurdish Iraqi, and Turkish volunteers resident in Germany, according to the guidelines of the Declaration of Helsinki, and approved by the Institutional Review Board of the Faculty of Medicine, University of Cologne, Germany, reference no. 17-416 (dated 16 May 2018).

Informed Consent Statement: Informed consent was obtained from all subjects involved in the study.

Data Availability Statement: All data generated in these studies, except the cross-validation likelihoods, are included in the Files.

Acknowledgments: STRUCTURE and ADMIXTURE runs were performed by the FinisTerrae II supercomputer at the Centro de Supercomputación de Galicia, Santiago de Compostela (CESGA), Spain.

Conflicts of Interest: The authors declare no conflict of interest.

Appendix A

Centres and investigators of the VISible Attributes through GEnomics (VISAGE) Consortium, Website: http://www.visage-h2020.eu/ (accessed on 20 August 2021).

- Erasmus University Medical Center Rotterdam, Rotterdam, The Netherlands: Manfred Kayser, Vivian Kalamara, Arwin Ralf, Athina Vidaki
- Jagiellonian University, Krakow, Poland: Wojciech Branicki, Ewelina Pośpiech, Aleksandra Pisarek
- Universidade de Santiago de Compostela, Santiago de Compostela, Spain: Ángel Carracedo, Maria Victoria Lareu, Christopher Phillips, Ana Freire-Aradas, Ana Mosquera-Miguel, María de la Puente
- Medizinische Universität Innsbruck, Innsbruck, Austria: Walther Parson, Catarina Xavier, Antonia Heidegger, Harald Niederstätter
- Universität zu Köln, Cologne, Germany: Michael Nothnagel, Maria-Alexandra Katsara, Tarek Khellaf
- King's College London, London, UK: Barbara Prainsack, Gabrielle Samuel
- Klinikum der Universität zu Köln, Cologne, Germany: Peter M. Schneider, Theresa E. Gross, Jan Fleckhaus, Elaine Cheung.
- Bundeskriminalamt, Wiesbaden, Germany: Ingo Bastisch, Nathalie Schury, Jens Teodoridis, Martina Unterländer
- Institut National de Police Scientifique, Lyon, France: François-Xavier Laurent, Caroline Bouakaze, Yann Chantrel, Anna Delest, Clémence Hollard, Ayhan Ulus, Julien Vannier
- Netherlands Forensic Institute, The Hague, Netherlands: Titia Sijen, Kris van der Gaag, Marina Ventayol-Garcia
- National Forensic Centre, Swedish Police Authority, Linköping, Sweden: Johannes Hedman, Klara Junker, Maja Sidstedt
- Metropolitan Police Service, London, United Kingdom: Shazia Khan, Carole E. Ames, Andrew Revoir
- Centralne Laboratorium Kryminalistyczne Policji, Warsaw, Poland: Magdalena Spólnicka, Ewa Kartasinska, Anna Woźniak

References

1. Phillips, C. Forensic genetic analysis of bio-geographical ancestry. *Forensic Sci. Int. Genet.* **2015**, *18*, 49–65. [CrossRef]
2. Kayser, M. Forensic DNA Phenotyping: Predicting human appearance from crime scene material for investigative purposes. *Forensic Sci. Int. Genet.* **2015**, *18*, 33–48. [CrossRef] [PubMed]
3. Freire-Aradas, A.; Phillips, C.; Lareu, M.V. Forensic individual age estimation with DNA: From initial approaches to methylation tests. *Forensic Sci. Rev.* **2017**, *29*, 121–144. [PubMed]
4. King, T.E.; Fortes, G.G.; Balaresque, P.; Thomas, M.G.; Balding, D.; Delser, P.M.; Neumann, R.; Parson, W.; Knapp, M.; Walsh, S.; et al. Identification of the remains of King Richard III. *Nat. Commun.* **2014**, *5*, 5631. [CrossRef]
5. Walsh, S.; Liu, F.; Ballantyne, K.N.; van Oven, M.; Lao, O.; Kayser, M. IrisPlex: A sensitive DNA tool for accurate prediction of blue and brown eye colour in the absence of ancestry information. *Forensic Sci. Int. Genet.* **2011**, *5*, 170–180. [CrossRef]
6. Walsh, S.; Liu, F.; Wollstein, A.; Kovatsi, L.; Ralf, A.; Kosiniak-Kamysz, A.; Branicki, W.; Kayser, M. The HIrisPlex system for simultaneous prediction of hair and eye colour from DNA. *Forensic Sci. Int. Genet.* **2013**, *7*, 98–115. [CrossRef] [PubMed]
7. Walsh, S.; Chaitanya, L.; Breslin, K.; Muralidharan, C.; Bronikowska, A.; Pospiech, E.; Koller, J.; Kovatsi, L.; Wollstein, A.; Branicki, W.; et al. Global skin colour prediction from DNA. *Hum. Genet.* **2017**, *136*, 847–863. [CrossRef]
8. Phillips, C.; Parson, W.; Lundsberg, B.; Santos, C.; Freire-Aradas, A.; Torres, M.; Eduardoff, M.; Børsting, C.; Johansen, P.; Fondevila, M.; et al. Building a forensic ancestry panel from the ground up: The EUROFORGEN Global AIM-SNP set. *Forensic Sci. Int. Genet.* **2014**, *11*, 13–25. [CrossRef]
9. Phillips, C.; Freire Aradas, A.; Kriegel, A.K.; Fondevila, M.; Bulbul, O.; Santos, C.; Serrulla Rech, F.; Perez Carceles, M.D.; Carracedo, A.; Schneider, P.M.; et al. *Eurasiaplex*: A forensic SNP assay for differentiating European and South Asian ancestries. *Forensic Sci. Int. Genet.* **2013**, *7*, 359–366. [CrossRef]
10. Carvalho Gontijo, C.; Porras-Hurtado, L.G.; Freire-Aradas, A.; Fondevila, M.; Santos, C.; Salas, A.; Henao, J.; Isaza, C.; Beltrán, L.; Nogueira Silbiger, V.; et al. PIMA: A population informative multiplex for the Americas. *Forensic Sci. Int. Genet.* **2020**, *44*, 102200. [CrossRef]
11. Santos, C.; Phillips, C.; Fondevila, M.; Daniel, R.; van Oorschot, R.A.H.; Burchard, E.G.; Schanfield, M.S.; Souto, L.J.; Uacyisrael, J.; Via, M.; et al. Pacifiplex: An ancestry-informative SNP panel centred on Australia and the Pacific region. *Forensic Sci. Int. Genet.* **2016**, *20*, 71–80. [CrossRef] [PubMed]
12. Phillips, C.; McNevin, D.; Kidd, K.K.; Lagacé, R.; Wootton, S.; de la Puente, M.; Freire-Aradas, A.; Mosquera-Miguel, A.; Eduardoff, M.; Gross, T.; et al. MAPlex-A massively parallel sequencing ancestry analysis multiplex for Asia-Pacific populations. *Forensic Sci. Int. Genet.* **2019**, *42*, 213–226. [CrossRef]
13. Breslin, K.; Wills, B.; Ralf, A.; Ventayol Garcia, M.; Kukla-Bartoszek, M.; Pospiech, E.; Freire-Aradas, A.; Xavier, C.; Ingold, S.; de La Puente, M.; et al. HIrisPlex-S system for eye, hair, and skin color prediction from DNA: Massively parallel sequencing solutions for two common forensically used platforms. *Forensic Sci. Int. Genet.* **2019**, *43*, 102152. [CrossRef] [PubMed]
14. Al-Asfi, M.; McNevin, D.; Mehta, B.; Power, D.; Gahan, M.E.; Daniel, R. Assessment of the Precision ID Ancestry Panel. *Int. J. Legal. Med.* **2018**, *132*, 1581–1594. [CrossRef]
15. The 1000 Genomes Project Consortium; Auton, A.; Brooks, L.D.; Durbin, R.M.; Garrison, E.P.; Kang, H.M.; Korbel, J.O.; Marchini, J.L.; McCarthy, S.; McVean, G.A.; et al. A global reference for human genetic variation. *Nature* **2015**, *526*, 68–74.
16. Bergström, A.; McCarthy, S.A.; Hui, R.; Almarri, M.A.; Ayub, Q.; Danecek, P.; Chen, Y.; Felkel, S.; Hallast, P.; Kamm, J.; et al. Insights into human genetic variation and population history from 929 diverse genomes. *Science* **2020**, *367*, 1339–1349. [CrossRef]
17. Byrska-Bishop, M.; Evani, U.S.; Zhao, X.; Basile, A.O.; Abel, H.J.; Regier, A.A.; André Corvelo, A.; Clarke, W.E.; Musunuri, R.; Nagulapalli, K.; et al. High Coverage Whole Genome Sequencing of the Expanded 1000 Genomes Project Cohort Including 602 trios. Available online: https://www.internationalgenome.org/data-portal/data-collection/30x-grch38; http://ftp.1000genomes.ebi.ac.uk/vol1/ftp/data_collections/1000G_2504_high_coverage/working/20190425_NYGC_GATK/ (accessed on 20 June 2021).
18. Xavier, C.; de la Puente, M.; Phillips, C.; Eduardoff, M.; Heidegger, A.; Mosquera-Miguel, A.; Freire-Aradas, A.; Lagace, R.; Wootton, S.; Power, D.; et al. Forensic evaluation of the Asia Pacific ancestry-informative MAPlex assay. *Forensic Sci. Int. Genet.* **2020**, *48*, 102344. [CrossRef]
19. Cheung, E.Y.Y.; Phillips, C.; Eduardoff, M.; Lareu, M.V.; McNevin, D. Performance of ancestry-informative SNP and microhaplotype markers. *Forensic Sci. Int. Genet.* **2019**, *43*, 102141. [CrossRef] [PubMed]
20. Phillips, C.; Amigo, J.; Tillmar, A.O.; Peck, M.A.; de la Puente, M.; Ruiz-Ramírez, J.; Bittner, F.; Idrizbegović, Š.; Wang, Y.; Parsons, T.J.; et al. A compilation of tri-allelic SNPs from 1000 Genomes and use of the most polymorphic loci for a large-scale human identification panel. *Forensic Sci. Int. Genet.* **2020**, *46*, 102232. [CrossRef]
21. Galanter, J.M.; Fernandez-Lopez, J.C.; Gignoux, C.R.; Barnholtz-Sloan, J.; Fernandez-Rozadilla, C.; Via, M.; Hidalgo-Miranda, A.; Contreras, A.V.; Figueroa, L.U.; Raska, P.; et al. Development of a panel of genome-wide ancestry informative markers to study admixture throughout the Americas. *PLoS Genet.* **2012**, *8*, e1002554. [CrossRef] [PubMed]
22. Kidd, K.K.; Speed, W.C.; Pakstis, A.J.; Furtado, M.R.; Fang, R.; Madbouly, A.; Maiers, M.; Middha, M.; Friedlaender, F.R.; Kidd, J.R. Progress toward an efficient panel of SNPs for ancestry inference. *Forensic Sci. Int. Genet.* **2014**, *10*, 23–32. [CrossRef]
23. Pereira, V.; Freire-Aradas, A.; Ballard, D.; Børsting, C.; Diez, V.; Pruszkowska-Przybylska, P.; Ribeiro, J.; Achakzai, N.M.; Aliferi, A.; Bulbul, O.; et al. Development and validation of the EUROFORGEN NAME (North African and Middle Eastern) ancestry panel. *Forensic Sci. Int. Genet.* **2019**, *42*, 260–267. [CrossRef] [PubMed]

24. Mao, X.; Bigham, A.W.; Mei, R.; Gutierrez, G.; Weiss, K.M.; Brutsaert, T.D.; Leon-Velarde, F.; Moore, L.G.; Vargas, E.; McKeigue, P.M.; et al. A genomewide admixture mapping panel for Hispanic/Latino populations. *Am. J. Hum. Genet* **2007**, *80*, 1171–1178. [CrossRef] [PubMed]

25. Available online: http://mathgene.usc.es/Snipper/ (accessed on 20 June 2021).

26. Phillips, C.; Amigo, J.; McNevin, D.; de la Puente, M.; Cheung, E.Y.Y.; Lareu, M.V. Online population data resources for forensic SNP analysis with Massively Parallel Sequencing: An overview of online population data for forensic purposes. In *Forensic DNA Analysis: Technological Development and Innovative Applications*; Pilli, E., Berti, A., Eds.; CRC Press: Boca Raton, FL, USA, 2021.

27. Mallick, S.; Li, H.; Lipson, M.; Mathieson, I.; Gymrek, M.; Racimo, F.; Zhao, M.; Chennagiri, N.; Nordenfelt, S.; Tandon, A.; et al. The Simons Genome Diversity Project: 300 genomes from 142 diverse populations. *Nature* **2016**, *538*, 201–206. [CrossRef]

28. Pagani, L.; Lawson, D.J.; Jagoda, E.; Mörseburg, A.; Eriksson, A.; Mitt, M.; Clemente, F.; Hudjashov, G.; DeGiorgio, M.; Saag, L.; et al. Genomic analyses inform on migration events during the peopling of Eurasia. *Nature* **2016**, *538*, 238–242. [CrossRef]

29. Xavier, C.; de la Puente, M.; Mosquera-Miguel, A.; Freire-Aradas, A.; Kalamara, V.; Vidaki, A.; Gross, T.; Revoir, A.; Pośpiech, E.; Kartasińska, E.; et al. Development and validation of the VISAGE AmpliSeq Basic Tool to predict appearance and ancestry from DNA. *Forensic Sci. Int. Genet.* **2020**, *48*, 102336. [CrossRef]

30. Pritchard, J.K.; Stephens, M.; Donnelly, P. Inference of population structure using multilocus genotype data. *Genetics* **2000**, *155*, 945–959. [CrossRef]

31. Evanno, G.; Regnaut, S.; Goudet, J. Detecting the number of clusters of individuals using the software STRUCTURE: A simulation study. *Mol. Ecol.* **2005**, *14*, 2611–2620. [CrossRef]

32. Kopelman, N.M.; Mayzel, J.; Jakobsson, M.; Rosenberg, N.A.; Mayrose, I. Clumpak: A program for identifying clustering modes and packaging population structure inferences across K. *Mol. Ecol. Resour.* **2015**, *15*, 1179–1191. [CrossRef] [PubMed]

33. R: A Language and Environment for Statistical Computing. Available online: http://www.r-project.org/ (accessed on 20 June 2021).

34. Paradis, E. Pegas: An R package for population genetics with an integrated-modular approach. *Bioinformatics* **2010**, *26*, 419–420. [CrossRef]

35. Alexander, D.; Novembre, J.; Lange, K. Fast model-based estimation of ancestry in unrelated individuals. *Genome Res.* **2009**, *19*, 1655–1664. [CrossRef] [PubMed]

36. Cheung, E.Y.Y.; Gahan, M.E.; McNevin, D. Prediction of biogeographical ancestry from genotype: A comparison of classifiers. *Int. J. Legal Med.* **2017**, *131*, 901–912. [CrossRef] [PubMed]

37. Palencia-Madrid, L.; Xavier, C.; de la Puente, M.; Hohoff, C.; Phillips, C.; Kayser, M.; Parson, W. on behalf of the VISAGE Consortium, Evaluation of the VISAGE Basic Tool for Appearance and Ancestry Prediction Using PowerSeq Chemistry on the MiSeq FGx System. *Genes* **2020**, *11*, 708. [CrossRef] [PubMed]

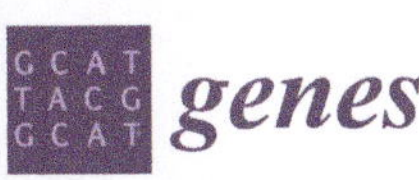

genes

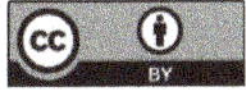

Review

On the Identification of Body Fluids and Tissues: A Crucial Link in the Investigation and Solution of Crime

Titia Sijen [1,2,*] and SallyAnn Harbison [3,4]

1   Division Human Biological Traces, Netherlands Forensic Institute, Laan van Ypenburg 6,
    2497 GB The Hague, The Netherlands
2   Swammerdam Institute for Life Sciences, University of Amsterdam, Science Park 904,
    1098 XH Amsterdam, The Netherlands
3   Institute of Environmental Science and Research Limited, Private Bag 92021, Auckland 1142, New Zealand;
    sallyann.harbison@esr.cri.nz
4   Department of Statistics, University of Auckland, Private Bag 92019, Auckland 1142, New Zealand
*   Correspondence: t.sijen@nfi.nl; Tel.: +31-70-888-6666

Abstract: Body fluid and body tissue identification are important in forensic science as they can provide key evidence in a criminal investigation and may assist the court in reaching conclusions. Establishing a link between identifying the fluid or tissue and the DNA profile adds further weight to this evidence. Many forensic laboratories retain techniques for the identification of biological fluids that have been widely used for some time. More recently, many different biomarkers and technologies have been proposed for identification of body fluids and tissues of forensic relevance some of which are now used in forensic casework. Here, we summarize the role of body fluid/ tissue identification in the evaluation of forensic evidence, describe how such evidence is detected at the crime scene and in the laboratory, elaborate different technologies available to do this, and reflect real life experiences. We explain how, by including this information, crucial links can be made to aid in the investigation and solution of crime.

Keywords: forensic; review; body fluid; organ; tissue; identification; mRNA; DNA methylation; activity level

Citation: Sijen, T.; Harbison, S. On the Identification of Body Fluids and Tissues: A Crucial Link in the Investigation and Solution of Crime. *Genes* **2021**, *12*, 1728. https://doi.org/ 10.3390/genes12111728

Academic Editor: Niels Morling

Received: 12 October 2021
Accepted: 26 October 2021
Published: 28 October 2021

1. Activity-Level Evaluations: The Context of Body Fluid and Tissue Identification

Body fluid and tissue identification can add evidence in criminal investigations by establishing a crucial link between the donor, the cell type and the activities that occurred. In this review, we first provide the forensic context of body fluid and tissue identification which resides in activity-level evaluations, then we discuss methods to locate body fluids at the scene or in the laboratory, which is followed by the major marker methodologies to analyze them. One of these methods is mRNA profiling, and we take a retrospective look at casework details and verdicts for mRNA cases in the Netherlands. This leads us to a criminalistic view on targets that can be accommodated in assays and the interpretation of cell typing results for instance, in mixed stains, which needs a very different approach from the interpretation of DNA results. Lastly, we consider possible other marker types that have been suggested, and practical aspects when introducing cell typing into a forensic laboratory.

1.1. Prosecution and Defense Scenario

Increasingly, cases come to court in which the presence of cellular material of a person is not disputed but the activity that caused the deposition is. The debate then centers around the question 'how did his/her DNA get there'? Forensic scientists approach such questions by performing activity-level evaluations [1–8]. Figure 1 shows activity-level evaluation in the context of forensic human biology analyses. Generalizing, activity-level evaluations weigh the likelihood of the forensic evidence under one scenario (hypothesis 1; H1, also known as prosecution scenario) versus an alternative scenario (hypothesis 2; H2, also known as defense scenario). The two hypotheses need to be formulated well, describe the alleged activities and be mutually exclusive. In the evaluation, the probability of the findings given the propositions is considered (not the probability of the propositions themselves) [1].

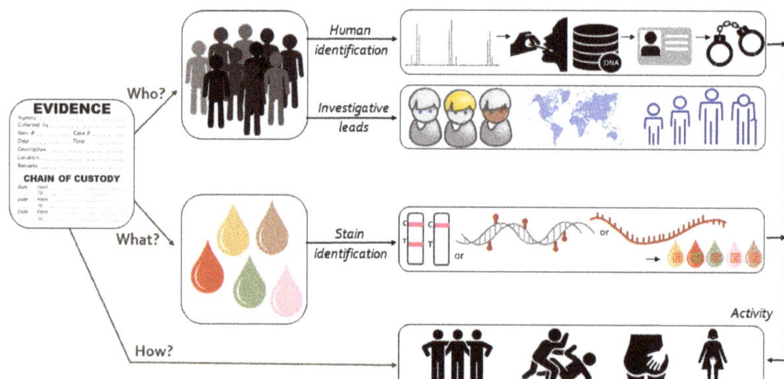

Figure 1. Stain identification in the context of the forensic process showing the link between 'who', 'what' and 'how'.

The 'findings' in the case can relate to cellular material matching victim or suspect which under H1 is indicative of an offensive activity (e.g., blood matching the victim on the blade of a knife indicative of the victim being stabbed; cellular material matching the suspect on the handle of a knife supporting the proposition that the suspect carried out the stabbing). Under H2, this questioned cellular material on the evidentiary item may result from a number of scenarios: (1) the cellular material was deposited not during the offense but at an earlier or later time (the suspect did not stab but picked up the knife after the stabbing); (2) the cellular material was not deposited by direct contact but was the result of secondary (or tertiary or further) transfer (the suspect shook hands with the real perpetrator who then handled the knife in the stabbing); (3) the item on which the cellular material was deposited belongs to the suspect but was used in the offense by another person (the knife (owned by the suspect who uses it to cut food) was handled by the real perpetrator in the stabbing); (4) the cellular material was deposited on the knife in a different way (the victim fell into the knife).

1.2. Addressing Alternative Scenarios

Forensic studies aim to develop approaches to assist in addressing offensive and alternative scenarios. To address deposition during the offense or during an earlier or later encounter, inferring the time since deposition (TSD) may be helpful. For bloodstains, various spectroscopic and chemometric TSD methods have been proposed that rely foremost on changes to hemoglobin [9–13]. An approach that would be applicable to more body fluids than blood is based on differences in the degradation over time of distinct RNA molecules outside the human body. Determining relative expression ratios may allow inference of TSD, although robustness is not yet at the level needed for forensic casework [14–19]. Recently, microbes were explored for TSD purposes of saliva samples with some success, but the high inter-individual variation can surpass the time-dependent variation [20].

To address the question of primary deposition or secondary transfer, TPPR (transfer, prevalence, persistence and recovery) issues are studied [21–31]. The aspect of transfer appears the most complex among TPPR issues and many studies have gained information on transfer rates, and the various aspects that influence transfer rates such as wet or dried state, application of friction and pressure, smooth or rough surface and size of the stain [32–38]. Generally, probabilistic frameworks are used to guide the evaluation, and Bayesian networks are appreciated for their graphical strength in this evaluative process [39,40].

Inferring the body fluid(s) present in stains is, in the context of secondary (or more) transfer, important for two reasons: (1) to assess the cellular content of the primary stain in relation to the DNA recovered from the evidentiary sample as some fluids have very high cellular content (for example nasal secretion), whilst others contain much fewer cells (for instance urine) and (2) to assess whether the body fluid involved is likely to occur in what is suggested) to be the primary location [41]. For example, intimate body fluids (vaginal cellular material, menstrual secretion, semen) can be found in underpants of the wearer, but are less expected on hands or touched items [42–44]. Saliva and nasal secretion, on the other hand, can reside on hands or items, and blood could occur when people have (small) wounds. Organ tissues (for instance, CNS (central nervous system), heart, or adipose tissue), on the other hand, are not expected on hands or on items.

The scenario that another person and not the suspect utilized an item (belonging to the suspect) on which cellular material was deposited in the offense, can relate to objects (e.g., a knife used for stabbing or a bottle that was inserted vaginally) or clothing/ shoes that appear to have been worn during the offense for instance because blood spatter or organ tissue matching the victim found on them. Cell typing of samples from such items may provide the crucial link of the evidentiary item to the alleged crime (the knife carries muscle tissue matching the victim on the blade; the bottle contains vaginal material matching the victim on the bottle neck; the shoe carries CNS tissue matching the head-kicked victim), but the link to the perpetrator needs to be provided by other means. This may be addressed for instance through fingerprint analysis (e.g., on the bottom of the bottle or the handle of the knife), DNA-analysis (e.g., of the shoelaces or the insides of the neck and collar areas of the sweater) or CCTV-footage or witness reports on the suspect acting in the stabbing or wearing the shoes or clothing at the time of the attack.

When a different way for the deposition of the cellular material is proposed (e.g., shooting out of self-defense, intercourse with consent), the evaluation is often at the offense level, which means the domain of the court [2,45,46]. With such scenarios, DNA nor cell typing add value in most of the cases.

1.3. Contextualizing Evidentiary Traces

Not only the type of body fluid or organ tissue, but also the location, pattern and amount of cellular material can be relevant for activity-level evaluations or contextualizing the scene. For example, trousers of a suspect may carry multiple bloodstains matching the DNA profile of a deceased person. Bloodstain pattern analysis may reveal a mist-like pattern and diluted bloodstains. RNA analysis of multiple stains could indicate the presence of blood, saliva, and nasal mucosa in various combinations. Together, the location, pattern, amount, and type of detected body fluids indicate expirated blood. Pathology may reveal injuries to the lungs or airways, which could have triggered the victim to expel blood mixed with air from the lungs through the nose or mouth. The combination of identified body fluids, location/ pattern and amounts would support the suspect being in the vicinity of the dying victim expelling blood and would provide less support for a scenario in which the suspect would visit the scene of the crime a day later.

2. Locating Biological Forensic Evidence

Locating and identifying body fluids and tissues is important for two main reasons: (1) to find traces related to the alleged crime which can then be collected and from which the identity of the perpetrator may be revealed by further testing; (2) to contextualize the traces as explained in Section 1.3 to provide information about what activities may have taken place. This can be done at the scene, where time is limited, using techniques that are mostly presumptive and visual in nature, or in a forensic laboratory (using samples and items collected at the scene) where more detailed analysis is possible.

2.1. At the Scene of the Crime

Here we describe technologies for locating latent biological evidence for use at the scene that can also be used in the laboratory. These include chemiluminescent sprays such as those based on luminol, safer and non-invasive alternative light sources and spectroscopic methods using handheld instruments. Handheld devices, and technologies that are non-destructive to the sample offer the greatest potential as these can be used to rapidly direct investigations and the collection of evidence.

2.1.1. Chemical Sprays for Blood and Semen

Sometimes blood at crime scenes is difficult to see, perhaps there is a very small quantity of diluted blood (cleaning may have taken place), the blood is on a surface that makes it difficult to find (like a dark substrate or upon repainting) or there is a trail of blood-stained shoeprints leading from the scene which are no longer visible. Luminol and the more user-friendly, luminol-derived Bluestar (Bluestar Forensic, Monaco) reagent [47], are often used to detect haemoglobin and its derivatives resulting in a blue fluorescence which is captured by photography [48]. One disadvantage of such methods includes that the luminescence produced can be faint and short-lived, and in the case of luminol the visualization must be carried out in near darkness [48]. Different formulations exist and those that maximise the brightness and longevity of the fluorescence and that have few adverse effects on subsequent tests for blood or on DNA profiling are preferred [48–51]. A more recent development is the proposed use of a click reaction [52] between serum albumin and tetraphenylethene maleimide. The reaction is less harsh than that of luminol and BlueStar and produces a stable and sensitive response and shows promise for further development.

To locate semen, alternative light sources (ALS; see Section 2.1.2) and acid phosphatase tests are used that suffer from limitations in sensitivity and toxicity, respectively. In 2017, STK Sperm Tracker™ was introduced to the market by AXO Science (Lyon, France) as a human semen-specific test [53]. Sperm Tracker is available as a spray for crime scene use and in impregnated sheets for use on larger items. Detection requires a UV light source, that the room or space be darkened, and it must be used before luminol or BlueStar.

2.1.2. Alternative Light Sources

ALS refers to the use of light of different wavelengths, including infrared, to detect forensic evidence in a non-destructive manner, and are often used to assist in the reconstruction of events. The detection of biological evidence is possible because they contain autofluorescent components which allow them to be visualized when illuminated at specific wavelengths.

An early study comparing different laser and ultraviolet light sources for the detection of biological fluids [54] has been followed by the development of many commercially available light sources such as the Polilight® series (Rofin Australia Pty Ltd., Melbourne, VIC, Austraila) and the LED-based Crime-lite® series (Foster and Freeman Ltd., Evesham, UK). A selection of illustrative articles is presented here.

In an examination of the utility of the Polilight® [55] stains of blood, semen and saliva, not visible to the eye, were able to be detected and Polilight® performed well when compared to other presumptive screening tests.

As different body fluids and substrates fluoresce at different wavelengths, selecting the best combination of lightsource (wavelength) and filter used for detection is important. By comparing results obtained from five body fluids applied to 29 different materials, the Lumatec Superlight 410 (Lumatec GMBH, Deisenhofen, Germany) was used on fresh stains [56] and the same stains after two years [57] using different filters. Their findings show that for every combination of substrate, fluid, light source, and filter, except one, there was a specific combination that was best. In general though, stains could still be visualised two years later, using a light source between 415 nm and 460 nm in combination with a yellow or orange filter.

To improve the utility of light sources and photography at crime scenes, a study was conducted [51] combining a blue Crime-lite XL light source in combination with a 360° camera to capture semen and saliva stains on a number of different substrates. This study was carried out in a mock crime scene indoor setting using volunteers to examine the images and locate the stains. The colour of the substrate was found to have an effect on the ability to see the stains, however, in general, the combination of light source and camera was effective.

A side by side comparison of the Crime-lite® 82S, Polilight® PL400 and Polilight® PL500 [58] was recently carried out, comparing the sensitivity and performance of each on dilutions of saliva and semen on different fabrics. The LED light source used in the Crime-lite® 82S provided better detection of dilutions of saliva and overall performed better as a screening tool.

Recent developments include combined handheld, UV/Vis/IR multi-wavelength light sources and camera combined, with automatic filter selection all controlled from an integrated touch screen for example the Crime-lite AUTO. This handheld instrument appears to offer a number of advantages for crime scene use, the most obvious of which is the combined handheld unit. See also Section 2.2.3 for an alternative.

2.1.3. Spectroscopic Methods at the Scene

Spectroscopic techniques for locating and identifying body fluids are available, with handheld devices for crime scene use as well as methods requiring laboratory-based equipment [59]. Handheld NIR (near infrared) spectrometers have been tested [60] with blood and potential applications to other fluids including age estimation [13]. NIR spectroscopy is quick and non-destructive with no sample preparation and background fluorescence encountered with [61]. In the most recent example [60], the instrument is paired with a mobile phone and software containing the necessary tools to train a variety of statistical models to interpret test data based on machine learning. The best of these models could correctly identify blood in 94% of cases, albeit with a false positive rate of 14% for blood-like substances such as red wine, tomato sauce, and coffee.

Hyperspectral imaging (HSI) is also a non-destructive spectroscopic technique and can be used to "map" large geographical areas as well as smaller items [62]. HSI records, as a continuous measurement, electromagnetic spectra over a wide range of wavelengths for every pixel in an image, and from this creates unique spectra. Since 2012 when first proposed as a tool to characterise forensic evidence [63,64] HIS has emerged as a potential tool for bloodstain detection.

The identification of blood by HIS is based upon the visualisation of haemoglobin and its components in the 400 to 700 nm range. Changes in the Soret peak observed at 415 nm are used to detect aging of the sample. In a set of fingerprints, aged over a 30 day period, HSI enabled the identification of the blood as well as aging of the prints [65].

When comparing a Crime-lite® ML2 ALS instrument (Foster and Freeman Ltd., Evesham, UK) and HIS-NIR imaging using an SWIR3 hyperspectral camera working in the 1000–2500 nm spectral range (Specim Ltd., Oulu, Finland) [66], the resultant images obtained from the HIS-NIR imaging were shown to be superior at revealing the location of body fluid staining in known reference samples, simulated casework samples and on unknown staining on forensic exhibits. Using blood samples and different substrates, spectra were generated [67] that were used to train different classifiers to detect aged bloodstains and most recently a "blood detection dataset" was produced [68] specifically to assist in the challenging task of algorithm development for this new technology.

2.2. At the Forensic Laboratory

In the previous section, we described approaches for locating biological evidence at crime scenes, particularly latent evidence that may not be visible to the naked eye.

These methods can also be employed in a forensic laboratory when transportable items are involved. In the remainder of this section, we discuss methods that are primarily laboratory-based for locating biological fluids. These chemical, immunological, and spectroscopic tests are often used to presumptively identify biological fluids before conducting further, more specific testing where necessary.

2.2.1. Chemical and Immunochromatographic Tests

With the exception of microscopic identification of spermatozoa, forensic scientists often rely on sensitive but non-specific chemical tests, based primarily on the activity of enzymes in the target body fluid. Although easy to use, they are not human-specific and are largely presumptive in nature with many examples of false positive reactions reported. For reviews covering this area, see [69–71].

To supplement these chemical tests, laboratories may use immunochromatographic assays, which include tests for saliva, semen, urine, blood and menstrual blood. Despite advantages of speed, cost and ease of use, these assays are not as suitable for crime scene deployment as they require an extract of a sample to be made and are not an integral part of the DNA profiling process. To date, there is only one report of combining such tests into a format amenable to detecting body fluids in mixtures [72]. The more recent emergence of proteomics in the forensic literature (see Section 7.1.2) and the identification of new candidate markers [73] is likely to drive the development of immunologically-based assays based on multiplexing in a single assay that may be amenable for use at the crime scene.

Immunochromatographic methods can also be used to detect DNA amplicons and direct PCR of *Streptococcus sanguinis* and *Streptococcus salivarius* specific to saliva has been successfully integrated with an immunochromatographic strip detection method [74].

Improvements to the technology for detection have allowed for the development of a protein microarray sensor [75] for the detection of semen and vaginal cellular material. Antibodies to semenogelin-2 and anti-17 beta estradiol were immobilised on an array surface. To enhance the signal achieved and increase the sensitivity of the assay, a metal enhanced fluorescence (MEF) approach was taken. The sample containing body fluids was itself labelled with a fluorescent dye and after hybridisation and washing steps the fluorescence signals are detected.

2.2.2. Spectroscopic Techniques

Raman spectroscopy, for which less sensitive handheld devices are available, relies upon the scattering of light by biological compounds. The outputs are complex spectra built up of the multiple components of each fluid. Statistical tools are available and needed to determine the unique spectroscopic profile of the molecular structure of each. Such profiles have been determined for a range of body fluids and tissues of forensic interest, such as blood [76], semen, saliva, vaginal fluid and sweat [77,78].

Early evaluations [76] considered factors of forensic interest such as the substrate, within-person variability and time since deposition in blood samples. Blood was able to be detected on luminescent fabrics by first removing the stained area from the substrate. Variability was observed as bloodstains aged and also between and within people. The changes in spectra as a bloodstain ages were further explored [79] over a period of 2 years with age predicted with an accuracy of approximately 70%. Statistical models were further improved [80] to accommodate environmental factors.

Fourier transform infrared (FT-IR) spectroscopy, routinely used in forensic chemistry, has also been evaluated for biological fluids with an important consideration that any environmental contamination is accounted for. Attenuated total reflectance (ATF) FT-IR spectroscopy [81,82] has been used to characterise a number of body fluids, accommodating the age of the stain and excluding unexpected non-target components. Similar studies have also been undertaken on semen [83,84], with methods developed to identify and avoid interference from a number of environmental factors; on dried urine [85] where the gender of the donor was able to be deciphered; and to distinguish between menstrual and peripheral blood [86]. The alternative modification, external reflection FT-IR spectroscopy, has also been proposed [59] to specifically identify body fluids associated with sexual assault. The effects of different fabric colours and commonly used household substances on identification were also assessed. These instruments are not handheld and, therefore, not compatible with examinations at the crime scene.

2.2.3. A Practical Example

The utility of combining ALS detection with an immunochromatographic test for the presence of prostate-specific antigen (PSA, also known as gamma-seminoprotein, kallikrein-3 or P-30 antigen), on laundered clothing [87] followed by DNA profiling has been demonstrated. In this example, semen stains were located using a Forenscope Mobile Multispectral UV-VIS-IR Imaging System® (Grimed Ltd., Voor, The Netherlands) which, like the Crime Lite AUTO described in Section 2.1.2, combines light source, filters, camera and software in one handheld instrument. Semen stains could be detected and confirmed using both the Forenscope system and the PSA test. High washing temperatures had the biggest impact on the ALS detection, polyester fabric had the biggest detrimental impact on the PSA test. DNA profiling however was successful on all semen samples regardless of washing temperature, detergent or fabric.

3. Major Types of Markers and Technologies Employed to Detect Them

3.1. RNA Markers

RNA is the link between the genome and protein content of each cell and its expression or its effect on expression of cell type-specific proteins has been widely adopted as a laboratory-based approach for body fluid identification [69,71,88] for forensic purposes. Alongside mRNA, small non-coding RNAs have generated significant interest [89] to date, which will be described in Section 7.1.1. RNA analysis has also been suggested for other forensic applications such as post mortem interval and age of a stain determination [17,19,90].

3.1.1. Messenger RNA

There are many examples, over more than twenty years, of messenger RNA (mRNA) being proposed as a confirmatory test for body fluid and tissue identification with an early example being the identification of menstrual blood [91]. A selection of the numerous papers published are included here and will assist in directing the reader to further studies.

The stability of RNA in stains of forensic interest was described in 1999 [92] with a demonstration of the detection of skin epithelial cells in dried blood cells. This was followed by studies describing stability studies in vaginal swabs, blood, semen and saliva stains [93], stains up to 23 years old [94] and transcriptome studies showing the persistence of regions of RNA of interest in samples deliberately degraded [95–97].

To minimise sample loss during testing and optimise the efficiency of the laboratory process, it is important to recover DNA and RNA from the same sample [98–100]. A recent paper compared a number of different approaches [101] and found methods with small modifications to [98,99] remained the best. Equally important in minimising sample loss and optimising the laboratory process is the creation of multiplex assays each containing mRNA markers of known specificity [98,102–107] that can be selected from the literature and online databases [98,107] and whole genome expression analysis [108–110]. Once these factors are considered, then casework and casework applications follow [111–115].

Most of the published work depends upon the detection of mRNA markers by reverse transcription PCR (RT PCR) and capillary electrophoresis (CE) [92,102,103,106,116]. Real time PCR (qPCR) has also been used [116,117] but is somewhat limited by the number of markers that can be multiplexed together (restricted by the availability of fluorescent dyes) and the difficulty in identifying appropriate housekeeping genes, applicable to all included body fluids of interest. More recently, massively parallel sequencing (MPS) has been used to detect multiplexed markers [118–120] reflecting a shift towards this technology in forensic science [121]. The main advantages of MPS is the high multiplexing capacity, that amplicons can have overlapping (small) sizes and that nucleotide variation is detected. These first two features are of importance with forensic traces as they are often of minute amounts and suffer from degradation due to external factors. The forensic importance of analysing sequence variation in RNA amplicons will be discussed in Section 6.4. Other techniques for detecting markers are given in Section 3.1.3.

3.1.2. Circular RNA

Circular RNAs (circRNAs) are highly expressed [122,123] and as they share sequence with the mRNA equivalent to which they are related can also be body fluid/ tissue-specific [124]. Because these molecules are closed circular structures, they are very stable and this makes them promising candidates for body fluid identification. In the first report [125] of their inclusion for forensic application, microarray expression profiles of circRNAs of venous blood, semen, saliva, vaginal cellular material and menstrual blood samples were produced. Although semen, saliva and venous blood could be distinguished from each other vaginal cellular material and menstrual blood could not.

A further study [126] combined mRNA markers with circRNA markers for the same genes (ALAS2 and MMP7), which were markers already used for body fluid identification [106,127,128], and demonstrated improvements in the sensitivity and stability of the assay compared to mRNA alone. This was also found in a similar study of circRNA markers in blood, menstrual blood, saliva, semen, urine and vaginal cellular material, using gene targets well known in the mRNA profiling community (for example HTN3 for saliva and CYP2B7P1 for vaginal material) [129]. Further investigation resulted in an 18 plex multiplex assay combining circRNAs, mRNAs and housekeeping genes, with good sensitivity and specificity and the potential to identify fluids in degraded samples due to the stability of the circRNA molecules [129].

3.1.3. Alternative Techniques to Analyse RNA Markers

Many of the methods and much of the research described above use either RT PCR and CE, qPCR and/or increasingly RNA sequencing to detect the markers under study. These have been described in more detail in a recent review [88]. Some examples of newly proposed techniques follow.

Loop mediated isothermal amplification (LAMP) [130] can provide higher specificity than PCR because of the use of multiple primers and the higher temperatures at which amplification occurs. In 2015, the first reports of applying LAMP to mRNA body fluid identification [131] detected hemoglobin beta as a marker for blood and was followed by similar studies using a direct RT LAMP method to detect the expression of the statherin gene in saliva [132] The same markers and the TGM4 gene marker for semen were targeted in the design of an assay for the identification of blood, semen and saliva [133]. Extending the format to include vaginal cellular material and azoospermatic semen in a microtitre plate with a metal dye indicator and colorimetric detection, significantly improved the utility of the approach and may make it more suitable to laboratory requiring a higher throughput [134].

High resolution melt (HRM) curve analysis measures the melting temperature (Tm) and generates a distinct and characteristic melt curve for each amplicon in a sample. It has been proposed for a number of applications such as a detection method for SNPs [135], to detect sequence differences in the hypervariable regions of mtDNA [136], to characterise the oral microbiome of different people using 16SrRNA [137], as a technique to analyse methylation sensitive sites for body fluid determination [138] and as a method to identify mRNA markers in body fluids [139] in a multiplex format due to the high resolution of each distinct melt curve for each amplicon.

Since two publications some time ago [108,140], the NanoStringR nCounter system (nanoString, Seattle, WA, USA) [141] has received little forensic interest. This is somewhat surprising given the strengths of the platform that include a direct assay not involving PCR and measurement of gene expression of up to 800 mRNA candidates in a single multiplex reaction in a semi-automated fashion. These studies successfully tested 18 and 23 markers for body fluids, respectively. [108,140]

Similarly, HyBeacon probes [142], used for the detection of SNPs and STRs in areas such as clinical diagnostics and food authentication, have received some but not extensive interest. The ParaDNA Body Fluid ID test comprising RT PCR and melt curve detection was successfully evaluated for the detection of mRNA in body fluids of forensic interest [143] in combination with the now withdraw/ unavailable ParaDNA system (LGC Forensics Teddington, Middlesex, UK) [144] for STR detection.

3.2. Epigenetic Markers

Body fluid identification can also be accomplished at the DNA level by examining epigenetic modifications to specific sites on the genome, primarily methylation at the $5'$ position of cytosine in a CpG dinucleotide. These sites are known as tissue-based differentially methylated regions (tDMRs) and have been specifically examined for body fluids of forensic interest such as blood, semen, saliva, skin, urine, and vaginal secretions.

Whilst the initial application of epigenetics in forensic science was the identification of body fluids and tissues, methylation analysis has also been proposed for age estimation and differentiation of twins [145–147]. A range of methods have been applied for identifying appropriate markers, detecting the epigenetic modifications, and assessing the results. A comprehensive review [146], describes many of these approaches in more detail.

3.2.1. Marker Selection and Assay Design

With the increasing availability of freely available methylation data, researchers can assess many thousands of CpG sites simultaneously to find candidate markers. For example, the human methylation bead array system (Illumina) was used to screen over 450,000 CpG sites in samples of blood, saliva, and vaginal cellular material [148,149]. More recently, overexpressed genes in genome wide expression datasets were combined with heavily methylated gene body CpG islands (CGI) from methylation datasets [150]. Further *in silico* analysis of one of these datasets [149] was undertaken and four new markers able to discriminate blood (2 markers), vaginal cellular material (1 marker) and buccal cells (1 marker) were found [151].

Once identified, primers are designed and ideally markers are multiplexed enabling the simultaneous identification of different fluids/tissues. An example is a PCR multiplex combining CpG sites in the DACT1, USP49, PFN3, and PRMT2 genes to identify spermatozoa and differentiate between menstrual blood and vaginal cellular material from blood and saliva [148,152]. This multiplex has been extended to include amplicons for the 16S rRNA gene of bacteria specific oral and vaginal origin, *Veillonella atypica* and/or *Streptococcus salivarius*, and *Lactobacillus crispatus* and/or *Lactobacillus gasseri* respectively [153].

3.2.2. Techniques to Analyse Epigenetic Modifications

Early research focused on the use of methylation-sensitive/ dependent restriction enzymes followed by PCR and CE [154]. The advantage of this approach was the ability to co-amplify STRs at a similar level of sensitivity, but drawbacks included incomplete restriction and template degradation, which can distort the methylation ratios that are critical to the interpretation of the results, which was particularly pronounced in low template samples. More recent assays [155], therefore, use amplicons with multiple restriction sites.

There are multiple methods to determine the relative methylation levels achieved, and they all start with bisulfite conversion of the DNA and amplification using primers designed to anneal to the converted DNA. Examples are qPCR with HRM [138,151] often confirmed with pyrosequencing [156], sequencing of cloned products [150] and changes in mobility of the PCR amplicons [157]. A multiplex methylation SNaPshot approach has been used to identify blood, saliva, semen and vaginal cellular material, and produced successful DNA methylation profiles in aged and mixed samples [148]. In a separate study it was successful in the identification of semen, saliva, venous blood and menstrual blood in body fluid mixtures and in crime scene stains [158]. Methylation state specificity was achieved using the single-base extension primers of the SNaPshot assay. Amplification refractory mutation system-PCR (ARMS-PCR), otherwise known as allele-based PCR [159], in combination with CE was used as an alternative method to test 22 possible markers for venous blood, saliva, semen, menstrual blood, and vaginal cellular material in multiplexes [160]. A random forest model was employed and performed well in predicting single source body fluids with high prediction accuracy (99.66%).

The multistep process of bisulfite conversion, PCR and detection by CE or sequencing is vulnerable to variation due to poor sample quality and quantity and especially degradation during the bisulfite conversion step. A new multiplex quantitative RT PCR method to measure the amount of genomic and bisulfite-converted DNA, and the degradation level of the conversion step as well as the conversion efficiency has been described [161]. Besides, natural variation in methylation status has been found between individuals, and some tissue-specific differentially methylated regions are susceptible to change due to environmental factors and age. For example, methylation of a CpG site in PRMT2 in blood samples was found to be an age-associated marker, whereas no significant difference based on age was observed for three spermatozoa-specific hypomethylated markers DACT1, USP49, and PRMT2 in men of different ages [149,152]. Others have demonstrated that within-person variation in methylation ratios was not observed, but variation was observed between people in an assay designed to identify vaginal cellular material [157].

3.3. Microbial Markers

Microbiomes are comprised of the bacterial, archaeal, viral and fungal microbial taxa communities present in/on a location of interest, such as the human body. Microbes have an advantage of high abundance and stability. Microbiomes can be considered as a whole (the human microbiome) or more specifically relating to a more defined location, for example the skin microbiome of humans where different bodily locations (moist armpit, sebaceous facial areas, dry forearm) can be dominated by different species [162]. A subset of markers and target organisms can be chosen to represent the fluid/ body site of choice [153,163] but it should be noted that different species may perform the same biological function (such as the production of lactic acid in the vagina) and may not function in all individuals [164,165]. Even human blood, previously considered to be sterile in a healthy person, may not be so [166].

More routine analysis of microbiomes has been made possible by developments in sequencing and related technology. Despite early promise, some challenges remain in adopting this technology for forensic science. In addition to variations between and within people [164,167–170] a key consideration is that microbial communities are strongly influenced by many external factors such as geography, time, season, health, diet, genetic factors, anti-inflammatory drugs and lifestyle [171–176], and even the presence of pets [177]. Consideration of these factors is necessary for any evaluation of microbiomes whether they "match" or not. Many of these factors relating to the human skin microbiome are neatly summarized in [178,179] and can be directly applied to all microbiome research and applications. In particular, the potential effects of the presence of contamination in the reagents and consumables used has been highlighted [180].

3.3.1. Microbial Markers for Body Fluid Identification

Many possible applications of the analysis of microbiomes are described in a recent review [181]. These include the identification of people [182–184]; establishing links with personal possessions such as phones and shoes [185–187]; forensic botany (including environmental DNA), in which analysis of the phyllosphere and soil can provide links between people and crime scene locations [171,188–190]; and the identification of microflora specific to different body locations such as saliva [191].

Many studies have focused on specific body sites/ fluids for example the microbiomes of saliva [192,193], faeces [194], the vagina [164,195] with recent publications focusing on distinguishing between different sources of blood (menstrual, venous, fingerpick and nasal) [196,197] and semen [198]. *Lactobacillus* species have been incorporated into mRNA multiplexes and collaborative exercises [163,199] and in multiplexed methylation -sensitive restriction enzyme PCR assays [153]. Interpretation of the presence of such markers should proceed with care as microorganisms can be detected on non-target body locations, probably either from their high abundance and/or carry-over [104].

Unsurprisingly, vaginal samples and menstrual blood are unable to be distinguished and share metagenomic profiles [196,200], and in one study, samples taken from the penis the vaginal markers responded while no female DNA was detected [168].

In an extension from simply identifying bacteria representative of the oral cavity, it was [201] recognized that identifying them could be used to distinguish between expirated bloodstains (such as those forced by airflow out of the nose or mouth) and impact spatter, providing what could be an additional crucial piece of information for an investigation (see Section 1.3).

3.3.2. Technologies to Analyze Microbial Markers

For the identification of microbial profiles specific to body locations, sequencing of the 16S rRNA gene is typically carried out, with the profiles found to be diagnostic of the area sampled. Saliva, skin, peripheral blood, menstrual blood, faeces and semen have all been tested in this way [169,200,202]. Whole genome shotgun sequencing has been suggested to outperform 16S rRNA analysis because of higher accuracy [203], but this comes with higher costs.

Not all assays are based on the 16S rRNA gene or on sequencing. For example microarrays targeting multiple genes across a range of known microorganisms have been described [164,168] and a qPCR assay [193] has been developed to detect three bacteria (*Streptococcus salivarius*, *Streptococcus sanguinis*, and *Neisseria subflava*) known to be present in the oral cavity. A similar microarray-based method has been described [194] for targeting the 16S rRNA, GroEL and 18S rRNA genes of a number of microorganisms present in faeces and other forensically relevant fluids.

4. Retrospective Analysis of RNA Typing in Forensic Casework

4.1. Requests and Results for RNA Typing in Casework

Forensic casework comes in great diversity, and questions can be put forward that cannot be addressed with existing methodologies. This feeds the development of new methods, like RNA typing assays which were especially triggered by the limitations for the tests for vaginal cellular material and menstrual secretion [72,204–207] and the difficulties to apply immunohistochemical staining for organ tissues to samplings from bullets where the tissue tends to reside in the grooves [208]. It is interesting to reflect, in a retrospective manner, on which forensic questions RNA typing assays are applied in actual forensic casework, and whether this corresponds to the questions that initially triggered the development of the assays.

RNA typing has been applied regularly at the Netherlands Forensic Institute since 2012. RNA was extracted in 452 cases and in 238 of these cases, RNA typing was performed (in the other 214 cases, RNA was extracted but RNA typing was not (yet) requested by police or prosecution). In 178 cases (75%) body fluid typing was performed and in 60 cases (25%) organ typing. On average, RNA is extracted for four samples per case. To study the context and details of cases in which RNA typing was performed, the details of 27 body fluid cases analyzed in 2020 were examined. All 27 cases were sexual assaults, of which 25 questioned the presence of vaginal cellular material (note that at the NFI presumptive tests are used to assess the presence of blood, saliva, and seminal fluid). The 26th case aimed to discern menstrual or peripheral blood in a vaginal sampling of an assaulted female and the 27th case questioned the presence of semen or seminal fluid on the genitals of an adolescent female (generally the presence of semen is not assessed through RNA typing but microscopic analysis and differential extraction is used). Thus, in the Netherlands, RNA body fluid typing is mostly applied in sexual assault cases to assess the presence of vaginal cellular material.

In the 25 cases that assessed vaginal cellular material, 56 samples were analyzed of which 19 resulted in vaginal cellular material detected (13 cases). In nine samples (four cases), saliva was detected (one of these samples, a penile swab, was also positive for vaginal cellular material; the other saliva-positive samples were all finger/nail dirt samplings). The corresponding DNA profiles of 53 of these 56 samples were mixed male/female profiles, while three showed no male (amelogenin Y) DNA and a full female profile (samplings from paper tissue, condom, or finger). The male/female ratio at the amelogenin locus in these mixed samples varied from 0.8 to 178, but this bore no relation to whether vaginal cellular material was seen or not. This is not unexpected as these are casework specimens, not ground truth data, and the female component may derive from other cells, for example skin cells, which are no longer included in the NFI body fluid RNA assay used in 2020.

4.2. RNA Typing Results in Verdicts

The ultimate value of RNA typing is best assessed by regarding verdicts after trial procedures (the proof is in the pudding). In the Dutch registry of verdicts [209], 21 cases can be found in which RNA typing was actively considered in the verdict by the judge (note that not all verdicts are taken up in the registry and that the judge decided on the use of the RNA results in the context of all evidence presented, in most cases without data on prevalence of such RNA results in alternative scenarios).

Ten cases were sexual assaults and 11 cases were not. For the sexual assaults, in nine cases the presence of vaginal cellular material was of importance; in one case menstrual secretion. These body fluids were found four times on a penis, three times on a finger/nail dirt, once in underpants of a male, once on the outside of a condom and once on an inserted item (in this case a piece of ginger; a cultural punishment by a father). In eight of these ten cases, the defense presented alternative scenarios: once the timing of deposition was questioned ("the forensic report does not state when the menstrual secretion was deposited on the penis"). In six cases, secondary transfer was suggested: Three times vaginal material was supposedly picked up from either an item carrying vaginal material, or from being nearby the victim's vagina or from an unspecified source and then transferred to the penis. Vaginal cells on fingers of the suspect were suggested to originate from the victim touching her vagina and then shaking hands with the suspect, or from an unspecified activity. Vaginal cells in male underpants were suggested to originate from assisting the victim during vomiting after which her cellular material was transferred to his penis and underpants after a toilet visit (RNA typing was performed much later so the alternative scenario focused on explaining the female DNA). For a case with the presence of vaginal cells on the outside of a condom, the alternative scenario was that the father masturbated using a condom and that the results of vaginal cells and DNA-match with the adolescent daughter should be ignored as the mother was not included in the comparison (note that the DNA-profile fully matched the daughter).

These alternative scenarios follow three of the four general scenarios proposed in Section 1.1. These were: (1) 'time of deposition', (2) 'secondary transfer' and (3) 'innocent explanation'; 'another person performed the crime' was not proposed. This makes sense as most of the evidentiary items involved body parts such as finger/nail dirt or penis.

In the remaining 11 verdicts considering RNA typing results, the evidentiary items included two bullets, two knives, a baseball bat, five pieces of clothing and a bed sheet. The cellular material found on these items matched the victim(s) in all 11 cases. Of the 11 cases, nine cases were analyzed for organ tissues and two for body fluids. Both multiplexes contain markers for blood, and in all 11 cases, blood was present in the stains analyzed. In four cases, CNS tissue was found as well (not necessarily in all evidentiary stains analyzed within a case; all four cases involved samplings taken from clothing). In five cases, skeletal muscle was detected (both cases that involved a knife, one of the cases involving a bullet and two cases involving clothing: for these latter two cases, CNS was observed in stains analyzed within the case as well). In one of the two cases analyzed for body fluids, besides blood, saliva was found in a mist-like pattern indicating expirated blood (this case was analyzed using a body fluid assay not yet carrying nasal mucosa markers).

The alternative scenarios put forward by the defense fall into three categories: once the time of deposition was questioned (this was for the case in which expirated blood was implied; the suspect was suggested to have visited the scene a day later when the victims had already died). Five times it was suggested that another person was involved (twice handling the knife, three times wearing the clothing that contained CNS material matching the victim). Five times another explanation was given (the suspect shot at a car not at the victim; the victim started shooting first so it was self-defense; the victim fell of the stairs (for the case in which blood was found on a baseball bat); the injuries were self-inflicted and the large puddles of blood on the bed sheets were staged by using animal or menstrual blood (this was the second case analyzed by body fluid typing); the CNS and blood on the clothing of the suspect are not shown to be the result of violence (no suggestion was given how CNS did end up on trousers and a shirt).

For these cases, the alternative scenarios follow three of the four general scenarios proposed in Section 1.1. These were: (1) 'time of deposition', (2) 'another person performed the crime' and (3) 'innocent explanation'; 'secondary transfer' was not proposed. This makes sense, as in these cases, generous amounts of cellular material matching the victim(s) were found for which it is more difficult to invoke secondary transfer.

5. A Criminalistic View on Targets to Be Included in a Cell Typing Assay

Basically, there are two main reasons to include markers for a body fluid or an organ tissue in a cell typing assay: (1) the cell type can be questioned in forensic cases and (2) the cell type can be informative to an alternative, innocent explanation.

5.1. Cell Types Questioned in Forensic Cases

From the case descriptions in Section 4.1, it is evident that in sexual assault allegations, most often the presence of vaginal cellular material and menstrual secretions is questioned.

Semen (spermatozoa and/or seminal fluid) can be involved as well, generally in three circumstances: (1) as questioned body fluid in a sample in which semen is expected to be the predominant body fluid such as in a ejaculation stain on the body or clothing of the victim or inside a condom; (2) as a questioned body fluid in a sample containing a surplus amount of other cellular material such as in a vaginal, oral or rectal sample taken from the victim; or (3) as a background body fluid in a penile swab or finger/nail dirt sample that is examined for the presence of, for example, vaginal cellular material.

Under circumstance (1), semen will be the predominant cell type, and, in most cases, microscopic analysis will suffice to show presence of spermatozoa and generate a DNA profile for the semen donor. In circumstance (2), when a surplus amount of cellular material of the victim is present, differential extraction (DE), (in which a mild lysis to extract nucleic acids from non-spermatozoa cells, followed by a strong lysis to extract nucleic acids of the spermatozoa) is likely performed. Since the presence of semen is questioned, most often this DE method will suffice and produce a sperm fraction from which a DNA profile informative for the semen donor is derived. When confirmation of the presence of spermatozoa in the sperm fraction is needed, various methods can be applied such as microscopic analysis or MSRE analysis [154,155,210,211] on DNA extracted from the sperm fraction [212]

This is different in circumstance (3), where semen may be present in such amounts that it masks the presence of other body fluids. Here, it would be useful to apply a DE method that not only extracts DNA but also RNA and analyze the non-sperm RNA fraction for cell types other than spermatozoa (note that seminal fluid RNA will end up in this non-sperm RNA fraction as well). However, DE is hard to combine with RNA extraction as RNases are active during the mild lysis step unless an ample amount of strong RNase inhibitors is used [104].

Other body fluids of which the presence may be questioned, are saliva and peripheral blood. For blood, molecular analyses are mostly applied for discerning peripheral blood and menstrual secretion. Saliva may be assessed in allegations of licking, which means that often body locations are sampled (breasts, genitals, mouth), and mixed DNA profiles are expected.

To assess allegations of anal penetration, the identification of a rectal mucosa marker was described recently [213]. A rectal mucosa marker is to be preferred over markers for fecal matter as rectal mucosa provides a more direct link to invasive activities. Finding a marker specific for rectal mucosa is challenging since many body cavities and tubular organs in the human body are lined by mucous membranes (for instance, along the respiratory, digestive, and urogenital tract), an epithelial tissue that secretes mucus. Thus, specificity of mucous membrane genes may be an issue, they may prove general mucosa markers or cross-react with some other body fluid derived from a mucous membrane [98,214].

5.2. Cell Types Informing on an Alternative Scenario

The second reason to include markers for a specific body fluid in a cell typing assay is to inform an alternative, innocent explanation for the findings. Nasal secretion has a high cellular content and may therefore leave detectable amounts after secondary transfer, which may be proposed as an alternative scenario (H1: vaginal penetration by penis; H2: victim sneezes in hand, shakes hand of the suspect, suspect touches his penis during toilet visit). Thus, nasal secretion markers have been identified and included in body fluid typing assays [104,215]. In addition, the presence of nasal secretion and blood in a sample may indicate nosebleed blood, that can be a spontaneous occurrence not connected to a crime. Occasionally, nasal secretion may be among the questioned body fluid such as in case of expiration of blood (here saliva markers will also be informative) or when a nosebleed is caused in a fight.

Other body fluids for which markers have been identified are urine and sweat [128,216–218]. These two body fluids have a relatively low cellular amount and are likely of limited importance. Urine may contribute some cellular material in underpants; sweat can be deposited together with skin. Skin was one of the earlier cell types for which mRNA markers were identified [98,219–222], probably because contact traces are frequently submitted for forensic analyses. However, forensic practice in the Netherlands has shown that there is hardly any value in showing the presence of skin, as skin residues reside in almost all submitted samples. The presence of skin and DNA of a person of interest may be regarded mistakenly as an indication of direct contact, and due to the abundance of epithelial material in public and private items [42], secondary transfer is within the bound of possibility.

For the assessment of cases of violence, various tissue types can be included. CNS tissue (brain and spinal cord) is highly important to include in the assays because of the often-lethal consequences. Other organs such as liver, heart, kidney, lung, trachea, intestine, stomach, spleen can be included for chest and abdominal injuries, but blood, muscular tissue and/or adipose are informative for injuries anywhere on a body [223–225].

5.3. Fluids and Tissues Carry Multiple Cell Types

In a human body, there are ~210 cell types [226], and body fluids and organs contain several types of cells (semen may be an exception as semen carries besides spermatozoa only few other cell types).

As evidentiary stains may be minute, not all cell types may be represented in a sample, so it can be opportune to include markers for various cell types from one tissue or fluid in an assay. For example, CNS tissue comprises two major tissues: grey matter and white matter. Grey matter (~10% of the tissue in the brain volume) consists mainly of neuronal cell bodies (and unmyelinated axons and glial cells), while white matter (the deeper layer) mainly contains myelinated axons (and astrocytes and oligodendrocytes that produce myelin) [227]. Whether an evidentiary stain carries predominantly grey or white matter, will affect which markers can respond.

With body fluids, samplings may have a more even distribution of cell types, due to the liquid constitution. These have different biological functions that affect their localization. For example, red blood cells function within the blood (amongst others for carriage of oxygen) while white blood cells act mostly outside of the bloodstream (immune system). As a consequence, white blood cells crawl into the lymphatic system by a process denoted extravasation [228]). The lymphatic system is an extensive drainage network and several other forensically relevant body fluids may thereby carry white blood cells (e.g., nasal secretion [228]).

It is crucial to understand the biological function and performance on other body fluids or tissues for markers included in a cell typing assay.

6. Interpretation of Cell Typing Results

Generally, an evidentiary stain that is subjected for cell type analysis is also submitted for DNA profiling as one wishes to infer what cell type is donated by which person. This invokes a three-way interpretation: (1) the DNA profile; (2) the cell typing data and 3) the combination aiming to associate donor and cell type. The interpretation of DNA profiles has progressed tremendously through the application of probabilistic software [229–233] that use information on the number of contributors, allele frequencies, peak height, drop-in, dropout, degradation and more to provide a weight of evidence in the form of a likelihood ratio (LR). The LR includes a person of interest under H1 (H2 generally calculates the likelihood for an unknown, unrelated person). With the interpretation of cell typing data, several issues are to be considered: (1) limitations in sensitivity; (2) constraints for specificity; (3) degradation in evidentiary stains; (4) complications in case of a mixture of cell types and (5) providing an evidential value. These issues are discussed below, followed by developments on the association of donor and cell type.

6.1. Sensitivity, Specificity and Degradation Issues Affecting Interpretation

Ideally, a cell typing method has similar sensitivity for all cell types assessed in an assay, and a similar sensitivity as DNA profiling so that for all donors that give DNA information cell type information is derived as well. Over time, DNA profiling has become more and more sensitive and a full DNA profile can be generated from DNA amounts that equate to a few cells. The sensitivity of cell typing depends greatly on the type of marker that is used. DNA-based markers (those assessing methylation status) will at best be as sensitive as DNA profiling as both analyze features of the two genomic DNA copies. MSRE analysis [154,155,210,211] indeed approaches the sensitivity of DNA profiling, but methods that rely on a bisulfite conversion are much less sensitive as a large portion of DNA is lost during the conversion [146,147].

RNA and protein/ enzyme markers are expressed and translated from DNA and may be several folds more abundant than DNA although expression levels can vary highly for different genes, and abundance is further influenced by stability/ turnover rates. Environmental and physiological factors may cause variation between people and over time (an infection will increase the number of white blood cells and the mRNAs these cells contain). Thus, it appears inevitable that the sensitivity of markers targeting either the same or different body fluids will vary [121] despite careful marker selection and assay optimization. An extreme example is semen from an azoospermic male, which will provide RNA and proteins for seminal fluid but little DNA (or spermatozoa mRNAs/ proteins). Thorough validation by which understanding of marker performance is obtained is of pivotal importance.

Specificity issues can relate to human-specificity or tissue-specificity [234]. Methods that analyze nucleic acids, can most often be designed to be human (or at least primate)-specific, which is less feasible for tests based on enzyme activity or antibodies. Processes such as readthrough or spurious transcription giving rise to non-specific background expression of mRNAs may result in signals above the detection threshold for the assay, especially when samples are over-amplified (by using too much input or too many amplification cycles). Technological imperfections can also cause non-specific signals like remnants of DNA in RNA assays (this is only an issue when it is not possible to design cDNA-specific amplicons with for instance one primer spanning an exon-exon boundary) or incomplete bisulfite conversion in methylation-based assays. The most difficult form of non-specificity is when markers cross-react with cell types other than the intended cell type. This occurs more with body fluids than with organs. For instance, saliva, nasal secretion and vaginal material are produced in body cavities (oral, nasal, vaginal) that are all lined with mucous membranes. These can, as previously mentioned, give rise to expression of the same mucous markers in these body fluids (denoted general mucosa markers [98]). These non-specific responses can show inter-individual variation: mRNA vaginal markers were detected in nasal secretions in many donors, with no relation to gender or having a cold [104]. As with sensitivity, thorough validation with different donors is highly important to understand marker performance.

Outside the human body, factors such as high humidity, UV radiation and/or high temperature can invoke degradation of nucleic acids, especially when stains have not fully dried. DNA is more resistant to hydrolysis than RNA, as the 2′-OH group can attack the 3′-phosphate, leading to hydrolytic cleavage of the phosphodiester bond, which may lead to samples providing a DNA but no or hardly an RNA profile [97]. Amplicons in RNA assays are therefore generally shorter (preferably under ~150 base pairs) than in DNA typing (up to ~450 base pairs). Intramolecular base pairing within RNA molecules (not only G:C and A:U but also G:U) may result in secondary and tertiary structures that provide more stability to certain regions, and amplicons targeting such stable RNA regions (StaRs) [95,235] may enhance RNA profiling. DNA methylation assays have the advantage of using the same nucleic acid as used for DNA profiling, so there is no difference in stability (the methylation marks remain stable also in body fluids deposited outside a human body [236]).

6.2. Interpretation of Mixed Samples

RNA casework has shown that most evidentiary samples contain multiple fluids/tissues, particularly with body fluid typing and less so with organ typing. One cause is that many samplings are taken from body locations (penis, fingers) or fabrics (clothing, bedding) that are likely to carry skin and other body fluid depositions. Moreover, the contributions may be highly unbalanced. To work on mixtures, markers should best respond in on-off modus meaning that a signal is obtained when the body fluid is present and not when a body fluid is absent. This can be achieved with RNA-based assays when markers are selected that show a large difference in expression between target and non-target tissues. Over-amplification needs to be avoided and detection thresholds need to be set.

For methylation-based assays, application to mixtures depends on the technology that is chosen. With MSRE, CpG targets are selected that are only methylated in the target tissue (this does not need to be a 100% methylation). PCR product can only be generated when the restriction enzyme is unable to cut the DNA due to methylation of the restriction site [237].

When methylation levels are assessed quantitively, for instance by sequencing bisulfite-converted DNA, it is highly complex to set interpretation guidelines for mixed samples. For example, when a chosen marker shows on average a 50% methylation rate in vaginal mucosa and 10% in other cell types, a 20% methylation level for the marker in an evidentiary sample can occur in different ways: (1) no vaginal mucosa is present and the methylation level of the other cell types (skin and/or semen) turns out higher than the average of 10%; (2) vaginal mucosa is present and no other cell types and the 20% methylation rate is an outlier for vaginal mucosa; (3) vaginal mucosa is mixed with other cell types for which a ratio of 1:3 would nicely explain the methylation rate of 20%. In this example, the DNA profile may be informative as a female donor will correspond to vaginal mucosa and the male donor to semen (if detected), but assumptions may need to made, for example, that no saliva from either one of the donors is present. When choosing a methodology for casework application, its suitability for mixed samples needs to be considered to enable appropriate interpretation.

6.3. Reporting Cell Typing Results

In expert reports, cell typing results are generally given as 'indication for the presence of' when genetic markers or tests for a body fluid or organ tissue are observed. With RNA typing, interpretation thresholds are applied as both drop-in and dropout may occur, due to limitations in sensitivity and specificity described above. These interpretation thresholds can include a numerical scoring [238], or a strategy of using replicates and a 50% rule in which at least half of the markers over all replicates need to be detected [111]. All have the drawback that they represent a 'fall-of-the-cliff' method, which means that the detection of one marker more or less may change the interpretation of the results.

Nowadays, the general trend in forensic reporting is to provide an evidential value, for example by presenting a likelihood ratio; the probability of the evidence given two competing hypotheses, H1 and H2. Formulating H1 can be straightforward ('the sample contains vaginal cellular material'); formulating H2 is more complex as it could be 'the sample does not contain vaginal cellular material' or 'the sample contains another body fluid'. These hypotheses follow the simplifying assumption of one body fluid per sample. More realistic hypotheses consider mixtures and could be formulated as H1: 'the sample contains vaginal cellular material, and possibly other body fluids' and H2: 'the sample does not contain vaginal cellular material, but other body fluids' (note that one could also specify these other body fluids). Conditioning on cellular material assumed to be present (for instance, because the sample is a penile swab) would generate hypotheses like H1: 'the sample contains vaginal cellular material, and penile skin and possibly other body fluids' and H2: 'the sample does not contain vaginal cellular material, but penile skin and possibly other body fluids'.

Some statistical approaches have been proposed for body fluid typing; for organ typing, a multivariate statistical model was trained [120,239–242]. The basis of such models is an experimental dataset consisting of ground truth data, that should be casework representative. This is challenging as casework includes a wide range of samples for which the true composition is not known. It is not trivial to prepare such a dataset, and the LR should be calibrated to suit the size of the dataset (note that for DNA datasets the allele frequencies are used, while with RNA datasets an RNA profile is considered in its entirety). Reporting the LR in a verbal scale rather than a numerical value, seems more appropriate. Clearly, further development is needed, although the developments are promising.

6.4. Associating Donor and Body Fluid

A challenge for any forensic RNA typing method is the association of donor and body fluid. Complications are that one body fluid can be given by multiple donors and/or one donor can give multiple body fluids. Even with simple mixtures of two donors each giving one body fluid, it was shown that peak heights in DNA and RNA profiles cannot be used straightforwardly [97]. Only with gender-specific body fluids (vaginal cellular material and semen) and the involvement (or assumption) of one donor of that gender, is association of donor and body fluid possible. This introduces the risk of an association fallacy [2,243]. Thus, alternative procedures are being developed like SNPs (single nucleotide polymorphisms) in transcribed regions (RNA-SNPs) [242,244–246]. The concept is that the RNA indicates which cell type is present and that, as the RNA is transcribed from DNA, the genetic variation within this transcribed region provides information on the identity of the donor. First, which cell types are present is assessed, then the genotype for the RNA-SNPs of the donors that are assumed to be present are derived by genotyping their reference DNA (since this is DNA, there is no need to provide the body fluid questioned) and lastly the RNA of the stain is sequenced to see what SNPs are present in the transcribed mRNA to see if/ who of the donors matches this sequence.

This is a developing area with multiple challenges at hand: (1) SNPs can affect the stability or transcription level of RNAs, so the genotypes at the DNA and RNA level may not align (for instance one appears heterozygous at the DNA level but since the presence of a SNP affects RNA stability or expression level, one appears homozygous at the RNA level; (2) linked SNPs should be regarded according to their genetic phase (equivalent to a microhaplotype), which may be complicated when different SNPs reside in different amplicons; (3) the approach is only to be explored for samples in which all donors can be assumed as there is no clear strategy/consensus yet on how to deal with unknown donors. It is probably best to limit the approach initially to two-person mixtures.

CpG-SNPs (SNPs nearby CpGs indicative of cell types) have also been described [247,248]. Methods not depending on bisulfite conversion (such as MSRE) may be most practical to use to detect these as the bisulfite conversion will affect all non-methylated cytosines complicating SNP detection and primer design. A MS-HRM assay targeting DACT1 that is hypomethylated in semen was used [249] to determine if it was possible to associate semen with a DNA profile in a mixture. Some progress was made, and it was possible to determine whether the semen compromised the majority, almost half, or was in the minority of the components in a mixed fluid.

7. Further Considerations
7.1. Other Marker Types and Technologies That Have Been Explored
7.1.1. Non-Coding RNAs

Various non-coding RNAs have been explored as markers for body fluid and tissue identification.

miRNAs are a class of small RNA molecules, 18–25 nucleotides in length, which are involved in the regulation (repression) of mRNA translation and stability [69,71]. with various forensic applications including body fluid identification [250].

Adult-specific roles for miRNAs (adult physiology, cancer development or suppression) have been described in various stem cell populations [251] and show continuous/ steady expression. This means these markers may be less specific for body fluid and tissue identification than might be suggested by the highly specific expression patterns seen in embryos [252]. Additionally, since human miRNAs generally interact through limited base pairing of only a few bases in the 5′ part of the miRNA, a miRNA can bind to many targets. Conversely, an mRNA may be targeted by several (different) miRNAs. For these reasons, a key limitation of miRNAs is their specificity. Nonetheless, many studies have proposed miRNAs for body fluids such as blood, saliva, menstrual blood and semen [253–257] and body tissues including brain, liver, skeletal muscle and skin [258]. miRNAs are stable [259] and have been shown to be detectable in forensic-like samples when treated to a range of environmental conditions [218,260] after laundering [261].

Methods to analyze miRNAs primarily include miRNA expression profiles to identify candidate markers, followed by qPCR to test specificity [253,255,256,258,262]. Some approaches include the extraction and analysis of miRNA and DNA together [263] and multiplexed miRNA panels [264] able to discriminate between venous blood, menstrual blood, semen, and saliva. High throughput sequencing of miRNAs from body fluid samples has also been used to identify new candidates [265]. Statistical methods and reference (endogenous) miRNA markers [262] are needed to measure miRNA expression with qPCR. Recently classification algorithms have been applied to the interpretation of miRNA profiles as detection is not a simple yes–no answer [259].

The longest known class of small non-coding RNA are the piwi-interacting RNA (piRNA), 26–31 nucleotides in length. Their role is in the transcriptional and post-transcriptional silencing of transposable elements which may be differentially expressed in different body fluids making them suitable candidates for identifying body fluids (although transposon silencing is foremost important in the germline where piRNAs were initially found [266]).

Two papers [267,268] describe the characterization by RNA sequencing of piRNA expression profiles and the selection of three piRNA markers (piR-hsa-27622, piR-hsa-1207 and piR-hsa-27493) that distinguish between venous blood and menstrual blood and a further two (piR-hsa-27493 and piR-hsa-26591) to distinguish between saliva and vaginal material, implemented as TaqMan RT-qPCR assays.

Short interfering RNA (siRNA) are another class of small non-coding RNA with a role in gene expression [269]. To date there are no reports of their use as markers in forensic science, perhaps because their role is to interfere with the expression of specific genes, by degrading RNA after transcription, rather than to promote the expression or modification of specific transcripts.

Long non-coding RNAs (lncRNAs) are RNA transcripts not translated into proteins that appear to be involved in the regulation of gene expression. Approximately 78% of them are tissue-based compared to approximately 18% of mRNA transcripts. One of the best studied is the X-inactive-based transcript (XIST) involved in X-chromosome inactivation [270,271]. To date, XIST has been incorporated into an assay [272] to positively identify male and female cell material in forensic samples with a second study [273] further testing the assay on forensic type samples.

7.1.2. Proteome

All body fluids and tissues contain unique proteomes, derived from the expression of mRNAs (see Section 3.1.1) in turn derived from the genome. In the past, unique proteins of each body fluid or tissue type have been detected and presumptively identified by determination of the enzyme activity (acid phosphatase for example) or immunological properties (RSID tests (Independent Forensics, Lombard, IL, USA) for example). More recently technological developments in proteomics, as for genomics, have highlighted potential benefits for forensic identification purposes and useful reviews of the forensic potential have been published [274–276].

Mass spectrometry (MS) is the analytical method of choice with advantages including high sensitivity and specificity [277]. Generally, candidate markers are found by *de novo* analysis or from reference proteomes, then validated by testing on known samples. By detecting multiple peptides in a single assay from more than one protein per fluid, the assay can be considered not only confirmatory but also human-based and suitable for mixtures. Sensitive and specific assays have been developed including blood, semen, seminal fluid, saliva, vaginal/ menstrual fluid and urine [277–280] using methods such as matrix-assisted laser desorption/ionization (MALDI) MS [277], quadrupole time-of-flight MS [278,279] MALDI MS Profiling and Imaging [281] and MALDI time-of-flight MS [282] from samples as diverse as blood-stained finger marks [281] and blood and vaginal cellular material under fingernails [282], although difficulties in identifying urine recovered from substrates and semen samples that had been mixed with lubricants were found [280]. A challenge to be addressed is that the protein content of each fluid/ tissue varies considerably, and whilst it is possible to detect very small amounts of blood in saliva, the opposite was not true [277–279].

MS methods tend to be destructive to the sample, however in a recent report [283] a new approach, sheath-flow probe electrospray ionisation MS was used, which allows stains to be sampled with no preparation or sample destruction bar the initial small amount taken. In the research which examined blood, saliva and urine, alterations were observed in the spectra over time suggesting that this approach could also be used to age a stain.

The relationship between the proteome and the genome offers the possibility for proteomic "genotyping" [284,285] in a similar manner to the suggested RNA SNP and CpG SNP approaches described in Section 6.4. This has clear advantages when DNA in a sample is compromised in quality and quantity such as in a hair shaft, as proteins are more stable and resistant to damage and decay than DNA. Genetic variations in human DNA can be linked to mutations found in hair proteins (genetically variant peptides (GVPs) referred to as single amino acid polymorphisms, SAPs, which in turn can be associated with their DNA counterparts (missense SNPs). GVPs containing SAPs can be identified by mapping these peptide sequences using MS and results have been obtained from short lengths of human hair [275,286]. Not only could this approach be used to "identify" and link individuals, but it can also be used to infer ancestry as SNP profiles varied between ancestral groups.

7.1.3. Aptamers

Aptamers are single-stranded oligonucleotides or peptides that are selected using SELEX (systematic evolution of ligands by exponential enrichment) in a sequential process to bind their target molecules in a highly specific and sensitive manner. Initial studies used RNA aptamers [287,288], with the first description of a DNA aptamer in 1992 [289] and the first XNA aptamer capable of binding to a small molecule (ochratoxin A) in 2018 [290]. Aptamers have a number of advantages over assays such as the immunochromatogenic-based methods described in Section 2.2.1. Consistent aptamer synthesis methods, more straightforward functionalization, equivalent binding affinities and cheaper long term and stable production are all factors.

Aptamers are now widely used as biosensors in a large number of fields [291,292] with significant and recent examples seen for the rapid detection of SARS-CoV-2 [293,294] and have potential for the use in forensic science [295]. Aptamers have been developed to detect PSA [296], hemoglobin [297] and more recently, aptamers to detect spermatozoa have been described using a combination of Cell-SELEX and massively parallel sequencing technologies [295]. Once suitably specific and sensitive aptamers are obtained, they can be built into a range of sensors for detection many of them suitable for field deployment.

8. Concluding Remarks

Preferably, body fluid typing and DNA profiling (to answer the what and the who question) are analyzed on the exact same sample. This can be achieved when the DNA extract is used for cell type inference (as with methylation analysis) or when RNA is extracted from a fraction normally discarded during DNA extraction (like a flow through fraction when binding DNA to a silica column). Case reports have been published for both methylation [298] and RNA-based assays [299]. The advantage of using DNA for body fluid typing is that no additional extraction procedure is needed; the disadvantage is that less DNA remains for further analyses such as Y-STR profiling, mtDNA analysis or the prediction of age, ancestry, appearance. Microbiome analysis can use either DNA or RNA. The global COVID-19 pandemic has stimulated the development of assays that may find their use in forensic analysis such as multiplexed and extraction-free amplification assays [300], which may provide RNA-based tests prior to DNA extraction and analysis that may present the opportunity of triage. Such extraction-free methods [301] present pioneering opportunities beyond advancements such as one-step RT-PCR methods that simplify current methodology [302].

Introducing cell typing methodologies in a forensic laboratory requires extensive validation, implementation of interpretation and reporting, and explaining results for judiciary. This comes with additional costs (also because the technique itself may ask quite some hands-on laboratory work) and it has been suggested that it is best performed or outsourced to specialized laboratories.

Author Contributions: S.H. and T.S. both wrote sections of the original draft (S.H. Sections 2, 3 and 7; T.S. Sections 1 and 4–6). Reviewing and editing was performed by both S.H. and T.S. The authors apologize that not all literature could be referenced. All authors have read and agreed to the published version of the manuscript.

Funding: This research received no external funding.

Acknowledgments: We thank Margreet van den Berge (NFI) and Stephanie Opperman (ESR) for critical reading of parts of the manuscript.

Conflicts of Interest: The authors declare no conflict of interest.

References

1. Taylor, D.; Kokshoorn, B.; Biedermann, A. Evaluation of Forensic Genetics Findings given Activity Level Propositions: A Review. *Forensic Sci. Int. Genet.* **2018**, *36*, 34–49. [CrossRef]
2. Meakin, G.E.; Kokshoorn, B.; Oorschot, R.A.H.; Szkuta, B. Evaluating Forensic DNA Evidence: Connecting the Dots. *WIREs Forensic Sci.* **2021**, *3*, e1404. [CrossRef]
3. Gill, P.; Hicks, T.; Butler, J.M.; Connolly, E.; Gusmão, L.; Kokshoorn, B.; Morling, N.; van Oorschot, R.A.H.; Parson, W.; Prinz, M.; et al. DNA Commission of the International Society for Forensic Genetics: Assessing the Value of Forensic Biological Evidence—Guidelines Highlighting the Importance of Propositions: Part I: Evaluation of DNA Profiling Comparisons given (Sub-) Source Propositions. *Forensic Sci. Int. Genet.* **2018**, *36*, 189–202. [CrossRef]
4. Gill, P.; Hicks, T.; Butler, J.M.; Connolly, E.; Gusmão, L.; Kokshoorn, B.; Morling, N.; van Oorschot, R.A.H.; Parson, W.; Prinz, M.; et al. DNA Commission of the International Society for Forensic Genetics: Assessing the Value of Forensic Biological Evidence—Guidelines Highlighting the Importance of Propositions. Part II: Evaluation of Biological Traces Considering Activity Level Propositions. *Forensic Sci. Int. Genet.* **2020**, *44*, 102186. [CrossRef]
5. Jackson, G.; Biedermann, A. "Source" or "Activity" What Is the Level of Issue in a Criminal Trial? *Significance* **2019**, *16*, 36–39. [CrossRef]
6. Pope, S.; Biedermann, A. Editorial: The Dialogue Between Forensic Scientists, Statisticians and Lawyers About Complex Scientific Issues for Court. *Front. Genet.* **2020**, *11*, 704. [CrossRef]
7. Puch-Solis, R.; Pope, S. Interpretation of DNA Data within the Context of UK Forensic Science—Evaluation. *Emerg. Top. Life Sci.* **2021**, *5*, 405–413. [CrossRef]
8. Pope, S.; Puch-Solis, R. Interpretation of DNA Data within the Context of UK Forensic Science—Investigation. *Emerg. Top. Life Sci.* **2021**, *5*, 395–404. [CrossRef] [PubMed]
9. Lin, H.; Zhang, Y.; Wang, Q.; Li, B.; Huang, P.; Wang, Z. Estimation of the Age of Human Bloodstains under the Simulated Indoor and Outdoor Crime Scene Conditions by ATR-FTIR Spectroscopy. *Sci. Rep.* **2017**, *7*, 13254. [CrossRef]
10. Stotesbury, T.; Cossette, M.-L.; Newell-Bell, T.; Shafer, A.B.A. An Exploratory Time Since Deposition Analysis of Whole Blood Using Metrics of DNA Degradation and Visible Absorbance Spectroscopy. *Pure Appl. Geophys.* **2021**, *178*, 735–743. [CrossRef]
11. Weber, A.R.; Lednev, I.K. Crime Clock—Analytical Studies for Approximating Time since Deposition of Bloodstains. *Forensic Chem.* **2020**, *19*, 100248. [CrossRef]
12. Bremmer, R.H.; Nadort, A.; van Leeuwen, T.G.; van Gemert, M.J.C.; Aalders, M.C.G. Age Estimation of Blood Stains by Hemoglobin Derivative Determination Using Reflectance Spectroscopy. *Forensic Sci. Int.* **2011**, *206*, 166–171. [CrossRef] [PubMed]
13. Edelman, G.; van Leeuwen, T.G.; Aalders, M.C.G. Hyperspectral Imaging for the Age Estimation of Blood Stains at the Crime Scene. *Forensic Sci. Int.* **2012**, *223*, 72–77. [CrossRef] [PubMed]
14. Alshehhi, S.; Haddrill, P.R. Estimating Time since Deposition Using Quantification of RNA Degradation in Body Fluid-Specific Markers. *Forensic Sci. Int.* **2019**, *298*, 58–63. [CrossRef]
15. Alshehhi, S.; Haddrill, P.R. Evaluating the Effect of Body Fluid Mixture on the Relative Expression Ratio of Blood-Specific RNA Markers. *Forensic Sci. Int.* **2020**, *307*, 110116. [CrossRef]
16. Fu, J.; Allen, R.W. A Method to Estimate the Age of Bloodstains Using Quantitative PCR. *Forensic Sci. Int. Genet.* **2019**, *39*, 103–108. [CrossRef]
17. Heneghan, N.; Fu, J.; Pritchard, J.; Payton, M.; Allen, R.W. The Effect of Environmental Conditions on the Rate of RNA Degradation in Dried Blood Stains. *Forensic Sci. Int. Genet.* **2021**, *51*, 102456. [CrossRef]
18. Weinbrecht, K.D.; Fu, J.; Payton, M.E.; Allen, R.W. Time-Dependent Loss of mRNA Transcripts from Forensic Stains. *Res. Rep. Forensic Med. Sci.* **2017**, *7*, 1–12. [CrossRef]
19. Salzmann, A.P.; Russo, G.; Kreutzer, S.; Haas, C. Degradation of Human mRNA Transcripts over Time as an Indicator of the Time since Deposition (TsD) in Biological Crime Scene Traces. *Forensic Sci. Int. Genet.* **2021**, *53*, 102524. [CrossRef]
20. Díez López, C.; Kayser, M.; Vidaki, A. Estimating the Time Since Deposition of Saliva Stains With a Targeted Bacterial DNA Approach: A Proof-of-Principle Study. *Front. Microbiol.* **2021**, *12*, 1102. [CrossRef]
21. Gill, P.; Bleka, Ø.; Roseth, A.; Fonneløp, A.E. An LR Framework Incorporating Sensitivity Analysis to Model Multiple Direct and Secondary Transfer Events on Skin Surface. *Forensic Sci. Int. Genet.* **2021**, *53*, 102509. [CrossRef] [PubMed]
22. Puliatti, L.; Handt, O.; Taylor, D. The Level of DNA an Individual Transfers to Untouched Items in Their Immediate Surroundings. *Forensic Sci. Int. Genet.* **2021**, *54*, 102561. [CrossRef]
23. Saric, N.; Fabien, L.; Fischer, J.; Hermelin, A.; Massonnet, G.; Burnier, C. A Preliminary Investigation of Transfer of Condom Lubricants in the Vaginal Matrix. *Forensic Sci. Int.* **2021**, *325*, 110847. [CrossRef]
24. Kelly, P.; Connolly, E. The Prevalence and Persistence of Saliva in Vehicles. *Forensic Sci. Int. Genet.* **2021**, *53*, 102530. [CrossRef]
25. Reither, J.B.; Gray, E.; Durdle, A.; Conlan, X.A.; van Oorschot, R.A.H.; Szkuta, B. Investigation into the Prevalence of Background DNA on Flooring within Houses and Its Transfer to a Contacting Surface. *Forensic Sci. Int.* **2021**, *318*, 110563. [CrossRef]
26. Thornbury, D.; Goray, M.; van Oorschot, R.A.H. Indirect DNA Transfer without Contact from Dried Biological Materials on Various Surfaces. *Forensic Sci. Int. Genet.* **2021**, *51*, 102457. [CrossRef]
27. Tanzhaus, K.; Reiß, M.-T.; Zaspel, T. "I've Never Been at the Crime Scene!"—Gloves as Carriers for Secondary DNA Transfer. *Int. J. Legal Med.* **2021**, *135*, 1385–1393. [CrossRef]

28. Burrill, J.; Kombara, A.; Daniel, B.; Frascione, N. Exploration of Cell-Free DNA (CfDNA) Recovery for Touch Deposits. *Forensic Sci. Int. Genet.* **2021**, *51*, 102431. [CrossRef] [PubMed]

29. Schyma, C.; Madea, B.; Müller, R.; Zieger, M.; Utz, S.; Grabmüller, M. DNA-Free Does Not Mean RNA-Free—The Unwanted Persistence of RNA. *Forensic Sci. Int.* **2021**, *318*, 110632. [CrossRef]

30. Ménard, H.; Cole, C.; Gray, A.; Mudie, R.; Klu, J.K.; Nic Daéid, N. Creation of a Universal Experimental Protocol for the Investigation of Transfer and Persistence of Trace Evidence: Part 1—From Design to Implementation for Particulate Evidence. *Forensic Sci. Int. Synerg.* **2021**, *3*, 100165. [CrossRef] [PubMed]

31. Samie, L.; Taroni, F.; Champod, C. Estimating the Quantity of Transferred DNA in Primary and Secondary Transfers. *Sci. Justice J. Forensic Sci. Soc.* **2020**, *60*, 128–135. [CrossRef] [PubMed]

32. van Oorschot, R.A.H.; Szkuta, B.; Meakin, G.E.; Kokshoorn, B.; Goray, M. DNA Transfer in Forensic Science: A Review. *Forensic Sci. Int. Genet.* **2019**, *38*, 140–166. [CrossRef] [PubMed]

33. Goray, M.; Eken, E.; Mitchell, R.J.; van Oorschot, R.A.H. Secondary DNA Transfer of Biological Substances under Varying Test Conditions. *Forensic Sci. Int. Genet.* **2010**, *4*, 62–67. [CrossRef] [PubMed]

34. Goray, M.; van Oorschot, R.A.H.; Mitchell, J.R. DNA Transfer within Forensic Exhibit Packaging: Potential for DNA Loss and Relocation. *Forensic Sci. Int. Genet.* **2012**, *6*, 158–166. [CrossRef]

35. Verdon, T.J.; Mitchell, R.J.; van Oorschot, R.A.H. The Influence of Substrate on DNA Transfer and Extraction Efficiency. *Forensic Sci. Int. Genet.* **2013**, *7*, 167–175. [CrossRef]

36. Szkuta, B.; Harvey, M.L.; Ballantyne, K.N.; van Oorschot, R.A.H. DNA Transfer by Examination Tools—A Risk for Forensic Casework? *Forensic Sci. Int. Genet.* **2015**, *16*, 246–254. [CrossRef]

37. McColl, D.L.; Harvey, M.L.; van Oorschot, R.A.H. DNA Transfer by Different Parts of a Hand. *Forensic Sci. Int. Genet. Suppl. Ser.* **2017**, *6*, e29–e31. [CrossRef]

38. Lehmann, V.J.; Mitchell, R.J.; Ballantyne, K.N.; van Oorschot, R.A.H. Following the Transfer of DNA: How Far Can It Go? *Forensic Sci. Int. Genet. Suppl. Ser.* **2013**, *4*, e53–e54. [CrossRef]

39. Taylor, D.; Biedermann, A.; Samie, L.; Pun, K.-M.; Hicks, T.; Champod, C. Helping to Distinguish Primary from Secondary Transfer Events for Trace DNA. *Forensic Sci. Int. Genet.* **2017**, *28*, 155–177. [CrossRef]

40. Taylor, D.; Samie, L.; Champod, C. Using Bayesian Networks to Track DNA Movement through Complex Transfer Scenarios. *Forensic Sci. Int. Genet.* **2019**, *42*, 69–80. [CrossRef]

41. Bouzga, M.M.; Dørum, G.; Gundersen, K.; Kohler, P.; Hoff-Olsen, P.; Fonneløp, A.E. Is It Possible to Predict the Origin of Epithelial Cells?—A Comparison of Secondary Transfer of Skin Epithelial Cells versus Vaginal Mucous Membrane Cells by Direct Contact. *Sci. Justice* **2020**, *60*, 234–242. [CrossRef]

42. van den Berge, M.; Ozcanhan, G.; Zijlstra, S.; Lindenbergh, A.; Sijen, T. Prevalence of Human Cell Material: DNA and RNA Profiling of Public and Private Objects and after Activity Scenarios. *Forensic Sci. Int. Genet.* **2016**, *21*, 81–89. [CrossRef] [PubMed]

43. Van den Berge, M.; van de Merwe, L.; Sijen, T. DNA Transfer and Cell Type Inference to Assist Activity Level Reporting: Post-Activity Background Samples as a Control in Dragging Scenario. *Forensic Sci. Int. Genet. Suppl. Ser.* **2017**, *6*, e591–e592. [CrossRef]

44. Burrill, J.; Daniel, B.; Frascione, N. Illuminating Touch Deposits through Cellular Characterization of Hand Rinses and Body Fluids with Nucleic Acid Fluorescence. *Forensic Sci. Int. Genet.* **2020**, *46*, 102269. [CrossRef]

45. Cook, R.; Evett, I.W.; Jackson, G.; Jones, P.J.; Lambert, J.A. A Model for Case Assessment and Interpretation. *Sci. Justice* **1998**, *38*, 151–156. [CrossRef]

46. Evett, I.W.; Jackson, G.; Lambert, J.A. More on the Hierarchy of Propositions: Exploring the Distinction between Explanations and Propositions. *Sci. Justice* **2000**, *40*, 3–10. [CrossRef]

47. Blum, L.J.; EsperanÇA, P.; Rocquefelte, S. A New High-Performance Reagent and Procedure for Latent Bloodstain Detection Based on Luminol Chemiluminescence. *Can. Soc. Forensic Sci. J.* **2006**, *39*, 81–99. [CrossRef]

48. Quinones, I.; Sheppard, D.; Harbison, S.; Elliot, D. Comparative Analysis of Luminol Formulations. *Can. Soc. Forensic Sci. J.* **2007**, *40*, 53–63. [CrossRef]

49. Finnis, J.; Lewis, J.; Davidson, A. Comparison of Methods for Visualizing Blood on Dark Surfaces. *Sci. Justice* **2013**, *53*, 178–186. [CrossRef]

50. Patel, G.; Hopwood, A. An Evaluation of Luminol Formulations and Their Effect on DNA Profiling. *Int. J. Leg. Med.* **2013**, *127*, 723–729. [CrossRef] [PubMed]

51. Sheppard, K.; Cassella, J.P.; Fieldhouse, S.; King, R. The Adaptation of a 360° Camera Utilising an Alternate Light Source (ALS) for the Detection of Biological Fluids at Crime Scenes. *Sci. Justice J. Forensic Sci. Soc.* **2017**, *57*, 239–249. [CrossRef] [PubMed]

52. Wang, Z.; Zhang, P.; Liu, H.; Zhao, Z.; Xiong, L.; He, W.; Kwok, R.T.K.; Lam, J.W.Y.; Ye, R.; Tang, B.Z. Robust Serum Albumin-Responsive AIEgen Enables Latent Bloodstain Visualization in High Resolution and Reliability for Crime Scene Investigation. *ACS Appl. Mater. Interfaces* **2019**, *11*, 17306–17312. [CrossRef]

53. Borges, E.; Degiuli, A.; Desrentes, S.; Popielarz, C.; Blum, L.J.; Marquette, C.A. Evaluation of the SPERM TRACKER™ for Semen Stains Localization on Fabrics. *J. Forensic Res.* **2017**, *8*. [CrossRef]

54. Auvdel, M.J. Comparison of Laser and Ultraviolet Techniques Used in the Detection of Body Secretions. *J. Forensic Sci.* **1987**, *32*, 326–345. [CrossRef] [PubMed]

55. Vandenberg, N.; van Oorschot, R.A.H. The Use of Polilight® in the Detection of Seminal Fluid, Saliva, and Bloodstains and Comparison with Conventional Chemical-Based Screening Tests. *J. Forensic Sci.* **2006**, *51*, 361–370. [CrossRef] [PubMed]

56. Sterzik, V.; Panzer, S.; Apfelbacher, M.; Bohnert, M. Searching for Biological Traces on Different Materials Using a Forensic Light Source and Infrared Photography. *Int. J. Leg. Med.* **2016**, *130*, 599–605. [CrossRef]

57. Sterzik, V.; Hinderberger, P.; Panzer, S.; Bohnert, M. Visualizing Old Biological Traces on Different Materials without Using Chemicals. *Int. J. Leg. Med.* **2018**, *132*, 35–41. [CrossRef]

58. Tay, J.; Joudo, J.; Tran, T.; Ta, H.; Botting, J.; Liew, Y.; Cooper, P.; Rye, M. Comparison of Crime-Lite® 82S, Polilight® PL400 and Polilight® PL500 for the Detection of Semen and Saliva Stains. *Aust. J. Forensic Sci.* **2020**, *53*, 483–493. [CrossRef]

59. Zapata, F.; de la Ossa, M.Á.F.; García-Ruiz, C. Differentiation of Body Fluid Stains on Fabrics Using External Reflection Fourier Transform Infrared Spectroscopy (FT-IR) and Chemometrics. *Appl. Spectrosc.* **2016**, *70*, 654–665. [CrossRef]

60. Morillas, A.V.; Gooch, J.; Frascione, N. Feasibility of a Handheld near Infrared Device for the Qualitative Analysis of Bloodstains. *Talanta* **2018**, *184*, 1–6. [CrossRef] [PubMed]

61. Pereira, J.F.Q.; Silva, C.S.; Vieira, M.J.L.; Pimentel, M.F.; Braz, A.; Honorato, R.S. Evaluation and Identification of Blood Stains with Handheld NIR Spectrometer. *Microchem. J.* **2017**, *133*, 561–566. [CrossRef]

62. Edelman, G.J.; van Leeuwen, T.G.; Aalders, M.C.G. Hyperspectral Imaging of the Crime Scene for Detection and Identification of Blood Stains. In Proceedings of the Algorithms and Technologies for Multispectral, Hyperspectral, and Ultraspectral Imagery XIX, Baltimore, MD, USA, 18 May 2013; Volume 8743, pp. 47–53.

63. Edelman, G.; Manti, V.; Ruth, S.; van Leeuwen, T.; Aalders, M.C.G. Identification and Age Estimation of Blood Stains on Colored Backgrounds by near Infrared Spectroscopy. *Forensic Sci. Int.* **2012**, *220*, 239–244. [CrossRef]

64. Edelman, G.; Gaston, E.; van Leeuwen, T.; Cullen, P.J.; Aalders, M.C.G. Hyperspectral Imaging for Non-Contact Analysis of Forensic Traces. *Forensic Sci. Int.* **2012**, *223*, 28–39. [CrossRef] [PubMed]

65. Cadd, S.; Li, B.; Beveridge, P.; O'Hare, W.T.; Islam, M. Age Determination of Blood-Stained Fingerprints Using Visible Wavelength Reflectance Hyperspectral Imaging. *J. Imaging* **2018**, *4*, 141. [CrossRef]

66. Malegori, C.; Alladio, E.; Oliveri, P.; Manis, C.; Vincenti, M.; Garofano, P.; Barni, F.; Berti, A. Identification of Invisible Biological Traces in Forensic Evidences by Hyperspectral NIR Imaging Combined with Chemometrics. *Talanta* **2020**, *215*, 120911. [CrossRef]

67. Zulfiqar, M.; Ahmad, M.; Sohaib, A.; Mazzara, M.; Distefano, S. Hyperspectral Imaging for Bloodstain Identification. *Sensors* **2021**, *21*, 3045. [CrossRef] [PubMed]

68. Romaszewski, M.; Głomb, P.; Sochan, A.; Cholewa, M. A Dataset for Evaluating Blood Detection in Hyperspectral Images. *Forensic Sci. Int.* **2021**, *320*, 110701. [CrossRef]

69. Sijen, T. Molecular Approaches for Forensic Cell Type Identification: On mRNA, MiRNA, DNA Methylation and Microbial Markers. *Forensic Sci. Int. Genet.* **2015**, *18*, 21–32. [CrossRef]

70. Sakurada, K.; Watanabe, K.; Akutsu, T. Current Methods for Body Fluid Identification Related to Sexual Crime: Focusing on Saliva, Semen, and Vaginal Fluid. *Diagnostics* **2020**, *10*, 693. [CrossRef]

71. Harbison, S.A.; Fleming, R.I. Forensic Body Fluid Identification: State of the Art. *Res. Rep. Forensic Med. Sci.* **2016**, *6*, 11–23. [CrossRef]

72. Holtkötter, H.; Schwender, K.; Wiegand, P.; Peiffer, H.; Vennemann, M. Improving Body Fluid Identification in Forensic Trace Evidence—Construction of an Immunochromatographic Test Array to Rapidly Detect up to Five Body Fluids Simultaneously. *Int. J. Leg. Med.* **2018**, *132*, 83–90. [CrossRef] [PubMed]

73. de Beijer, R.P.; de Graaf, C.; van Weert, A.; van Leeuwen, T.G.; Aalders, M.C.G.; van Dam, A. Identification and Detection of Protein Markers to Differentiate between Forensically Relevant Body Fluids. *Forensic Sci. Int.* **2018**, *290*, 196–206. [CrossRef]

74. Lee, J.W.; Jung, J.Y.; Lim, S.-K. Simple and Rapid Identification of Saliva by Detection of Oral Streptococci Using Direct Polymerase Chain Reaction Combined with an Immunochromatographic Strip. *Forensic Sci. Int. Genet.* **2018**, *33*, 155–160. [CrossRef]

75. Abbas, N.; Lu, X.; Badshah, M.A.; In, J.B.; Heo, W.I.; Park, K.Y.; Lee, M.-K.; Kim, C.H.; Kang, P.; Chang, W.-J.; et al. Development of a Protein Microarray Chip with Enhanced Fluorescence for Identification of Semen and Vaginal Fluid. *Sensors* **2018**, *18*, 3874. [CrossRef]

76. Boyd, S.; Bertino, M.F.; Seashols, S.J. Raman Spectroscopy of Blood Samples for Forensic Applications. *Forensic Sci. Int.* **2011**, *208*, 124–128. [CrossRef] [PubMed]

77. Virkler, K.; Lednev, I.K. Raman Spectroscopic Signature of Semen and Its Potential Application to Forensic Body Fluid Identification. *Forensic Sci. Int.* **2009**, *193*, 56–62. [CrossRef]

78. Casey, T.; Mistek, E.; Halámková, L.; Lednev, I.K. Raman Spectroscopy for Forensic Semen Identification: Method Validation vs. Environmental Interferences. *Vib. Spectrosc.* **2020**, *109*, 103065. [CrossRef]

79. Doty, K.C.; Muro, C.K.; Lednev, I.K. Predicting the Time of the Crime: Bloodstain Aging Estimation for up to Two Years. *Forensic Chem.* **2017**, *5*, 1–7. [CrossRef]

80. Rosenblatt, R.; Halámková, L.; Doty, K.C.; de Oliveira, E.A.C.; Lednev, I.K. Raman Spectroscopy for Forensic Bloodstain Identification: Method Validation vs. Environmental Interferences. *Forensic Chem.* **2019**, *16*, 100175. [CrossRef]

81. Takamura, A.; Watanabe, K.; Akutsu, T.; Ozawa, T. Soft and Robust Identification of Body Fluid Using Fourier Transform Infrared Spectroscopy and Chemometric Strategies for Forensic Analysis. *Sci. Rep.* **2018**, *8*, 8459. [CrossRef] [PubMed]

82. Orphanou, C.-M. The Detection and Discrimination of Human Body Fluids Using ATR FT-IR Spectroscopy. *Forensic Sci. Int.* **2015**, *252*, e10–e16. [CrossRef]

83. Sharma, S.; Chophi, R.; Singh, R. Forensic Discrimination of Menstrual Blood and Peripheral Blood Using Attenuated Total Reflectance (ATR)-Fourier Transform Infrared (FT-IR) Spectroscopy and Chemometrics. *Int. J. Leg. Med.* **2020**, *134*, 63–77. [CrossRef]

84. Zha, S.; Wei, X.; Fang, R.; Wang, Q.; Lin, H.; Zhang, K.; Zhang, H.; Liu, R.; Li, Z.; Huang, P.; et al. Estimation of the Age of Human Semen Stains by Attenuated Total Reflection Fourier Transform Infrared Spectroscopy: A Preliminary Study. *Forensic Sci. Res.* **2020**, *5*, 119–125. [CrossRef]

85. Takamura, A.; Halamkova, L.; Ozawa, T.; Lednev, I.K. Phenotype Profiling for Forensic Purposes: Determining Donor Sex Based on Fourier Transform Infrared Spectroscopy of Urine Traces. *Anal. Chem.* **2019**, *91*, 6288–6295. [CrossRef]

86. Mistek-Morabito, E.; Lednev, I.K. Discrimination of Menstrual and Peripheral Blood Traces Using Attenuated Total Reflection Fourier Transform-Infrared (ATR FT-IR) Spectroscopy and Chemometrics for Forensic Purposes. *Anal. Bioanal. Chem.* **2021**, *413*, 2513–2522. [CrossRef]

87. Karadayi, S.; Moshfeghi, E.; Arasoglu, T.; Karadayi, B. Evaluating the Persistence of Laundered Semen Stains on Fabric Using a Forensic Light Source System, Prostate-Specific Antigen Semiquant Test and DNA Recovery-Profiling. *Med. Sci. Law* **2020**, *60*, 122–130. [CrossRef] [PubMed]

88. Lynch, C.; Fleming, R. RNA-Based Approaches for Body Fluid Identification in Forensic Science. *WIREs Forensic Sci.* **2021**, *3*, e1407. [CrossRef]

89. El-Mogy, M.; Lam, B.; Haj-Ahmad, T.A.; McGowan, S.; Yu, D.; Nosal, L.; Rghei, N.; Roberts, P.; Haj-Ahmad, Y. Diversity and Signature of Small RNA in Different Bodily Fluids Using next Generation Sequencing. *BMC Genom.* **2018**, *19*, 408. [CrossRef] [PubMed]

90. Na, J.-Y. Estimation of the Post-Mortem Interval Using MicroRNA in the Bones. *J. Forensic Leg. Med.* **2020**, *75*, 102049. [CrossRef] [PubMed]

91. Bauer, M.; Patzelt, D. Evaluation of Mrna Markers for the Identification of Menstrual Blood. *J. Forensic Sci.* **2002**, *47*, 1278–1282. [CrossRef]

92. Bauer, M.; Kraus, A.; Patzelt, D. Detection of Epithelial Cells in Dried Blood Stains by Reverse Transcriptase-Polymerase Chain Reaction. *J. Forensic Sci.* **1999**, *44*, 1232–1236. [CrossRef]

93. Setzer, M.; Juusola, J.; Ballantyne, J. Recovery and Stability of RNA in Vaginal Swabs and Blood, Semen, and Saliva Stains. *J. Forensic Sci.* **2008**, *53*, 296–305. [CrossRef]

94. Kohlmeier, F.; Schneider, P.M. Successful mRNA Profiling of 23 Years Old Blood Stains. *Forensic Sci. Int. Genet.* **2012**, *6*, 274–276. [CrossRef]

95. Lin, M.-H.; Jones, D.F.; Fleming, R. Transcriptomic Analysis of Degraded Forensic Body Fluids. *Forensic Sci. Int. Genet.* **2015**, *17*, 35–42. [CrossRef] [PubMed]

96. Salzmann, A.P.; Russo, G.; Aluri, S.; Haas, C. Transcription and Microbial Profiling of Body Fluids Using a Massively Parallel Sequencing Approach. *Forensic Sci. Int. Genet.* **2019**, *43*, 102149. [CrossRef] [PubMed]

97. Harteveld, J.; Lindenbergh, A.; Sijen, T. RNA Cell Typing and DNA Profiling of Mixed Samples: Can Cell Types and Donors Be Associated? *Sci. Justice* **2013**, *53*, 261–269. [CrossRef]

98. Lindenbergh, A.; de Pagter, M.; Ramdayal, G.; Visser, M.; Zubakov, D.; Kayser, M.; Sijen, T. A Multiplex (m)RNA-Profiling System for the Forensic Identification of Body Fluids and Contact Traces. *Forensic Sci. Int. Genet.* **2012**, *6*, 565–577. [CrossRef] [PubMed]

99. Bowden, A.; Fleming, R.; Harbison, S. A Method for DNA and RNA Co-Extraction for Use on Forensic Samples Using the Promega DNA IQ™ System. *Forensic Sci. Int. Genet.* **2011**, *5*, 64–68. [CrossRef]

100. Alvarez, M.; Juusola, J.; Ballantyne, J. An mRNA and DNA Co-Isolation Method for Forensic Casework Samples. *Anal. Biochem.* **2004**, *335*, 289–298. [CrossRef]

101. Wang, S.; Shanthan, G.; Bouzga, M.M.; Dinh, H.M.T.; Haas, C.; Fonneløp, A.E. Evaluating the Performance of Five Up-to-Date DNA/RNA Co-Extraction Methods for Forensic Application. *Forensic Sci. Int.* **2021**, *328*, 110996. [CrossRef] [PubMed]

102. Juusola, J.; Ballantyne, J. Multiplex mRNA Profiling for the Identification of Body Fluids. *Forensic Sci. Int.* **2005**, *152*, 1–12. [CrossRef]

103. Akutsu, T.; Watanabe, K.; Takamura, A.; Sakurada, K. Evaluation of Skin- or Sweat-Characteristic mRNAs for Inferring the Human Origin of Touched Contact Traces. *Leg. Med.* **2018**, *33*, 36–41. [CrossRef]

104. van den Berge, M.; Bhoelai, B.; Harteveld, J.; Matai, A.; Sijen, T. Advancing Forensic RNA Typing: On Non-Target Secretions, a Nasal Mucosa Marker, a Differential Co-Extraction Protocol and the Sensitivity of DNA and RNA Profiling. *Forensic Sci. Int. Genet.* **2016**, *20*, 119–129. [CrossRef] [PubMed]

105. Cossu, C.; Germann, U.; Kratzer, A.; Bär, W.; Haas, C. How Specific Are the Vaginal Secretion mRNA-Markers HBD1 and MUC4? *Forensic Sci. Int. Genet. Suppl. Ser.* **2009**, *2*, 536–537. [CrossRef]

106. Richard, M.L.L.; Harper, K.A.; Craig, R.L.; Onorato, A.J.; Robertson, J.M.; Donfack, J. Evaluation of mRNA Marker Specificity for the Identification of Five Human Body Fluids by Capillary Electrophoresis. *Forensic Sci. Int. Genet.* **2012**, *6*, 452–460. [CrossRef]

107. Fleming, R.I.; Harbison, S. The Development of a mRNA Multiplex RT-PCR Assay for the Definitive Identification of Body Fluids. *Forensic Sci. Int. Genet.* **2010**, *4*, 244–256. [CrossRef]

108. Park, J.-L.; Park, S.-M.; Kim, J.-H.; Lee, H.-C.; Lee, S.-H.; Woo, K.-M.; Kim, S.-Y. Forensic Body Fluid Identification by Analysis of Multiple RNA Markers Using NanoString Technology. *Genom. Inform.* **2013**, *11*, 277–281. [CrossRef]

109. Hanson, E.; Ingold, S.; Haas, C.; Ballantyne, J. Targeted Multiplexed next Generation RNA Sequencing Assay for Tissue Source Determination of Forensic Samples. *Forensic Sci. Int. Genet. Suppl. Ser.* **2015**, *5*, e441–e443. [CrossRef]

110. Zubakov, D.; Hanekamp, E.; Kokshoorn, M.; van IJcken, W.; Kayser, M. Stable RNA Markers for Identification of Blood and Saliva Stains Revealed from Whole Genome Expression Analysis of Time-Wise Degraded Samples. *Int. J. Leg. Med.* **2008**, *122*, 135–142. [CrossRef]

111. Lindenbergh, A.; Maaskant, P.; Sijen, T. Implementation of RNA Profiling in Forensic Casework. *Forensic Sci. Int. Genet.* **2013**, *7*, 159–166. [CrossRef]

112. Tozzo, P.; Nespeca, P.; Spigarolo, G.; Caenazzo, L. The Importance of Distinguishing Menstrual and Peripheral Blood in Forensic Casework: A Case Report. *Am. J. Forensic Med. Pathol.* **2018**, *39*, 337–340. [CrossRef]

113. Fabbri, M.; Venturi, M.; Talarico, A.; Inglese, R.; Gaudio, R.M.; Neri, M. mRNA Profiling: Application to an Old Casework. *Forensic Sci. Int. Genet. Suppl. Ser.* **2017**, *6*, e380–e382. [CrossRef]

114. Fox, A.; Gittos, M.; Harbison, S.A.; Fleming, R.; Wivell, R. Exploring the Recovery and Detection of Messenger RNA and DNA from Enhanced Fingermarks in Blood. *Sci. Justice* **2014**, *54*, 192–198. [CrossRef]

115. Lux, C.; Schyma, C.; Madea, B.; Courts, C. Identification of Gunshots to the Head by Detection of RNA in Backspatter Primarily Expressed in Brain Tissue. *Forensic Sci. Int.* **2014**, *237*, 62–69. [CrossRef] [PubMed]

116. Haas, C.; Klesser, B.; Maake, C.; Bär, W.; Kratzer, A. mRNA Profiling for Body Fluid Identification by Reverse Transcription Endpoint PCR and Realtime PCR. *Forensic Sci. Int. Genet.* **2009**, *3*, 80–88. [CrossRef] [PubMed]

117. Nussbaumer, C.; Gharehbaghi-Schnell, E.; Korschineck, I. Messenger RNA Profiling: A Novel Method for Body Fluid Identification by Real-Time PCR. *Forensic Sci. Int.* **2006**, *157*, 181–186. [CrossRef]

118. Ingold, S.; Dørum, G.; Hanson, E.; Berti, A.; Branicki, W.; Brito, P.; Elsmore, P.; Gettings, K.B.; Giangasparo, F.; Gross, T.E.; et al. Body Fluid Identification Using a Targeted mRNA Massively Parallel Sequencing Approach—Results of a EUROFORGEN/EDNAP Collaborative Exercise. *Forensic Sci. Int. Genet.* **2018**, *34*, 105–115. [CrossRef]

119. Hanson, E.; Ingold, S.; Haas, C.; Ballantyne, J. Messenger RNA Biomarker Signatures for Forensic Body Fluid Identification Revealed by Targeted RNA Sequencing. *Forensic Sci. Int. Genet.* **2018**, *34*, 206–221. [CrossRef]

120. Dørum, G.; Ingold, S.; Hanson, E.; Ballantyne, J.; Snipen, L.; Haas, C. Predicting the Origin of Stains from next Generation Sequencing mRNA Data. *Forensic Sci. Int. Genet.* **2018**, *34*, 37–48. [CrossRef] [PubMed]

121. Haas, C.; Neubauer, J.; Salzmann, A.P.; Hanson, E.; Ballantyne, J. Forensic Transcriptome Analysis Using Massively Parallel Sequencing. *Forensic Sci. Int. Genet.* **2021**, *52*, 102486. [CrossRef] [PubMed]

122. Salzman, J.; Gawad, C.; Wang, P.L.; Lacayo, N.; Brown, P.O. Circular RNAs Are the Predominant Transcript Isoform from Hundreds of Human Genes in Diverse Cell Types. *PLoS ONE* **2012**, *7*, e30733. [CrossRef]

123. Guo, J.U.; Agarwal, V.; Guo, H.; Bartel, D.P. Expanded Identification and Characterization of Mammalian Circular RNAs. *Genome Biol.* **2014**, *15*, 409. [CrossRef]

124. Salzman, J.; Chen, R.E.; Olsen, M.N.; Wang, P.L.; Brown, P.O. Cell-Type Specific Features of Circular RNA Expression. *PLOS Genet.* **2013**, *9*, e1003777. [CrossRef]

125. Song, F.; Luo, H.; Xie, M.; Zhu, H.; Hou, Y. Microarray Expression Profile of Circular RNAs in Human Body Fluids. *Forensic Sci. Int. Genet. Suppl. Ser.* **2017**, *6*, e55–e56. [CrossRef]

126. Zhang, Y.; Liu, B.; Shao, C.; Xu, H.; Xue, A.; Zhao, Z.; Shen, Y.; Tang, Q.; Xie, J. Evaluation of the Inclusion of Circular RNAs in mRNA Profiling in Forensic Body Fluid Identification. *Int. J. Leg. Med.* **2018**, *132*, 43–52. [CrossRef]

127. Juusola, J.; Ballantyne, J. mRNA Profiling for Body Fluid Identification by Multiplex Quantitative RT-PCR *. *J. Forensic Sci.* **2007**, *52*, 1252–1262. [CrossRef] [PubMed]

128. Liu, B.; Yang, Q.; Meng, H.; Shao, C.; Jiang, J.; Xu, H.; Sun, K.; Zhou, Y.; Yao, Y.; Zhou, Z.; et al. Development of a Multiplex System for the Identification of Forensically Relevant Body Fluids. *Forensic Sci. Int. Genet.* **2020**, *47*, 102312. [CrossRef]

129. Baonian, L.; Song, F.; Yang, Q.; Zhou, Y.; Chengchen, S.; Shen, Y.; Zhao, Z.; Tang, Q.; Hou, Y.; Xie, J. Characterization of Tissue-Specific Biomarkers with the Expression of CircRNAs in Forensically Relevant Body Fluids. *Int. J. Leg. Med.* **2019**, *133*, 1321–1331. [CrossRef]

130. Notomi, T.; Okayama, H.; Masubuchi, H.; Yonekawa, T.; Watanabe, K.; Amino, N.; Hase, T. Loop-Mediated Isothermal Amplification of DNA. *Nucleic Acids Res.* **2000**, *28*, e63. [CrossRef] [PubMed]

131. Su, C.-W.; Li, C.-Y.; Lee, J.C.-I.; Ji, D.-D.; Li, S.-Y.; Daniel, B.; Syndercombe-Court, D.; Linacre, A.; Hsieh, H.-M. A Novel Application of Real-Time RT-LAMP for Body Fluid Identification: Using HBB Detection as the Model. *Forensic Sci. Med. Pathol.* **2015**, *11*, 208–215. [CrossRef]

132. Tsai, L.-C.; Su, C.-W.; Lee, J.C.-I.; Lu, Y.-S.; Chen, H.-C.; Lin, Y.-C.; Linacre, A.; Hsieh, H.-M. The Detection and Identification of Saliva in Forensic Samples by RT-LAMP. *Forensic Sci. Med. Pathol.* **2018**, *14*, 469–477. [CrossRef]

133. Satoh, T.; Kouroki, S.; Ogawa, K.; Tanaka, Y.; Matsumura, K.; Iwase, S. Development of MRNA-Based Body Fluid Identification Using Reverse Transcription Loop-Mediated Isothermal Amplification. *Anal. Bioanal. Chem.* **2018**, *410*, 4371–4378. [CrossRef]

134. Jackson, K.R.; Layne, T.; Dent, D.A.; Tsuei, A.; Li, J.; Haverstick, D.M.; Landers, J.P. A Novel Loop-Mediated Isothermal Amplification Method for Identification of Four Body Fluids with Smartphone Detection. *Forensic Sci. Int. Genet.* **2020**, *45*, 102195. [CrossRef]

135. Mehta, B.; Daniel, R.; McNevin, D. HRM and SNaPshot as Alternative Forensic SNP Genotyping Methods. *Forensic Sci. Med. Pathol.* **2017**, *13*, 293–301. [CrossRef] [PubMed]

136. Rocha, A.D.S.; De Amorim, I.S.S.; Simão, T.D.A.; Fonseca, A.D.S.; Garrido, R.G.; Mencalha, A.L. High-Resolution Melting (HRM) of Hypervariable Mitochondrial DNA Regions for Forensic Science. *J. Forensic Sci.* **2018**, *63*, 536–540. [CrossRef]

137. Wang, S.; Song, F.; Wang, Y.; Huang, Y.; Xie, B.; Luo, H. High Resolution Melting Analysis (HRM) Based on 16SrRNA as a Tool for Personal Identification with the Human Oral Microbiome. *Forensic Sci. Int. Genet. Suppl. Ser.* **2019**, *7*, 161–163. [CrossRef]

138. Alghanim, H.; Balamurugan, K.; McCord, B. Development of DNA Methylation Markers for Sperm, Saliva and Blood Identification Using Pyrosequencing and QPCR/HRM. *Anal. Biochem.* **2020**, *611*, 113933. [CrossRef]

139. Hanson, E.K.; Ballantyne, J. Rapid and Inexpensive Body Fluid Identification by RNA Profiling-Based Multiplex High Resolution Melt (HRM) Analysis. *F1000Research* **2014**, *2*, 281. [CrossRef]

140. Danaher, P.; White, R.L.; Hanson, E.K.; Ballantyne, J. Facile Semi-Automated Forensic Body Fluid Identification by Multiplex Solution Hybridization of NanoString® Barcode Probes to Specific MRNA Targets. *Forensic Sci. Int. Genet.* **2015**, *14*, 18–30. [CrossRef]

141. Malkov, V.A.; Serikawa, K.A.; Balantac, N.; Watters, J.; Geiss, G.; Mashadi-Hossein, A.; Fare, T. Multiplexed Measurements of Gene Signatures in Different Analytes Using the Nanostring Ncounter™ Assay System. *BMC Res. Notes* **2009**, *2*, 80. [CrossRef] [PubMed]

142. French, D.J.; Archard, C.L.; Brown, T.; McDowell, D.G. HyBeaconTM Probes: A New Tool for DNA Sequence Detection and Allele Discrimination. *Mol. Cell. Probes* **2001**, *15*, 363–374. [CrossRef] [PubMed]

143. Blackman, S.; Stafford-Allen, B.; Hanson, E.K.; Panasiuk, M.; Brooker, A.-L.; Rendell, P.; Ballantyne, J.; Wells, S. Developmental Validation of the ParaDNA® Body Fluid ID System—A Rapid Multiplex MRNA-Profiling System for the Forensic Identification of Body Fluids. *Forensic Sci. Int. Genet.* **2018**, *37*, 151–161. [CrossRef] [PubMed]

144. Blackman, S.; Dawnay, N.; Ball, G.; Stafford-Allen, B.; Tribble, N.; Rendell, P.; Neary, K.; Hanson, E.K.; Ballantyne, J.; Kallifatidis, B.; et al. Developmental Validation of the ParaDNA® Intelligence System—A Novel Approach to DNA Profiling. *Forensic Sci. Int. Genet.* **2015**, *17*, 137–148. [CrossRef]

145. Hong, S.R.; Jung, S.-E.; Lee, E.H.; Shin, K.-J.; Yang, W.I.; Lee, H.Y. DNA Methylation-Based Age Prediction from Saliva: High Age Predictability by Combination of 7 CpG Markers. *Forensic Sci. Int. Genet.* **2017**, *29*, 118–125. [CrossRef] [PubMed]

146. Vidaki, A.; Kayser, M. Recent Progress, Methods and Perspectives in Forensic Epigenetics. *Forensic Sci. Int. Genet.* **2018**, *37*, 180–195. [CrossRef]

147. Kader, F.; Ghai, M.; Olaniran, A.O. Characterization of DNA Methylation-Based Markers for Human Body Fluid Identification in Forensics: A Critical Review. *Int. J. Leg. Med.* **2020**, *134*, 1–20. [CrossRef]

148. Lee, H.Y.; An, J.H.; Jung, S.-E.; Oh, Y.N.; Lee, E.Y.; Choi, A.; Yang, W.I.; Shin, K.-J. Genome-Wide Methylation Profiling and a Multiplex Construction for the Identification of Body Fluids Using Epigenetic Markers. *Forensic Sci. Int. Genet.* **2015**, *17*, 17–24. [CrossRef] [PubMed]

149. Park, J.-L.; Kwon, O.-H.; Kim, J.H.; Yoo, H.-S.; Lee, H.-C.; Woo, K.-M.; Kim, S.-Y.; Lee, S.-H.; Kim, Y.S. Identification of Body Fluid-Specific DNA Methylation Markers for Use in Forensic Science. *Forensic Sci. Int. Genet.* **2014**, *13*, 147–153. [CrossRef]

150. Ghai, M.; Naidoo, N.; Evans, D.L.; Kader, F. Identification of Novel Semen and Saliva Specific Methylation Markers and Its Potential Application in Forensic Analysis. *Forensic Sci. Int. Genet.* **2020**, *49*, 102392. [CrossRef]

151. Antunes, J.; Gauthier, Q.; Aguiar-Pulido, V.; Duncan, G.; McCord, B. A Data-Driven, High-Throughput Methodology to Determine Tissue-Specific Differentially Methylated Regions Able to Discriminate Body Fluids. *Electrophoresis* **2021**, *42*, 1168–1176. [CrossRef]

152. An, J.H.; Choi, A.; Shin, K.-J.; Yang, W.I.; Lee, H.Y. DNA Methylation-Specific Multiplex Assays for Body Fluid Identification. *Int. J. Leg. Med.* **2013**, *127*, 35–43. [CrossRef]

153. Choi, A.; Shin, K.-J.; Yang, W.I.; Lee, H.Y. Body Fluid Identification by Integrated Analysis of DNA Methylation and Body Fluid-Specific Microbial DNA. *Int. J. Leg. Med.* **2014**, *128*, 33–41. [CrossRef] [PubMed]

154. Frumkin, D.; Wasserstrom, A.; Budowle, B.; Davidson, A. DNA Methylation-Based Forensic Tissue Identification. *Forensic Sci. Int. Genet.* **2011**, *5*, 517–524. [CrossRef] [PubMed]

155. Liu, K.-L.; Tsai, L.-C.; Lin, Y.-C.; Huang, N.-E.; Yang, L.-J.; Su, C.-W.; Lee, J.C.-I.; Linacre, A.; Hsieh, H.-M. Identification of Spermatozoa Using a Novel 3-Plex MSRE-PCR Assay for Forensic Examination of Sexual Assaults. *Int. J. Leg. Med.* **2020**, *134*, 1991–2004. [CrossRef]

156. Vidaki, A.; Giangasparo, F.; Court, D.S. Discovery of Potential DNA Methylation Markers for Forensic Tissue Identification Using Bisulphite Pyrosequencing. *Electrophoresis* **2016**, *37*, 2767–2779. [CrossRef]

157. Doi, M.; Nishimukai, H.; Asano, M. Application of Fragment Analysis Based on Methylation Status Mobility Difference to Identify Vaginal Secretions. *Sci. Justice* **2021**, *61*, 384–390. [CrossRef]

158. Holtkötter, H.; Beyer, V.; Schwender, K.; Glaub, A.; Johann, K.S.; Schürenkamp, M.; Sibbing, U.; Banken, S.; Wiegand, P.; Pfeiffer, H.; et al. Independent Validation of Body Fluid-Specific CpG Markers and Construction of a Robust Multiplex Assay. *Forensic Sci. Int. Genet.* **2017**, *29*, 261–268. [CrossRef]

159. Newton, C.R.; Graham, A.; Heptinstall, L.E.; Powell, S.J.; Summers, C.; Kalsheker, N.; Smith, J.C.; Markham, A.F. Analysis of Any Point Mutation in DNA. The Amplification Refractory Mutation System (ARMS). *Nucleic Acids Res.* **1989**, *17*, 2503–2516. [CrossRef]

160. Tian, H.; Bai, P.; Tan, Y.; Li, Z.; Peng, D.; Xiao, X.; Zhao, H.; Zhou, Y.; Liang, W.; Zhang, L. A New Method to Detect Methylation Profiles for Forensic Body Fluid Identification Combining ARMS-PCR Technique and Random Forest Model. *Forensic Sci. Int. Genet.* **2020**, *49*, 102371. [CrossRef] [PubMed]

161. Hong, S.R.; Shin, K.-J. Bisulfite-Converted DNA Quantity Evaluation: A Multiplex Quantitative Real-Time PCR System for Evaluation of Bisulfite Conversion. *Front. Genet.* **2021**, *12*, 173. [CrossRef]

162. Schommer, N.N.; Gallo, R.L. Structure and Function of the Human Skin Microbiome. *Trends Microbiol.* **2013**, *21*, 660–668. [CrossRef]

163. Fleming, R.I.; Harbison, S. The Use of Bacteria for the Identification of Vaginal Secretions. *Forensic Sci. Int. Genet.* **2010**, *4*, 311–315. [CrossRef]

164. Benschop, C.C.G.; Quaak, F.C.A.; Boon, M.E.; Sijen, T.; Kuiper, I. Vaginal Microbial Flora Analysis by next Generation Sequencing and Microarrays; Can Microbes Indicate Vaginal Origin in a Forensic Context? *Int. J. Leg. Med.* **2012**, *126*, 303–310. [CrossRef]

165. Ravel, J.; Gajer, P.; Abdo, Z.; Schneider, G.M.; Koenig, S.S.K.; McCulle, S.L.; Karlebach, S.; Gorle, R.; Russell, J.; Tacket, C.O.; et al. Vaginal Microbiome of Reproductive-Age Women. *Proc. Natl. Acad. Sci. USA* **2011**, *108*, 4680–4687. [CrossRef]

166. Castillo, D.J.; Rifkin, R.F.; Cowan, D.A.; Potgieter, M. The Healthy Human Blood Microbiome: Fact or Fiction? *Front. Cell. Infect. Microbiol.* **2019**, *9*, 148. [CrossRef]

167. Huse, S.M.; Ye, Y.; Zhou, Y.; Fodor, A.A. A Core Human Microbiome as Viewed through 16S RRNA Sequence Clusters. *PLoS ONE* **2012**, *7*, e34242. [CrossRef] [PubMed]

168. Quaak, F.C.A.; van Duijn, T.; Hoogenboom, J.; Kloosterman, A.D.; Kuiper, I. Human-Associated Microbial Populations as Evidence in Forensic Casework. *Forensic Sci. Int. Genet.* **2018**, *36*, 176–185. [CrossRef] [PubMed]

169. Hanssen, E.N.; Avershina, E.; Rudi, K.; Gill, P.; Snipen, L. Body Fluid Prediction from Microbial Patterns for Forensic Application. *Forensic Sci. Int. Genet.* **2017**, *30*, 10–17. [CrossRef]

170. Human Microbiome Project Consortium. Structure, Function and Diversity of the Healthy Human Microbiome. *Nature* **2012**, *486*, 207–214. [CrossRef]

171. Ishak, S.; Dormontt, E.; Young, J.M. Microbiomes in Forensic Botany: A Review. *Forensic Sci. Med. Pathol.* **2021**, *17*, 297–307. [CrossRef] [PubMed]

172. Damaso, N.; Mendel, J.; Mendoza, M.; von Wettberg, E.J.; Narasimhan, G.; Mills, D. Bioinformatics Approach to Assess the Biogeographical Patterns of Soil Communities: The Utility for Soil Provenance. *J. Forensic Sci.* **2018**, *63*, 1033–1042. [CrossRef] [PubMed]

173. Cho, H.-W.; Eom, Y.-B. Forensic Analysis of Human Microbiome in Skin and Body Fluids Based on Geographic Location. *Front. Cell. Infect. Microbiol.* **2021**, *11*, 695191. [CrossRef] [PubMed]

174. Badgley, A.J.; Jesmok, E.M.; Foran, D.R. Time Radically Alters Ex Situ Evidentiary Soil 16S Bacterial Profiles Produced Via Next-Generation Sequencing. *J. Forensic Sci.* **2018**, *63*, 1356–1365. [CrossRef] [PubMed]

175. Signoretto, C.; Bianchi, F.; Burlacchini, G.; Sivieri, F.; Spratt, D.; Canepari, P. Drinking Habits Are Associated with Changes in the Dental Plaque Microbial Community. *J. Clin. Microbiol.* **2010**, *48*, 347–356. [CrossRef] [PubMed]

176. Rogers, M.A.M.; Aronoff, D.M. The Influence of Non-Steroidal Anti-Inflammatory Drugs on the Gut Microbiome. *Clin. Microbiol. Infect.* **2016**, *22*, 178.e1. [CrossRef]

177. Kates, A.E.; Jarrett, O.; Skarlupka, J.H.; Sethi, A.; Duster, M.; Watson, L.; Suen, G.; Poulsen, K.; Safdar, N. Household Pet Ownership and the Microbial Diversity of the Human Gut Microbiota. *Front. Cell. Infect. Microbiol.* **2020**, *10*, 73. [CrossRef] [PubMed]

178. Neckovic, A.; van Oorschot, R.A.H.; Szkuta, B.; Durdle, A. Challenges in Human Skin Microbial Profiling for Forensic Science: A Review. *Genes* **2020**, *11*, 1015. [CrossRef]

179. Kim, D.; Hofstaedter, C.E.; Zhao, C.; Mattei, L.; Tanes, C.; Clarke, E.; Lauder, A.; Sherrill-Mix, S.; Chehoud, C.; Kelsen, J.; et al. Optimizing Methods and Dodging Pitfalls in Microbiome Research. *Microbiome* **2017**, *5*, 52. [CrossRef]

180. Salter, S.J.; Cox, M.J.; Turek, E.M.; Calus, S.T.; Cookson, W.O.; Moffatt, M.F.; Turner, P.; Parkhill, J.; Loman, N.J.; Walker, A.W. Reagent and Laboratory Contamination Can Critically Impact Sequence-Based Microbiome Analyses. *BMC Biol.* **2014**, *12*, 87. [CrossRef]

181. Robinson, J.M.; Pasternak, Z.; Mason, C.E.; Elhaik, E. Forensic Applications of Microbiomics: A Review. *Front. Microbiol.* **2021**, *11*, 3455. [CrossRef]

182. Schmedes, S.E.; Woerner, A.E.; Novroski, N.M.M.; Wendt, F.R.; King, J.L.; Stephens, K.M.; Budowle, B. Targeted Sequencing of Clade-Specific Markers from Skin Microbiomes for Forensic Human Identification. *Forensic Sci. Int. Genet.* **2018**, *32*, 50–61. [CrossRef]

183. Woerner, A.E.; Novroski, N.M.M.; Wendt, F.R.; Ambers, A.; Wiley, R.; Schmedes, S.E.; Budowle, B. Forensic Human Identification with Targeted Microbiome Markers Using Nearest Neighbor Classification. *Forensic Sci. Int. Genet.* **2019**, *38*, 130–139. [CrossRef] [PubMed]

184. Fierer, N.; Lauber, C.L.; Zhou, N.; McDonald, D.; Costello, E.K.; Knight, R. Forensic Identification Using Skin Bacterial Communities. *Proc. Natl. Acad. Sci. USA* **2010**, *107*, 6477–6481. [CrossRef]

185. Meadow, J.F.; Altrichter, A.E.; Green, J.L. Mobile Phones Carry the Personal Microbiome of Their Owners. *PeerJ* **2014**, *2*, e447. [CrossRef] [PubMed]

186. Goga, H. Comparison of Bacterial DNA Profiles of Footwear Insoles and Soles of Feet for the Forensic Discrimination of Footwear Owners. *Int. J. Leg. Med.* **2012**, *126*, 815–823. [CrossRef]

187. Lax, S.; Hampton-Marcell, J.T.; Gibbons, S.M.; Colares, G.B.; Smith, D.; Eisen, J.A.; Gilbert, J.A. Forensic Analysis of the Microbiome of Phones and Shoes. *Microbiome* **2015**, *3*, 21. [CrossRef]

188. Young, J.M.; Linacre, A. Massively Parallel Sequencing Is Unlocking the Potential of Environmental Trace Evidence. *Forensic Sci. Int. Genet.* **2021**, *50*, 102393. [CrossRef]
189. Allwood, J.S.; Fierer, N.; Dunn, R.R. The Future of Environmental DNA in Forensic Science. *Appl. Environ. Microbiol.* **2020**, *86*, e01504-19. [CrossRef] [PubMed]
190. Giampaoli, S.; Berti, A.; Di Maggio, R.M.; Pilli, E.; Valentini, A.; Valeriani, F.; Gianfranceschi, G.; Barni, F.; Ripani, L.; Spica, V.R. The Environmental Biological Signature: NGS Profiling for Forensic Comparison of Soils. *Forensic Sci. Int.* **2014**, *240*, 41–47. [CrossRef]
191. Costello, E.K.; Lauber, C.L.; Hamady, M.; Fierer, N.; Gordon, J.I.; Knight, R. Bacterial Community Variation in Human Body Habitats across Space and Time. *Science* **2009**, *326*, 1694–1697. [CrossRef]
192. Leake, S.L.; Pagni, M.; Falquet, L.; Taroni, F.; Greub, G. The Salivary Microbiome for Differentiating Individuals: Proof of Principle. *Microbes Infect.* **2016**, *18*, 399–405. [CrossRef]
193. Jung, J.Y.; Yoon, H.K.; An, S.; Lee, J.W.; Ahn, E.-R.; Kim, Y.-J.; Park, H.-C.; Lee, K.; Hwang, J.H.; Lim, S.-K. Rapid Oral Bacteria Detection Based on Real-Time PCR for the Forensic Identification of Saliva. *Sci. Rep.* **2018**, *8*, 10852. [CrossRef]
194. Quaak, F.C.A.; de Graaf, M.-L.M.; Weterings, R.; Kuiper, I. Microbial Population Analysis Improves the Evidential Value of Faecal Traces in Forensic Investigations. *Int. J. Leg. Med.* **2017**, *131*, 45–51. [CrossRef]
195. Akutsu, T.; Motani, H.; Watanabe, K.; Iwase, H.; Sakurada, K. Detection of Bacterial 16S Ribosomal RNA Genes for Forensic Identification of Vaginal Fluid. *Leg. Med.* **2012**, *14*, 160–162. [CrossRef] [PubMed]
196. Díez López, C.; Montiel González, D.; Haas, C.; Vidaki, A.; Kayser, M. Microbiome-Based Body Site of Origin Classification of Forensically Relevant Blood Traces. *Forensic Sci. Int. Genet.* **2020**, *47*, 102280. [CrossRef]
197. López, C.D.; Vidaki, A.; Ralf, A.; González, D.M.; Radjabzadeh, D.; Kraaij, R.; Uitterlinden, A.G.; Haas, C.; Lao, O.; Kayser, M. Novel Taxonomy-Independent Deep Learning Microbiome Approach Allows for Accurate Classification of Different Forensically Relevant Human Epithelial Materials. *Forensic Sci. Int. Genet.* **2019**, *41*, 72–82. [CrossRef] [PubMed]
198. Yao, T.; Han, X.; Guan, T.; Wang, Z.; Zhang, S.; Liu, C.; Liu, C.; Chen, L. Effect of Indoor Environmental Exposure on Seminal Microbiota and Its Application in Body Fluid Identification. *Forensic Sci. Int.* **2020**, *314*, 110417. [CrossRef]
199. Haas, C.; Hanson, E.; Anjos, M.J.; Ballantyne, K.N.; Banemann, R.; Bhoelai, B.; Borges, E.; Carvalho, M.; Courts, C.; De Cock, G.; et al. RNA/DNA Co-Analysis from Human Menstrual Blood and Vaginal Secretion Stains: Results of a Fourth and Fifth Collaborative EDNAP Exercise. *Forensic Sci. Int. Genet.* **2014**, *8*, 203–212. [CrossRef]
200. Dobay, A.; Haas, C.; Fucile, G.; Downey, N.; Morrison, H.G.; Kratzer, A.; Arora, N. Microbiome-Based Body Fluid Identification of Samples Exposed to Indoor Conditions. *Forensic Sci. Int. Genet.* **2019**, *40*, 105–113. [CrossRef] [PubMed]
201. Donaldson, A.E.; Taylor, M.C.; Cordiner, S.J.; Lamont, I.L. Using Oral Microbial DNA Analysis to Identify Expirated Bloodspatter. *Int. J. Leg. Med.* **2010**, *124*, 569–576. [CrossRef]
202. Giampaoli, S.; Berti, A.; Valeriani, F.; Gianfranceschi, G.; Piccolella, A.; Buggiotti, L.; Rapone, C.; Valentini, A.; Ripani, L.; Spica, V.R. Molecular Identification of Vaginal Fluid by Microbial Signature. *Forensic Sci. Int. Genet.* **2012**, *6*, 559–564. [CrossRef]
203. Ranjan, R.; Rani, A.; Metwally, A.; McGee, H.S.; Perkins, D.L. Analysis of the Microbiome: Advantages of Whole Genome Shotgun versus 16S Amplicon Sequencing. *Biochem. Biophys. Res. Commun.* **2016**, *469*, 967–977. [CrossRef] [PubMed]
204. Holtkötter, H.; Dierig, L.; Schürenkamp, M.; Sibbing, U.; Pfeiffer, H.; Vennemann, M. Validation of an Immunochromatographic D-Dimer Test to Presumptively Identify Menstrual Fluid in Forensic Exhibits. *Int. J. Leg. Med.* **2015**, *129*, 37–41. [CrossRef]
205. Holtkötter, H.; Filho, C.R.D.; Schwender, K.; Stadler, C.; Vennemann, M.; Pacheco, A.C.; Roca, G. Forensic Differentiation between Peripheral and Menstrual Blood in Cases of Alleged Sexual Assault—Validating an Immunochromatographic Multiplex Assay for Simultaneous Detection of Human Hemoglobin and D-Dimer. *Int. J. Leg. Med.* **2018**, *132*, 683–690. [CrossRef] [PubMed]
206. Giampaoli, S.; Alessandrini, F.; Berti, A.; Ripani, L.; Choi, A.; Crab, R.; De Vittori, E.; Egyed, B.; Haas, C.; Lee, H.Y.; et al. Forensic Interlaboratory Evaluation of the ForFLUID Kit for Vaginal Fluids Identification. *J. Forensic Leg. Med.* **2014**, *21*, 60–63. [CrossRef] [PubMed]
207. Hausmann, R.; Pregler, C.; Schellmann, B. The Value of the Lugol's Iodine Staining Technique for the Identification of Vaginal Epithelial Cells. *Int. J. Leg. Med.* **1994**, *106*, 298–301. [CrossRef]
208. Nichols, C.A.; Sens, M.A. Recovery and Evaluation by Cytologic Techniques of Trace Material Retained on Bullets. *Am. J. Forensic Med. Pathol.* **1990**, *11*, 17–34. [CrossRef] [PubMed]
209. Uitspraken. Available online: https://www.rechtspraak.nl/Uitspraken/Paginas/default.aspx (accessed on 12 September 2021).
210. Lin, Y.-C.; Tsai, L.-C.; Lee, J.C.-I.; Liu, K.-L.; Tzen, J.T.-C.; Linacre, A.; Hsieh, H.-M. Novel Identification of Biofluids Using a Multiplex Methylation-Specific PCR Combined with Single-Base Extension System. *Forensic Sci. Med. Pathol.* **2016**, *12*, 128–138. [CrossRef]
211. Wasserstrom, A.; Frumkin, D.; Davidson, A.; Shpitzen, M.; Herman, Y.; Gafny, R. Demonstration of DSI-Semen—A Novel DNA Methylation-Based Forensic Semen Identification Assay. *Forensic Sci. Int. Genet.* **2013**, *7*, 136–142. [CrossRef]
212. Iwasaki, M.; Kubo, S.-I.; Ogata, M.; Nakasono, I. A Demonstration of Spermatozoa on Vaginal Swabs after Complete Destruction of the Vaginal Cell Deposits. *J. Forensic Sci.* **1989**, *34*, 659–664. [CrossRef]
213. Bamberg, M.; Dierig, L.; Kulstein, G.; Kunz, S.N.; Schmidt, M.; Hadrys, T.; Wiegand, P. Development and Validation of an MRNA-Based Multiplex Body Fluid Identification Workflow and a Rectal Mucosa Marker Pilot Study. *Forensic Sci. Int. Genet.* **2021**, *54*, 102542. [CrossRef] [PubMed]

214. Zubakov, D.; Kokshoorn, M.; Kloosterman, A.; Kayser, M. New Markers for Old Stains: Stable MRNA Markers for Blood and Saliva Identification from up to 16-Year-Old Stains. *Int. J. Leg. Med.* **2009**, *123*, 71–74. [CrossRef] [PubMed]
215. Chirnside, O.; Lemalu, A.; Fleming, R. Identification of Nasal Mucosa Markers for Forensic MRNA Body Fluid Determination. *Forensic Sci. Int. Genet.* **2020**, *48*, 102317. [CrossRef]
216. Xu, Y.; Xie, J.; Cao, Y.; Zhou, H.; Ping, Y.; Chen, L.; Gu, L.; Hu, W.; Bi, G.; Ge, J.; et al. Development of Highly Sensitive and Specific MRNA Multiplex System (XCYR1) for Forensic Human Body Fluids and Tissues Identification. *PLoS ONE* **2014**, *9*, e100123. [CrossRef] [PubMed]
217. Sakurada, K.; Akutsu, T.; Fukushima, H.; Watanabe, K.; Yoshino, M. Detection of Dermcidin for Sweat Identification by Real-Time RT-PCR and ELISA. *Forensic Sci. Int.* **2010**, *194*, 80–84. [CrossRef]
218. Layne, T.R.; Green, R.A.; Lewis, C.A.; Nogales, F.; Cruz, T.C.D.; Zehner, Z.E.; Seashols-Williams, S.J. MicroRNA Detection in Blood, Urine, Semen, and Saliva Stains After Compromising Treatments. *J. Forensic Sci.* **2019**, *64*, 1831–1837. [CrossRef]
219. Visser, M.; Zubakov, D.; Ballantyne, K.N.; Kayser, M. MRNA-Based Skin Identification for Forensic Applications. *Int. J. Leg. Med.* **2011**, *125*, 253–263. [CrossRef]
220. Hanson, E.; Haas, C.; Jucker, R.; Ballantyne, J. Identification of Skin in Touch/Contact Forensic Samples by Messenger RNA Profiling. *Forensic Sci. Int. Genet. Suppl. Ser.* **2011**, *3*, e305–e306. [CrossRef]
221. Haas, C.; Hanson, E.; Banemann, R.; Bento, A.M.; Berti, A.; Carracedo, Á.; Courts, C.; Cock, G.D.; Drobnic, K.; Fleming, R.; et al. RNA/DNA Co-Analysis from Human Skin and Contact Traces—Results of a Sixth Collaborative EDNAP Exercise. *Forensic Sci. Int. Genet.* **2015**, *16*, 139–147. [CrossRef]
222. van den Berge, M.; Carracedo, A.; Gomes, I.; Graham, E.A.M.; Haas, C.; Hjort, B.; Hoff-Olsen, P.; Maroñas, O.; Mevåg, B.; Morling, N.; et al. A Collaborative European Exercise on MRNA-Based Body Fluid/Skin Typing and Interpretation of DNA and RNA Results. *Forensic Sci. Int. Genet.* **2014**, *10*, 40–48. [CrossRef]
223. Lindenbergh, A.; van den Berge, M.; Oostra, R.-J.; Cleypool, C.; Bruggink, A.; Kloosterman, A.; Sijen, T. Development of a MRNA Profiling Multiplex for the Inference of Organ Tissues. *Int. J. Leg. Med.* **2013**, *127*, 891–900. [CrossRef]
224. Hanson, E.; Ballantyne, J. Human Organ Tissue Identification by Targeted RNA Deep Sequencing to Aid the Investigation of Traumatic Injury. *Genes* **2017**, *8*, 319. [CrossRef]
225. Euteneuer, J.; Courts, C. Ten Years of Molecular Ballistics—a Review and a Field Guide. *Int. J. Leg. Med.* **2021**, *135*, 1121–1136. [CrossRef]
226. Alberts, B.; Johnson, A.; Lewis, J.; Raff, M.; Roberts, K.; Walter, P. *Molecular Biology of the Cell*, 4th ed.; Garland Science: New York, NY, USA, 2002; ISBN 978-0-8153-3218-3.
227. Mathiesen, C.; Thomsen, K.; Lauritzen, M. Integrated Measurements of Electrical Activity, Oxygen Tension, Blood Flow, and Ca2+-Signaling in Rodents In Vivo. In *Brain Energy Metabolism. Neuromethods*; Hirrlinger, J., Waagepetersen, H., Eds.; Humana Press: New York, NY, USA, 2014; Volume 90. [CrossRef]
228. Jackson, D.G. Leucocyte Trafficking via the Lymphatic Vasculature—Mechanisms and Consequences. *Front. Immunol.* **2019**, *10*, 471. [CrossRef]
229. Slagter, M.; Kruise, D.; van Ommen, L.; Hoogenboom, J.; Steensma, K.; de Jong, J.; Hovers, P.; Parag, R.; van der Linden, J.; Kneppers, A.L.J.; et al. The DNAxs Software Suite: A Three-Year Retrospective Study on the Development, Architecture, Testing and Implementation in Forensic Casework. *Forensic Sci. Int. Rep.* **2021**, *3*, 100212. [CrossRef]
230. McNevin, D.; Wright, K.; Barash, M.; Gomes, S.; Jamieson, A.; Chaseling, J. Proposed Framework for Comparison of Continuous Probabilistic Genotyping Systems amongst Different Laboratories. *Forensic Sci.* **2021**, *1*, 33–45. [CrossRef]
231. Bleka, Ø.; Storvik, G.; Gill, P. EuroForMix: An Open Source Software Based on a Continuous Model to Evaluate STR DNA Profiles from a Mixture of Contributors with Artefacts. *Forensic Sci. Int. Genet.* **2016**, *21*, 35–44. [CrossRef]
232. Bright, J.-A.; Cheng, K.; Kerr, Z.; McGovern, C.; Kelly, H.; Moretti, T.R.; Smith, M.A.; Bieber, F.R.; Budowle, B.; Coble, M.D.; et al. STRmix™ Collaborative Exercise on DNA Mixture Interpretation. *Forensic Sci. Int. Genet.* **2019**, *40*, 1–8. [CrossRef] [PubMed]
233. Coble, M.D.; Bright, J.-A. Probabilistic Genotyping Software: An Overview. *Forensic Sci. Int. Genet.* **2019**, *38*, 219–224. [CrossRef]
234. van den Berge, M.; Sijen, T. Extended Specificity Studies of MRNA Assays Used to Infer Human Organ Tissues and Body Fluids. *Electrophoresis* **2017**, *38*, 3155–3160. [CrossRef] [PubMed]
235. Lin, M.-H.; Albani, P.P.; Fleming, R. Degraded RNA Transcript Stable Regions (StaRs) as Targets for Enhanced Forensic RNA Body Fluid Identification. *Forensic Sci. Int. Genet.* **2016**, *20*, 61–70. [CrossRef] [PubMed]
236. Sasaki, A.; Kim, B.; Murphy, K.E.; Matthews, S.G. Impact of Ex Vivo Sample Handling on DNA Methylation Profiles in Human Cord Blood and Neonatal Dried Blood Spots. *Front. Genet.* **2020**, *11*, 224. [CrossRef]
237. Lin, Y.-C.; Tsai, L.-C.; Lee, J.C.-I.; Su, C.-W.; Tzen, J.T.-C.; Linacre, A.; Hsieh, H.-M. Novel Identification of Biofluids Using a Multiplex Methylation Sensitive Restriction Enzyme-PCR System. *Forensic Sci. Int. Genet.* **2016**, *25*, 157–165. [CrossRef] [PubMed]
238. Roeder, A.D.; Haas, C. MRNA Profiling Using a Minimum of Five MRNA Markers per Body Fluid and a Novel Scoring Method for Body Fluid Identification. *Int. J. Leg. Med.* **2013**, *127*, 707–721. [CrossRef] [PubMed]
239. Iacob, D.; Fürst, A.; Hadrys, T. A Machine Learning Model to Predict the Origin of Forensically Relevant Body Fluids. *Forensic Sci. Int. Genet. Suppl. Ser.* **2019**, *7*, 392–394. [CrossRef]
240. de Zoete, J.; Curran, J.; Sjerps, M. A Probabilistic Approach for the Interpretation of RNA Profiles as Cell Type Evidence. *Forensic Sci. Int. Genet.* **2016**, *20*, 30–44. [CrossRef] [PubMed]

241. Ypma, R.J.F.; Wijk, P.A.M.; Gill, R.; Sjerps, M.; van den Berge, M. Calculating LRs for Presence of Body Fluids from MRNA Assay Data in Mixtures. *Forensic Sci. Int. Genet.* **2021**, *52*, 102455. [CrossRef]

242. Hanson, E.; Ingold, S.; Dorum, G.; Haas, C.; Lagace, R.; Ballantyne, J. Assigning Forensic Body Fluids to DNA Donors in Mixed Samples by Targeted RNA/DNA Deep Seqeuncing of Coding Region SNPs Using Ion Torrent Technology. *Forensic Sci. Int. Genet. Suppl. Ser.* **2019**, *7*, 23–24. [CrossRef]

243. Gill, P. Misleading DNA Evidence: Reasons for Miscarriages of Justice. *Int. Comment. Evid.* **2012**, *10*, 55–71. [CrossRef]

244. Wang, S.; Wang, Z.; Tao, R.; Song, F.; Hou, Y. Validating the Consistency of CSNPs Analysis Results between DNA and RNA Using SNaPshot Method. *Forensic Sci. Int. Genet. Suppl. Ser.* **2019**, *7*, 76–78. [CrossRef]

245. Ingold, S.; Dørum, G.; Hanson, E.; Ballantyne, J.; Haas, C. Assigning Forensic Body Fluids to Donors in Mixed Body Fluids by Targeted RNA/DNA Deep Sequencing of Coding Region SNPs. *Int. J. Leg. Med.* **2020**, *134*, 473–485. [CrossRef] [PubMed]

246. Ingold, S.; Haas, C.; Dørum, G.; Hanson, E.; Ballantyne, J. Association of a Body Fluid with a DNA Profile by Targeted RNA/DNA Deep Sequencing. *Forensic Sci. Int. Genet. Suppl. Ser.* **2017**, *6*, e112–e113. [CrossRef]

247. Li, Z.; Li, J.; Li, Y.; Liu, N.; Liu, F.; Ren, J.; Yun, K.; Yan, J.; Zhang, G. Development of a Multiplex Methylation-Sensitive Restriction Enzyme-Based SNP Typing System for Deconvolution of Semen-Containing Mixtures. *Int. J. Leg. Med.* **2021**, *135*, 1281–1294. [CrossRef] [PubMed]

248. Watanabe, K.; Taniguchi, K.; Akutsu, T. Development of a DNA Methylation-Based Semen-Specific SNP Typing Method: A New Approach for Genotyping from a Mixture of Body Fluids. *Forensic Sci. Int. Genet.* **2018**, *37*, 227–234. [CrossRef]

249. Fujimoto, S.; Hamano, Y.; Ichioka, K.; Manabe, S.; Hirai, E.; Ogawa, O.; Tamaki, K. Rapid Semen Identification from Mixed Body Fluids Using Methylation-Sensitive High-Resolution Melting Analysis of the DACT1 Gene. *Leg. Med.* **2021**, *48*, 101806. [CrossRef]

250. Rocchi, A.; Chiti, E.; Maiese, A.; Turillazzi, E.; Spinetti, I. MicroRNAs: An Update of Applications in Forensic Science. *Diagnostics* **2021**, *11*, 32. [CrossRef]

251. Sun, K.; Lai, E.C. Adult-Specific Functions of Animal MicroRNAs. *Nat. Rev. Genet.* **2013**, *14*, 535–548. [CrossRef]

252. Wienholds, E.; Kloosterman, W.P.; Miska, E.; Alvarez-Saavedra, E.; Berezikov, E.; de Bruijn, E.; Horvitz, H.R.; Kauppinen, S.; Plasterk, R.H.A. MicroRNA Expression in Zebrafish Embryonic Development. *Science* **2005**, *309*, 310–311. [CrossRef]

253. Omelia, E.J.; Uchimoto, M.L.; Williams, G. Quantitative PCR Analysis of Blood- and Saliva-Specific MicroRNA Markers Following Solid-Phase DNA Extraction. *Anal. Biochem.* **2013**, *435*, 120–122. [CrossRef]

254. Hanson, E.K.; Lubenow, H.; Ballantyne, J. Identification of Forensically Relevant Body Fluids Using a Panel of Differentially Expressed MicroRNAs. *Anal. Biochem.* **2009**, *387*, 303–314. [CrossRef]

255. Zubakov, D.; Boersma, A.W.M.; Choi, Y.; van Kuijk, P.F.; Wiemer, E.A.C.; Kayser, M. MicroRNA Markers for Forensic Body Fluid Identification Obtained from Microarray Screening and Quantitative RT-PCR Confirmation. *Int. J. Leg. Med.* **2010**, *124*, 217–226. [CrossRef] [PubMed]

256. Park, J.-L.; Park, S.-M.; Kwon, O.-H.; Lee, H.; Kim, J.; Seok, H.H.; Lee, W.S.; Lee, S.-H.; Kim, Y.S.; Woo, K.-M.; et al. Microarray Screening and QRT-PCR Evaluation of MicroRNA Markers for Forensic Body Fluid Identification. *Electrophoresis* **2014**, *35*, 3062–3068. [CrossRef]

257. Li, Z.; Bai, P.; Peng, D.; Wang, H.; Guo, Y.; Jiang, Y.; He, W.; Tian, H.; Yang, Y.; Huang, Y.; et al. Screening and Confirmation of MicroRNA Markers for Distinguishing between Menstrual and Peripheral Blood. *Forensic Sci. Int. Genet.* **2017**, *30*, 24–33. [CrossRef]

258. Sauer, E.; Extra, A.; Cachée, P.; Courts, C. Identification of Organ Tissue Types and Skin from Forensic Samples by MicroRNA Expression Analysis. *Forensic Sci. Int. Genet.* **2017**, *28*, 99–110. [CrossRef] [PubMed]

259. Liu, Y.; He, H.; Xiao, Z.-X.; Ji, A.; Ye, J.; Sun, Q.; Cao, Y. A Systematic Analysis of miRNA Markers and Classification Algorithms for Forensic Body Fluid Identification. *Brief. Bioinform.* **2021**, *22*. [CrossRef]

260. Zhao, C.; Zhao, M.; Zhu, Y.; Zhang, L.; Zheng, Z.; Wang, Q.; Li, Y.; Zhang, P.; Zhu, S.; Ding, S.; et al. The Persistence and Stability of miRNA in Bloodstained Samples under Different Environmental Conditions. *Forensic Sci. Int.* **2021**, *318*, 110594. [CrossRef] [PubMed]

261. Mayes, C.; Houston, R.; Seashols-Williams, S.; LaRue, B.; Hughes-Stamm, S. The Stability and Persistence of Blood and Semen MRNA and miRNA Targets for Body Fluid Identification in Environmentally Challenged and Laundered Samples. *Leg. Med.* **2019**, *38*, 45–50. [CrossRef]

262. Sirker, M.; Fimmers, R.; Schneider, P.M.; Gomes, I. Evaluating the Forensic Application of 19 Target MicroRNAs as Biomarkers in Body Fluid and Tissue Identification. *Forensic Sci. Int. Genet.* **2017**, *27*, 41–49. [CrossRef]

263. Van der Meer, D.; Uchimoto, M.L.; Williams, G. Simultaneous Analysis of Micro-RNA and DNA for Determining the Body Fluid Origin of DNA Profiles. *J. Forensic Sci.* **2013**, *58*, 967–971. [CrossRef] [PubMed]

264. Mayes, C.; Seashols-Williams, S.; Hughes-Stamm, S. A Capillary Electrophoresis Method for Identifying Forensically Relevant Body Fluids Using miRNAs. *Leg. Med.* **2018**, *30*, 1–4. [CrossRef] [PubMed]

265. Seashols-Williams, S.; Lewis, C.; Calloway, C.; Peace, N.; Harrison, A.; Hayes-Nash, C.; Fleming, S.; Wu, Q.; Zehner, Z.E. High-Throughput miRNA Sequencing and Identification of Biomarkers for Forensically Relevant Biological Fluids. *Electrophoresis* **2016**, *37*, 2780–2788. [CrossRef]

266. Parhad, S.S.; Theurkauf, W.E. Rapid Evolution and Conserved Function of the PiRNA Pathway. *Open Biol.* **2019**, *9*, 180181. [CrossRef] [PubMed]

267. Wang, S.; Wang, Z.; Tao, R.; He, G.; Liu, J.; Li, C.; Hou, Y. The Potential Use of Piwi-Interacting RNA Biomarkers in Forensic Body Fluid Identification: A Proof-of-Principle Study. *Forensic Sci. Int. Genet.* **2019**, *39*, 129–135. [CrossRef]

268. Wang, S.; Wang, Z.; Tao, R.; Wang, M.; Liu, J.; He, G.; Yang, Y.; Xie, M.; Zou, X.; Hou, Y. Expression Profile Analysis of Piwi-Interacting RNA in Forensically Relevant Biological Fluids. *Forensic Sci. Int. Genet.* **2019**, *42*, 171–180. [CrossRef]

269. Dana, H.; Chalbatani, G.M.; Mahmoodzadeh, H.; Karimloo, R.; Rezaiean, O.; Moradzadeh, A.; Mehmandoost, N.; Moazzen, F.; Mazraeh, A.; Marmari, V.; et al. Molecular Mechanisms and Biological Functions of SiRNA. *Int. J. Biomed. Sci. IJBS* **2017**, *13*, 48–57.

270. Staedtler, F.; Hartmann, N.; Letzkus, M.; Bongiovanni, S.; Scherer, A.; Marc, P.; Johnson, K.J.; Schumacher, M.M. Robust and Tissue-Independent Gender-Specific Transcript Biomarkers. *Biomarkers* **2013**, *18*, 436–445. [CrossRef] [PubMed]

271. Ng, K.; Pullirsch, D.; Leeb, M.; Wutz, A. *Xist* and the Order of Silencing. *EMBO Rep.* **2007**, *8*, 34–39. [CrossRef] [PubMed]

272. Van den Berge, M.; Sijen, T. A Male and Female RNA Marker to Infer Sex in Forensic Analysis. *Forensic Sci. Int. Genet.* **2017**, *26*, 70–76. [CrossRef]

273. Hassan, F.M.; Razik, H.A.A.; Wadie, M.S.; Abdelfattah, D.S. XIST and RPS4Y1 Long Non-Coding RNA Transcriptome as Sex Biomarkers in Different Body Fluids. *Egypt. J. Forensic Sci.* **2019**, *9*, 16. [CrossRef]

274. Merkley, E.D.; Wunschel, D.S.; Wahl, K.L.; Jarman, K.H. Applications and Challenges of Forensic Proteomics. *Forensic Sci. Int.* **2019**, *297*, 350–363. [CrossRef]

275. Merkley, E.D. *Applications in Forensic Proteomics: Protein Identification and Profiling*; ACS Symposium Series; American Chemical Society: Washington, DC, USA, 2020.

276. Parker, G.J.; McKiernan, H.E.; Legg, K.M.; Goecker, Z.C. Forensic Proteomics. *Forensic Sci. Int. Genet.* **2021**, *54*, 102529. [CrossRef]

277. Yang, H.; Zhou, B.; Deng, H.; Prinz, M.; Siegel, D. Body Fluid Identification by Mass Spectrometry. *Int. J. Leg. Med.* **2013**, *127*, 1065–1077. [CrossRef] [PubMed]

278. Legg, K.M.; Powell, R.; Reisdorph, N.; Reisdorph, R.; Danielson, P.B. Discovery of Highly Specific Protein Markers for the Identification of Biological Stains. *Electrophoresis* **2014**, *35*, 3069–3078. [CrossRef] [PubMed]

279. Legg, K.M.; Powell, R.; Reisdorph, N.; Reisdorph, R.; Danielson, P.B. Verification of Protein Biomarker Specificity for the Identification of Biological Stains by Quadrupole Time-of-Flight Mass Spectrometry. *Electrophoresis* **2017**, *38*, 833–845. [CrossRef]

280. McKiernan, H.E.; Danielson, P.B.; Brown, C.O.; Signaevsky, M.; Westring, C.G.; Legg, K.M. Developmental Validation of a Multiplex Proteomic Assay for the Identification of Forensically Relevant Biological Fluids. *Forensic Sci. Int.* **2021**, *326*, 110908. [CrossRef]

281. Bradshaw, R.; Bleay, S.; Clench, M.R.; Francese, S. Direct Detection of Blood in Fingermarks by MALDI MS Profiling and Imaging. *Sci. Justice* **2014**, *54*, 110–117. [CrossRef]

282. Kamanna, S.; Henry, J.; Voelcker, N.H.; Linacre, A.; Kirkbride, K.P. Direct Identification of Forensic Body Fluids Using Matrix-Assisted Laser Desorption/Ionization Time-of-Flight Mass Spectrometry. *Int. J. Mass Spectrom.* **2016**, *397–398*, 18–26. [CrossRef]

283. Rankin-Turner, S.; Ninomiya, S.; Reynolds, J.C.; Hiraoka, K. Sheath-Flow Probe Electrospray Ionization (SfPESI) Mass Spectrometry for the Rapid Forensic Analysis of Human Body Fluids. *Anal. Methods* **2019**, *11*, 3633–3640. [CrossRef]

284. Parker, G.J.; Leppert, T.; Anex, D.S.; Hilmer, J.K.; Matsunami, N.; Baird, L.; Stevens, J.; Parsawar, K.; Durbin-Johnson, B.P.; Rocke, D.M.; et al. Demonstration of Protein-Based Human Identification Using the Hair Shaft Proteome. *PLoS ONE* **2016**, *11*, e0160653. [CrossRef]

285. Goecker, Z.C.; Salemi, M.R.; Karim, N.; Phinney, B.S.; Rice, R.H.; Parker, G.J. Optimal Processing for Proteomic Genotyping of Single Human Hairs. *Forensic Sci. Int. Genet.* **2020**, *47*, 102314. [CrossRef] [PubMed]

286. Chu, F.; Mason, K.E.; Anex, D.S.; Jones, A.D.; Hart, B.R. Hair Proteome Variation at Different Body Locations on Genetically Variant Peptide Detection for Protein-Based Human Identification. *Sci. Rep.* **2019**, *9*, 7641. [CrossRef]

287. Tuerk, C.; Gold, L. Systematic Evolution of Ligands by Exponential Enrichment: RNA Ligands to Bacteriophage T4 DNA Polymerase. *Science* **1990**, *249*, 505–510. [CrossRef] [PubMed]

288. Ellington, A.D.; Szostak, J.W. In Vitro Selection of RNA Molecules That Bind Specific Ligands. *Nature* **1990**, *346*, 818–822. [CrossRef]

289. Bock, L.C.; Griffin, L.C.; Latham, J.A.; Vermaas, E.H.; Toole, J.J. Selection of Single-Stranded DNA Molecules That Bind and Inhibit Human Thrombin. *Nature* **1992**, *355*, 564–566. [CrossRef] [PubMed]

290. Rangel, A.E.; Chen, Z.; Ayele, T.M.; Heemstra, J.M. In Vitro Selection of an XNA Aptamer Capable of Small-Molecule Recognition. *Nucleic Acids Res.* **2018**, *46*, 8057–8068. [CrossRef] [PubMed]

291. Bunka, D.H.J.; Stockley, P.G. Aptamers Come of Age—At Last. *Nat. Rev. Microbiol.* **2006**, *4*, 588–596. [CrossRef]

292. Song, S.; Wang, L.; Li, J.; Fan, C.; Zhao, J. Aptamer-Based Biosensors. *TrAC Trends Anal. Chem.* **2008**, *27*, 108–117. [CrossRef]

293. Chen, Z.; Wu, Q.; Chen, J.; Ni, X.; Dai, J. A DNA Aptamer Based Method for Detection of SARS-CoV-2 Nucleocapsid Protein. *Virol. Sin.* **2020**, *35*, 351–354. [CrossRef]

294. Abrego-Martinez, J.C.; Jafari, M.; Chergui, S.; Pavel, C.; Che, D.; Siaj, M. Aptamer-Based Electrochemical Biosensor for Rapid Detection of SARS-CoV-2: Nanoscale Electrode-Aptamer-SARS-CoV-2 Imaging by Photo-Induced Force Microscopy. *Biosens. Bioelectron.* **2022**, *195*, 113595. [CrossRef]

295. Gooch, J.; Tungsirisurp, S.; Costanzo, H.; Napier, R.; Frascione, N. Generating Aptamers towards Human Sperm Cells Using Massively Parallel Sequencing. *Anal. Bioanal. Chem.* **2021**, *413*, 5821–5834. [CrossRef] [PubMed]

296. Satoh, T.; Kouroki, S.; Kitamura, Y.; Ihara, T.; Matsumura, K.; Iwase, S. Detection of Prostate-Specific Antigen in Semen Using DNA Aptamers: An Application of Nucleic Acid Aptamers in Forensic Body Fluid Identification. *Anal. Methods* **2020**, *12*, 2703–2709. [CrossRef] [PubMed]
297. Lin, H.-I.; Wu, C.-C.; Yang, C.-H.; Chang, K.-W.; Lee, G.-B.; Shiesh, S.-C. Selection of Aptamers Specific for Glycated Hemoglobin and Total Hemoglobin Using On-Chip SELEX. *Lab. Chip* **2015**, *15*, 486–494. [CrossRef] [PubMed]
298. Choung, C.M.; Lee, J.W.; Park, J.H.; Kim, C.H.; Park, H.-C.; Lim, S.-K. A Forensic Case Study for Body Fluid Identification Using DNA Methylation Analysis. *Leg. Med.* **2021**, *51*, 101872. [CrossRef]
299. Cortellini, V.; Brescia, G.; Cerri, N.; Verzeletti, A. Simultaneous DNA and RNA Profiling in a Case of Sexual Assault in a 3-Year-Old Child: Forensic Genetics Solves the Crime. *Leg. Med.* **2020**, *47*, 101727. [CrossRef]
300. Byrnes, S.A.; Gallagher, R.; Steadman, A.; Bennett, C.; Rivera, R.; Ortega, C.; Motley, S.T.; Jain, P.; Weigl, B.H.; Connelly, J.T. Multiplexed and Extraction-Free Amplification for Simplified SARS-CoV-2 RT-PCR Tests. *Anal. Chem.* **2021**, *93*, 4160–4165. [CrossRef] [PubMed]
301. Verheij, S.; Harteveld, J.; Sijen, T. A Protocol for Direct and Rapid Multiplex PCR Amplification on Forensically Relevant Samples. *Forensic Sci. Int. Genet.* **2012**, *6*, 167–175. [CrossRef] [PubMed]
302. Yang, Q.; Liu, B.; Zhou, Y.; Yao, Y.; Zhou, Z.; Li, H.; Shao, C.; Sun, K.; Xu, H.; Tang, Q.; et al. Evaluation of One-Step RT-PCR Multiplex Assay for Body Fluid Identification. *Int. J. Leg. Med.* **2021**, *135*, 1727–1735. [CrossRef] [PubMed]

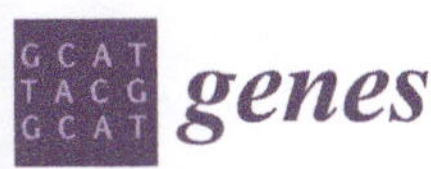

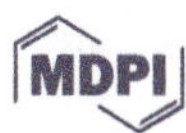

Review

Review of the Forensic Applicability of Biostatistical Methods for Inferring Ancestry from Autosomal Genetic Markers

Torben Tvedebrink [1,2]

1   Department of Mathematical Sciences, Aalborg University, DK-9220 Aalborg, Denmark; tvede@math.aau.dk
2   Section of Forensic Genetics, Department of Forensic Medicine, Faculty of Health and Medical Sciences, University of Copenhagen, DK-1165 Copenhagen, Denmark

Abstract: The inference of ancestry has become a part of the services many forensic genetic laboratories provide. Interest in ancestry may be to provide investigative leads or identify the region of origin in cases of unidentified missing persons. There exist many biostatistical methods developed for the study of population structure in the area of population genetics. However, the challenges and questions are slightly different in the context of forensic genetics, where the origin of a specific sample is of interest compared to the understanding of population histories and genealogies. In this paper, the methodologies for modelling population admixture and inferring ancestral populations are reviewed with a focus on their strengths and weaknesses in relation to ancestry inference in the forensic context.

Keywords: ancestry; biostatistics; clustering; classification; distance based; likelihood; hypothesis tests

Citation: Tvedebrink, T. Review of the Forensic Applicability of Biostatistical Methods for Inferring Ancestry from Autosomal Genetic Markers. *Genes* **2022**, *13*, 141. https://doi.org/10.3390/genes13010141

Academic Editor: David Caramelli

Received: 14 December 2021
Accepted: 11 January 2022
Published: 14 January 2022

Publisher's Note: MDPI stays neutral with regard to jurisdictional claims in published maps and institutional affiliations.

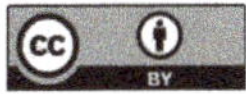

1. Ancestry Informative Markers

The increased availability of whole human genome sequences in the public domain is an invaluable data resource in many genomics, biomedical, and anthropological research areas. In particular, the data repositories focusing on the genomic diversity among human populations (e.g., HapMap Project [1], 1000 Genomes Project [2], Simons Genome Diversity Project [3], and more recently curated in the Genome Aggregation Database Project, gnomAD [4]) have contributed to the understanding of human evolution, migration histories, waves, and patterns.

Typically, genetic samples from populations with different geographical locations, cultural backgrounds, tribal memberships, and linguistic groups constitute the data used to identify genomic differences among the derived populations. These genomic differences are the result of a mixture of causes: mutations, recombination, genetic drift, selection, and migration [5]. The variations in the human genome can be observed both in tandemly repeated DNA sequences (e.g., short tandem repeats, STRs) and in single-nucleotide polymorphisms (SNPs) but are also manifested in sequence variations in lineage markers (e.g., Y-chromosome and mitochondrial DNA) and structural variations (e.g., copy-number variation) [6].

The geography of human populations (ancestry) and genetic polymorphisms are closely related [7–12]. Hence, identifying ancestry informative markers (AIMs) can be accomplished by analysing the publicly available genome sequences. Several measures of informativeness has been derived in order to rank candidate markers [13,14].

In forensic genetics, STRs are presently the standard markers used for identification and relationship testing. Furthermore, variation in allele frequencies may be used to infer an individual's ancestry [15,16]. Other types of AIMs are microhaplotypes [17], which are groups of closely located SNPs (often positioned within 500 bp), and insertion–deletion polymorphisms (indels) [18,19]. However, SNPs are more commonly used for ancestry analysis [20,21], where several commercial assays have been developed for ancestry investigations. The selection of SNPs to be included in commercial kits depends both on their biochemical properties (e.g., allele balances and primer site location) and their informativeness regarding specific continental and regional populations. Hence, the companies focused on specific population structures (e.g., intracontinental differences) may result in poor resolution in other regions and among populations of close proximity. Consequently, all results obtained from the genotyping and subsequent analysis are conditioned on the specific SNPs included in the analysis. This is important to bear in mind when interpreting the results of an analysis, as general patterns and expectations to population variability may not be contained on a narrowly selected set of markers.

2. Biostatistical Methods

The study of population structure from genomic data has a long history within the genetic and statistical literature. The increasing complexity and availability of data from ancestry informative markers on multiple populations have required the development of appropriate methodologies to model and capture the subtle genetic structures in the data: from the first studies of a few hundred markers and individuals to more recent studies with thousands of individuals genotyped on highly dense assays or from whole genome sequences.

This progress, driven by biotechnological advances, has been challenging not only from a methodological point of view but increasingly so from a computational perspective. Where independence between the markers was ensured by their genetic distance, the closer proximity of genetic markers results in statistical dependence (e.g., due to linkage disequilibrium, LD). This increases the complexity of the analysis since such dependencies must be adequately modelled and their dependence structure learned from the data. Some methods incorporate the structure into their modelling framework, either by identifying stretches supposedly inherited as a complete block (e.g., [22]) or attempts to learn the association structure using graphical models [23]. Others operate by removing the dependence among markers by pruning or thinning the data based on LD (e.g., [24]) or using the residual signal after successively regressing the markers on each other (e.g., [25]).

The most widely used methodologies for analysing genetic structure can broadly be divided into four different groups: principal components analysis, model-based clustering, classification and likelihood-based, and hypothesis test-based methods. In addition, tree-based and distance/dissimilarity clustering methods are used but not included in this review. Most of the development in the study of population structures is driven by interests in medical genetics or population genetics, where controlling for population stratification may be vital for some applications or where the study of population dynamics on its own is the main purpose. Hence, few methods have been developed with the applications of forensic genetics in mind. In the subsequent sections, the various methodologies are discussed with references to key publications in their domain.

To demonstrate and visualise the results from the various methods, data from [26] are used in the following sections. The data consist of samples from six reference metapopulations (comprised by a total of $n_{ref} = 3453$ samples) and $n_{test} = 517$ test samples all genotyped on the 164 ancestry informative SNPs included in the Precision ID Ancestry Panel (excluding marker rs10954737 due to a high degree of missingness). The reference samples are known to originate from the indicated metapopulation, are of high sequencing quality, and used to estimate the metapopulation's allele frequencies. The 517 test samples were harvested online, where their alleged metapopulation of origin was derived from the sampling location and other available meta information [26]. Both the reference and test samples originated from six regional areas, where the regional specific n_{ref}/n_{test} counts are: Sub-Saharan Africa (668/37), North Africa (283/49), Europe (1014/173), Middle East (377/52), South/Central Asia (489/85), and East Asia (622/121).

2.1. Principal Components Analysis

Principal components analysis (PCA) has a long history of application in the study of population structure. The usage of PCA in the analysis of population structure was pioneered by [27], as an efficient way to capture the underlying structure for visualisation purposes. PCA is able to capture continuous admixture between populations, implying that admixed populations typically falls on the *lines* between its *parental* populations. More recent PCA-based methods for inference include SMARTPCA [25] and EIGENSTRAT [28]. These methodologies provide further insight as to how many PCs are required to capture detectable population structures by the use of hypothesis testing on the magnitude of the PCA's eigenvalues. For the reference samples (cf. above) from [26], there are four significant PCs according to EIGENSTRAT. The first three PCs are plotted in Figure 1 (plots including the fourth PC do not visually separate the metapopulations). The often detected *triangle* spanned by Sub-Saharan Africa, Europe, and East Asia is cleary visible in the plot of PC1 and PC2.

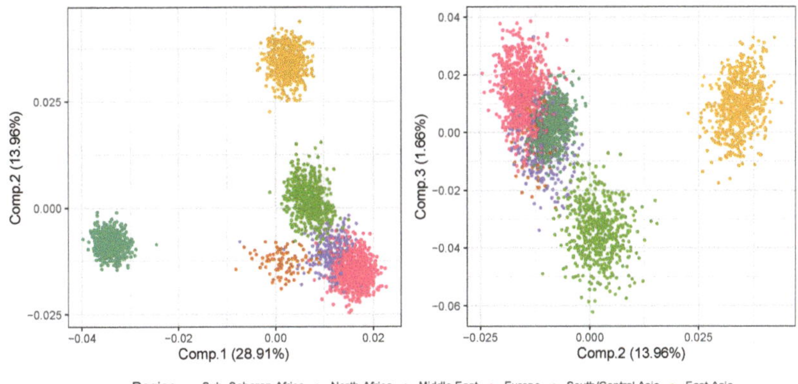

Figure 1. Plot of the first three PCs from the PCA of the reference samples.

Besides being an efficient tool for visualising high-dimensional (genetic) data, PCA also yields the best linear low-dimensional approximation of the data in terms of Euclidean distance. This, together with the orthogonality of the principal components (PCs), implies that population substructures can be detected by the discriminant analysis of the PCs, DAPC [29]. Primarily relying on linear algebra, DAPCis computationally much faster than STRUCTURE and gives comparable results. However, several papers discuss some of the known pitfalls when using PCA [30–33]. The most important issue to be aware of is PCA's sensitivity to the sampling of individuals and populations. An unbalanced sampling of some populations forces the PCs to account for the variation caused by the majority groups. Since most models and methods try to minimise a *loss function*, this implies that in the estimation of the unknown quantities (e.g., model parameters, here, the PCs) emphasis is given to the majority groups in the data [30,31]. The loss function is typically proportional to the deviation between the observed data and the model's predictions (or expectation), e.g., measured by the model's likelihood or squared distance of the residuals. For PCA, the loss function is inversely proportional to the fraction of explained variance of the first PCs, with DAPC's loss also depending on the intracluster variances as a function of the numbers of cluster K (measured by a Bayesian Information Criterion, BIC). Another property shared by several methods and statistical models is that they provide a *compression* of the data, in the sense that the methods are trying to retrieve as much information from the data as possible and discard a nonsignal as noise. Taken a bit further, one may interpret the model output and parameter estimates as *data summaries* (some more informative, advanced, and interpretable than others). Consequently, some of these summaries (e.g., the PCs and STRUCTURE as discussed next) are similar or even identical for different population genealogies [31].

2.2. Model-Based Clustering Methods

The seminal STRUCTURE paper [34] introduced a population genetics methodology based on a statistical finite mixture model. Using a Bayesian approach, the posterior probabilities for cluster memberships and cluster-specific allele frequencies are estimated using an MCMC-algorithm (MCMC: Markov chain Monte Carlo). STRUCTURE has been used in numerous studies and has, according to Google Scholar, more than 30,000 citations, which indicates its enormous influence in the field of population genetics [35]. Forensic applications were mentioned as one of motivations for STRUCTURE ([34], p. 945) in order to identify cryptic population structures and assess their influence on the detection of immigrants and calculation of match probabilities [36–38]. In essence, the initial STRUCTURE model is a simple Hardy–Weinberg model with the relaxation that subpopulations have different allele frequencies and individuals may inherit alleles from several subpopulations, i.e., being admixed [35]. Following the initial publication, several modifications both on the population genetic model (allowing for, e.g., linked markers and null alleles) [22,39] and computational aspects (faster and more efficient algorithmic schemes) [40–42] have been suggested. See [35,43] for further references and remarks.

Despite the many successful applications of STRUCTURE (including variants and similar methodologies, e.g., FRAPPE [40] and ADMIXTURE [41]), to population genetic data and research questions, no model is better or more general than its underlying assumptions. Similar stories apply to simple linear regression models, where the assessment and evaluation of the residuals is part of any analysis. However, because of STRUCTURE's complexity, it is harder to conduct the assessment of the model fit. A recently published instructive tutorial [44] provides a critical view on how to assess the outcome of STRUCTURE analysis using the tools badMIXTURE [45], GLOBETROTTER [46], fineSTRUCTURE, and CHROMOPAINTER [47]. In particular, the authors highlighted the fact that different population scenarios (e.g., recent admixture, bottleneck, and admixture contribution from untyped populations) result in similar STRUCTURE barplots [7,48] (the typical data summary from a STRUCTURE analysis). Supplementing the STRUCTURE analysis by residual plots based on badMIXTURE, patterns were detected enabling these scenarios to be distinguished [44]. Similar to PCA, STRUCTURE is sensitive toward biased sampling and population sample sizes. Specifically, imbalances between the analysed populations may influence how and which of the sampled populations that exhibit patterns of population admixture ([44], Case Study 3, pp. 5–8). However, choosing the appropriate (or in a sense, *correct*) value for K, the number of population clusters, is not a well-defined problem, i.e., only heuristic methods exist for guiding the specification of K [34,35,43,44]. Different choices of K may result in rather different results and interpretations of the population stratification and history.

In Figure 2, the estimated STRUCTURE admixture components, $q = (q^{(1)}, \ldots, q^{(K)})$, for the reference samples (cf. above) are shown for $K = 4$. There is a clear visual distinction in the distribution of q_i across the 3453 reference samples.

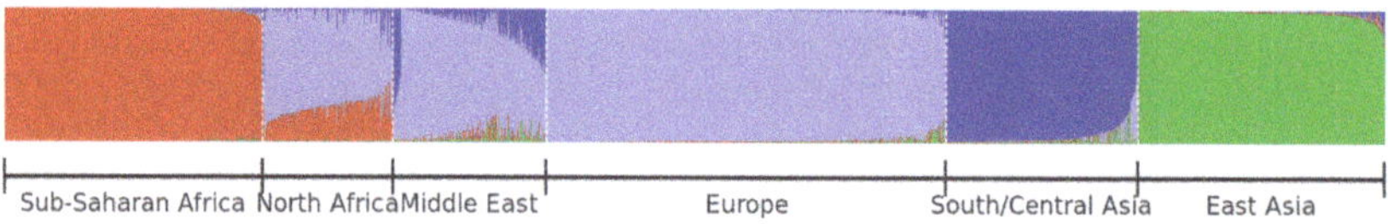

Figure 2. Barplots of the STRUCTURE admixture components ($K = 4$) for the reference samples from six metapopulations. There is a clear visual difference between the admixture components for the six metapopulations

The four clusters of Figure 2, $K = 4$, may be associated with Sub-Saharan African, European, South/Central Asian, and East Asian components. The samples from North African and Middle Eastern regions show the strongest admixture of these four components.

2.3. Classification and Likelihood-Based Methods

The statistical problem solved by STRUCTURE [34] and the related methodologies (e.g., ADMIXTURE [41]) is a rather complex one: Assign individuals to populations while estimating the unknown populations' unknown allele frequencies. As discussed above (Section 2.2), this is performed by finite mixture models, where the assignment of individuals and updating of population allele frequencies are conducted iteratively (either by Bayesian MCMC methods [34] or using efficient variants of expectation–maximisation algorithms [41]). However, if analysis of population structure is not the purpose and the allele frequencies are known for a set of populations, the assignment of individuals is simpler.

In this case, the assignment of nonadmixed individuals can be conducted by a Bayes classifier, where the individual is assigned to the most probable population among the ones included in the reference database. As such, the population assignment problem can be solved by several types of classification algorithms known from the machine learning literature (e.g., classification trees, random forest, support vector machines, multinomial regression, partial least squares, discriminant analysis, nearest neighbours, gradient boosting, and other ensemble learners). Common to most of these methods is their ability to account for interaction effects between the explanatory variables on the outcome (here, the marker interactions when predicting the population of origin). Furthermore, similar to the methods of Sections 2.1 and 2.2 (e.g., PCA and STRUCTURE), sample sizes and imbalanced training data typically influence the tuning and therefore performance of the machine learning methods. When training a classification algorithm on a specific dataset, the objective is to drive the overall loss function downwards. Typically, the loss function in classification contexts decreases with more samples being accurately classified (e.g., the misclassification rate or smooth functions, thereof). However, if some populations have low proportions in the sample, the classifier gains little from classifying these correct compared to the frequently occurring populations. Hence, the relative composition of the populations in the data may impact the trained classifier quite substantially. In the context of forensic genetics, the risk of incomplete AIMs profiles obtained from, e.g., crime scenes, makes some methods less applicable to samples with some or more untyped markers (e.g., due to low signals or marker drop-out). Some methods (e.g., naïve Bayes classifiers and classification trees using *surrogate splits*) may readily deal with partial profiles, whereas in particular regression, models are susceptible to missing data.

From a forensic perspective evaluating the weight of the evidence is typically conducted using the likelihood ratio principle. For multiple propositions (in this case, multiple populations), this approach generalises to several ratios assessing the pairwise agreement between data and the alleged populations of origin. The predicted population of origin is the population where the profile is most probable. The likelihood function typically assumes a specific population genetic model, e.g., within each population assuming Hardy–Weinberg equilibrium and independent genetic markers. This corresponds to a naïve Bayes classifier assuming a Binomial distribution for each marker given the population specific allele frequencies. Two forensically relevant implementations including several reference populations and AIMs panels are freely available online (FROG-kb (http://frog.med.yale.edu/FrogKB/, accessed on 13 December 2021) [49,50] and Snipper (http://mathgene.usc.es/snipper, accessed on 13 December 2021) [51]). Other approaches toward classification have been considered and compared (e.g., multinomial regression and genetic distances) [52]. These methods are in particular relevant in the case of admixed individuals, where the single population likelihoods do not suffice [53,54].

2.4. Hypothesis Test-Based Methods

An underlying and important assumption for both clustering and classification is that of *exhaustive* populations. This means that for clustering the admixture components *must* sum to one, indicating that *all* the genetic admixture of an individual can be explained by contributions from the K clusters. However, the *Ghost admixture* example of ([44],

p. 3) shows that the noninclusion of important branches of a genealogy may result in misleading results. In that case, the contribution from the unsampled reference population to the admixture was replaced by the reference population most similar to the unsampled one. This scenario may easily occur in the forensic setting, where only major populations are included in the reference material, but where conclusions are wanted on a finer (sub)population scale.

For classifications, an underlying assumption is that an observation belongs to *exactly* one class (i.e., one and only one). Hence, this *forced* classification means that even when all the possible classes are (highly) unlikely, the DNA profile under classification *must* be assigned to precisely one of the populations (typically the *least unlikely* population).

This issue was the main motivation for the derivation of the GenoGeographer methodology [55,56]. Rather than forcing an observation to be classified to any of the prespecified populations in the reference material, it was assessed whether the sample could originate from each of the reference populations. Logically, this implied that the sample was tested for being an outlier in each of the possible populations, and this was formally conducted by testing the hypothesis of the DNA profile sample and database sample originated from the same underlying population or not [55]. This outlier test is equivalent to a Fisher's exact test and thus enjoys many of the same statistical properties, e.g., increasing power with increasing sample size and robustness toward missing observations. Other hypothesis-based methodologies include a likelihood ratio test for recent admixture [57].

For each reference sample $i = 1, \ldots, 3453$, STRUCTURE estimates the admixture components, $\boldsymbol{q}_i = (q_i^{(1)}, \ldots, q_i^{(K)})$, where $\sum_{k=1}^{K} q_i^{(k)} = 1$ by definition. From these, the average admixture component is calculated for each of the reference metapopulations, by the average over the admixture components for reference samples belonging to this metapopulation:

$$\bar{\boldsymbol{q}}_j = (\bar{q}_j^{(1)}, \ldots, \bar{q}_j^{(K)}), \quad \text{with} \quad \bar{q}_j^{(k)} = n_j^{-1} \sum_{i \in R_j} q_i^{(k)}, \quad k = 1, \ldots, K,$$

where R_j is the set of the n_j samples from metapopulation j.

As for the training samples STRUCTURE admixture components $\boldsymbol{q}_l$ was calculated for the test samples, $l = 1, \ldots, 517$. The closer $\boldsymbol{q}_l$ is to $\bar{\boldsymbol{q}}_j$ for some test sample l and referece metapopulation j, the more likely it is to assume l to originate from metapopulation j. However, how (dis)similar should these admixture components be to declare l (not) to originate from j? Moreover, how should this similarity be measured? One possible measure of proximity could be to use a Brier-like score, B_{lj}, which is the sum of squared admixture components differences between test sample l and reference metapopulation j:

$$B_{lj} = \frac{1}{K} \sum_{k=1}^{K} (q_l^{(k)} - \bar{q}_j^{(k)})^2.$$

The closer B_{lj} is 0, the more similar is sample l to metapopulation j in terms of STRUCTURE admixture components [Supplementary materials of 26]. The maximal value of B_{lj} is $2/K$, which happens if $q_l^{(k)} = 1$ and $\bar{q}_j^{(k')} = 1$ for $k \neq k'$. In Figure 3, the boxplots of the Brier scores for each of six metapopulations are grouped according to the test samples' status inferred by the GenoGeographer methodology (in colours) [55]. Added to plot in grey boxplots are the Brier scores for the reference samples, which are the samples used to compute $\bar{q}_j$. Thus, the grey boxplots are expected to show lower Brier scores compared to those of the coloured boxplots.

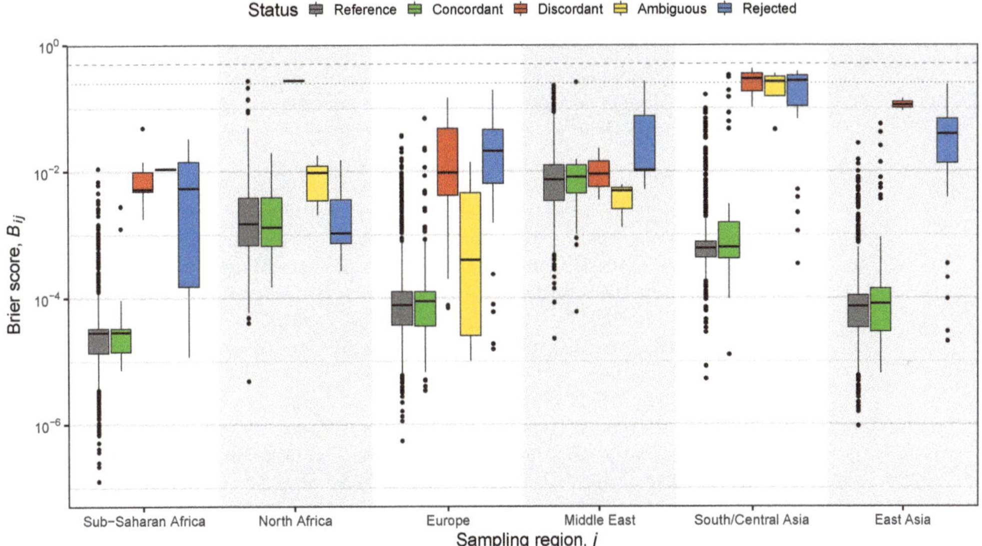

Figure 3. Boxplots of the Brier scores, B_{ij}, with $K = 4$ in the STRUCTURE analysis and j running through the metapopulations of [58]. *Reference:* Samples constituting the metapopulations (and used to calculate $\bar{q}_j$). *Concordant:* A sample is accepted in the metapopulation coinciding with its sampling region (with a likelihood value significantly larger than any other metapopulation). *Discordant:* A sample is accepted in a metapopulation different than its sampling region (with a likelihood value significantly larger than any other metapopulation). *Ambiguous:* A sample's likelihood value is not significantly different in two or more of the accepted metapopulations. *Rejected:* A sample is rejected in all metapopulations. The concordant test samples (green) have similar Brier scores as those of the reference samples (grey). Discordant samples (red) tend to have the largest Brier scores, followed by the rejected samples (blue) with the ambiguous (yellow) in between (see text for definitions). The horizontal dashed and dotted lines in the top of the plot indicates $B_{ij} = 0.5$ and 0.25, respectively ([26], inspired by Supplementary Figure 8).

The Brier scores, B_{ij}, in Figure 3, tend to be larger for discordant, ambiguous, and rejected samples (see definitions in caption of Figure 3). However, from the visual inspection of the STRUCTURE barplots (data not shown), it is often rather hard to judge when a sample deviates substantially from a given metapopulation to declare it extreme compared to the other samples. The advantage of GenoGeographer is that such visual inspections or *ad hoc* defined thresholds for dissimilarity (e.g., using a Brier score) are not required. The conclusions are based solely on a hypothesis test and a predefined significance level.

The model formulation of STRUCTURE implies that any spurious and complex type of admixture can be modelled. For the GenoGeographer framework, however, only specific admixtures can be assessed. Currently, first-order admixtures can be accounted for [56], but the admixture approach can be generalised to handle outlier tests for higher-order admixtures (e.g., second-order where the parents themselves may be admixed). However, the ancestry SNPs may not be sufficiently informative to distinguish between certain admixture configurations (e.g., two pedigrees with different founder populations may be equally likely).

One solution to this may be to use linked markers as these typically are more informative for pedigree analyses [59]. In order to handle linked markers in the framework of hypothesis tests, e.g., microhaplotypes [17], the interactions between the markers was modelled using decomposable graphical models, where association structures between the

SNPs could be different among the reference populations [23] (e.g., the linkage between SNPs was allowed to be different between continental regions). For a microhaplotype with K biallelic SNPs, there exist 2^K different alleles, implying that many samples are needed to obtain accurate allele frequency estimates for moderate values of K. By exploiting the conditional independence structures, the framework of graphical models provides a more data efficient modelling of the microhaplotype frequencies and thus requires fewer samples.

3. Discussion

STRUCTURE remains to be a valuable methodology and approach for analysing population structure in forensic genetics. There exist several guides and tutorials for how to prepare the population data and choosing parameter settings for STRUCTURE (e.g., [60,61], with some emphasis on forensic applications). However, as warned by [44], the resulting barplots should not be overinterpreted. The badMIXTURE approach [45] provides the means to reduce the risk of being mislead by the summaries provided by STRUCTURE and supporting software (e.g., [7,48]).

However, STRUCTURE's popularity in the field of population genetics to study population structure is well deserved. It complemented PCA with a quantitative method that assigns sample specific weights to each of the K populations specified in the study. This is a powerful way to summarise the data in terms of cluster membership probabilities and the estimated allele frequencies for the identified populations. Both PCA and STRUCTURE are valuable for exploratory analysis, where encoding errors (e.g., of missing data) and warnings about misspecification of origin may be detected by visual inspections of the results. From a forensic point of view, the results from both PCA and STRUCTURE are hard to report in terms of a weight of evidence calculation. The similarity (or dissimilarity) between the sample and reference materials can be reported but typically only in terms of their visual appearance. By contrast, classification and likelihood-based methods are able to give weight to the evidence. This may be in terms of a posterior probability or likelihood ratio, where the assignment would be to the most probable population. However, none of these methods take into account the risk of assigning the profile to the *least unlikely* population in the case where none of the populations are representative for the true population of origin.

Inferring a DNA profile's geographic region or population of origin has been an active field of research in forensic genetics for several years. The vast collections of publicly available databases of whole-genome sequences provide a unique resource for researchers. Rather than spending time and consumables on collecting samples, these DNA profiles can now be harvested online. However, in doing so, one relies on the quality of the data provided by others, which includes the genetic typing and base calling but also the metadata regarding sampling location and ethnic information.

In the case of forensic genetics, the finer resolutions are often of interest. In order to increase the specificity, it may be necessary to supplement the selected AIMs with more locally informative markers, specific to separating the local and often related populations of interest. In the search for such markers, the publicly available datasets are of immense importance as they can be used to screen for candidate AIMs. In particular, the samples from regions close to the specific populations of interest are essential for selecting potential markers.

Combining the flexibility of STRUCTURE with the appealing visual features of PCA (e.g., using EIGENSTRAT to determine the number of significant components) is essential in the exploratory phase of ancestry inference. However, the forensic questions related to ancestry is typically different from those of population genetics, where the focus may be on *population* specific patterns (e.g., bottleneck and expansion events or migration). The typical forensic use case focuses on a specific *individual* (or human remains), for which the most likely population of origin needs to be identified. In such cases, likelihood ratio or classification methods can be used. However, the fundamental assumption of the existence of an appropriate population in the reference material may very often be violated. Hence,

DNA profiles are assigned to the population that is most similar to the sample, which due to human evolution and history may geographically and culturally be very far away from the true population. The GenoGeographer methodology attempts to overcomes this logical problem by using statistically based outlier tests.

Funding: This research received no external funding.

Institutional Review Board Statement: Not applicable.

Informed Consent Statement: Not applicable.

Data Availability Statement: Not applicable.

Acknowledgments: The author would like to thank two anonymous reviewers for instructive comments that improved the final version of the manuscript

Conflicts of Interest: The author declares no conflict of interest.

References

1. International HapMap Consortium. The International HapMap Project. *Nature* **2003**, *426*, 789–796. [CrossRef] [PubMed]
2. The 1000 Genomes Project Consortium. A global reference for human genetic variation. *Nature* **2015**, *526*, 68–74. [CrossRef] [PubMed]
3. Mallick, S.; Li, H.; Lipson, M.; Mathieson, I.; Gymrek, M.; Racimo, F.; Zhao, M.; Chennagiri, N.; Nordenfelt, S.; Tandon, A.; et al. The Simons Genome Diversity Project: 300 genomes from 142 diverse populations. *Nature* **2016**, *538*, 201–206. [CrossRef] [PubMed]
4. Karczewski, K.J.; Francioli, L.C.; Tiao, G.; Cummings, B.B.; Alföldi, J.; Wang, Q.; Collins, R.L.; Laricchia, K.M.; Ganna, A.; Birnbaum, D.P.; et al. The mutational constraint spectrum quantified from variation in 141,456 humans. *Nature* **2020**, *581*, 434–443. [CrossRef]
5. Cavalli-Sforza, L.L.; Menozzi, P.; Piazza, A. *The History and Geography of Human Genes*; Princeton Universily Press: Princeton, NJ, USA, 1994.
6. Jobling, M.A.; Hollox, E.; Hurles, M.; Kivisild, T.; Tyler-Smith, C. *Human Evolutionary Genetics*, 2nd ed.; Garland Science, Taylor & Francis Group: New York, NY, USA, 2014.
7. Rosenberg, N.A.; Pritchard, J.K.; Weber, J.L.; Cann, H.M.; Kidd, K.K.; Zhivotovsky, L.A.; Feldman, M.W. Genetic structure of human populations. *Science* **2002**, *298*, 2381–2384. [CrossRef] [PubMed]
8. Cavalli-Sforza, L.L.; Feldman, M.W. The application of molecular genetic approaches to the study of human evolution. *Nat. Genet. (Suppl.)* **2003**, *33*, 266–275. [CrossRef]
9. Serre, D.; Pääbo, S. Evidence for gradients of human genetic diversity within and among continents. *Genome Res.* **2004**, *14*, 1679–1685. [CrossRef]
10. Manica, A.; Prugnolle, F.; Balloux, F. Geography is a better determinant of genetic differentiation than ethnicity. *Hum. Genet.* **2005**, *118*, 366–371. [CrossRef]
11. Novembre, J.; Johnson, T.; Bryc, K.; Kutalik, Z.; Boyko, A.R.; Auton, A.; Indap, A.; King, K.S.; Bergmann, S.; Nelson, M.R.; et al. Genes mirror geography within Europe. *Nature* **2008**, *456*, 98–101. [CrossRef]
12. Wang, C.; Zöllner, S.; Rosenberg, N. A quantitative comparison of the similarity between genes and geography in worldwide human populations. *PLoS Genet.* **2012**, *8*, e1002886. [CrossRef]
13. Rosenberg, N.; Li, L.; Ward, R.; Pritchard, J. Informativeness of genetic markers for inference of ancestry. *Am. J. Hum. Genet.* **2003**, *73*, 1402–1422. [CrossRef]
14. Rosenberg, N.A. Algorithms for Selecting Informative Marker Panels for Population Assignment. *J. Comput. Biol.* **2005**, *12*, 1183–1201. [CrossRef] [PubMed]
15. Brinkmann, B.; Junge, A.; Meyer, E.; Wiegand, P. Population Genetic Diversity in Relation to Microsatellite Heterogeneity. *Hum. Mut.* **1998**, *11*, 135–44. [CrossRef]
16. Alladio, E.; Della Rocca, C.; Barni, F.; Dugoujon, J.M.; Garofano, P.; Semino, O.; Berti, A.; Novelletto, A.; Vincenti, M.; Cruciani, F.; et al. A multivariate statistical approach for the estimation of the ethnic origin of unknown genetic profiles in forensic genetics. *Forensic Sci. Int. Genet.* **2020**, *45*, 102209. [CrossRef]
17. Oldoni, F.; Kidd, K.K.; Podini, D. Microhaplotypes in forensic genetics. *Forensic Sci. Int. Genet.* **2019**, *38*, 54–69. [CrossRef]
18. Yang, N.; Li, H.; Criswell, L.A.; Gregersen, P.K.; Alarcon-Riquelme, M.E.; Kittles, R.; Shigeta, R.; Silva, G.; Patel, P.I.; Belmont, J.W.; et al. Examination of ancestry and ethnic affiliation using highly informative diallelic DNA markers: Application to diverse and admixed populations and implications for clinical epidemiology and forensic medicine. *Hum. Genet.* **2005**, *118*, 382–392. [CrossRef]
19. Moriot, A.; Santos, C.; Freire-Aradas, A.; Phillips, C.; Hall, D. Inferring biogeographic ancestry with compound markers of slow and fast evolving polymorphisms. *Eur. J. Hum. Genet.* **2018**, *26*, 1697–1707. [CrossRef]
20. Phillips, C. Forensic genetic analysis of bio-geographical ancestry. *Forensic Sci. Int. Genet.* **2015**, *18*, 49–65. [CrossRef] [PubMed]

21. Phillips, C.; Santos, C.; Fondevila, M.; Carracedo, Á.; Lareu, M.V. Inference of Ancestry in Forensic Analysis I: Autosomal Ancestry-Informative Marker Sets. In *Forensic DNA Typing Protocols*; Methods in Molecular Biology; Goodwin, W., Ed.; Springer: Berlin/Heidelberg, Germany, 2016; Volume 1420, pp. 234–253.

22. Falush, D.; Stephens, M.; Pritchard, J.K. Inference of Population Structure Using Multilocus Genotype Data: Linked Loci and Correlated Allele Frequencies. *Genetics* **2003**, *164*, 1567–1587. [CrossRef]

23. Lindskou, M.; Eriksen, P.S.; Tvedebrink, T. Outlier detection in contingency tables using decomposable graphical models. *Scand. J. Stat.* **2020**, *47*, 347–360. [CrossRef]

24. Purcell, S.; Neale, B.; Todd-Brown, K.; Thomas, L.; Ferreira, M.A.; Bender, D.; Maller, J.; Sklar, P.; de Bakker, P.I.; Daly, M.J.; et al. PLINK: A Tool Set for Whole-Genome Association and Population-Based Linkage Analyses. *Am. J. Hum. Genet.* **2007**, *81*, 559–575. [CrossRef]

25. Patterson, N.; Price, A.L.; Reich, D. Population Structure and Eigenanalysis. *PLoS Genet.* **2006**, *2*, e190. [CrossRef]

26. Mogensen, H.S.; Tvedebrink, T.; Børsting, C.; Pereira, V.; Morling, N. Ancestry prediction efficiency of the software GenoGeographer using a z-score method and the ancestry informative markers in the Precision ID Ancestry Panel. *Forensic Sci. Int. Genet.* **2020**, *44*, 102154. [CrossRef]

27. Menozzi, P.; Piazza, A.; Cavalli-Sforza, L.L. Synthetic maps of human gene frequencies in Europeans. *Science* **1978**, *201*, 786–792. [CrossRef] [PubMed]

28. Price, A.L.; Patterson, N.J.; Plenge, R.M.; Weinblatt, M.E.; Shadick, N.A.; Reich, D. Principal components analysis corrects for stratification in genome-wide association studies. *Nat. Genet.* **2006**, *38*, 904–909. [CrossRef] [PubMed]

29. Jombart, T.; Devillard, S.; Balloux, F. Discriminant analysis of principal components: A new method for the analysis of genetically structured populations. *BMC Genet.* **2010**, *11*, 94. [CrossRef] [PubMed]

30. Novembre, J.; Stephens, M. Interpreting principal component analyses of spatial population genetic variation. *Nat. Genet.* **2008**, *40*, 646–649. [CrossRef]

31. McVean, G. A Genealogical Interpretation of Principal Components Analysis. *PLoS Genet.* **2009**, *5*, 1–10. [CrossRef]

32. Wangkumhang, P.; Hellenthal, G. Statistical methods for detecting admixture. *Curr. Opin. Genet. Dev.* **2018**, *53*, 121–127. [CrossRef]

33. Miller, J.M.; Cullingham, C.I.; Peery, R.M. The influence of a priori grouping on inference of genetic clusters: Simulation study and literature review of the DAPC method. *Heredity* **2020**, *125*, 269–280. [CrossRef]

34. Pritchard, J.K.; Stephens, M.; Donnelly, P.J. Inference of population structure using multilocus genotype data. *Genetics* **2000**, *155*, 945–959. [CrossRef] [PubMed]

35. Novembre, J. Pritchard, Stephens, and Donnelly on Population Structure. *Genetics* **2016**, *204*, 391–393. [CrossRef] [PubMed]

36. Rannala, B.; Mountain, J.L. Detecting immigration by using multilocus genotypes. *Proc. Natl. Acad. Sci. USA* **1997**, *94*, 9197–9201. [CrossRef] [PubMed]

37. Foreman, L.; Smith, A.; Evett, I. Bayesian analysis of DNA profiling data in forensic identification applications. *J. R. Stat. Soc. A* **1997**, *160*, 429–469. [CrossRef]

38. Roeder, K.; Escobar, M.; Kadane, J.B.; Balazs, I. Measuring heterogeneity in forensic databases using hierarchical Bayes models. *Biometrika* **1998**, *85*, 269–287. [CrossRef]

39. Falush, D.; Stephens, M.; Pritchard, J.K. Inference of population structure using multilocus genotype data: Dominant markers and null alleles. *Mol. Ecol. Notes* **2007**, *7*, 574–578. [CrossRef]

40. Tang, H.; Peng, J.; Wang, P.; Risch, N. Estimation of Individual Admixture: Analytical and Study Design Considerations. *Genet. Epidemiol.* **2005**, *28*, 289–301. [CrossRef]

41. Alexander, D.H.; Novembre, J.; Lange, K. Fast model-based estimation of ancestry in unrelated individuals. *Genome Res.* **2009**, *19*, 1655–1664. [CrossRef]

42. Raj, A.; Stephens, M.; Pritchard, J.K. fastSTRUCTURE: Variational Inference of Population Structure in Large SNP Data Sets. *Genetics* **2014**, *197*, 573–589. [CrossRef]

43. Novembre, J. Variations on a Common STRUCTURE: New Algorithms for a Valuable Model. *Genetics* **2014**, *197*, 809–811. [CrossRef]

44. Lawson, D.J.; van Dorp, L.; Falush, D. A tutorial on how not to over-interpret STRUCTURE and ADMIXTURE bar plots. *Nat. Commun.* **2018**, *9*, 3258. [CrossRef]

45. Lawson, D. *badMIXTURE: Validating Structure With Chromosome Painting*; R Package Version 0.0.0.9000; 2018. Available online: https://github.com/danjlawson/badMIXTURE (accessed on 13 December 2021).

46. Hellenthal, G.; Busby, G.B.J.; Band, G.; Wilson, J.F.; Capelli, C.; Falush, D.; Myers, S. A Genetic Atlas of Human Admixture History. *Science* **2014**, *343*, 747–751. [CrossRef]

47. Lawson, D.J.; Hellenthal, G.; Myers, S.; Falush, D. Inference of Population Structure using Dense Haplotype Data. *PLoS Genet.* **2012**, *8*, 1–16. [CrossRef] [PubMed]

48. Jakobsson, M.; Rosenberg, N.A. CLUMPP: A cluster matching and permutation program for dealing with label switching and multimodality in analysis of population structure. *Bioinformatics* **2007**, *23*, 1801–1806. [CrossRef]

49. Cheung, K.H.; Osier, M.V.; Kidd, J.R.; Pakstis, A.J.; Miller, P.L.; Kidd, K.K. ALFRED: An allele frequency database for diverse populations and DNA polymorphisms. *Nucleic Acids Res.* **2000**, *28*, 361–363. [CrossRef]

50. Pakstis, A.; Kang, L.; Liu, L.; Zhang, Z.; Jin, T.; Grigorenko, E.L.; Wendt, F.R.; Budowle, B.; Hadi, S.; Qahtanif, M.S.A.; et al. Increasing the reference populations for the 55 AISNP panel: The need and benefits. *Int. J. Legal Med.* **2017**, *131*, 913–917. [CrossRef]

51. Phillips, C.; Prieto, L.; Fondevila, M.; Salas, A.; Gomez-Tato, A.; Alvarez-Dios, J.; Alonso, A.; Blanco-Verea, A.; Brion, M.; Montesino, M.; et al. Ancestry analysis in the 11-M Madrid bomb attack investigation. *PLoS ONE* **2009**, *4*, e6583. [CrossRef] [PubMed]

52. Cheung, E.Y.; Gahan, M.E.; McNevin, D. Prediction of biogeographical ancestry from genotype: A comparison of classifiers. *Int. J. Legal Med.* **2017**, *131*, 901–912. [CrossRef]

53. McNevina, D.; Santos, C.; Gómez-Tato, A.; Álvarez-Dios, J.; Casares de Cal, M.; Daniel, R.; Phillips, C.; Lareu, M.V. Anassessment of Bayesian and multinomial logistic regression classification systems to analyse admixed individuals. *Forensic Sci. Int. Genet. Suppl. Ser.* **2013**, *4*, e63–e64. [CrossRef]

54. Cheung, E.Y.Y.; Gahan, M.E.; McNevin, D. Prediction of biogeographical ancestry in admixed individuals. *Forensic Sci. Int. Genet.* **2018**, *36*, 104–111. [CrossRef]

55. Tvedebrink, T.; Eriksen, P.S.; Mogensen, H.S.; Morling, N. Weight of the Evidence of Genetic Investigations of Ancestry Informative Markers. *Theor. Popul. Biol.* **2018**, *120*, 1–10. [CrossRef]

56. Tvedebrink, T.; Eriksen, P.S. Inference of admixed ancestry with Ancestry Informative Markers. *Forensic Sci. Int. Genet.* **2019**, *42*, 147–153. [CrossRef]

57. Pfaffelhuber, P.; Sester-Huss, E.; Baumdicker, F.; Naue, J.; Lutz-Bonengel, S.; Staubach, F. Inference of recent admixture using genotype data. *Forensic Sci. Int. Genet.* **2021**, *56*, 102593. [CrossRef]

58. Tvedebrink, T.; Eriksen, P.S.; Mogensen, H.S.; Morling, N. GenoGeographer—A tool for genogeographic inference. *Forensic Sci. Int. Genet. Suppl. Ser.* **2017**, *6*, e463–e465. [CrossRef]

59. Kling, D.; Tillmar, A.; Egeland, T.; Mostad, P. A general model for likelihood computations of genetic marker data accounting for linkage, linkage disequilibrium, and mutations. *Int. J. Legal Med.* **2015**, *129*, 943–954. [CrossRef]

60. Porras-Hurtado, L.; Ruiz, Y.; Santos, C.; Phillips, C.; Carracedo, Á.; Lareu, M. An overview of STRUCTURE: Applications, parameter settings, and supporting software. *Front. Genet.* **2013**, *4*, 98. [CrossRef]

61. Santos, C.; Phillips, C.; Gomez-Tato, A.; Alvarez-Dios, J.; Carracedo, Á.; Lareu, M.V. Inference of Ancestry in Forensic Analysis II: Analysis of Genetic Data. In *Forensic DNA Typing Protocols*; Methods in Molecular Biology; Goodwin, W., Ed.; Springer: Berlin/Heidelberg, Germany, 2016; Volume 1420, pp. 255–285.

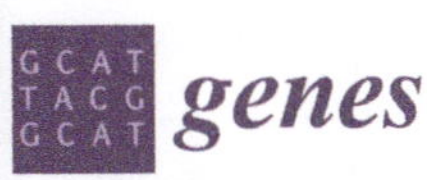

genes

Article

Ethics as Lived Practice. Anticipatory Capacity and Ethical Decision-Making in Forensic Genetics

Matthias Wienroth [1,*], Rafaela Granja [2], Veronika Lipphardt [3], Emmanuel Nsiah Amoako [4] and Carole McCartney [5]

1 Centre for Crime and Policing, Department of Social Sciences, Northumbria University, Newcastle upon Tyne NE1 8ST, UK
2 Communication and Society Research Centre, University of Minho, 4710-057 Braga, Portugal; r.granja@ics.uminho.pt
3 University College Freiburg, Albert-Ludwigs-Universität, 79098 Freiburg, Germany; veronika.lipphardt@ucf.uni-freiburg.de
4 Department of Applied Sciences, University of the West of England, Bristol BS16 1QY, UK; emmanuel.nsiahamoako@uwe.ac.uk
5 Science & Justice Research Interest Group, Law School, Northumbria University, Newcastle upon Tyne NE1 8ST, UK; carole.mccartney@northumbria.ac.uk
* Correspondence: matthias.wienroth@northumbria.ac.uk

Abstract: Greater scrutiny and demands for innovation and increased productivity place pressures on scientists. Forensic genetics is advancing at a rapid pace but can only do so responsibly, usefully, and acceptably within ethical and legal boundaries. We argue that such boundaries require that forensic scientists embrace 'ethics as lived practice'. As a starting point, we critically discuss 'thin' ethics in forensic genetics, which lead to a myopic focus on procedures, and to seeing 'privacy' as the sole ethical concern and technology as a mere tool. To overcome 'thin' ethics in forensic genetics, we instead propose understanding ethics as an intrinsic part of the lived practice of a scientist. Therefore, we explore, within the context of three case studies of emerging forensic genetics technologies, ethical aspects of decision-making in forensic genetics research and in technology use. We discuss the creation, curation, and use of databases, and the need to engage with societal and policing contexts of forensic practice. We argue that open communication is a vital ethical aspect. Adoption of 'ethics as lived practice' supports the development of anticipatory capacity—empowering scientists to understand, and act within ethical and legal boundaries, incorporating the operational and societal impacts of their daily decisions, and making visible ethical decision making in scientific practice.

Keywords: ethics; forensic genetics; ethics as lived practice; decision-making; genetic databasing; forensic DNA phenotyping; forensic genealogy; forensic epigenetics; communication; database

Citation: Wienroth, M.; Granja, R.; Lipphardt, V.; Nsiah Amoako, E.; McCartney, C. Ethics as Lived Practice. Anticipatory Capacity and Ethical Decision-Making in Forensic Genetics. *Genes* **2021**, *12*, 1868. https://doi.org/10.3390/genes12121868

Academic Editor: Niels Morling

Received: 1 November 2021
Accepted: 23 November 2021
Published: 24 November 2021

Publisher's Note: MDPI stays neutral with regard to jurisdictional claims in published maps and institutional affiliations.

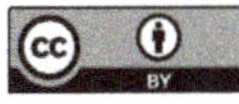

1. Introduction

Ethical principles and their application in practice have come to matter to many individual forensic geneticists, working to ensure that, while the scientific foundation of the techniques they are developing and deploying for casework is reliable, they are also contributing to a just society. Yet forensic genetics as a discipline and a community of practice—research scientists, laboratory practitioners, journals, industry, professional bodies, and users of forensic genetic analyses in policing and elsewhere—continue to face scrutinize new and emerging forensic genetic technologies for their social, ethical, and legal ramifications, alongside their scientific and technical dimensions. For example, the German Government led an inquiry into forensic DNA phenotyping and biogeographic ancestry testing between 2017 and 2019, leading to the legalisation of the former in 2019, but not of the latter, due to concerns around racial profiling [1]. The Law Commission of New Zealand reported on new and emergent forensic genetics in 2020, recommending the comprehensive revision of legislation; increased oversight; and greater consideration of concerns surrounding privacy and discrimination [2]. The Law Commission of Ontario reviewed Artificial Intelligence (AI) and probabilistic genotyping DNA tools in June 2021, suggesting that inherent biases in these technologies challenge the notion of DNA profiling as a "gold standard" and requires that there is continuous scrutiny as well as new legislation [3]. The Scottish Government and the UK House of Lords have commenced parallel enquiries into developments in technologies for policing in 2021 [4,5], scoping opportunities, and challenges arising for policing from new technologies.

While these enquiries are undertaken, reports published, and debates held, demand continues for the utility of databases (including genetic ones) to be maximised, and the promise of forensic genetics—often portrayed as the greatest crime-fighting tool since fingerprinting—be realised and capitalised upon. Meanwhile, new techniques are being developed and debated. Despite remaining contentious, internationally, the use of genetic 'phenotyping' in police investigations is growing. The Swiss Parliament is the latest to prepare legislation to allow for forensic DNA phenotyping amidst, both, supportive and critical debate [6]. Similarly, since 2018, forays into forensic genetic genealogy have been spreading since the successful detection of the perpetrator with the help of the technique in the 'Golden State Killer' case in the USA [7–10].

In these areas, as well as generally, forensic scientists face institutional pressures, both from casework and their scientific community (including employers/funders), which must be met with scientific professionalism and ethical practice. Yet it was not long ago that scientists themselves conceded that forensic science 'is not sufficiently well developed as a profession' (p. 523, [11]). Within the scientific community, there is increased scrutiny regarding the way that data are sourced and shared, informing both forensic research and casework analysis [12]. The intensification of external scrutiny, and productivity pressures demand the highest levels of professionalism, which must include a strong, internalized code of ethics that has not yet been proven to be universal [13].

In some parts of the world, forensic genetics research and casework have become an important aspect of policing, criminal justice, and victim identification. In multiple ways, forensic genetics contributes to rendering these domains more agile vis-à-vis existing and emerging demands and challenges. Novel technologies are developed in response to scientific insights and practical problems while remaining subject to the same responsibilities that scientists and users have towards their specific institutions, disciplines, and to society as a whole.

Therefore, in this paper, we offer an approach through which the forensic genetics community can reflect on their daily decisions in both scientific research and casework as part of their professional and ethical forensic practice. While we cannot, nor do we aim to, provide technical or legal solutions, we offer a framework for ethical conduct. We consider the problem of 'thin' ethics in forensic genetics and propose understanding ethics as an intrinsic part of the lived practice of a scientist. We aim to support scientists in developing anticipatory capacity [14]—to understand the wider operational and societal impacts of their daily decisions around forensic genetics—by making visible the ethical decisions in both their scientific practice and in the application and implementation of forensic technologies. We do so by exploring ethical aspects of decision-making in forensic genetics and illustrating the discussion by way of three case studies of emerging forensic genetics technologies.

2. Materials and Methods

This paper builds on literature analysed in three previous reviews of social and ethical aspects of scientific, technological, and operational developments in forensic genetics [15–17], adding consideration of scholarship published since 2017, and focusing on three technologies currently being debated: forensic DNA phenotyping (FDP), forensic genetic genealogy (FGG), and forensic epigenetics (FEpi). In this endeavour, the concept of the "social life of DNA," proposed by Corinna Kruse [18], which captures the different social relationships observed in the processing of DNA as it moves from crime scene to courtroom, resonates. As such, we analyse the different life stages of advanced forensic

DNA technologies. While DNA profiling is a relatively widely accepted technology, having stabilized and been implemented across different contexts, the three technologies we focus on are yet to reach such a point of stability. In reviewing these examples, we highlight key ethical concerns to assist forensic practitioners in expanding their anticipatory capacity and thus work towards ethically sound decision making. By anticipatory capacity, we refer to antecedent considerations in science, and in real-world application of science, set within a wider context of liberal-democratic social and cultural norms and values. These three technologies were selected, firstly, due to controversy concerning their utility and reliability/validity specifically, and their ethics more generally [19,20]. Secondly, these technologies present opportunities to engage with ethics as lived practice, as they pose ethical dilemmas. Thirdly, debates are ongoing over their use, and measures in place to regulate these technologies differ across countries. Finally, each of these technologies is currently at different life stages. Forensic DNA phenotyping, although still the subject of complex politics of legitimation and contestation [20–23], is currently regulated and applied in some countries such as Slovakia and Germany. Forensic genetic genealogy is under intense scrutiny in many jurisdictions and upcoming regulation can be expected (see for example recent initiatives in the USA and in Australia). Forensic epigenetics is being developed and has not (yet) been considered widely with respect to regulation and/or application.

3. The Limitations of "Thin" Ethics in Forensic Genetics

Controversies surrounding advances in forensic genetics could (at least in part) be a consequence of a structural deficiency in comprehensive, systematic understandings of what ethics is—or should be—in forensic genetics and related technological innovations. Let us explain what we mean by a "thin" understanding of ethics.

Firstly, forensic geneticists will encounter ethics as part of an administrative process to be followed to enable research, innovation, and implementation: following codes of practice, completing forms, attending training, and submitting authorizations to some form of the institutional oversight body. Such administrative tasks and tools are clearly essential in ensuring forensic scientists navigate the most basic rules of research and technology use. However, the main thrust of this 'procedural ethics' [24] is to comply with administrative and legal procedural requirements, with ethics conceived of as 'passive', lending itself to the interpretation of ethics as a hurdle to research, innovation, and (positive) societal impact that forensic genetics could otherwise make. Consequently, exclusive adherence to this "thin" procedural ethics can extinguish the light that a (pro-)active approach can shine on the complex environment within which forensic work takes place. It also 'disengages' forensic geneticists (both in research and casework) from ethics to the detriment of forensic genetics, and more widely to science in the criminal justice system.

Secondly, within this "thin" understanding of ethics, 'privacy' tends to be perceived as an interpretable legal concept, addressed by compliance with the law. Moreover, 'data protection' is often used as a proxy for 'privacy', whereby observance with principles of data protection will suffice, yet 'privacy' is far more expansive and manifold than mere data protection (pp. 33–50, [25,26]). A reductionist understanding of ethics as privacy obscures other vital aspects of ethical practice, including attending to justice and fairness, human dignity (and its cultural values, see, e.g., recommendations by the Law Commission of New Zealand vis-a-vis forensic genetics and the Māori), and the physical and informational integrity of a person and/or a group of persons (community). A focus on privacy also misdirects debate into a cul-de-sac of arguments over balancing 'personal privacy' with 'public security' since this dichotomy is erroneous; privacy and security are symbiotic [27,28].

Thirdly, technology may be perceived as a mere tool, process, or method. However, as several years of consolidated scientific research have shown (particularly in social studies of science and technology in health research, and more recently in the social studies of forensic science), technology is a product of social, cultural, and moral facets of society. Technology is always technology-in-practice [29] resulting from, and shaping social interactions and the organisation of social life. As Greenhalgh and Swinglehurst (p. 3, [30]) suggest, considering technology as social practices "moves us on from studying either people or technologies" towards a rich, inclusive analysis of technology as an aspect of social life, considering technology-in-use as well as the discourses and practices of technology [31].

Reducing technology to its instrumental aspects conceals many ethical decisions that shape technology, from its conception to application and maintenance as well as to its oversight. Thus, we consider "thin" or 'procedural ethics' insufficient in forensic research and application, with privacy as just one ethical concern. Nor is technology a mere tool or method but should be viewed as social practice. Thus, we propose an approach to ethics as intrinsic to the lived practice of forensic geneticists, making deliberate decisions about daily practices and procedures, acting in light of these decisions, while continually reflecting upon their broader impacts now and in the future.

4. Ethics as Lived Practice

Ethics as lived practice extends throughout the life cycle of science: from development and implementation to regulation and oversight. Regardless, then, of the role(s) that professionals fulfil—whether as research scientist engaged with the laboratory-based development of forensic applications; as a forensic practitioner working on criminal cases; as an expert advising on casework or giving evidence in court—ethical engagement is inalienably part of professional practice. Such ethical engagement is inescapable because (i) the development of forensic technologies will affect human beings; (ii) those conducting forensic casework, and working with forensic data and information, are, as all other human beings, subjective, open to influence, and fallible; and (iii) forensic casework builds upon and contributes to selecting, categorising, and curating data and data repositories as reference points, thus making choices that will affect future forensic research and casework, and as such, many more humans.

Our understanding of ethics as lived practice stands in contrast to the notion of ethics as a necessary evil and to the "thin" ethics discussed above—where ethics only arise at bounded points in time when the ethics 'hurdle' is jumped. Ethics as lived practice, instead, recognises that decision-making is ongoing, and an intrinsic part of the practice. Continual reflection, then, becomes central: taking time, sometimes briefly, sometimes for a longer period; alone or as a team; discipline; or community, to (re)consider the basis and motivations on which decisions are being taken, as well as their consequences. This also calls for serious engagement with others, including those from outside the laboratory (such as criminal investigators, social scientists, policymakers forging legislation and regulation, as well as the civil society), to discuss research, analysis, and future application, within their wider social and cultural contexts. We call upon the forensic genetics community to build on emerging strengths here by making ethical reflection—as a way of building anticipatory capacity—an integral part of forensic genetics work.

The remarkable potential of forensic science, to not only contribute to the pursuit of justice, but to shape and direct society, is highly valued, but comes with enormous responsibility. Acknowledgment of the wider impact of forensic work means that ethics ought to be reflected in scientists' and practitioners' training, in their daily decision-making, and in contributions to scientific and public debates about forensics. Guillemin and Guillam [24] explain that ethics work occurs in researchers' daily practice beyond procedural ethics. Such a practice-related understanding of ethics has been suggested as a way of incorporating principle-based reflections about the impact and implications of scientific design and work into everyday decisions [32]. Furthermore, Guillemin and Guillam suggest that researchers may encounter ethically relevant moments, where the approach taken or decision made has important ethical ramifications, but where researchers do not necessarily feel themselves to be on the horns of a dilemma. In fact, in some cases, it might be clear how the researcher should respond or proceed, and yet there is still something ethically important at stake (p. 265, [24]). While the scientist or practitioner might not perceive this moment as particularly vital or difficult, the decisions made at this moment can have significant long-term implications and impacts: on the person making the decision and their forensic specialism; on forensic science more widely and its perception among users, policy and publics; on the domains using forensic science services; and, via these domains, on ethical issues such as: social justice; equality; equity; dignity; privacy; integrity, and so forth. In these 'ethical moments' (for a look at ethical moments in forensic genetics, see e.g., [33]) different perspectives are brought together, to identify and resolve disagreements, making visible ethical reasoning about scientific practice and the use of scientific knowledge [20].

Consider, for example, the forensic scientist tracing a partial DNA match indicative of a familial relationship between a suspect DNA profile and that of a dragnet/mass test volunteer. If permitted by law, the modus operandi is clear, and the practitioner should always follow what the law prescribes. However, the law does not, and cannot, provide for every situation practitioners will come across in their daily practice. If the law has not explicitly provided for a situation, there is a significant decision to be made: should the expert report a partial match and thus a potential familial relationship, even though familial searching is not explicitly regulated in their jurisdiction? In pursuit of a perpetrator, it may be legitimate to report, even if such analyses are not formally accepted practice (e.g., not regulated by law, nor a laboratory accredited for), thus shifting the ultimate ethical decision to others, such as the investigating judge (in predominantly inquisitorial systems) or the police and prosecution (in more adversarial systems). Nonetheless, the forensic geneticist is required to make an ethical decision about their practice at this point, and procedures to support them in doing so—perhaps by calling on them to reflect upon their decision—may often be non-existent or very limited. This example, like many others occurring daily in forensic genetics, clearly demonstrates that ethics cannot be limited to an initial passing of a procedural ethical hurdle, but relies on many decisions around reliability, utility, and legitimacy [20] that an individual or their team take in forensic research and casework.

Ethics as lived practice demands more attention, while a "thin" understanding of ethics, anchored, for example, in 'procedural ethics', is insufficient for responsible (and as such also accountable) forensic genetics practice. We argue that ethics as lived practice, therefore, means that forensic researchers and practitioners identify and understand the need to address opportunities as well as limitations of their work set within an institutional and societal context—e.g., in criminal justice, migration management, or disaster victim identification. In the next section, we discuss ethical decision-making in forensic genetics practice using the example of data repositories because their creation, curation, and use are vital to forensic genetics research and can play a significant role in investigative work and law enforcement.

5. Building upon Strong Foundations: Ethical Decision-Making in Genetic Databasing

Central to forensic genetics is the data collected from individuals from diverse groups and curated for use by the scientific community. However, as we show in the example of forensic genetic genealogy below, data collected and curated for non-forensic purposes are also increasingly of interest to forensic geneticists and law enforcement agencies. Data collection and curation in repositories form a key life stage of genetic data and ethical considerations in forensic genetics, as with any human genetics field, therefore begin with the sampling design for DNA data for research and for databases such as EMPOP or YHRD. Since some forensic genetics services depend on population data, genetic data from diverse populations have been widely collected from individuals across the globe for decades. Since the 1970s, the fields of human and medical genetics have developed and adopted a number of ethical standards and procedures, including, most notably, requirements for informed consent and approval by ethics committees [34]. Such processes have been continuously refined and upgraded, and yet ethical debates around genetic data continue [35–39].

In contrast, the forensic genetics community's leading journal, Forensic Science International: Genetics, introduced statements about these basic ethical standards (informed consent and ethics approval) as a publication requirement as late as 2010 [40]. In 2020, guidelines were updated and extended, with a specific focus on population data from minorities or indigenous communities [38]. Until 2010, there were no ethical standards for authors to meet when publishing DNA data; and data collected before 2010 without informed consent and ethical approval is still used, shared, and uploaded. Furthermore, forensic genetic databases usually require the publication of data in peer-reviewed journal articles before such data can be uploaded, along with ethical approval and/or evidence of informed consent. However, in some databases, data can be uploaded without meeting these criteria [41]. Notably, such databases are not only used for research, but also for investigation by law enforcement authorities. Ethical debates around these databases have only now begun.

In human genetics, the demands of obtaining consent for samples from sufficiently large numbers of individuals requires the building of an ethical regime of institutional and personal infrastructures in order to enable the legal and ethical use of samples and profiles (e.g., [42]). Numerous ethical decisions, consciously or not, are inevitably made when recruiting donors: whom to include or exclude, how to frame the research to donors about why samples and data are requested, what to give back to donors and their community, and so forth. In forensic genetics the stakes are higher, as persuading individuals to donate their DNA is challenging. Willingness to donate DNA for forensic purposes used to be considerably lower than for health purposes [43]; albeit more recently there has been an increase in voluntary offers of existing genetic profiles or donation of new genetic data to enable the forensic use of ancestry, health, and research databases [8]. Such donations place a particular responsibility upon researchers and analysts to be very clear about the potential uses of such data, not only at the time of sample collection but also afterwards, as data moves along different life stages.

For such data repositories to serve law enforcement, data acquisition needs to be as extensive as possible to represent diverse populations. Previous resolutions to this problem have attracted criticism: E.g. some forensic practitioners have argued that over-representation of marginalised minorities on databases means they are more likely to be exonerated, but this theory has yet to be supported with evidence while emerging database uses for biogeographic ancestry testing and capacities to de-anonymize profiles increase the riskiness of overrepresentation [12]. Another example is that in China, but also in numerous other countries, police and security forces have been involved in collection efforts, nullifying any supposed 'consent' [1,41,44,45]. Recent discussions focus upon the reuse of data and samples previously collected under unclear ethical conditions, or without any demonstrable adherence to ethical principles [1,12]. Some of these datasets have been obtained from vulnerable populations and shared by, and between researchers from forensic, medical, and population genetics, raising serious questions about whether such data transfers violate general ethical standards.

Even if data have been sampled ethically and safely stored in databases, to be used as training and test data in calibration exercises, or as reference data for criminal investigative application, social and ethical issues may still arise. A key issue is whether the data is representative of the 'target' population [1]. Yet rarely discussed are potential problems arising from non-representative data collection. For example, if the training data for an FDP application has been sampled too selectively (e.g., [46]) and hence is very homogeneous, probability calculations might be overly optimistic. Then, in a criminal investigation, the technology will overestimate its own reliability against the backdrop of a local population that is not as homogeneous as the training data. In biogeographic ancestry testing (BGA), so-called "mixed populations" in training and reference data lead to erroneous test results and overly optimistic reliability estimates [47]. However, "mixed ancestries" will most likely be more commonplace in real life but, in a worst-case scenario, the technology will produce erroneously high probability estimates, and yet these are more likely to be trusted than other evidence-based on perceptions of scientific objectivity and DNA's standing as "biological witness"—and thus risk leading investigations astray [45].

It is critical, therefore, that ethics as lived practice commences at the very first life stages of DNA data: when collecting and curating data and establishing repositories. As this DNA data is then utilised by forensic practitioners within the context of the criminal justice system, the next vital life stage of forensic genetic data, further ethical decision-making is required.

6. Challenges of Context and Communication: Ethical Decision-Making as Forensic Expert

Forensic DNA technologies have been framed by metaphorical affirmations of DNA as representing a "truth machine" [48] or the "gold standard" of evidence [49], reflecting high expectations based upon unrivalled (alleged) levels of validity, certainty, reliability, and objectivity. Besides disregarding issues arising during the "social life of DNA" [18], as it moves from crime scene (or database) to court, such metaphors eclipse the challenges of communicating probabilistic DNA evidence to non-experts [50,51]. These challenges occur at many different contact points: in the regulatory process leading up to new or amended laws or regulations; in the training of geneticists and investigators; in public communications during police investigations; during and after a trial; and in the aftermath of a solved case when the efficiency of different investigative tools is compared and highlighted. In addition, as DNA analysis becomes more sensitive (entailing the analysis of mixed traces, DNA transfer, etc.), and more open to interpretation, it becomes yet more challenging to report [52], with scientists deciding whether to apply a probative value to a result, or provide an inconclusive result that neither includes or excludes the suspect [53].

A rational assessment of what advanced DNA profiling techniques can bring to a police investigation is essential but rare. For example, in the UK, 'familial searching' has been available since 2012 and utilised in 120 cases, with just nine reported 'successes' [54], perhaps challenging proportionality equations over its use. A realistic appraisal must particularly consider how 'results', once outside of a laboratory or research setting such as in forensic validation, are applied during real-life criminal investigations. A host of confounding variables and diverse considerations come into play during the criminal process, which may distort or nullify laboratory results: "while a forensic technique may have a valid scientific basis and prove reliable in a laboratory setting, how can it be ascertained that it remains reliable when applied in the present case? What are the error rates associated with the technique, and are there any pertinent factors that could jeopardise the reliability of the testing in this particular instance?" (p. 240, [13]). A forensic scientist engaged in ethics as the lived practice may be required to inform these more 'realistic' appreciations of what forensic genetics can and cannot achieve within the context of police investigations, particularly when asked to deploy advanced techniques. Both law enforcement and the public should not be 'oversold' benefits that may never be realised outside of a research laboratory [33,55]. Our three case studies below address intelligence-related uses of forensic genetics in investigations, when arguably, the dangers of over-selling capacities by forensic scientists and service providers as well as the ready acceptance of such leads by investigators in order to progress a complex case, are high.

Assuming that DNA science moves from investigation onto a later life stage: forensic intelligence from genetic genealogy, but perhaps also from other techniques, may lead to requests by police for arrest warrants. This potential outcome would require such forensic intelligence to be carefully articulated and to take into account the context in which it may be used, including institutional policing cultures and wider political debates, e.g., about migration and criminality. In inquisitorial systems (but highly unlikely ever in adversarial systems), forensic intelligence may even make it into the report submitted to the investigating judge. At some point, if rarely, forensic experts may be called as witnesses to explain the intelligence.

We know for forensic evidence that the judge may be required to take on a "gatekeeper" role to ensure that "junk science" remains inadmissible at trial. This role and its fulfilment has been highly criticized already for adversarial systems where mechanisms are in place for contestation [56,57], with conclusions drawn that "scientific illiteracy on the part of the legal profession, when coupled with the flaws in forensic science, forms a 'toxic combination'" (p. 82, [56]). The trial process rarely affords even the scientifically literate much opportunity to interpret and apply 'correctly' complex tests (assuming there is a 'correct' application) for whether scientific evidence is 'sufficiently reliable' [58]. In addition, such admissibility testing may come too late in the criminal process. Consider, too, that in the inquisitorial system forensic expertise is very rarely challenged. Even where challenges to scientific information exist, decisions to admit such information at trial can appear arbitrary, or inconsistent, with decisions based upon non-scientific criteria [59].

Scientists, in providing intelligence as well as in giving testimony, are called upon to make ethical decisions about which information to present and how it should be best communicated. Much work has gone into, e.g., developing verbal scales as equivalents of reporting numerical values and effectively interpreting probabilities [60–62]. Forensic geneticists' adherence to ethical principles and practices in giving testimony, is a key aspect of their responsibility as practitioners (see, e.g., [63]), yet can be complicated by different scientific, investigative, and juridical pressures and demands on the scientific expert. A key responsibility is avoiding 'over-egging the pudding'. As such, scientific experts have personal and disciplinary responsibility for their communication, and thus at least in part, a wider responsibility for the role of intelligence in investigations and for scientific evidence in court.

In response to the exposure of mistakes, misrepresentations, and misunderstandings of DNA evidence that have led to failed investigations or miscarriages of justice, there have been efforts to regulate forensic science [64]. Political crises induced by a wrongful conviction or scandal have most often proven necessary to provoke regulatory intervention, but this may come too late for an individual who cannot be adequately compensated for their loss of liberty or diverse publics whose trust in the administration of justice is irreparably damaged. In addition, the implementation of such regulation, including the writing of standards and operating procedures not underpinned by rigorous research, has been criticised [65]. It also remains the case that error rates and limitations of techniques often remain sufficiently unarticulated, or even undetermined. Yet even assuming extra resources are provided to produce robust error rates, it is questionable whether risks can be meaningfully quantified, given the inherently contextual nature of forensic DNA evidence. As we argue, many questions are not purely scientific but include ethical considerations from the very outset of the social life of DNA. Acceptability of DNA evidence thus turns, in part, upon the criminal justice system's values and public tolerance of error, but classic regulatory risk analysis typically takes little (if any) account of sociological, economic, ethical, or even legal considerations. The countervailing difficulty of encouraging innovation and development within regulatory parameters, demands innovative solutions operating within an 'ethics as lived practice' framework. This will require embedded ethical practice, as well as regulatory flexibility and pluralism, to avoid stagnation, and setting forensic science 'in aspic' [66].

Such flexibility to innovate is especially critical when also facing the challenges of commercialization, leading to the confluence of competition and profit-oriented practices with those of scientific endeavour and of the criminal justice system. This confluence can lead most obviously to conflicts of interest, which can affect the portrayal of validity/reliability and utility of forensic technologies, but also directly impact the quality of forensic analyses undertaken; the reporting of these forensic analyses, and also the scientifically robust development of existing and emerging forensic technologies [67–69]. Forensic scientists constantly make ethical decisions in this context, as discussed above for scientific and evidentiary reasons. In the commercial context, additionally, forensic practitioners make ethical decisions around accreditation for services; negotiating access to contracts; customer satisfaction; access to material and financial means in order to conduct research; contestations around other service providers, etc. [33]. Many scientists work together with companies in developing forensic technologies, equipment, and also at times, services. They may be delivering services for commercial providers, or they may be in direct competition. Due to the potential conflicts of interest, the commercial context makes it even more important for forensic scientists and practitioners to reflect on their decision-making in order to ensure responsible and accountable delivery of forensic genetics analyses and interpretations.

7. Case Studies

Our call to adopt ethics as lived practice in decision-making processes throughout key stages in the life of forensic DNA is underscored by three case studies. These vignettes explore ethical decision-making in forensic DNA phenotyping, forensic (or: investigative) genetic genealogy, and forensic epigenetics. The three fields share a common basis: they are presented by forensic scientists and users as providing intelligence for investigations without apparent leads by generating data on a group of suspects, and they are portrayed to facilitate even cold case investigations, based on probability calculations and human (epi)genetics.

7.1. Forensic DNA Phenotyping (FDP) and Biogeographic Ancestry Testing (BGA)

FDP and BGA have provided intelligence to criminal investigations that, at times, have resulted in the detection of suspects. To date, in the USA, hundreds of investigations have drawn on intelligence from FDP and BGA analyses since 2015. In Europe, these techniques (especially BGA), have found application in cases since at least 1999, including in the Marianne Vaatstra case [70]; the investigation of the Madrid train bombings of 2004 [71]; the Phantom of Heilbronn investigation in 2008 [72]; and the detection of the murder of Eva Blanco Puig in Spain in 2015. In the Vaatstra case in 1999, an early form of BGA was used to the effect of taking public pressure off asylum seekers who had been considered prime suspects. In the Madrid investigation, the BGA analysis contributed some intelligence to the investigation. In the case of the Phantom of Heilbronn, the results did not contribute to the detection of perpetrators; rather, they seemed to fuel the bias of investigators. While the case of the Phantom was widely debated, unsuccessful applications of FDP or BGA tend not to be discussed publicly. Yet insight into limitations can assist the wider forensic genetics community of scientists and users, but also the public, in understanding the effective parameters of these techniques.

A more recent case is the rape and murder of Maria Ladenburger, on 16 October 2016, in the German city of Freiburg im Breisgau, Germany. At the start of the investigation, suspicion quickly fell on the large migrant community of approximately one million people who had come to Germany in 2015/16. Representatives from politics, policing and forensic genetics suggested that expanded DNA technologies would contribute to faster detection of the perpetrator if only analyses of the perpetrator's (1) appearance, using FDP, and (2) continental origin, via BGA, would have been permitted. While many German experts, including the German Spurenkommission (trace commission), initially argued that the Ladenburger murder would have been an ideal test case for application of FDP in a criminal investigation, senior German forensic geneticists working on FDP later commented that this specific case would not have benefitted from its use [73–75]. Yet, the raised expectations of audiences and investigators remained unrealistically high, leading to the legalization of FDP in Germany in 2019. Yet the Maria Ladenburger case was solved through traditional police investigative techniques, resulting in the arrest of Hussein Khavari, an Afghan migrant, previously convicted in Greece.

The discussion of FDP and BGA, in this case, has raised several questions, specifically around the communication of the utility and reliability of these emerging technologies, but also about the implications of using technology that aims to identify categories of people rather than individuals [20,76]. Overall, FDP and BGA raise a number of ethical questions for forensic scientists, questions that need to be reflected upon time and again in order to deliver responsible and accountable science. While we focus on the estimation of externally visible characteristics in this case study, we do acknowledge that the testing of biogeographic ancestry (BGA) has its own technical and ethical pitfalls, some of which it shares with FDP and some of which are specific to BGA. For example, there are significant incongruities between 'population' labels used by the forensic laboratory and those used by police forces which risk miscommunications, while opening up casework to being highly susceptible to bias (e.g., [72]).

First, FDP works on the basis of attribution rather than identification. However, defining visible/external attributes, e.g., hair/eye/skin colour, must be couched in ambiguity because they are subject to individual evaluation, e.g., colour perception, but also culturally informed perception of such traits (see further [15]). These individual attributions are then compared to non-uniform standards. Here also, as mentioned earlier, the choice of reference data has a fundamental influence, requiring forensic scientists to reflect on the biases that go into defining reference data. In many cases, DNA analysis results might be meaningless or even misleading. Articulating such crucial limitations and distinctions to users is central to ensuring the reliability and utility of FDP in an investigation, even if reporting forms seem to leave scant space for such important information. Space and time must be made for communicating these aspects since they can significantly impact the understanding investigators develop of intelligence generated via FDP analyses.

Second, the investigative value of forensic genetics arises from the capacity of technology to either deliver evidence or intelligence to detect crimes and perpetrators. In the case of FDP, intelligence is produced only in as far as the genetic analysis can either point towards (or away from) a group of shared attributes/characteristics a perpetrator may have. FDP is about shared characteristics and as such applies suspicion to groups, collectivising suspicion [77]. However, since FDP deals in probabilities, the extent to which a group can be excluded can never be 100% certain. A key issue here is that the technology works best on minority groups (of an appearance distinctly different to that of a majority population) to deliver on its aim of directing the next steps in an investigation (e.g., [78]). It is thus vital to reflect when using technologies such as FDP, on their investigative value, which is reduced when the analysis points towards a majority group as then the expected 'reduction' in suspect populations is not achieved. Effectively, this may lead to minority groups being implicated in active investigations more often because the investigative tools work less well in the case of majority populations [79]. At the same time, forensic technologies such as FDP do not work in isolation from policing practices and institutional cultures [21]. Therefore, forensic scientists need to reflect on the discriminatory power of the technology that lies at its heart-both at policing and at public levels. This was the case in the Ladenburger investigation where non-European migrants were associated with criminal behaviour because of the way that FDP was, for a long period of time, communicated as the key technological solution to violent crime investigations.

Third, and this may be the most apparent element to forensic scientists, FDP remains an emerging technology. While pigmentation analyses may be well advanced for darker and lighter aspects of the continuum, medium levels of pigmentation remain more difficult to test for reliably (e.g., [80]). Furthermore, public debates between politicians, police, and scientists around the Ladenburger case confused the technology readiness level of FDP: while scientists were talking about lab-based levels of testing and aspirations for future analytical capacities, perhaps even up to "facial composites", publics, politicians and police representatives perceived of these capacities as already realised and ready for use. Key messages around the reliability and utility of FDP were mixed up. This may yet result in a significant loss of trust in the technology and forensic science in policing should its legalisation in Germany in 2019 not lead to any significant positive results in investigations in the near future.

7.2. Forensic Genetic Genealogy (FGG)

From 1974 to 1986 in California, USA, crimes including murder and rape, were committed by the same unknown individual. In 2018, investigators uploaded genetic information derived from crime scenes onto the public-access genetic ancestry database, GEDmatch. This database aggregates genetic information from citizens who upload the results of their direct-to-consumer genetic tests from genealogy companies, such as AncestryDNA, 23andMe, MyHeritage, and FamilyTreeDNA. Investigators found partial DNA matches assumed to belong to distant relatives, which enabled the creation of a 'family tree', primarily based on online genealogy database records, and including information from sources such as social media and other records. The data of these records sit outside of the forensic domain, and their use in policing raises a number of legal and ethical questions, including on the level of appropriate consent; dual/unintended use of data; and whether the capacity exists or can be introduced for blocking or deleting data from such sources if data subjects disagree with law enforcement uses of their data. Consequently, Joseph James DeAngelo, 72 years old, was identified as a suspect, and his "abandoned" DNA collected to facilitate confirmatory DNA analysis. Although the Golden State Killer was not the first case in which this technique has been used, it has become what Prainsack and Toom [81] term a "founding myth" and is being enthusiastically explored by police globally, and several cases have now been solved through FGG internationally. According to Kling et al. [82], FGG has been used to generate investigative leads in nearly 200 cold cases and some active investigations (see also [10,83,84]). In Sweden, prosecutors have allowed investigators to use consumer genealogy databases to solve cold cases: missing persons and a criminal case [85]. In Canada, two cold cases have been solved through forensic genealogy [8]. In the UK, a study has assessed the likely effectiveness of long-range familial searches through GEDmatch [86]. The Golden State Killer also sparked interest in this procedure among citizens and the companies offering these services, with existing databases now allowing for and, in some cases, encouraging law enforcement searches, as in the case with GEDmatch (recently acquired by commercial forensic service provider Verogen which raises further ethical issues which we do not have the space to explore here) and FamilyTreeDNA. In addition, services exclusively dedicated to law enforcement searches, e.g., DNASolves, DNA.Land, Geneanet, and Geni, are emerging [82] and some law enforcement agencies are setting up their own FGG services.

The ethical implications of FGG are wide-ranging. First, this technique increases acutely the amount of information that can be garnered from DNA data, as it makes use of a significant number of markers and uses SNPs, instead of a relatively reduced number of markers and STRs, as used in 'traditional' forensic DNA testing and databases. Genetic genealogy also allows users to identify distant relatives [34,35] and disease predispositions.

Second, FGG challenges the notion of what constitutes a DNA database used for law enforcement. Until recently, forensic DNA databases were solely constituted of DNA profiles of individuals with some degree of involvement with the criminal justice system [36]. Yet suspects are now being searched for in databases consisting of voluntarily uploaded genetic data from citizens who wish to know more about their health, ancestry, and/or search for relatives: a clear example of 'function creep'. Such repurposing of DNA data requires a discussion of (informed) consent [33], data ownership, and the accountability of genealogy companies and law enforcement in relation to human rights.

Third, the genetic databases being used/created for FGG usually have a significantly different composition than "traditional" forensic databases, the latter over-representing groups that are most likely to interact with the criminal justice system, such as racial and ethnic minorities [87] while genetic genealogy databases are mainly composed of an economically privileged and a European-descent population [51]. This leads to the expansion of affected populations as involvement with the criminal justice system is no longer a prerequisite to inclusion in law enforcement searches and follows broader patterns of surveillance expansion that encompasses ever more citizens. FGG, therefore, brings individuals whose profiles are in a recreational DNA database, under the 'genetic surveillance' gaze, making them suspects by association [88]. This 'function creep' illustrates the potential for wider ramifications of decisions that are particularly risky when impacts cannot be known and their diffusion across society remains uncharted. However, it should be noted that different databases have varying policies in terms of making genetic data available for law enforcement searches [89] GEDmatch and FamilyTreeDNA encourage such searches. GEDmatch offers users to opt-in while FamilyTreeDNA, in 2019, instituted an opt-out policy that automatically opens up users' data to law enforcement searches. However, under the jurisdiction of the European Union's General Data Protection Regulation (GDPR), users from current and recent European Union member states who have profiles on FamilyTreeDNA have been automatically opted out. This means that European Union citizens must opt-in if they wish to have their DNA profile included for criminal investigation purposes [8,54]. Adopting a different stance, companies such as AncestryDNA and 23andMe have categorically denied access for law enforcement agents to such data, unless subpoenaed by a court order to do so [89].

7.3. Forensic Epigenetics/-Genomics (FEpi)

Imagine: A woman is found dead, and DNA samples collected from crime scenes do not provide any investigative leads. After making a genetic estimation of appearance traits and biogeographic ancestry (see case 1), it is decided to conduct epigenetic prediction of chronological age [90], as well as epigenomic prediction of lifestyle and environmental factors through the DNA samples. Results indicate that the presumed suspect is approximately twenty years old, smokes tobacco, has a high alcohol intake, and probably belongs to a specific "socioeconomic status"(p. 7, [91]). Based on these results, police investigative work will be prioritised towards a more specific suspect pool. While hypothetical, this is the aspiration of forensic epigenetics.

Until recently, despite the enormous interest in post-genomics research, forensic applications of epigenetics were mainly restricted to body fluid identification, differentiating between monozygotic twins, and age prediction [90,92,93]. The potential uses of epigenetics in forensic research have only recently expanded, with expectations that the understanding of how environmental factors impact our DNA might be useful 'intelligence', by identifying suspects' lifestyle, such as smoking habits, alcohol intake, other drug use, diet, body shape and size, physical exercise, zone of residence, and socioeconomic status [91,94]. As with FGG, the potential ramifications of FEpi are extensive and impossible to fully predict, when technology is still in an embryonic life stage. It is thus critical that potential consequences are contemplated to develop anticipatory capacity.

First, revealing lifestyle and environmental characteristics directly interferes with the right to privacy of individuals and populations. Despite arguments—already expressed and disputed [15]—that "the genetic prediction of obvious appearance traits [such as smoking] because their external visibility cannot be considered private" (p. 8, [91]), it is clear that inferring smoking, drinking and drug and food consumption habits indirectly correlates with health information and medical conditions, further blurring the distinction between forensic and medical uses of genetic data.

Second, we might question how useful information about smoking and drinking habits might be for investigators since the indication that a suspect smokes and/or consumes alcohol does not significantly advance a criminal investigation without any suspects. Similar to FDP (case 1) and FGG (case 2), FEpi casts suspicion across entire groups by clustering 'suspect' populations that share certain lifestyles.

Third, epigenetic markers are, to a considerable extent, established in early development, potentially transmissible to subsequent generations, and sensitive to environmental factors and lifestyles [95–97]. If we look back to the hypothetical criminal case and focus upon the information that the presumed suspect is approximately twenty years old, smokes, has a significant alcohol intake, we must take into consideration (i) that maternal smoking and alcohol consumption during pregnancy could cause epigenetic changes in the offspring; (ii) passive smoking also might impact the epigenome; (iii) alcohol-dependent epigenetic signatures are partly reversible upon abstinence [91,94]. This suggests that the variability of epigenetic markers does not constitute reliable or consistent predictors for identifying suspects. Although FEpi is still being developed in terms of scientific validation, an approach that is anchored in ethics as lived practice implies that issues around reliability, utility, and legitimacy [20] must be considered focal points to be addressed and discussed.

8. Concluding Remarks

As science is afforded a particularly powerful role in knowledge production and meaning-making in the criminal justice system, could this lead to a 'technological tyranny' [98] in which individuals and communities have to prove their innocence against probabilities? Might forensic scientists inadvertently contribute to creating new kinds of inequalities and insecurity when it comes to policing and criminal justice? (p. 365, [99]). In response to such questions, particularly facing forensic geneticists, in this paper we propose a move from the dominant "thin" ethics approach, to one of ethics as lived practice. We argue that forensic scientists are ethical agents, that is, they make ethical decisions daily and not just at procedural moments such as requesting ethics approval or reporting to an institutional review board. Rather, they have the agency and power to make decisions with far-reaching impacts. Such decision-making can be more apparent at some points than others and must go some way to building 'anticipatory capacity' for the governance of reliable and responsible forensic genetics. In this paper, we have articulated some of the key stages in the life of forensically relevant (epi)genetic data at which ethical decision-making takes place, and where it is vital to take the time to reflect on ethical principles and practices. Our aim has been to raise awareness of the need for continuous reflection upon ethical decisions and to articulate some of those key instances in which such reflection is clearly vital.

Key lessons:

1. Anticipatory capacity and ethics as lived practice are vital components of the work of forensic scientists. This implies the need to be able to anticipate how technology use will impact individuals and groups of people potentially drawn into investigations, as well as wider community relationships, and criminal justice more generally. Our first key point is that forensic geneticists need to engage with ethics in all stages of the sample and data life cycle.

2. There is an urgent need to address the power of forensic (epi)genetics to cast suspicion over a wide range of individuals and communities who may share visual characteristics, common family ancestry, and/or lifestyle habits. This poses several issues that forensic genetics should be aware of when developing and/or applying such technologies, as we move towards a society where individuals and even communities are increasingly called upon to prove their innocence. Our second key point, therefore, is that forensic geneticists need to be aware of the active role that their research and technologies can play in either strengthening or threatening such fundamental legal principles as the presumption of innocence, equality of arms, and the legal burden of proof.

3. Our third key point is that clarity and open communication about real-world capacities of technologies such as FDP, FGG, and FEpi (as well as BGA which is not discussed in depth in this paper) must be at the core of discussions around their use. Their reliability and effectiveness outside the laboratory, and their utility for specific cases, must be reflected upon, and openly and clearly articulated to users and commissioners of such technologies in order to build legitimacy, including public trust, responsible innovation and practice, and accountability.

Author Contributions: M.W. conceptualised the paper, and all authors contributed equally to writing its content. All authors have read and agreed to the published version of the manuscript.

Funding: An aspect of this work is supported by the Portuguese Foundation for Science and Technology (FCT) under project UIDB/00736/2020 and contract CEECINST/00157/2018 (attributed to Rafaela Granja).

Institutional Review Board Statement: Not applicable.

Informed Consent Statement: Not applicable.

Data Availability Statement: Not applicable.

Acknowledgments: Our thanks go to the guest editor of this Special Issue, Niels Morling, for inviting us to contribute, and to the two anonymous reviewers for their comments. We appreciate the many opportunities we have had over the years, to engage with colleagues in forensic genetics, in policing, policy, and governance, as well as in the social sciences and humanities, about the use of DNA in policing. These collaborative opportunities of learning have enabled us to discuss and explore ethics as lived practice in this paper. We dedicate the paper to the forensic genetics' community of learning.

Conflicts of Interest: The authors declare no conflict of interest.

References

1. Lipphardt, V.; Rappold, G.; Surdu, M. Representing vulnerable populations in genetic studies: The case of the Roma. *Sci. Context* **2020**. (Preprint). [CrossRef]
2. The Law Commission. *The Use of DNA in Criminal Investigations*; The Law Commission: Wellington, New Zealand, 2020; ISBN 978-1-877569-96-8.
3. Presser, J.R.; Robertson, K. *AI Case Study: Probabilistic Genotyping DNA Tools in Canadian Criminal Courts*; Law Commission of Ontario: Toronto, ON, Canada, 2021.
4. Call for Evidence Launched on New Technologies in Law Enforcement—Committees—UK Parliament. Available online: https://committees.parliament.uk/committee/519/justice-and-home-affairs-committee/news/156778/call-for-evidence-launched-on-new-technologies-in-law-enforcement/ (accessed on 14 October 2021).
5. Independent Advisory Group on Emerging Technologies in Policing: Call for Evidence. Available online: http://www.gov.scot/publications/independent-advisory-group-on-emerging-technologies-in-policing-call-for-evidence/ (accessed on 14 October 2021).
6. Kienzle, T. Draft DNA Phenotyping Law Set to Go before Swiss Parliament. Available online: https://www.swissinfo.ch/eng/draft-dna-phenotyping-law-set-to-go-before-swiss-parliament/46204608 (accessed on 14 October 2021).
7. Murphy, E. Law and policy oversight of familial searches in recreational genealogy databases. *Forensic Sci. Int.* **2018**, *292*, e5–e9. [CrossRef]
8. Granja, R. Long-range familial searches in recreational DNA databases: Expansion of affected populations, the participatory turn, and the co-production of biovalue. *New Genet. Soc.* **2021**, *40*, 331–352. [CrossRef]
9. Samuel, G.; Kennett, D. The impact of investigative genetic genealogy: Perceptions of UK professional and public stakeholders. *Forensic Sci. Int. Genet.* **2020**, *48*, 102366. [CrossRef] [PubMed]
10. Kennett, D. Using genetic genealogy databases in missing persons cases and to develop suspect leads in violent crimes. *Forensic Sci. Int.* **2019**, *301*, 107–117. [CrossRef]
11. Willis, S. Forensic science, ethics and criminal justice. In *Handbook of Forensic Science*; Fraser, J., Williams, R., Eds.; Willan: London, UK, 2009; ISBN 978-1-84392-732-7.
12. Schiermeier, Q. Forensic database challenged over ethics of DNA holdings. *Nature* **2021**, *594*, 320–322. [CrossRef] [PubMed]
13. McCartney, C. The forensic science paradox. In *Counter-Terrorism, Constitutionalism and Miscarriages of Justice: A Festschrift for Professor Clive Walker*; Lennon, G., King, C., McCartney, C., Eds.; Hart Publishing: Oxford, UK, 2018; pp. 227–248, ISBN 978-1-5099-1575-0.
14. Guston, D.H. Understanding "anticipatory governance". *Soc. Stud. Sci.* **2014**, *44*, 218–242. [CrossRef]
15. Toom, V.; Wienroth, M.; M'charek, A.; Prainsack, B.; Williams, R.; Duster, T.; Heinemann, T.; Kruse, C.; Machado, H.; Murphy, E. Approaching ethical, legal and social issues of emerging forensic DNA phenotyping (FDP) technologies comprehensively: Reply to 'Forensic DNA phenotyping: Predicting human appearance from crime scene material for investigative purposes' by Manfred Kayser. *Forensic Sci. Int. Genet.* **2016**, *22*, e1–e4. [CrossRef] [PubMed]
16. Williams, R.; Wienroth, M. Social and Ethical Aspects of Forensic Genetics: A Critical Review. *Forensic Sci. Rev.* **2017**, *29*, 145–169.
17. Williams, R.; Wienroth, M. Identity, mass fatality and forensic genetics. *New Genet. Soc.* **2014**, *33*, 257–276. [CrossRef]
18. Kruse, C. *The Social Life of Forensic Evidence*; University of California Press: Oakland, CA, USA, 2015; ISBN 978-0-520-28839-3.
19. Granja, R.; Machado, H. Ethical controversies of familial searching: The views of stakeholders in the United Kingdom and in Poland. *Sci. Technol. Hum. Values* **2019**, *44*, 1068–1092. [CrossRef]
20. Wienroth, M. Value beyond scientific validity: Let's RULE (Reliability, Utility, LEgitimacy). *J. Responsible Innov.* **2020**, *7*, 92–103. [CrossRef]
21. Skinner, D. Forensic genetics and the prediction of race: What is the problem? *BioSocieties* **2020**, *15*, 329–349. [CrossRef]
22. Wienroth, M. Governing anticipatory technology practices. Forensic DNA phenotyping and the forensic genetics community in Europe. *New Genet. Soc.* **2018**, *37*, 137–152. [CrossRef]
23. Granja, R.; Machado, H. Forensic DNA phenotyping and its politics of legitimation and contestation: Views of forensic geneticists in Europe. *Soc. Stud. Sci.* **2020**, 1–19, (ePub ahead of Print). [CrossRef]
24. Guillemin, M.; Gillam, L. Ethics, reflexivity, and "ethically important moments" in research. *Qual. Inq.* **2004**, *10*, 261–280. [CrossRef]
25. Kahn, J. Privacy as a legal principle of identity maintenance. *Seton Hall Law Rev.* **2002**, *33*, 371.
26. Presidential Commission for the Study of Bioethical Issues. *Privacy and Progress in Whole Genome Sequencing*; US Department of Health & Human Services: Washington, DC, USA, 2012; p. 154.

27. Evans, J. Personal Privacy vs. Public Security. Available online: https://techcrunch.com/2018/05/06/personal-privacy-vs-public-security-fight/ (accessed on 14 October 2021).

28. Orrù, E.; Porcedda, M.G.; Weydner-Volkmann, S. *Rethinking Surveillance and Control. Beyond the "Security vs. Privacy" Debate;* Nomos: Baden-Baden, Germany, 2017.

29. Timmermans, S.; Berg, M. The practice of medical technology. *Sociol. Health Illn.* **2003**, *25*, 97–114. [CrossRef]

30. Greenhalgh, T.; Swinglehurst, D. Studying technology use as social practice: The untapped potential of ethnography. *BMC Med.* **2011**, *9*, 45. [CrossRef]

31. Suchman, L.; Blomberg, J.; Orr, J.E.; Trigg, R. Reconstructing technologies as social practice. *Am. Behav. Sci.* **1999**, *43*, 392–408. [CrossRef]

32. Hunt, M.R.; Godard, B. Beyond procedural ethics: Foregrounding questions of justice in global health research ethics training for students. *Glob. Public Health* **2013**, *8*, 713–724. [CrossRef] [PubMed]

33. Wienroth, M. Socio-technical disagreements as ethical fora: Parabon NanoLab's forensic DNA Snapshot[TM] service at the intersection of discourses around robust science, technology validation, and commerce. *BioSocieties* **2020**, *15*, 28–45. [CrossRef]

34. The World Medical Association (WMA). *WMA Declaration of Helsinki—Ethical Principles for Medical Research Involving Human Subjects;* The World Medical Association (WMA): Helsinki, Finland, 1964.

35. Gaille, M.; Horn, R. The ethics of genomic medicine: Redefining values and norms in the UK and France. *Eur. J. Hum. Genet.* **2021**, *29*, 780–788. [CrossRef]

36. Alpaslan-Roodenberg, S.; Anthony, D.; Babiker, H.; Bánffy, E.; Booth, T.; Capone, P.; Deshpande-Mukherjee, A.; Eisenmann, S.; Fehren-Schmitz, L.; Frachetti, M.; et al. Ethics of DNA research on human remains: Five globally applicable guidelines. *Nature* **2021**, *599*, 41–46. [CrossRef] [PubMed]

37. Claw, K.G.; Anderson, M.Z.; Begay, R.L.; Tsosie, K.S.; Fox, K.; Garrison, N.A. A framework for enhancing ethical genomic research with Indigenous communities. *Nat. Commun.* **2018**, *9*, 2957. [CrossRef] [PubMed]

38. D'Amato, M.E.; Bodner, M.; Butler, J.M.; Gusmão, L.; Linacre, A.; Parson, W.; Schneider, P.M.; Vallone, P.; Carracedo, A. Ethical publication of research on genetics and genomics of biological material: Guidelines and recommendations. *Forensic Sci. Int. Genet.* **2020**, *48*, 102299. [CrossRef] [PubMed]

39. Fox, K. The illusion of inclusion—The "All of Us" research program and indigenous peoples' DNA. *N. Engl. J. Med.* **2020**, *383*, 411–413. [CrossRef] [PubMed]

40. Carracedo, Á.; Butler, J.M.; Gusmão, L.; Parson, W.; Roewer, L.; Schneider, P.M. Publication of population data for forensic purposes. *Forensic Sci. Int. Genet.* **2010**, *4*, 145–147. [CrossRef]

41. Moreau, Y. Crack down on genomic surveillance. *Nature* **2019**, *576*, 36–38. [CrossRef]

42. Kowal, E.; Radin, J. Indigenous biospecimen collections and the cryopolitics of frozen life. *J. Sociol.* **2015**, *51*, 63–80. [CrossRef]

43. Zieger, M.; Utz, S. About DNA databasing and investigative genetic analysis of externally visible characteristics: A public survey. *Forensic Sci. Int. Genet.* **2015**, *17*, 163–172. [CrossRef]

44. Forzano, F.; Genuardi, M.; Moreau, Y. ESHG warns against misuses of genetic tests and biobanks for discrimination purposes. *Eur. J. Hum. Genet.* **2021**, *29*, 894–896. [CrossRef]

45. Normile, D. Genetics papers from China face ethical scrutiny. *Science* **2021**, *373*, 727–728. [CrossRef] [PubMed]

46. Caliebe, A.; Walsh, S.; Liu, F.; Kayser, M.; Krawczak, M. Likelihood ratio and posterior odds in forensic genetics: Two sides of the same coin. *Forensic Sci. Int. Genet.* **2017**, *28*, 203–210. [CrossRef] [PubMed]

47. Pfaffelhuber, P.; Grundner-Culemann, F.; Lipphardt, V.; Baumdicker, F. How to choose sets of ancestry informative markers: A supervised feature selection approach. *Forensic Sci. Int. Genet.* **2020**, *46*, 102259. [CrossRef] [PubMed]

48. Lynch, M.; Cole, S.; Mcnally, R.; Jordan, K. *Truth Machine: The Contentious History of DNA Fingerprinting;* The University of Chicago Press: Chicago, IL, USA, 2008.

49. Lynch, M. God's signature: DNA profiling, the new gold standard in forensic science. *Endeavour* **2003**, *27*, 93–97. [CrossRef]

50. Amorim, A.; Crespillo, M.; Luque, J.A.; Prieto, L.; Garcia, O.; Gusmão, L.; Aler, M.; Barrio, P.A.; Saragoni, V.G.; Pinto, N. Formulation and communication of evaluative forensic science expert opinion—A GHEP-ISFG contribution to the establishment of standards. *Forensic Sci. Int. Genet.* **2016**, *25*, 210–213. [CrossRef] [PubMed]

51. Amelung, N.; Granja, R.; Machado, H. Communicating forensic genetics: "Enthusiastic" publics and the management of expectations. In *Exploring Science Communication: A Science and Technology Studies Approach;* SAGE Publishing: Thousand Oaks, CA, USA, 2020.

52. Lawless, C.J. The low template DNA profiling controversy: Biolegality and boundary work among forensic scientists. *Soc. Stud. Sci.* **2012**, *43*, 191–214. [CrossRef]

53. Gill, P.; Guiness, J.; Iveson, S. *The Interpretation of DNA Evidence (Including Low-Template DNA);* The Forensic Science Regulator: Birmingham, UK, 2012; pp. 1–27.

54. Jobling, M.; Syndercombe-Court, D. *Should We Be Making Use of Genetic Genealogy to Assist in Solving Crime?* A report on the feasibility of such methods in the UK; Government of the UK: London, UK, 2020; p. 16.

55. Amankwaa, A.O.; McCartney, C. The effectiveness of the current use of forensic DNA in criminal investigations in England and Wales. *WIREs Forensic Sci.* **2021**, *3*, e1414. [CrossRef]

56. Cassella, J.; McCartney, C. Lowering the drawbridges: Legal and forensic science education for the 21st century. *Forensic Sci. Policy Manag. Int. J.* **2011**, *2*, 81–93. [CrossRef]

57. Garrett, B.L.; Neufeld, P.J. Invalid forensic science testimony and wrongful convictions. *VA Law Rev.* **2009**, *95*, 1–97.
58. Edmond, G. Forensic science and the myth of adversarial testing. *Curr. Issues Crim. Justice* **2020**, *32*, 146–179. [CrossRef]
59. Edmond, G.; Hamer, D.; Cunliffe, E. A little ignorance is a dangerous thing: Engaging with exogenous knowledge not adduced by the parties. *Griffith Law Rev.* **2016**, *25*, 383–413. [CrossRef]
60. Kruse, C. The Bayesian approach to forensic evidence: Evaluating, communicating, and distributing responsibility. *Soc. Stud. Sci.* **2013**, *43*, 657–680. [CrossRef]
61. Taylor, D.; Kokshoorn, B.; Biedermann, A. Evaluation of forensic genetics findings given activity level propositions: A review. *Forensic Sci. Int. Genet.* **2018**, *36*, 34–49. [CrossRef] [PubMed]
62. Gill, P.; Hicks, T.; Butler, J.M.; Connolly, E.; Gusmão, L.; Kokshoorn, B.; Morling, N.; van Oorschot, R.A.H.; Parson, W.; Prinz, M.; et al. DNA commission of the International society for forensic genetics: Assessing the value of forensic biological evidence—Guidelines highlighting the importance of propositions. Part II: Evaluation of biological traces considering activity level propositions. *Forensic Sci. Int. Genet.* **2020**, *44*, 102186. [CrossRef]
63. Syndercombe-Court, D.; Reed, K.; Williams, R.; Wienroth, M. *A Guide to Legal and Ethical Principles and Practices in Forensic Genetics*; EUROFORGEN-NoE: Cologne, Germany, 2016; p. 73.
64. McCartney, C.; Amoako, E. The UK Forensic Science Regulator: A model for forensic science regulation? *GA State Univ. Law Rev.* **2018**, *34*, 945.
65. Nsiah Amoako, E.; McCartney, C. The UK forensic science regulator: Fit for purpose? *WIREs Forensic Sci.* **2021**, *3*, e1415. [CrossRef]
66. Brown, S.; Willis, S. Complexity in forensic science. *Forensic Sci. Policy Manag. Int. J.* **2010**, *1*, 192–198. [CrossRef]
67. Lawless, C.J.; Williams, R. Helping with inquiries or helping with profits? The trials and tribulations of a technology of forensic reasoning. *Soc. Stud. Sci.* **2010**, *40*, 731–755. [CrossRef]
68. Lawless, C. Policing markets: The contested shaping of neo-liberal forensic science. *Br. J. Criminol.* **2011**, *51*, 671–689. [CrossRef]
69. Roberts, P. What price a free market in forensic science services—The organization and regulation of science in the criminal process. *Br. J. Criminol.* **1996**, *36*, 37–60. [CrossRef]
70. M'charek, A. Silent witness, articulate collective: DNA evidence and the inference of visible traits. *Bioethics* **2008**, *22*, 519–528. [CrossRef] [PubMed]
71. Phillips, C.; Prieto, L.; Fondevila, M.; Salas, A.; Gómez-Tato, A.; Álvarez-Dios, J.; Alonso, A.; Blanco-Verea, A.; Brión, M.; Montesino, M.; et al. Ancestry analysis in the 11-M Madrid bomb attack investigation. *PLoS ONE* **2009**, *4*, e6583. [CrossRef]
72. Lipphardt, A. The invention of the Phantom of Heilbronn. *J. Eur. Ethnol. Cult. Anal.* **2020**, 49–69.
73. Science Media Center. *Press Briefing: DNA-Profiling und Die Wissenschaften: Wie Weit Kann Die Erweiterte DNA-Analyse Gehen?* Science Media Center: London, UK, 2017; p. 27.
74. Geuther, G.; Kazmierczak, L. Advanced DNA analysis: On the trail of the perpetrators. Deutschlandfunk, 20 June 2017. Available online: https://www.deutschlandfunk.de/erweiterte-dna-analyse-den-taetern-auf-der-spur-100.html (accessed on 23 November 2021).
75. Vogel, G. German law allows use of DNA to predict suspects' looks. *Science* **2018**, *360*, 841–842. [CrossRef]
76. Skinner, D. Race, Racism and identification in the era of technosecurity. *Sci. Cult.* **2020**, *29*, 77–99. [CrossRef]
77. Hopman, R.; M'charek, A. Facing the unknown suspect: Forensic DNA phenotyping and the oscillation between the individual and the collective. *BioSocieties* **2020**, *15*, 438–462. [CrossRef]
78. Kayser, M.; Knijff, P. de Improving human forensics through advances in genetics, genomics and molecular biology. *Nat. Rev. Genet.* **2011**, *12*, 179–192. [CrossRef]
79. M'charek, A.; Toom, V.; Jong, L. The trouble with race in forensic identification. *Sci. Technol. Hum. Values* **2020**, *45*, 804–828. [CrossRef]
80. Kayser, M. Forensic DNA phenotyping: Predicting human appearance from crime scene material for investigative purposes. *Forensic Sci. Int. Genet.* **2015**, *18*, 33–48. [CrossRef] [PubMed]
81. Prainsack, B.; Toom, V. Performing the Union: The Prüm decision and the European dream. *Stud. Hist. Philos. Sci. Part C Stud. Hist. Philos. Biol. Biomed. Sci.* **2013**, *44*, 71–79. [CrossRef] [PubMed]
82. Kling, D.; Phillips, C.; Kennett, D.; Tillmar, A. Investigative genetic genealogy: Current methods, knowledge and practice. *Forensic Sci. Int. Genet.* **2021**, *52*, 102474. [CrossRef] [PubMed]
83. Katsanis, S.H. Pedigrees and perpetrators: Uses of DNA and genealogy in forensic investigations. *Annu. Rev. Genomics Hum. Genet.* **2020**, *21*, 535–564. [CrossRef] [PubMed]
84. Greytak, E.M.; Moore, C.; Armentrout, S.L. Genetic genealogy for cold case and active investigations. *Forensic Sci. Int.* **2019**, *299*, 103–113. [CrossRef] [PubMed]
85. Tillmar, A.; Fagerholm, S.A.; Staaf, J.; Sjölund, P.; Ansell, R. Getting the conclusive lead with investigative genetic genealogy—A successful case study of a 16 year old double murder in Sweden. *Forensic Sci. Int. Genet.* **2021**, *53*, 102525. [CrossRef]
86. Thomson, J.; Clayton, T.; Cleary, J.; Gleeson, M.; Kennett, D.; Leonard, M.; Rutherford, D. An empirical investigation into the effectiveness of genetic genealogy to identify individuals in the UK. *Forensic Sci. Int. Genet.* **2020**, *46*, 102263. [CrossRef] [PubMed]
87. Skinner, D. 'The NDNAD Has No Ability in Itself to be Discriminatory': Ethnicity and the Governance of the UK National DNA Database. *Sociology* **2013**, *47*, 976–992. [CrossRef]

88. Granja, R.; Machado, H. Corpos relacionais, biofamília e suspeição por associação: O caso da pesquisa familiar em genética forense. In *Crime e Tecnologia: Desafios Culturais e Políticos para a Europa*; Machado, H., Ed.; Edições Afrontamento: Porto, Portugal, 2021; pp. 195–216, ISBN 978-972-36-1852-5.
89. Skeva, S.; Larmuseau, M.H.; Shabani, M. Review of policies of companies and databases regarding access to customers' genealogy data for law enforcement purposes. *Pers. Med.* **2020**, *17*, 141–153. [CrossRef] [PubMed]
90. Vidaki, A.; Daniel, B.; Court, D.S. Forensic DNA methylation profiling—Potential opportunities and challenges. *Forensic Sci. Int. Genet.* **2013**, *7*, 499–507. [CrossRef]
91. Vidaki, A.; Kayser, M. From forensic epigenetics to forensic epigenomics: Broadening DNA investigative intelligence. *Genome Biol.* **2017**, *18*, 238. [CrossRef] [PubMed]
92. Haddrill, P.R. Developments in forensic DNA analysis. *Emerg. Top. Life Sci.* **2021**, *5*, 381–393. [CrossRef] [PubMed]
93. Sabeeha, H.S.E. Forensic epigenetic analysis: The path ahead. *Med. Princ. Pract.* **2019**, *28*, 301–308. [CrossRef] [PubMed]
94. Vidaki, A.; Kayser, M. Recent progress, methods and perspectives in forensic epigenetics. *Forensic Sci. Int. Genet.* **2018**, *37*, 180–195. [CrossRef]
95. Hedlund, M. Epigenetic responsibility. *Med. Stud.* **2012**, *3*, 171–183. [CrossRef]
96. Loi, M.; Del Savio, L.; Stupka, E. Social epigenetics and equality of opportunity. *Public Health Ethics* **2013**, *6*, 142–153. [CrossRef]
97. Richardson, S. Maternal bodies in the postgenomic order: Gender and the explanatory landscape of epigenetics. In *Postgenomics: Perspectives on Biology after the Genome.*; Duke University Press: Durham, NC, USA, 2015.
98. Blake, E.T. Scientific and legal issues raised by DNA analysis. In *DNA Technology and Forensic Science*; Cold Spring Harbor Laboratory Press: New York, NY, USA, 1989.
99. Bowling, B. Transnational Criminology and the Globalization of Harm Production. In *What is Criminology?* Oxford University Press: Oxford, UK, 2011; ISBN 978-0-19-957182-6.

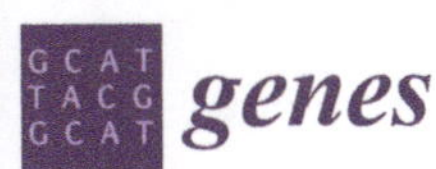

genes

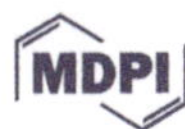

Article

Pushing the Boundaries: Forensic DNA Phenotyping Challenged by Single-Cell Sequencing

Marta Diepenbroek *, Birgit Bayer and Katja Anslinger

Department of Forensic Genetics, Institute of Legal Medicine, Ludwig Maximilian University of Munich, Nußbaumstraße 26, 80336 Munich, Germany; birgit.bayer@med.uni-muenchen.de (B.B.); katja.anslinger@med.uni-muenchen.de (K.A.)
* Correspondence: marta.diepenbroek@med.uni-muenchen.de

Abstract: Single-cell sequencing is a fast developing and very promising field; however, it is not commonly used in forensics. The main motivation behind introducing this technology into forensics is to improve mixture deconvolution, especially when a trace consists of the same cell type. Successful studies demonstrate the ability to analyze a mixture by separating single cells and obtaining CE-based STR profiles. This indicates a potential use of the method in other forensic investigations, like forensic DNA phenotyping, in which using mixed traces is not fully recommended. For this study, we collected single-source autopsy blood from which the white cells were first stained and later separated with the DEPArray™ N×T System. Groups of 20, 10, and 5 cells, as well as 20 single cells, were collected and submitted for DNA extraction. Libraries were prepared using the Ion AmpliSeq™ PhenoTrivium Panel, which includes both phenotype (HIrisPlex-S: eye, hair, and skin color) and ancestry-associated SNP-markers. Prior to sequencing, half of the single-cell-based libraries were additionally amplified and purified in order to improve the library concentrations. Ancestry and phenotype analysis resulted in nearly full consensus profiles resulting in correct predictions not only for the cells groups but also for the ten re-amplified single-cell libraries. Our results suggest that sequencing of single cells can be a promising tool used to deconvolute mixed traces submitted for forensic DNA phenotyping.

Keywords: forensic DNA phenotyping; FDP; HIrisPlex-S; DEPArray; ancestry prediction; phenotype prediction; massively parallel sequencing; next-generation sequencing; single-cell genomics; single-cell sequencing; mixture deconvolution; low template DNA; ltDNA

Citation: Diepenbroek, M.; Bayer, B.; Anslinger, K. Pushing the Boundaries: Forensic DNA Phenotyping Challenged by Single-Cell Sequencing. *Genes* **2021**, *12*, 1362. https://doi.org/10.3390/genes12091362

Academic Editor: Yutaka Suzuki

Received: 28 July 2021
Accepted: 27 August 2021
Published: 30 August 2021

Publisher's Note: MDPI stays neutral with regard to jurisdictional claims in published maps and institutional affiliations.

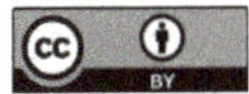

1. Introduction

A single human cell contains around six pg of DNA, which is translated to approximately 2×3.3 billion base pairs. Sequencing of this amount of genomic data became possible thanks to the rapid development of next-generation sequencing (NGS) [1]. The progress in the field has recently been called, by Nature, one of the technologies to watch in 2021 [2]. The efficacy of single-cell sequencing in medicine cannot be overestimated, and it demonstrates the possibility for implementation in forensics, where it is not commonly used. The main motivation behind introducing this technology into forensics is the potential to improve mixture deconvolution workflows and interpretation methods. If a trace is a mixture of different biological materials (for example, sperm and epithelium), there are methods to separate cell pools to investigate them separately [3–10]. Problems arise when the mixed trace is too complex or if it consists of the same cell type, such as blood-blood mixtures [11]. Implementing single-cell analyses can improve the efficacy of mixture deconvolution and, therefore, has already gained interest in the forensic community. A cell separation solution is the DEPArray™ N×T System from Menarini Silicon Biosystems, which is widely used in clinical research [12–15] and is suitable for forensic purposes. Current forensic studies focus on single cell separation followed by STR amplification and detection using capillary electrophoresis [11,16–19]. Mixtures are commonly analyzed with STR typing, but when using different, still new forensic applications, it requires a special approach. Since forensic DNA phenotyping (physical appearance and ancestry predictions) is becoming popular, as observed with legislation expansion in more countries [20], it is assumed that in some cases, a mixture might be the only trace submitted for phenotyping. Phenotyping workflows and prediction methods still need comprehensive research performed before they can be a fully recommended method for mixed trace analysis [20–23]. Here, we present an alternative approach to dealing with mixed traces submitted for forensic DNA phenotyping that introduces single-cell separation in order to deconvolute the mixture prior to genotyping and phenotyping.

2. Materials and Methods

For the study, a fresh blood sample (female) was collected during an autopsy performed in the Institute of Legal Medicine Munich. The sampling was approved by the Bioethical Commission from the Ludwig Maximilian University of Munich. The blood was used as a reference sample (1 ng DNA input, prepared as described in Section 2.3), for which the white blood cells were separated and used.

2.1. Staining and Counting the Cells

In order to conduct cell separation, the biological material was first stained with the DEPArray™ Forensic SamplePrep Kit (Menarini Silicon Biosystems, Bologna, Italy), which enables the staining of epithelial cells, leucocytes, and sperm cells. Following the manufacture's protocol, 5 µL of blood was used, from which the white blood cells were marked with PE (Phycoerythrin) conjugated CD45 antibody as well as with DAPI (4′,6-diamidino-2-phenylindole; to stain the nuclei). The maximum cell input for the DEPArray™ N×T System (Menarini Silicon Biosystems) is 6000 cells; therefore, the sample was analyzed with the Countess™ II FL (Thermo Fisher Scientific, Waltham, MA, USA) automated cell counter and diluted to the recommended concentration.

2.2. Sorting the Cells

The DEPArray™ N×T System's (Menarini Silicon Biosystems) forensic protocol was used to separate the white blood cells. Only highly evaluated (of typical size, morphology, and staining) cells were chosen for the experiment. The selected cells were moved automatically by the DEPArray™ platform and placed in dedicated tubes as follows: 5 groups of 20 cells, 10 groups of 10 cells, 10 groups of 5 cells, and 20 single cells (groups and single cells were collected in two separate experiments).

Preventing Contamination

Due to working with a special type of material (single cells), ensuring that there is no contamination is extremely important for the interpretation of the data. Since the DEPArray™ N×T System is a closed system, contamination within is not possible. In order to exclude its potential occurrence in the next stages of laboratory work, all steps were carried out with a negative control included.

2.3. Library Preparation and Sequencing

For all samples used in the study, genomic DNA (gDNA) was extracted with the DEPArray™ LysePrep Kit (Menarini Silicon Biosystems) directly from the cell separation tubes to make sure the input corresponds with the number of collected cells. All sample extracts were subjected to manual library preparation using the Precision ID Library Kit and IonCode™ barcode adapters using the validated Ion AmpliSeq™ PhenoTrivium Panel [24]. The amplification of the targets was carried out in the same tubes as the extraction to avoid changing the DNA input. The target amplification cycle number and annealing/extension time were 23 cycles and 4 min, respectively. Libraries prepared from cell groups and half of the collected single cells were quantified using the Ion Library TaqMan Quantitation Kit (Thermo Fisher Scientific), diluted (except for libraries of <30 pM concentration), and pooled equimolarly to 30 pM for template preparation on the Ion Chef using the Ion S5™ Precision ID Chef & Sequencing Kit (Thermo Fisher Scientific). The remaining half of the single-cell-based libraries were quantified and rescued by library amplification (see Section 2.3.1). A range of 12–24 libraries were pooled per 530 chip and sequenced on the Ion S5 [25].

2.3.1. Library Amplification

Half of the undiluted single-cell-based libraries were submitted for library amplification. A 25 µl sample of the previously eluted samples was combined with 72 µL of Platinum™ PCR SuperMix HiFi and 3 µL of Library Amplification Primer Mix from the Precision ID Library Kit (Thermo Fisher Scientific). The PCR products were purified in a two-round clean-up with the Agencourt™ AMPure™ XP Reagent according to the manufacturer's manual. The amplified libraries were quantified, diluted, and pooled for automated template preparation.

2.4. Data Analysis

Primary sequence analysis was performed on Torrent Suite™ Software (TSS) 5.10.1 (Thermo Fisher Scientific) with Torrent Mapping Alignment Program (TMAP) alignment of sample reads against the hg19 genome assembly. SNP genotyping and tertiary analysis, in the form of ancestry prediction, were performed using the HIDGenotyper–2.2 plugin and Converge v2.2 (Thermo Fisher Scientific). Low-quality results were double-checked by running VariantCaller v5.10.0.18 on TSS and reviewing the raw data in IGV 2.7 (Integrative Genomics Viewer) [26]. Tertiary analysis was separated into two parts: phenotype prediction (which cannot be performed within Converge v2.2) and ancestry prediction by the bootstrapping admixture analysis with Converge. For the cell groups, the coverage thresholds were adjusted as follows: for the SNPs corresponding with the HIrisPlex-S panel, the analytical coverage thresholds were set based on the HIrisPlex-S panel validation for MPS platforms [22]; for the remaining autosomal ancestry markers, the minimum coverage to call an SNP was set to 100 reads. For the single cells, the coverage threshold was lowered to 50 reads for all markers. The heterozygote balance threshold was set to 65%/35% for heterozygotes and 90%/10% for homozygotes.

2.4.1. Phenotype and Ancestry Prediction

For phenotype (HIrisPlex-S: eye, hair, and skin color) prediction, SNP genotypes were exported from Converge and used to manually generate single profiles, as described in Section 2.4.2, which were later converted into the input file format required by the HIrisPlex-S Webtool (https://hirisplex.erasmusmc.nl/ accessed date 29 April 2021). The HIrisPlex-S SNP set contains an indel SNP (rs796296176) in the form of an A insertion that was manually reviewed and called using IGV 2.7. Predictions were interpreted according to the PhenoTrivium validation paper [24]. For ancestry prediction, called genotypes were merged into a consensus single SNP profile using Converge, and the prediction was performed with the bootstrapping admixture analysis [27] feature of Converge using the 75% resampling size, 1000 replications, and the Precision ID Ancestry Panel Ancestry Frequency File v1.1. The PhenoTrivium Panel contains the 145 Precision ID Ancestry SNPs used for bootstrapping admixture analysis. In the bootstrapping admixture analysis feature of Converge, admixture predictions are made based on a maximum likelihood approach used to predict the most likely admixture proportions across seven root populations (herein referred to as the core admixture algorithm): Africa (AFR), East Asia (EA), South Asia (SA), Southwest Asia (SWA), Europe (EU), America (AME), and Oceania (OCE). The predictions are bootstrapped across a random subset of sequenced SNPs, specified by the user in %, with each bootstrapping replication ran through the core admixture algorithm N times using a different subset of SNPs for each replication to capture uncertainty in the predictions. The results are displayed as an average of the bootstrapping replications for each population group and a 95% confidence interval reflecting the probable range of variability of the estimated ethnicity percentages.

2.4.2. Interpretation Models

The consensus genotypes from cell groups and single cells were used to generate a single SNP profile for tertiary analysis. Two different interpretation models were used to build the profiles: "basic", which compromised genotypes detected at least twice, and "conservative", for which genotypes were included only if detected at least four times. The cell groups were interpreted using only the "basic" approach (following the interpretation pipeline from PhenoTrivium validation), and the profiles from the single cells were generated using both models. Additionally, the tertiary analysis was performed based on single profiles obtained from single cells with the highest coverage.

3. Results

3.1. Cell Groups

The cell groups were collected to evaluate the performance of the workflow combining single-cell separation using the DEPArray™ N×T System with Next Generation Sequencing using the Ion S5. The results obtained in this study were compared to the data from a previously performed validation study [24] of the PhenoTrivium assay. The collected cell groups approximately corresponded to 100, 50, and 25 pg DNA, which were similar to the DNA input used in the sensitivity study (125, 62, and 31 pg).

3.1.1. Coverage, Allele Frequency, and Genotype Calling

The study consisted of 5 groups of 20 cells, 9 groups of 10 cells (one sample was excluded due to a library prep error), and 10 groups of 5 cells, for a pool of 24 libraries total (one group of cells corresponds to one library), which was sequenced on a 530 Chip. Marker coverage across the 200 autosomal markers included in the panel ranged between 309,357 and 736,887 total reads for 20 cells, 216,401–549,980 reads for 10 cells, and 106,865–367,782 reads for 5 cells. The obtained values were comparable with the ones observed in the sensitivity study, where the total number of reads across the triplicates was 340,461–698,760, 374,692–637,041, and 94,120–395,664 for 125, 62, and 31 pg respectively [24]. The coverage for each marker is presented in Supplementary Materials, Table S1.

Allele frequencies were calculated for 43 out of 45 heterozygote loci. Markers rs1470608 and rs10756819 (from HIrisPlex-S) were not called among all the samples due to low coverage. Frequencies were calculated by dividing the number of reads obtained for the reference allele by the total number of reads per locus obtained for both reference and alternative allele. For 20 cells, the frequency varied between 45% and 57% (average 50%), for 10 cells between 47% and 55% (avg. 51%), and for 5 cells between 43% and 58% (avg. 50%). The allele frequency for loci classified as homozygote was between 92–100% for 20 cells (avg. 99.8%), between 90% and 100% for 10 cells (avg. 99.6%) and between 87% and 100% for 5 cells (avg. 99.5%).

Previously described coverage and heterozygote balance thresholds were used to call genotypes in Converge using the HID Genotyper-2.2 plugin. For 20 cells, between 94 and 99.5% of genotypes across all 200 autosomal loci met all the thresholds. For ten cells, the values were 84–98.5%, and for five cells, 64.5–98.5%. The percentage of called genotypes in the sensitivity study was 95–98.5% for 125 pg, 88.5–90% for 62 pg, and 72–81.5% for 31 pg. All the called genotypes were in concordance with the reference sample, no incorrect genotypes were observed. In comparison, the data from the previous study showed that allelic dropouts and drop-ins occurred among the replicates with a 31 pg DNA input, which caused incorrect genotype calling. The detailed genotyping results for all the samples are presented in the Supplementary Materials, Figure S1.

3.1.2. Phenotype and Ancestry Prediction

Phenotype and ancestry predictions were performed for the reference sample and for 'basic' consensus profiles generated for cell groups. From 41 markers associated with eye, hair, and skin color prediction, for all cell groups, 39 SNPs were recovered, and two loci were not called due to low coverage, namely rs1470608 and rs10756819 (similar as in the sensitivity study). Observed area under curve (AUC) accuracy loss (0.001 for very pale, 0.004 for pale, and 0.001 for intermediate skin) did not affect the final phenotype prediction, which was predicted to be the same as the reference, with the following p-values: brown eyes (0.998), black hair (0.661 for black and 0.995 for dark), and dark skin (0.696). From 145 markers used by Converge for ancestry analysis, the maximum number of SNPs was obtained from 5 cells while the profiles for 20 and 10 cells included one locus not called due to low coverage (rs2196051). The bootstrapping admixture analysis for all cell groups revealed an admixture of Southwest Asia and Europe (ratio ca. 70/30%), and the reported individual's place of birth was Iraq (no further details available). The detailed prediction results for all the samples are presented in Table 1.

Table 1. Phenotype and ancestry prediction summary for cell groups and consensus profiles from single cells. p-values and admixture proportions were compared with the results obtained for reference (ref.) sample (*italic* indicates identical values).

		Ref.	Cells–Consensus				
			20	10	5	1 "basic"	1 "conservative"
Eye color	blue	0.000			*0.000*		
	inter	0.002			*0.002*		
	brown	0.998			*0.998*		
Hair color and shade	blond	0.003			*0.003*		
	brown	0.337			*0.337*		
	red	0.000			*0.000*		
	black	0.661			*0.661*		
	light	0.005			*0.005*		
	dark	0.995			*0.995*		
	very pale	0.001			*0.001*		
Skin color	pale	0.008			*0.008*		
	inter	0.275			0.275		0.284
	dark	0.696			0.687		0.676
	dark to black	0.021			0.029		0.030
Admixture							

3.2. Single Cells

3.2.1. Coverage, allele frequency, base misincorporation rates, and genotype calling

For the unamplified libraries (NA), the number of mapped reads varied between 11,979 and 58,536, of which approximately 60% were on target (Figure 1a). Total coverage across all the markers analyzed in Converge ranged between 1891–26,400 (avg. 8889) reads, and the mean marker coverage ranged between 9 and 132 reads (avg. 44). For the amplified libraries (AMP), the number of mapped reads increased to a range of 44,445 to 186,402 reads, of which ca. 60% were on target (Figure 1b). This resulted in total coverage between 13,735 and 113,398 reads (avg. 49,642) and mean marker coverage between 69 and 567 reads (avg. 248). The coverage for each marker is presented in Supplementary Materials, Table S1. To visualize the coverage difference between the unamplified and amplified libraries, the percentage of amplicons with a very low and very high number of reads were compared (Figure 2).

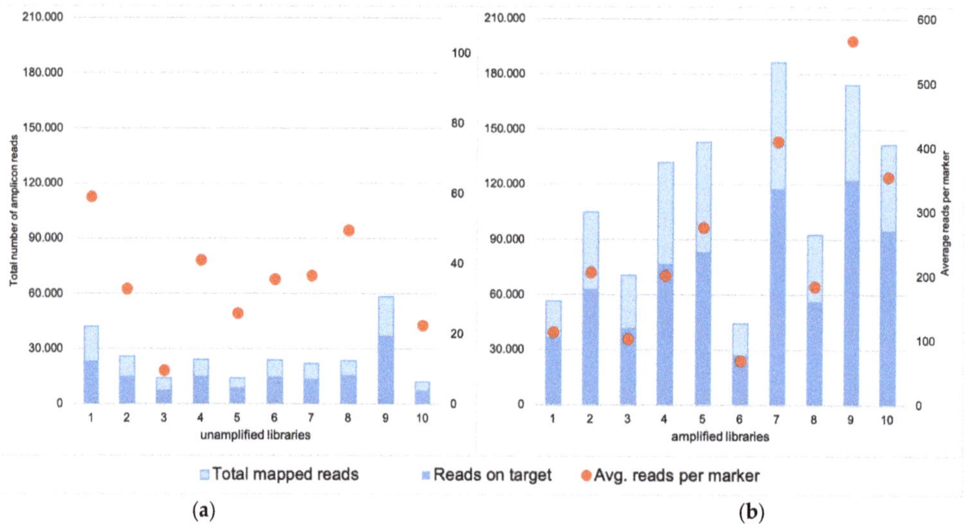

Figure 1. Comparison of the total mapped reads obtained for the unamplified (**a**) and amplified libraries (**b**), together with the number of the reads on target for both groups. The latter was comparable and reached around 60% for both unamplified and amplified libraries but the total number of mapped reads for the amplified libraries was much higher and therefore resulted in higher total coverage. Red dots represent the average coverage per marker for each sample (coverage threshold was set as 50 reads).

Due to a significant number of missing loci observed among the NA libraries, the allele frequency was estimated for the heterozygote loci (except for rs1470608 and rs10756819, which were not called due to low coverage) only among the AMP samples. The mean value per locus varied between 43% and 63%, and the detailed allele distribution across the loci is presented in Figure 3. For most of the markers, the mean heterozygote balance stayed between the accepted threshold of 35% and 65%, and only three markers (rs8035124, rs917115, rs4821004) showed imbalance. The average allele frequency for the remaining expected homozygotic loci was 100%, but for each sample, loci with frequencies below that were observed (Figure 4). The few loci per sample that did not meet the thresholds were marked as imbalanced, which did not result in an incorrect genotype being called.

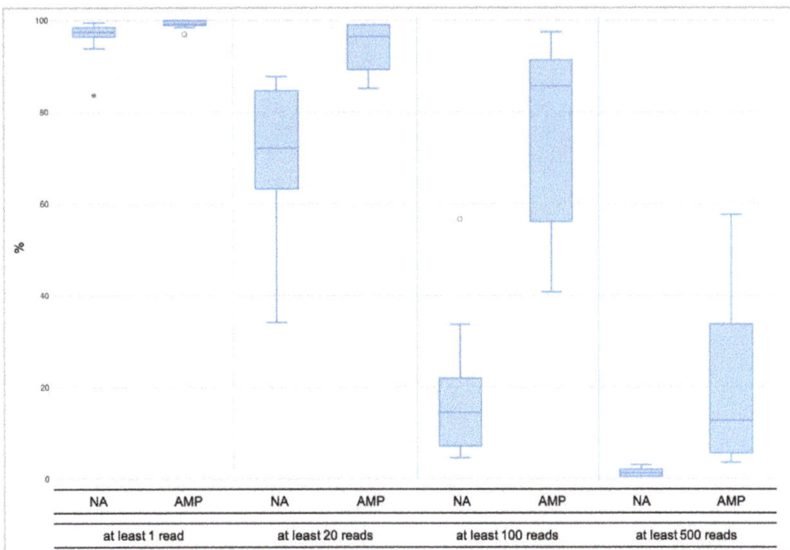

Figure 2. The minimal coverage of at least one read was observed for over 99% of all amplicons across the amplified libraries (AMP), whereas for unamplified libraries (NA), the value was 96%. At least 20 reads were reached by little less, namely 94% of the AMP libraries, while across the NA libraries, it was noticeably less, namely 70% of the amplicons. Over 75% of the amplicons across the AMP libraries had coverage of at least 100 reads, but less than 20% of the NA libraries reached the coverage. The 500X coverage was observed for almost 20% of the amplified libraries and 1% of the NA libraries.

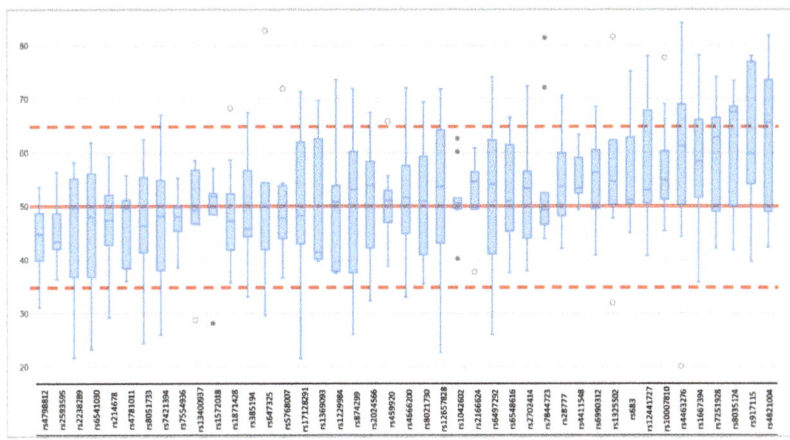

Figure 3. Allele frequency distribution across 43 heterozygote loci (rs1470608 and rs10756819 not called due to low coverage) among ten single-cell based libraries (AMP); red lines correspond to expected (50%), upper (65%), and lower (35%) thresholds.

Due to the special materials used, which were single cells, sequencing errors could be expected, like non-specific base misincorporation. When reviewing the genotypes in Converge, unexpected nucleotides were detected for two loci, namely rs7722456 (reference: C, variant: T, observed: A with maximum 20% frequency, resulting in incorrect genotyping) and rs8113143 (reference: C, variant: A, observed: G with maximum 3% frequency, discarded). The incorrect nucleotides were not observed after running the variantCaller plugin on Torrent Suite™ Software (TSS) 5.10.1 and when reviewing the raw data with IGV 2.7 (Integrative Genomics Viewer). Incorrect genotypes called in rs7722456 were discussed before [28] and can be explained by the homopolymer region flanking the SNP (as well as for the other SNP discussed, rs8113143). The genotypes for rs7722456 in Converge were called manually.

Previously described heterozygote balance and lowered coverage thresholds (50×) were used to call genotypes in Converge using the HIDGenotyper-2.2 plugin. For NA libraries, only between 2,5% and 48,5% (avg. 26%) genotypes across all 200 autosomal loci met all the thresholds, and for the AMP samples, the range was between 49,5% and 96% (avg. 78%) (Figure 5). Among the dropouts, most were loci with low coverage (78-185 loci for NA and 3-94 loci for AMP), and the remaining were imbalanced (max. 25 per sample for NA and 13 per sample for AMP). Across all samples, no genotype was called for one marker (rs10512572) despite passing the coverage threshold. After running the variantCaller plugin, the genotyping for this locus also failed. Upon reviewing the sequencing data in IGV 2.7, it was observed that leftover primer reads were misaligned, resulting in no call. Genotypes for this locus were called manually. Single incorrect genotypes were observed for both groups, all due to allelic dropouts. The detailed genotyping results for all the samples are presented in the Supplementary Materials, Figure S2.

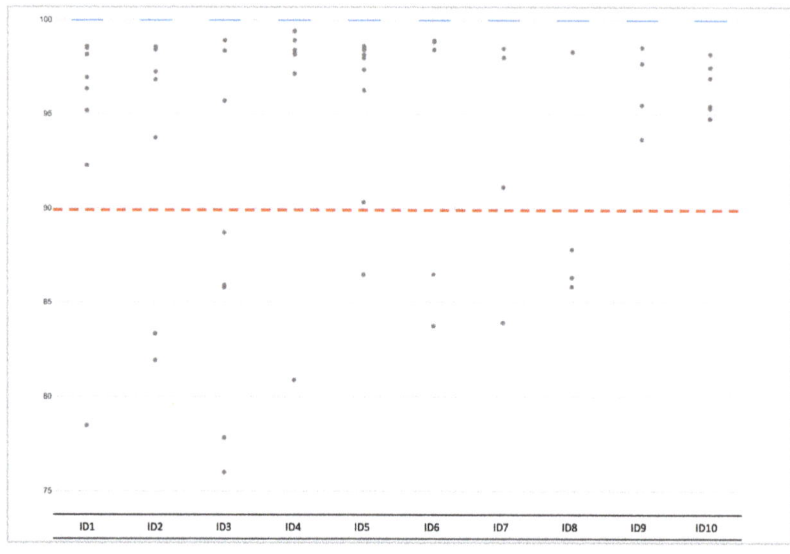

Figure 4. Allele frequency distribution across 155 homozygote loci among ten single-cell-based libraries (AMP). Grey dots represent the homozygotic loci with less than the expected 100% frequency, which is marked with blue lines. Red line corresponds to lowest (90%) accepted threshold. The minimum number of loci per sample below threshold was one; the maximum was five.

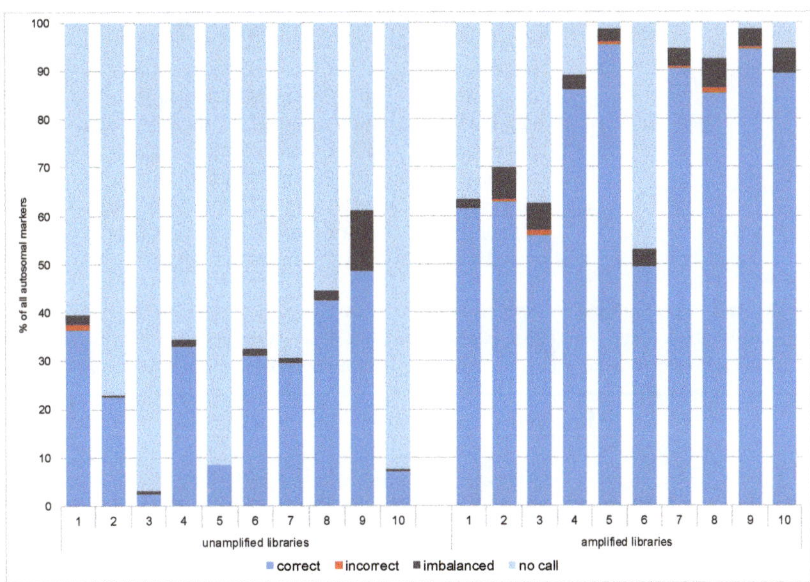

Figure 5. Genotyping rate per each sample across all 200 markers for unamplified and amplified single-cell-based libraries.

3.2.2. Data Interpretation–"Basic" and "Conservative" Models

Due to a significant number of missing loci observed among NA libraries (the Fisher exact test statistic value is < 0.00001), only the profiles from the AMP libraries were submitted for further interpretation. For the "basic" and "conservative" models, consensus profiles from a maximum of 41 phenotypes and 145 ancestry SNPs were generated as described in Section 2.4.1 and Section 2.4.2. All single cells had the same genotype called for 13 out of 41 phenotype-associated markers (concordant with the reference), while for ancestry, there were 50 out of 145 markers (Figure 6). Only three incorrect genotypes were observed across all the SNPs, all once per marker, which did not affect the prediction.

The final "basic" profile consisted of 39 phenotype SNPs (rs1470608 and rs10756819 not called due to low coverage) and 145 ancestry SNPs, which resulted in the same *p*-values for the phenotype prediction and the same admixture (calculated by Converge) as the cell groups (Table 1). The "conservative" model required a genotype to be called at least four times across all the single cells, which left 38 phenotypes and 139 ancestry markers used in the final profile. The one additional missing loci among the phenotype markers, namely rs1545397 (low coverage), caused an insignificant change in the *p*-values obtained for the skin color but overall did not affect the final phenotype prediction (Table 1). The ancestry analysis performed by Converge showed an admixture of Southwest Asia and Europe with a proportion of ca. 60/40%.

3.2.3. Data Interpretation-Single-Cell Based Predictions

From the ten sequenced single cells, six were selected for tertiary analysis due to their high genotype calling rate of ca. 90% (Figure 7). All profiles used for the phenotype prediction were partial with 33–38 SNPs; therefore, the obtained predictions were reported together with calculated AUC loss as recommended by prediction models [29] (Table 2). For eye color, all cells resulted in the correct brown color prediction, where one sample showed a slightly different *p*-value than expected. The correctness of eye color predictions is strongly dependent on the rs12913832 marker [30,31], and this locus was correctly genotyped among all the single cells. For hair color, the obtained *p*-values were identical or almost identical as for the reference for all except one cell. For the sample named ID4, the highest *p*-value was brown with 0.521, while black was 0.465. The profile missed the rs16891982 marker (imbalanced), for which the correct CC genotype is strongly associated with black hair color [32,33]. Despite the difference, the final prediction was black hair color for all samples. The biggest variance was observed for skin color due to several markers relevant for prediction missing. Furthermore, skin color is the most complex phenotypic trait to predict, and incomplete profiles make it even more difficult [34,35]. For only three cells, the final prediction would be the same as the reference, namely dark skin with 70% probability. For samples ID4, ID7, and ID10, the *p*-value for dark skin was only around 0.5, and for the last two samples (ID7 and ID10), the second-highest was dark to black, which would incorrectly suggest the skin color to be darker.

Table 2. Phenotype and ancestry prediction summary for selected single cells (with calling rate of at least 90%). *p*-values and admixture proportions were compared with the results obtained from reference (ref.) sample (*italic* indicates identical values; * indicates different values that affected the interpretation of the results). AUC-Area Under Curve.

		Ref.	Single Cells						AUC Loss					
			ID4	ID5	ID7	ID8	ID9	ID10	ID4	ID5	ID7	ID8	ID9	ID10
Eye color	blue	**0.000**	*0.000*						0.003	0.000				
	inter	**0.002**	0.012	*0.002*					0.012	0.000				
	brown	**0.998**	0.988	*0.998*					0.003	0.000				
Hair color and shade	blond	**0.003**	0.014	*0.003*					0.006	0.000				0.004
	brown	**0.337**	0.521 *	*0.337*		0.378	*0.337*	0.343	0.007	0.000				0.003
	red	**0.000**	*0.000*						0.028	0.000				0.027
	black	**0.661**	0.465 *	*0.661*		0.619	*0.661*	0.654	0.002	0.000		0.001	0.000	0.001
	light	**0.005**	0.018	*0.005*		0.003	*0.005*		0.001	0.000				
	dark	**0.995**	0.982	*0.995*		0.997	*0.995*		0.001	0.000				
Skin color	very pale	**0.001**	0.003	0.000	0.000	*0.001*			0.012	0.004	0.002	0.003	0.002	0.002
	pale	**0.008**	0.030	0.004	0.005	0.007	0.009	0.005	0.007	0.015	0.004	0.005	0.004	0.011
	inter	**0.275**	0.418 *	0.153	0.172	0.252	0.278	0.187	0.003	0.012	0.001	0.002	0.001	0.008
	dark	**0.696**	0.520 *	0.700	0.509 *	0.710	0.689	0.430 *	0.002	0.000	0.001	0.005	0.001	0.000
	dark to black	**0.021**	*0.029*	0.143	0.315 *	0.030	0.024	0.377*	0.001	0.001	0.002	0.001	0.000	0.002
Admixture	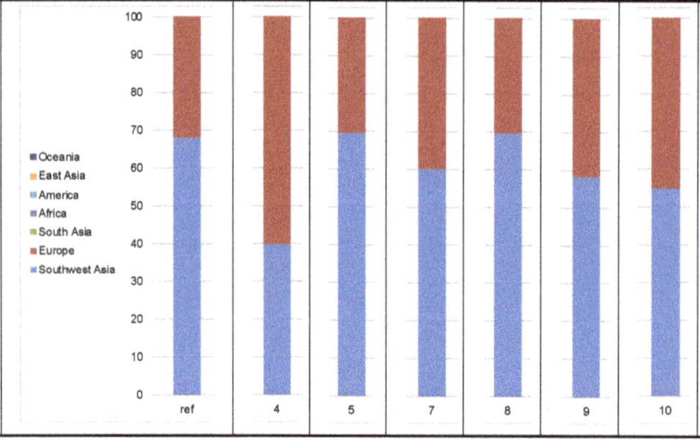													

The profiles used for ancestry prediction were also incomplete, which compromised 120 and 140 SNPs. For all the samples, the analysis performed by Converge revealed an admixture of Southwest Asia and Europe, and for all except one sample, the proportion was close to what was detected for the reference. The result obtained for sample ID4 suggested more European than Southwest Asian ancestry and was caused by missing genotypes for rs16891982 and rs2196051, which are strongly associated with South Asian, not European, populations.

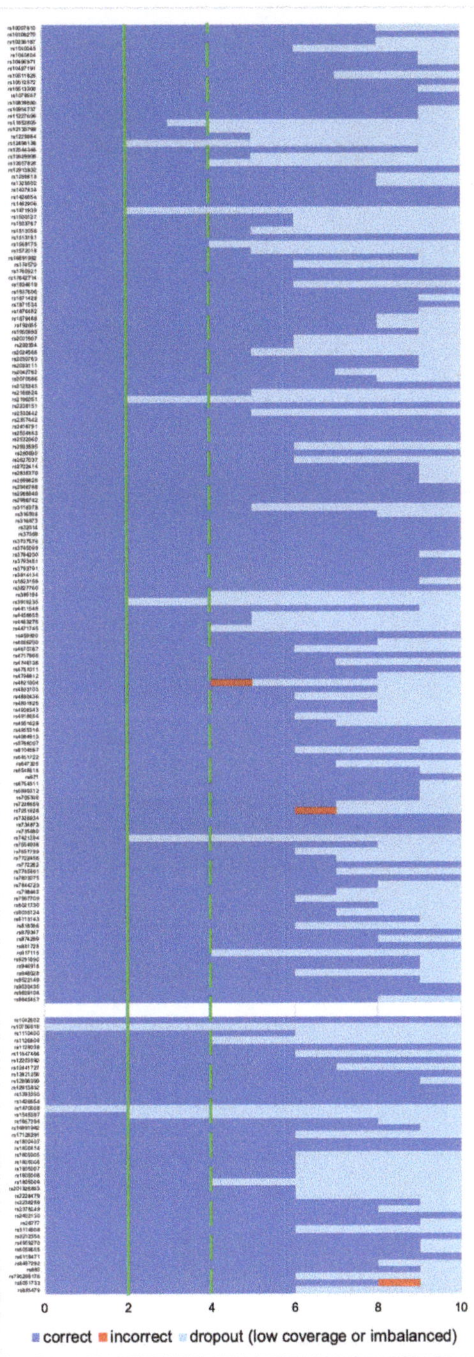

Figure 6. Genotyping rate per each locus used for ancestry prediction (max. 145 SNPs, upper part) and phenotype prediction (max. 41 SNPs, lower part). The x-axis shows the number of single cells with correct, incorrect or no genotype. Solid line: "basic" profile; dotted line: "conservative" profile.

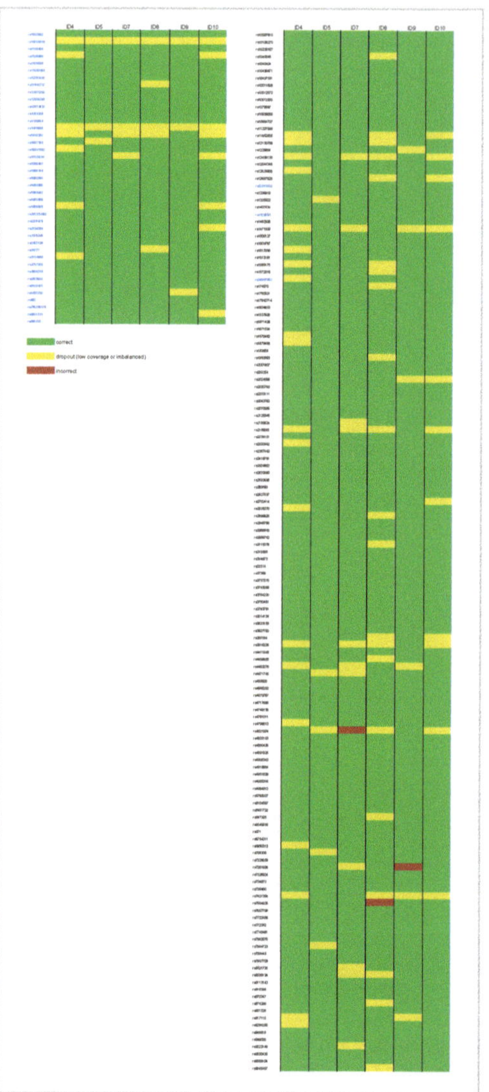

Figure 7. Genotyping summary for the selected single cells (with calling rate of at least 90%); left–41 SNPs used for the phenotype prediction, right–145 SNPs used for ancestry prediction.

4. Discussion

Mixture deconvolution is one of the most engaging topics in forensics. Over previous years different methods have been developed to assist the process, both prior to [3–10] and after, DNA typing of a mixed trace [36–38]. The DEPArray System, which uses a dielectrophoresis grid to isolate single cells, is a promising cell separation technology for forensic analysis. It was demonstrated that the DNA from the collected cells can successfully be processed with STR amplification kits and detected using capillary electrophoresis [11,17,18,39]. Single cells are considered ltDNA (low-template DNA), and handling such material is not uncommon in forensics, where specialists are often faced with low-quantity and low-quality DNA. Since such samples are treated with special lab protocols (e.g., increased number of PCR cycles), it makes them prone to stochastic effects (drop-ins and dropouts) and increased stutter ratios, the interpretation of ltDNA profiles is a common topic of discussion [40–45]. An alternative to traditional fragment analysis is to sequence the bi-allelic SNPs, which are less prone to artifacts and are characterized by smaller amplicons. The analysis of SNP markers is becoming more and more popular in forensics, especially thanks to the rapid development of massively parallel sequencing (MPS), which is not only more sensitive, but also features the use of high multiplex panels consisting of hundreds of markers. Successful single-cell-based STR experiments suggest additional applications in other forensic investigations. A combination of single-cell analysis and SNP sequencing could be especially useful for forensic DNA phenotyping and serve as an alternative solution for the analysis of mixed samples, for which the current interpretation of the phenotype and ancestry predictions can be complicated or impossible.

Panels containing SNPs associated with phenotype [22,46–48] and ancestry [21,49–51] have been introduced, and recently assays combining those have been published [23,24,52]. Forensic DNA phenotyping is now legislated in different European countries [20], and it is expected that police investigators will seek expert opinions on samples of interest. The desirable interpretation of phenotypic features should be based on traces derived from single individuals because mixed samples might not provide reliable results. The collection of single-source traces may not always be possible; therefore, published studies on phenotypic/ancestry SNPs should also discuss the analysis of mixtures. The first and basic indication of a mixed SNP profile is an overall increase in the number of heterozygotic loci [21,53]. This statement cannot easily be applied for individuals originating from admixed populations (or having biparental co-ancestry) where the number of heterozygotes is naturally higher. However, as presented in the study by Eduardoff et al. [21], the allele read frequencies (ARF) differ between unmixed and mixed samples. Mixtures exhibit a higher number of heterozygotes not meeting the balance threshold. Although the authors were able to successfully detect the major and minor contributors for all tested mixture ratios (from 1:1 to 1:9), they recommend careful data analysis, especially for extreme mixtures. The authors of the HirisPlex-S MPS validation paper [22] designed a calculator to aid an interpretation of 2-person mixtures, which is based on known major/minor contributor ratios obtained from STR typing done prior to SNP analysis. The ratios are used to separate read counts obtained during sequencing. The approach was tested on mixtures with different ratios (from 1:1 to 1:9) and using contributors with distinguishable genotypes and phenotypes. The exercise shows that the variants for 28 of the 41 SNPs included in the HirisPlex-S were successfully separated into individual profiles. The validation study of the comprehensive assay combining markers for appearance and ancestry predictions from the VISAGE consortium [23] also mentions mixture deconvolution, similarly of two contributors with different phenotypes and biogeographical ancestries, where the analysis was based on allele frequencies. A publication from Ralf and Kayser [54] presents the first actual crime scene trace of a mixed source submitted for phenotype prediction. The 2-person mixture sample of interest had almost 500 pg DNA. The phenotyping was done using the MPS-based HirisPlex-S Panel, and the sequencing included both the trace and reference material obtained from the victim. The authors were able to extract the probable suspect's genotype for all the SNP markers (one with an alternative genotype considered) and obtained distinguishable phenotypes with high probability values for all predicted traits. They also performed mixture deconvolution by using the aforementioned tool by Breslin et al. [22] and revealed concordance for 36/41 tested SNPs. The remaining genotypes were interpreted differently using both approaches. Overall, discussed studies show that the interpretation of the mixed samples must be made with caution, and the approach should be further evaluated, especially for low input samples or mixtures of individuals with indistinguishable phenotype/ancestry.

The advantage of implementing mixture deconvolution methods prior to the sequencing of the phenotypic/ancestry SNPs is being able to perform the predictions based on single-source profiles. In the case of single cells, the reliability of those predictions will depend on the quality of the obtained sequencing results. As already discussed before, the ltDNA requires careful and cautious analysis, and even though SNPs are less prone to stochastic effects, the following issues are expected when sequencing low template material: allelic drop-ins and dropouts, locus dropouts, imbalanced genotypes, and increased base misincorporation rates. The sensitivity studies of the large SNP assay suggest that the threshold for two of the most popular MPS platforms used in forensics, namely MiSeq FGx System and Ion S5, lies around 100 pg DNA [22–24,52]. In all studies, inputs as low as 5–7 pg were assessed, which roughly corresponds to one human cell. As expected, with such a low input, the obtained results consisted largely of no calls, drops in/out, and incorrect calls. Different forensically relevant SNP panels were tested for their efficacy in typing ltDNA, both using the golden forensic detection standard, namely capillary electrophoresis [55] and MPS [56,57]. Assuming that the DNA input is low, additional changes might be introduced to enhance the standard protocols to boost the coverage. The most common adjustment is to significantly increase the number of PCR cycles used to amplify the targets. The expected positive effect is a higher coverage, but some issues can also occur, like allelic drops in/out causing imbalances or incorrect calls [55,56]. When working with MPS and the AmpliSeq pipeline library, amplification might be applied in order to improve the read depth. The libraries which yielded low quants might be amplified with a high-fidelity PCR supermix. This step in the library preparation was previously implemented when using the AmpliSeq workflow in other molecular fields [58–61], but it does not seem to be a common practice in forensics. A study by Meiklejohn and Robertson mentions the amplification of libraries, but only in order to quantify them after using Qubit and Bioanalyzer [62]. The potential effect of the library amplification on the low-template samples is presented by Turchi et al. [63]. The authors performed a comprehensive validation of the Precision ID Identity Panel by Thermo Fisher Scientific by sequencing challenging forensic samples on the Ion PGM. The libraries from their study with less than 30 pM were amplified and again purified, similarly to our single cell-based libraries discussed in this paper. It was observed that the library amplification step helped to obtain a higher level of repeatability and improved the values of sequencing parameters. Our study shows that introducing this step resulted in over five times higher total coverage of the single cell-based libraries. The number of no-calls per sample decreased from an average of 70% for the unamplified libraries to 18% for the amplified ones. The highest number of imbalanced genotypes per sample was also half as low, and a maximum of two incorrect genotypes per sample were observed after the libraries were amplified.

The goal of sequencing a trace submitted for forensic DNA phenotyping is to obtain reliable genotypes which will be used for predictions. Incorrect phenotype and ancestry predictions might be caused by incorrect genotypes [64] and incomplete profiles [29,65]. The authors of the HirisPlex-S Panel explain that different genotypes missed from the profile will have different influences on the prediction model and that the incomplete data has to be reported as a probability of each trait predicted together with AUC (area under curve) accuracy loss [22,29,35]. We tested an approach of using incomplete single profiles generated by single cells to observe how they will affect the predictions. The calculated AUC loss would not be considered significant, but the missing genotypes resulted in p-values notably different than for the reference samples, causing even incorrect predictions for the skin color. In their paper, Cheung et al. tested how different percentages of genotypes missing from a profile will affect the ancestry prediction when analyzed with different classifiers [65]. Their study shows that an increasing number of missing markers can affect the predictions, especially in the case of admixed samples. Our method to perform the ancestry analysis was not mentioned in the paper, but our results show similar observations. We used bootstrapping admixture analysis based on a maximum likelihood approach to predict the most likely admixture proportions across seven root populations. The SNP profiles were bootstrapped using a varying number of replications, where each replication selected a random subset of SNPs to capture uncertainty in the predictions [27]. For the analysis of the single profiles obtained from the single cells, the number of SNPs available for bootstrapping differed between 123 and 139 out of 145. However, the number of markers missing had less impact than which markers were missing. For samples ID4 and ID8, almost the same number of SNPs were used for the analysis (123 and 125 respectively), but the prediction outcome was an admixture of Southwest Asia and Europe with a difference of 30%. For both phenotype and ancestry, the most accurate predictions in comparison to the reference sample were obtained for the "basic" consensus profile built from single cell-based libraries with the highest genotyping rate.

5. Conclusions

This study is a proof of concept demonstrating that single-cell sequencing can obtain the correct phenotype (HIrisPlex-S) and ancestry prediction, and therefore, can be considered a viable mixture deconvolution method for challenging samples submitted for forensic DNA phenotyping. The presented workflow combined single-cell separation with the DEPArray™ NxT System and sequencing of phenotype and ancestry-associated SNPs with the Ion S5 platform. The DNA typing was done using a previously validated custom Ion AmpliSeq™ PhenoTrivium Panel. The study was based on testing groups of 20, 10, and 5 cells, for which the results were comparable to DNA sensitivity tests performed in a previous validation study, showing the potential of the combined workflow. The number of tested single cells was 20, where half of the libraries were 'rescued' with library amplification prior to sequencing. Introducing this step helped to significantly increase the total coverage obtained for the 10 amplified libraries, which resulted in recovering more genotypes. More than half of the rescued single cells had a genotyping rate close to, or greater than, 90%. Additionally, different interpretation approaches were evaluated. The predictions for single cells were based on a "basic" and a "conservative" consensus profile (genotype called two or four times, respectively) and on single profiles themselves. The most reliable predictions were obtained when using the "basic" consensus profile, for which almost no dropouts were observed. The results suggest that collecting single cells from a mixed sample prior to forensic DNA phenotyping can be used as an alternative way of performing phenotype and ancestry predictions of the mixture's contributors. This approach will be further evaluated by sequencing mock mixtures with different ratios using contributors not only with distinguishable phenotype/ancestry but also similar ones. Additional changes to the workflow will also be evaluated, like increasing the number of PCR cycles prior to amplification, adjusting library inputs, and improving the genotyping.

Supplementary Materials: The following are available online at https://www.mdpi.com/article/10.3390/genes12091362/s1, Figure S1: Summary of genotype calling for all 200 autosomal markers across the cell groups; Figure S2: Summary of genotype calling for all 200 autosomal markers across the single cells, for both the unamplified and the amplified libraries; Table S1: Summary of coverage for all 200 autosomal markers across all tested samples.

Author Contributions: Conceptualization, M.D., B.B., and K.A.; validation, all authors; formal analysis, M.D.; investigation, M.D. and B.B.; writing—original draft preparation, M.D.; writing—review and editing, all authors. All authors have read and agreed to the published version of the manuscript.

Funding: This research received no external funding.

Institutional Review Board Statement: The study was conducted according to the guidelines of the Declaration of Helsinki and approved by the Ethics Committee of Ludwig Maximilian University of Munich (protocol code 18-870, approved on 19 March 2019).

Informed Consent Statement: Patient consent was waived due to the fact that they were deceased.

Data Availability Statement: No data to report.

Acknowledgments: We wish to thank J. Chang for reading and commenting on earlier manuscript versions.

Conflicts of Interest: The authors declare no conflict of interest.

References

1. Macaulay, I.C.; Voet, T. Single Cell Genomics: Advances and Future Perspectives. *PLoS Genet.* **2014**, *10*, e1004126. [CrossRef]
2. Seven Technologies to Watch in 2021. Available online: https://www.nature.com/articles/d41586-021-00191-z (accessed on 26 July 2021).
3. Elliott, K.; Hill, D.S.; Lambert, D.; Burroughes, T.R.; Gill, P. Use of laser microdissection greatly improves the recovery of DNA from sperm on microscope slides. *Forensic Sci. Int.* **2003**, *137*, 28–36. [CrossRef]
4. Verdon, T.J.; Mitchell, R.J.; Chen, W.; Xiao, K.; van Oorschot, R.A.H. FACS separation of non-compromised forensically relevant biological mixtures. *Forensic Sci. Int. Genet.* **2015**, *14*, 194–200. [CrossRef]
5. Stokes, N.A.; Stanciu, C.E.; Brocato, E.R.; Ehrhardt, C.J.; Greenspoon, S.A. Simplification of complex DNA profiles using front end cell separation and probabilistic modeling. *Forensic Sci. Int. Genet.* **2018**, *36*, 205–212. [CrossRef] [PubMed]
6. Dean, L.; Kwon, Y.J.; Philpott, M.K.; Stanciu, C.E.; Seashols-Williams, S.J.; Dawson Cruz, T.; Sturgill, J.; Ehrhardt, C.J. Separation of uncompromised whole blood mixtures for single source STR profiling using fluorescently-labeled human leukocyte antigen (HLA) probes and fluorescence activated cell sorting (FACS). *Forensic Sci. Int. Genet.* **2015**, *17*, 8–16. [CrossRef]
7. Auka, N.; Valle, M.; Cox, B.D.; Wilkerson, P.D.; Dawson Cruz, T.; Reiner, J.E.; Seashols-Williams, S.J. Optical tweezers as an effective tool for spermatozoa isolation from mixed forensic samples. *PLoS ONE* **2019**, *14*, e0211810. [CrossRef]
8. Horsman, K.M.; Barker, S.L.R.; Ferrance, J.P.; Forrest, K.A.; Koen, K.A.; Landers, J.P. Separation of sperm and epithelial cells in a microfabricated device: Potential application to forensic analysis of sexual assault evidence. *Anal. Chem.* **2005**, *77*, 742–749. [CrossRef]
9. Zhao, X.-C.; Wang, L.; Sun, J.; Jiang, B.-W.; Zhang, E.-L.; Ye, J. Isolating Sperm from Cell Mixtures Using Magnetic Beads Coupled with an Anti-PH-20 Antibody for Forensic DNA Analysis. *PLoS ONE* **2016**, *11*, e0159401. [CrossRef]
10. Huffman, K.; Hanson, E.; Ballantyne, J. Recovery of single source DNA profiles from mixtures by direct single cell subsampling and simplified micromanipulation. *Sci. Justice* **2021**, *61*, 13–25. [CrossRef]
11. Anslinger, K.; Bayer, B.; Graw, M. Deconvolution of blood-blood mixtures using DEPArrayTM separated single cell STR profiling. *Rechtsmedizin* **2019**, *29*, 30–40. [CrossRef]
12. Philippron, A.; Depypere, L.; Oeyen, S.; Laere, B.D.; Vandeputte, C.; Nafteux, P.; de Preter, K.; Pattyn, P. Evaluation of a marker independent isolation method for circulating tumor cells in esophageal adenocarcinoma. *PLoS ONE* **2021**, *16*, e0251052. [CrossRef]
13. Salvianti, F.; Gelmini, S.; Mancini, I.; Pazzagli, M.; Pillozzi, S.; Giommoni, E.; Brugia, M.; di Costanzo, F.; Galardi, F.; de Luca, F.; et al. Circulating tumour cells and cell-free DNA as a prognostic factor in metastatic colorectal cancer: The OMITERC prospective study. *Br. J. Cancer* **2021**, *125*, 94–100. [CrossRef]
14. Rossi, T.; Gallerani, G.; Angeli, D.; Cocchi, C.; Bandini, E.; Fici, P.; Gaudio, M.; Martinelli, G.; Rocca, A.; Maltoni, R.; et al. Single-Cell NGS-Based Analysis of Copy Number Alterations Reveals New Insights in Circulating Tumor Cells Persistence in Early-Stage Breast Cancer. *Cancers* **2020**, *12*, 2490. [CrossRef]
15. Boyer, M.; Cayrefourcq, L.; Garima, F.; Foulongne, V.; Dereure, O.; Alix-Panabières, C. Circulating Tumor Cell Detection and Polyomavirus Status in Merkel Cell Carcinoma. *Sci. Rep.* **2020**, *10*, 1612. [CrossRef]
16. Meloni, V.; Lombardi, L.; Aversa, R.; Barni, F.; Berti, A. Optimization of STR amplification down to single cell after DEPArrayTM isolation. *Forensic Sci. Int. Genet. Suppl. Ser.* **2019**, *7*, 711–713. [CrossRef]
17. Williamson, V.R.; Laris, T.M.; Romano, R.; Marciano, M.A. Enhanced DNA mixture deconvolution of sexual offense samples using the DEPArray™ system. *Forensic Sci. Int. Genet.* **2018**, *34*, 265–276. [CrossRef] [PubMed]
18. Watkins, D.R.L.; Myers, D.; Xavier, H.E.; Marciano, M.A. Revisiting single cell analysis in forensic science. *Sci. Rep.* **2021**, *11*, 7054. [CrossRef]
19. Fontana, F.; Rapone, C.; Bregola, G.; Aversa, R.; de Meo, A.; Signorini, G.; Sergio, M.; Ferrarini, A.; Lanzellotto, R.; Medoro, G.; et al. Isolation and genetic analysis of pure cells from forensic biological mixtures: The precision of a digital approach. *Forensic Sci. Int. Genet.* **2017**, *29*, 225–241. [CrossRef]
20. Schneider, P.M.; Prainsack, B.; Kayser, M. The use of forensic DNA phenotyping in predicting appearance and biogeographic ancestry. *Dtsch. Arztebl. Int.* **2019**, *116*, 873–880. [CrossRef]
21. Eduardoff, M.; Gross, T.E.; Santos, C.; de la Puente, M.; Ballard, D.; Strobl, C.; Børsting, C.; Morling, N.; Fusco, L.; Hussing, C.; et al. Inter-laboratory evaluation of the EUROFORGEN Global ancestry-informative SNP panel by massively parallel sequencing using the Ion PGM™. *Forensic Sci. Int. Genet.* **2016**, *23*, 178–189. [CrossRef]
22. Breslin, K.; Wills, B.; Ralf, A.; Garcia, M.V.; Kukla-Bartoszek, M.; Pospiech, E.; Freire-Aradas, A.; Xavier, C.; Ingold, S.; De La Puente, M.; et al. HIrisPlex-S system for eye, hair, and skin color prediction from DNA: Massively parallel sequencing solutions for two common forensically used platforms. *Forensic Sci. Int. Genet.* **2019**, *43*, 102152. [CrossRef]
23. Xavier, C.; De La Puente, M.; Mosquera-Miguel, A.; Freire-Aradas, A.; Kalamara, V.; Vidaki, A.; Gross, T.E.; Revoir, A.; Pośpiech, E.; Kartasińska, E.; et al. Development and validation of the VISAGE AmpliSeq basic tool to predict appearance and ancestry from DNA. *Forensic Sci. Int. Genet.* **2020**, *48*, 102336. [CrossRef]
24. Diepenbroek, M.; Bayer, B.; Schwender, K.; Schiller, R.; Lim, J.; Lagacé, R.; Anslinger, K. Evaluation of the Ion AmpliSeq™ PhenoTrivium Panel: MPS-Based Assay for Ancestry and Phenotype Predictions Challenged by Casework Samples. *Genes* **2020**, *11*, 1398. [CrossRef] [PubMed]

25. Precision ID SNP Panels with the HID Ion S5™/HID Ion GeneStudio™ S5 System Application Guide. Pub. No. MAN0017767. Available online: https://assets.thermofisher.com/TFS-Assets/LSG/manuals/MAN0017767_PrecisionID_SNP_Panels_S5_UG.pdf (accessed on 1 July 2021).

26. Thorvaldsdóttir, H.; Robinson, J.T.; Mesirov, J.P. Integrative Genomics Viewer (IGV): High-performance genomics data visualization and exploration. *Brief. Bioinform.* **2013**, *14*, 178–192. [CrossRef]

27. Wootton, S.; Vijaychander, S.; Hasegawa, R.; Deng, J.; Lackey, A.; Gabriel, M.; Lagacé, R.; Lim, J. Analytical Improvements in Biogeographic Ancestry Inference. Presented at the 28th Congress of the International Society for Forensic Genetics; Available online: https://www.thermofisher.com/de/de/home/products-and-services/promotions/isfg.html (accessed on 26 July 2021).

28. Pereira, V.; Mogensen, H.S.; Børsting, C.; Morling, N. Evaluation of the Precision ID Ancestry Panel for crime case work: A SNP typing assay developed for typing of 165 ancestral informative markers. *Forensic Sci. Int. Genet.* **2017**, *28*, 138–145. [CrossRef]

29. Liu, F.; van Duijn, K.; Vingerling, J.R.; Hofman, A.; Uitterlinden, A.G.; Cecile, A.; Janssens, J.W.; Kayser, M. Eye color and the prediction of complex phenotypes from genotypes. *Curr. Biol.* **2009**, *19*, 192–193. [CrossRef] [PubMed]

30. Meyer, O.S.; Lunn, M.M.B.; Garcia, S.L.; Kjærbye, A.B.; Morling, N.; Børsting, C.; Andersen, J.D. Association between brown eye colour in rs12913832:GG individuals and SNPs in TYR, TYRP1, and SLC24A4. *PLoS ONE* **2020**, *15*, e0239131. [CrossRef]

31. Meyer, O.S.; Salvo, N.M.; Kjærbye, A.; Kjersem, M.; Andersen, M.M.; Sørensen, E.; Ullum, H.; Janssen, K.; Morling, N.; Børstin, C.; et al. Prediction of Eye Colour in Scandinavians Using the EyeColour11 (EC11) SNP Set. *Genes* **2021**, *12*, 821. [CrossRef]

32. Branicki, W.; Brudnik, U.; Draus-Barini, J.; Kupiec, T.; Wojas-Pelc, A. Association of the SLC45A2 gene with physiological human hair colour variation. *J. Hum. Genet.* **2008**, *53*, 966–971. [CrossRef]

33. Lin, B.D.; Mbarek, H.; Willemsen, G.; Dolan, C.V.; Fedko, I.O.; Abdellaoui, A. Heritability and Genome-Wide Association Studies for Hair Color in a Dutch Twin Family Based Sample. *Genes* **2015**, *13*, 559–576. [CrossRef] [PubMed]

34. Walsh, S.; Chaitanya, L.; Breslin, K.; Muralidharan, C.; Bronikowska, A.; Pospiech, E.; Koller, J.; Kovatsi, L.; Wollstein, A.; Branicki, W.; et al. Global skin colour prediction from DNA. *Hum. Genet.* **2017**, *136*, 847–863. [CrossRef]

35. Chaitanya, L.; Breslin, K.; Zuñiga, S.; Wirken, L.; Pośpiech, E.; Kukla-Bartoszek, M.; Sijen, T.; De Knijff, P.; Liu, F.; Branicki, W.; et al. The HIrisPlex-S system for eye, hair and skin colour prediction from DNA: Introduction and forensic developmental validation. *Forensic Sci. Int. Genet.* **2018**, *35*, 123–135. [CrossRef]

36. Benschop, C.C.; Hoogenboom, J.; Hovers, P.; Slagter, M.; Kruise, D.; Parag, R.; Steensma, K.; Slooten, K.; Nagel, J.H.; Dieltjes, P.; et al. DNAxs/DNAStatistX: Development and validation of a software suite for the data management and probabilistic interpretation of DNA profiles. *Forensic Sci. Int. Genet.* **2019**, *42*, 81–89. [CrossRef]

37. Bleka, O.; Storvik, G.; Gill, P. EuroForMix: An open source software based on a continuous model to evaluate STR DNA profiles from a mixture of contributors with artefacts. *Forensic Sci. Int. Genet.* **2016**, *21*, 35–44. [CrossRef]

38. Bright, J.-A.; Cheng, K.; Kerr, Z.; McGovern, C.; Kelly, H.; Moretti, T.R.; Smith, M.A.; Bieber, F.R.; Budowle, B.; Coble, M.D.; et al. STRmix™ collaborative exercise on DNA mixture interpretation. *Forensic Sci. Int. Genet.* **2019**, *40*, 1–8. [CrossRef]

39. Anslinger, K.; Bayer, B.; von Mariassy, D. Application of DEPArrayTM technology for the isolation of white blood cells from cell mixtures in chimerism analysis. *Rechsmedizin* **2018**, *28*, 134–137. [CrossRef]

40. Balding, D.J. Evaluation of mixed-source, low-template DNA profiles in forensic science. *PNAS* **2013**, *110*, 12241–12246. [CrossRef]

41. Balding, D.J.; Buckleton, J. Interpreting low template DNA profiles. *Forensic Sci. Int. Genet.* **2009**, *4*, 1–10. [CrossRef]

42. Kanokwongnuwut, P.; Martin, B.; Taylor, D.; Kirkbride, K.P.; Linacre, A. How many cells are required for successful DNA profiling? *Forensic Sci. Int. Genet.* **2021**, *51*, 102453. [CrossRef]

43. Haned, H.; Slooten, K.; Gill, P. Exploratory data analysis for the interpretation of low template DNA mixtures. *Forensic Sci. Int. Genet.* **2012**, *6*, 762–774. [CrossRef]

44. Pfeifer, C.M.; Klein-Unseld, R.; Klintschar, M.; Wiegand, P. Comparison of different interpretation strategies for low template DNA mixtures. *Forensic Sci. Int. Genet.* **2012**, *6*, 716–722. [CrossRef]

45. Benschop, C.C.G.; Haned, H.; de Blaeij, T.J.P.; Meulenbroek, A.J.; Sijen, T. Assessment of mock cases involving complex low template DNA mixtures: A descriptive study. *Forensic Sci. Int. Genet.* **2012**, *6*, 697–707. [CrossRef]

46. Pośpiech, E.; Kukla-Bartoszek, M.; Karłowska-Pik, J.; Zieliński, P.; Woźniak, A.; Boroń, M.; Dąbrowski, M.; Zubańska, M.; Jarosz, A.; Grzybowski, T.; et al. Exploring the possibility of predicting human head hair greying from DNA using whole-exome and targeted NGS data. *BMC Genom.* **2020**, *21*, 538. [CrossRef] [PubMed]

47. Kukla-Bartoszek, M.; Pośpiech, E.; Woźniak, A.; Boroń, M.; Karłowska-Pik, J.; Teisseyre, P.; Zubańska, M.; Bronikowska, A.; Grzybowski, T.; Płoski, R.; et al. DNA-based predictive models for the presence of freckles. *Forensic Sci. Int. Genet.* **2019**, *42*, 252–259. [CrossRef]

48. Meyer, O.S.; Andersen, J.D.; Børsting, C. Presentation of the Human Pigmentation (HuPi) AmpliSeq™ custom panel. *Forensic Sci. Int. Genet. Suppl. Ser.* **2019**, *7*, 478–479. [CrossRef]

49. Xavier, C.; de la Puente, M.; Phillips, C.; Eduardoff, M.; Heidegger, A.; Mosquera-Miguel, A.; Freire-Aradas, A.; Lagace, R.; Wootton, S.; Power, D.; et al. Forensic evaluation of the Asia Pacific ancestry-informative MAPlex assay. *Forensic Sci. Int. Genet.* **2020**, *48*, 102344. [CrossRef]

50. Jia, J.; Wei, Y.-L.; Qin, C.-J.; Hu, L.; Wan, L.-H.; Li, C.-X. Developing a novel panel of genome-wide ancestry informative markers for bio-geographical ancestry estimates. *Forensic Sci. Int. Genet.* **2014**, *8*, 187–194. [CrossRef]

51. Pereira, R.; Phillips, C.; Pinto, N.; Santos, C.; Dos Santos, S.E.B.; Amorim, A.; Carracedo, A.; Gusmão, L. Straightforward Inference of Ancestry and Admixture Proportions through Ancestry-Informative Insertion Deletion Multiplexing. *PLoS ONE* **2012**, *7*, e29684. [CrossRef]

52. Palencia-Madrid, L.; Xavier, C.; de la Puente, M.; Hohoff, C.; Phillips, C.; Kayser, M.; Parson, W. Evaluation of the VISAGE Basic Tool for Appearance and Ancestry Prediction Using PowerSeq Chemistry on the MiSeq FGx System. *Genes* **2020**, *11*, 708. [CrossRef]

53. Eduardoff, M.; Santos, C.; de la Puente, M.; Gross, T.; Fondevila, M.; Strobl, C.; Sobrino, B.; Ballard, D.; Schneider, P.; Carracedo, A.; et al. Inter-laboratory evaluation of SNP-based forensic identification by massively parallel sequencing using the Ion PGM™. *Forensic Sci. Int. Genet.* **2015**, *17*, 110–121. [CrossRef] [PubMed]

54. Ralf, A.; Kayser, M. Investigative DNA analysis of two-person mixed crime scene trace in a murder case. *Forensic Sci. Int. Genet.* **2021**, *54*, 102557. [CrossRef]

55. Børsting, C.; Mogensen, H.S.; Morling, N. Forensic genetic SNP typing of low-template DNA and highly degraded DNA from crime case samples. *Forensic Sci. Int. Genet.* **2013**, *7*, 345–352. [CrossRef]

56. Elena, S.; Alessandro, A.; Ignazio, C.; Sharon, W.; Luigi, R.; Andrea, B. Revealing the challenges of low template DNA analysis with the prototype Ion AmpliSeq™ Identity panel v2.3 on the PGM™ Sequencer. *Forensic Sci. Int. Genet.* **2016**, *22*, 25–36. [CrossRef] [PubMed]

57. Butler Gettings, K.; Kiesler, K.M.; Vallone, P.M. Performance of a next generation sequencing SNP assay on degraded DNA. *Forensic Sci. Int. Genet.* **2015**, *19*, 1–9. [CrossRef]

58. Alessandrini, F.; Caucci, S.; Onofri, V.; Melchionda, F.; Tagliabracci, A.; Bagnarelli, P.; di Sante, L.; Turchi, C.; Menzo, S. Evaluation of the Ion AmpliSeq SARS-CoV-2 Research Panel by Massive Parallel Sequencing. *Genes* **2020**, *11*, 929. [CrossRef] [PubMed]

59. Siji, A.; Karthik, K.N.; Chhotusing Pardeshi, V.; Hari, P.S.; Vasudevan, A. Targeted gene panel for genetic testing of south Indian children with steroid resistant nephrotic syndrome. *BMC Med. Genet.* **2018**, *19*, 200. [CrossRef]

60. Kluska, A.; Balabas, A.; Paziewska, A.; Kulecka, M.; Nowakowska, D.; Mikula, M.; Ostrowski, J. New recurrent BRCA1/2 mutations in Polish patients with familial breast/ovarian cancer detected by next generation sequencing. *BMC Med. Genom.* **2015**, *8*, 19. [CrossRef]

61. Tavira, B.; Gómez, J.; Santos, F.; Gil, H.; Alvarez, V.; Coto, E. A labor- and cost-effective non-optical semiconductor (Ion Torrent) next-generation sequencing of the SLC12A3 and CLCNKA/B genes in Gitelman's syndrome patients. *J. Hum. Genet.* **2014**, *59*, 376–380. [CrossRef] [PubMed]

62. Meiklejohn, K.A.; Robertson, J.M. Evaluation of the Precision ID Identity Panel for the Ion Torrent ™ PGM ™ sequencer. *Forensic Sci. Int. Genet.* **2017**, *31*, 48–56. [CrossRef]

63. Turchi, C.; Previderè, C.; Bini, C.; Carnevali, E.; Grignani, P.; Manfredi, A.; Melchionda, F.; Onofri, V.; Pelotti, S.; Robino, C.; et al. Assessment of the Precision ID Identity Panel kit on challenging forensic samples. *Forensic Sci. Int. Genet.* **2020**, *49*, 102400. [CrossRef]

64. Santos, C.; Fondevila, M.; Ballard, D.; Banemann, R.; Bento, A.M.; Børsting, C.; Branicki, W.; Brisighelli, F.; Burrington, M.; Capal, T.; et al. Forensic ancestry analysis with two capillary electrophoresis ancestry informative marker (AIM) panels: Results of a collaborative EDNAP exercise. *Forensic Sci. Int. Genet.* **2015**, *19*, 56–67. [CrossRef] [PubMed]

65. Cheung, E.Y.Y.; Gahan, M.E.; McNevin, D. Prediction of biogeographical ancestry from genotype: A comparison of classifiers. *Int. J. Leg. Med.* **2017**, *131*, 901–912. [CrossRef] [PubMed]

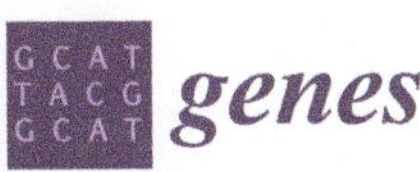 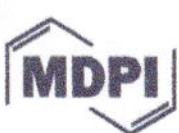

Article

Who Packed the Drugs? Application of Bayesian Networks to Address Questions of DNA Transfer, Persistence, and Recovery from Plastic Bags and Tape

Ane Elida Fonneløp [1,*,†], Sara Faria [2,†], Gnanagowry Shanthan [1] and Peter Gill [1,3]

[1] Department of Forensic Sciences, Oslo University Hospital, 0372 Oslo, Norway; rmgnsa@ous-hf.no (G.S.); peterd.gill@gmail.com (P.G.)
[2] Faculty of Sciences, University of Lisbon, 1749-016 Lisbon, Portugal; sarafaria1998@outlook.pt
[3] Department of Forensic Medicine, University of Oslo, 0315 Oslo, Norway
* Correspondence: rmanfo@ous-hf.no
† Contributed equally to this work.

Abstract: When DNA from a suspect is detected in a sample collected at a crime scene, there can be alternative explanations about the activity that may have led to the transfer, persistence and recovery of his/her DNA. Previous studies have shown that DNA can be indirectly transferred via intermediate surfaces and that DNA on a previously used object can persist after subsequent use of another individual. In addition, it has been shown that a person's shedder status may influence transfer, persistence, prevalence, and recovery of DNA. In this study we have investigated transfer persistence and recovery on zip-lock bags and tape, which are commonly encountered in drug cases and how the shedder status of the participants influenced the results. A probabilistic framework was developed which was based on a previously described Bayesian network with case-specific modifications. Continuous modelling of data was used to inform the Bayesian networks and two case scenarios were investigated. In the specific scenarios only moderate to low support for H_p was obtained. Applying a continuous model based on the profile quality can change the LRs.

Keywords: transfer; persistence; activity; Bayesian networks

Citation: Fonneløp, A.E.; Faria, S.; Shanthan, G.; Gill, P. Who Packed the Drugs? Application of Bayesian Networks to Address Questions of DNA Transfer, Persistence, and Recovery from Plastic Bags and Tape. *Genes* **2022**, *13*, 18. https://doi.org/10.3390/genes13010018

Academic Editor: Emiliano Giardina

Received: 8 December 2021
Accepted: 17 December 2021
Published: 22 December 2021

Publisher's Note: MDPI stays neutral with regard to jurisdictional claims in published maps and institutional affiliations.

1. Introduction

In criminal cases, when DNA from a suspect is detected in samples collected from drug wrappings, there can be alternative explanations about the activity that may have led to the transfer, persistence, and recovery of his/her DNA. Often these explanations involve indirect transfer from an object they have used (e.g., bag or clothing), or perhaps the suspect has been in contact with the object in a situation not related to the crime. The hierarchy of propositions describes the different levels of evaluation of the evidence given propositions at sub-source, source, activity, and offence level [1–3]. The guidelines from the International Society for Forensic Genetics (ISFG) DNA commission provide advice on evaluation and the formulation of propositions and recommend the evaluation of results at activity level in the light of the alternative propositions of the case and calculating a likelihood ratio (LR) [2]. A recommended tool to aid in the evaluation of evidence is Bayesian networks (BNs) [4] and examples of how they can be constructed and used are widely available [5,6]. To construct a BN, the relevant variables and their respective probabilities are required. Extensive research on transfer persistence, prevalence, and recovery (TPPR) of DNA has been conducted over the past 10 years [7], although knowledge bases that can be utilised for routine casework are currently lacking.

The indirect transfer of DNA is dependent upon several variables including: the amount of DNA present, time since initial contact, number of contacts and the type of surface of the objects involved [8–10]. DNA from a person who previously handled an object can be detected for some time after the object has been handed to a new user [10]. However, it is more likely that DNA from the most recent user of the object will become the major contributor over time [11,12]. Van Oorschot et al. [12] observed an average 50% drop in the DNA from the previous user immediately after handling by a new user when the surface was hard and non-porous. Mayuoni-Kirshenbaum et al. [13] studied the persistence of DNA from a person cutting aluminium foil when the foil was subsequently used for lock picking by another individual and only detected DNA from the cutter in 1/25 cases while the lock-picker was detected in 9/25 samples.

It has previously been demonstrated that individuals have a different propensity to transfer DNA to handled items (shedder status); shedder status is consistent over years, and it can influence transfer probabilities [14–16]. However, the classification method has been debated and a need to introduce an intermediate shedder category (between high and low) has been demonstrated [15–17].

The aim of this paper is to provide a dataset along with a probabilistic framework to interpret DNA evidence at activity level. We present two specific scenarios related to DNA evidence in drug related cases. The first considers direct and indirect transfer to a zip-lock drugs bag that has been stored in a personal bag, whilst the second considers the persistence of DNA from a previous user of tape which was used to pack drugs by a second individual (the cardboard drug wrap experiment). The results from both experiments were examined in the light of the participant's shedder status. A probabilistic framework was developed which was based on a previously described Bayesian network [5] with case-specific modifications. Previous work has usually applied discrete models to measure simple presence/absence of DNA that may be attributed to a person of interest (POI). A continuous model was demonstrated by Gill et al. [6], based upon sub-source likelihood ratios, and this was recently complemented with a method using mean $\overline{RFU}$ (peak height) instead of sub-source likelihood ratio [18]. Here we provide a demonstration of continuous modelling of indirect and direct transfer with two case examples. Continuous models are the preferred method with mixture analysis [19] because they take more information into account. It is natural that activity level assignments should take the same route.

The paper is structured as follows: in Sections 3.1–3.4 there is an empirical description of the data analysis, followed by probabilistic analysis using Bayesian networks of the zip-lock drugs bag experiment (Section 3.5.1), and the tape/cardboard drug wrap experiment (Section 3.5.2).

2. Materials and Methods

This project was approved by the data protection officer at Oslo University Hospital, all participants have given informed consent prior to participating in the experiments. Twenty participants were recruited and participated in all experiments.

2.1. Direct and Indirect Transfer to Zip-Lock Drugs Bags

Each participant was provided with a kit for the experiments containing two DNA-free (exposed to UV light for 10 min on each side) zip-lock bags (16.7 × 10 cm). One of the zip-lock bags contained a 15 mL centrifuge tube (VWR) filled with water to function as a weight.

2.1.1. Direct Transfer

Participants were instructed to wait at least one hour after washing hands/using antibacterial hand wash, after which they touched the upper surface of the zip-lock bag for about 30 s by opening and closing it. They were then asked to repeat this process with the same bag two more times (total of three handlings). When the procedure was completed, participants were instructed to place the zip-lock bag into a new labelled envelope. The dataset generated is labelled E1 and is available in the Supplementary Material S2.

2.1.2. Indirect Transfer

Participants were instructed to use their own personal bag/purse/backpack for this experiment. They were instructed to put on a pair of new disposable gloves before placing the zip-lock drugs bag containing the weight into their personal bag (which did not contain anything else during the experiment) and leave it there for 24 h; they were also instructed to move the personal bag during this period, e.g., carry it with them to work and home. After the 24 h had passed, the zip-lock drugs bag was removed, whilst wearing clean gloves, and placed into a new labelled envelope. The dataset generated is labelled E2 and is available in Supplementary Material S2.

2.2. Persistence and Detection of DNA from a Previous User of a Tape Roll

In this experiment participants were divided into pairs. Participant B was given a DNA-free (treated with UV light for 20 min on each side) roll of tape. The participants were instructed to wait at least 1 h after washing hands/using antibacterial liquid; then the tape was handled for 1 min by passing it from one hand to another, stroking the sides of the tape roll towards the palm of the hands; use of the tape was mimicked by tearing off a small piece. The roll of tape was placed in a labelled envelope and passed to participant A after a minimum 10 days in storage. Participant A was provided with a piece of clean cardboard (approx. 6 × 10 cm) (UV treated on each side for 20 min), to mimic a pack of drugs. He/she was instructed to wrap the piece of cardboard with the tape (previously handled by B). The "drug wrap" was placed in a new labelled envelope. Each of the 20 participants contributed twice to the experiments swapping the roles of A and B, giving a total of 20 wrapped cardboards. The data generated is available in Supplementary Material S2.

2.3. Shedder Status

Participants were asked to hold a plastic tube (15 mL centrifuge tube high performance tube, VWR) for 10 s in their dominant hand, at least one hour after washing hands/using antibacterial liquid. The experiments were repeated 3 times, with a new clean tube; there was a gap of at least three hours between each experiment. The data generated is available in Supplementary Material S2.

2.4. Sample Processing

Samples were collected with a moistened (one drop of water) swab (Tubed Sterile Dryswab, Medical Wire). The sampling was performed on: (a) zip-lock bags: the top 3 cm of the outside and inside (including lock) of the zip-lock bags; (b) wrapped cardboard: the full outside and edges of the tape around the cardboard; (c): tubes: the full body of the 15 mL centrifuge tubes (not lids). One negative control sample was collected from all items (tape, cardboard, zip-lock bag and tube). For the samples collected from zip-lock bags and wrapped cardboard, the tips of the swabs were cut, placed in 1.5 mL Eppendorf tube and stored at −20 °C until further processing to avoid degradation. Samples collected from tubes were stored in ventilated evidence bags to dry before the tips of the swabs were cut directly into single PCR-tubes for a direct PCR analysis.

Samples collected from zip-lock bags and wrapped cardboard were extracted by the 5% Chelex procedure [20] (no prior incubation with water) where 200 μL Chelex (Bio-Rad, Hercules, CA, USA) was added to swabs. All samples were quantified with PowerQuant (Promega, Madison, WI, USA) on the 7500 Real-Time PCR system (ThermoFisher, Waltham, MA, USA) using the manufacturers' recommendations. PCR amplification was carried out using the PowerPlex Fusion 6C System kit (Promega, Madison, WI, USA) as recommended by the manufacturer (1 ng template, 25 μL reaction volume and 29 amplification cycles). Samples that had lower concentrations than the recommended template amount were amplified with the maximum template volume of 15 μL. For the shedder experiment, the PCR reaction mix was added directly to the tube containing the swab tips. Amplification was carried out using a Veriti 96-Well Thermal Cycler (ThermoFisher, Waltham, MA, USA). Samples were injected on the Applied Biosystems 3500 xL Genetic Analyzer at 1.2 kV for 24 s. The results were analysed using the GeneMapper ID-X Software version 1.6 (ThermoFisher, Waltham, MA, USA). The analytical threshold (AT) for alleles was set to 100 RFU.

2.5. Data Analysis

Results were analysed using R version 4.0.3 with the package tidyverse version 1.3.0. Likelihood ratios and mixture proportions were calculated using EuroForMix version 3.2.0 using propositions shown in in Equation (1), where U corresponds to unknown contributors, necessary to explain all alleles present. The average RFU ($\overline{RFU}$) for a contributor was calculated by dividing the total RFU (RFU_{tot}) by the number (n) loci (23, except amelogenin), Equation (2). If the sample was a mixture, the contribution from the POI was found by multiplying $\overline{RFU}$ for the sample by the mixture proportion (M_x). If a sample was diluted then the result was multiplied by a dilution factor (d_l).

$$LR = \frac{\Pr(E|H_p : POI + U_1)}{\Pr(E|H_d : U_1 + U_2)} \tag{1}$$

$$\overline{RFU}_{POI} = M_x \times \frac{RFU_{tot}}{n} \times d_l \tag{2}$$

2.5.1. List of Variables

We follow the notation used by Gill et al. [6] (Section 4), summarised here:

t is the probability of direct transfer, persistence and recovery of DNA from the POI (under H_p only).

t' is the probability of direct transfer, persistence and recovery of DNA from an unknown contributor (under H_d only).

b is the probability of background DNA, based on observations, and is applied under both H_p and H_d. Background DNA is present from unknown sources and unknown activities. It can be described as "foreign" (non-self). For further details we refer to Section 3.2 in [6].

s is the probability of transfer, persistence and recovery; in experiment 1, this is indirect transfer under H_p and H_d, and in experiment 2, it is direct transfer under H_d only.

Suffixes are applied to described probabilities of an event given a particular contributor, e.g., t_A refers to the probability of direct transfer, persistence and recovery of DNA from contributor A.

2.5.2. Notation Relating to the Experiments

Experiment 1: zip-lock drugs bag

$E1_{dbag}$: Dataset from the zip-lock drugs bag; direct transfer

$E2_{pbag}$: Dataset from the personal bag experiment; indirect transfer

$\overline{RFU}_{E1dbag}$: Lognormal distribution of mean RFU from $E1_{dbag}$ data; direct transfer

$\overline{RFU}_{E2pbag}$: Lognormal distribution of mean RFU from $E2_{pbag}$ data; indirect transfer

Experiment 2: Tape/cardboard drug wraps

$C1_{pack}$: Dataset from drugs wrapper; direct transfer

$C2_{tape}$: Dataser from the tape handler; direct transfer

$\overline{RFU}_{C1pack}$: Lognormal distribution of mean RFU from $C1_{pack}$ data; direct transfer

$\overline{RFU}_{C2tape}$: Lognormal distribution of mean RFU from $C2_{tape}$ data; direct transfer

General

$\overline{RFU}_A$: the observed $\overline{RFU}$ value from contributor A

$\overline{RFU}_B$: the observed $\overline{RFU}$ value from contributor B

$\overline{RFU}_{unknown}$: the observed $\overline{RFU}$ value from an unknown contributor

2.5.3. Distribution Fitting

Log-normal distributions were fitted to the data using the R package *fitdistrplus* using function *lnorm*. The method is described in detail in Supplementary Material S1. The probability of background for experiment 1 was modelled using the same lognormal parameters calculated for indirect transfer data $\overline{RFU}_{E2pbag}$, as described in the Supplementary Material S1 (Section S4.4.1). To carry out sensitivity analysis, $1000\times$ bootstraps (with replacement) were taken of datasets (Supplementary Material S2). For each bootstrap, a new set of log-normal parameters (mean log and SD log) were calculated using the *fitdistrplus* R package using the *lnorm* function. The probability distributions were used to substantiate the Bayesian networks described in Sections 3.5.1 and 3.5.2. The programming of these networks was carried with R-code using the formulae described in Sections 3.5.1 and 3.5.2.

3. Results

3.1. Direct and Secondary Transfer to Zip-Lock Drugs Bags

The DNA from the POI could be detected in the samples collected after direct handling of a zip-lock drugs bag and after indirect transfer to the drugs bag from storage in a previously used personal bag. More alleles matching the POI along with higher DNA quantities were generally observed in the direct transfer experiment ($E1_{dbag}$) compared with indirect transfer from inside a personal bag ($E2_{pbag}$). Generally, the $\overline{RFU}_{POI}$ was higher in $E1_{dbag}$, but a few occurrences of higher $\overline{RFU}_{POI}$ were observed in $E2_{pbag}$ (Figure 1).

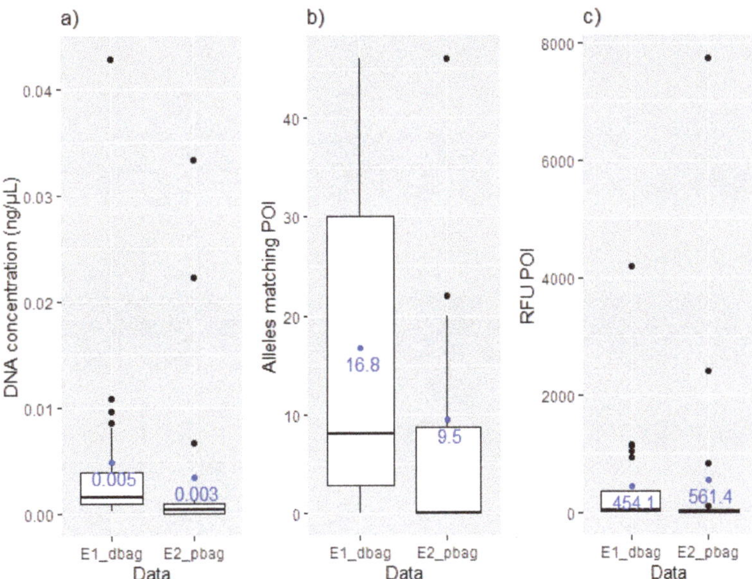

Figure 1. Boxplots displaying (**a**) the measured DNA concentrations (ng/μL in 200 μL), (**b**) the number of detected allele's matching the POI and (**c**) the $\overline{RFU}_{POI}$ for the samples in the $E1_{dbag}$ (direct) and $E2_{pbag}$ (indirect) data.

In the direct transfer experiment four full and seven partial profiles were detected, while six samples only displayed six or less alleles and four samples had no results. Only one sample contained (two) unknown alleles. From the indirect transfer experiment three full and two partial profiles corresponding to the POI were detected. Four samples only displayed five or less alleles and ten samples had no profiling results. One sample was a mixture with 21 unknown alleles, and one sample was a partial profile with alleles corresponding to a child of the participant. The most frequently used type of personal bag used was a backpack but a large proportion of these samples (7/11) had no results. The full dataset can be found in the Supplementary Material S2. The highest $\overline{RFU}$ values on the zip-lock drugs bags were observed after storage in a personal purse/handbag, (Figure 2).

A few participants (1 and 2, respectively) used a personal PC and shopping bag to store the zip-lock drugs bags. Most participants reported using the personal bag frequently or every day, while two participants reported rarely using their personal bags. No alleles were detected on zip lock bags after storage in rarely used personal bags.

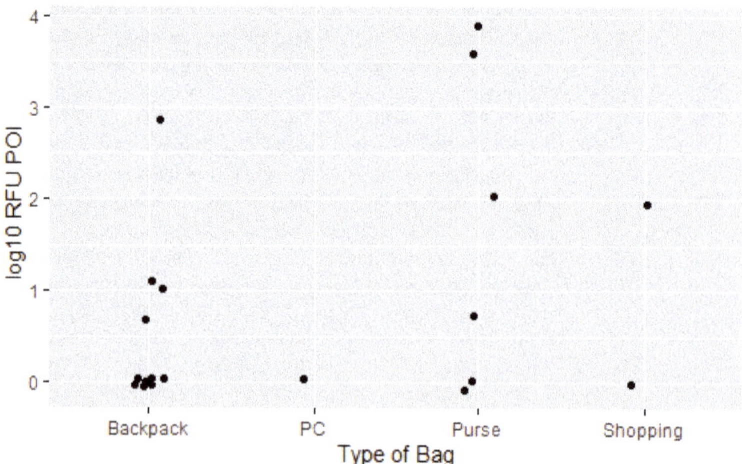

Figure 2. Dot plot displaying the $\log_{10}\overline{RFU}$ values detected in the samples collected from zip-lock drugs bags after storage in a previously used personal bag (backpack, PC bag, purse/handbag or shopping bag).

3.2. Persistence and Detection of DNA from a Previous User of a Tape Roll Used to Wrap Drugs

In samples collected from wrapped cardboard, DNA from both the person who previously handled the tape (C2$_{tape}$) and the person who packed the tape around the cardboard (C1$_{pack}$) could be detected. However, the quality of the profile, peak heights of detected alleles and mixture proportions varied between the cardboard wrapper and the tape handler (Figure 3).

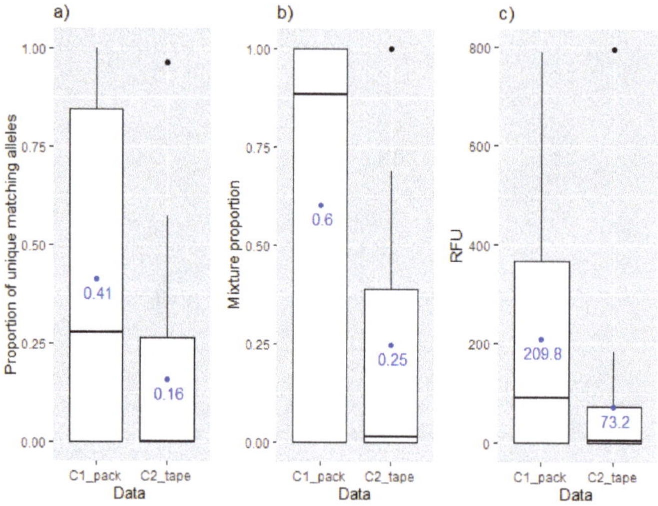

Figure 3. Boxplot displaying (**a**) proportion of unique alleles, (**b**) the mixture proportion and (**c**) $\overline{RFU}$ values corresponding to the wrapper (C1$_{pack}$) and the handler (C2$_{tape}$) of the tape.

Three samples had no profiling results and for an additional three samples only four alleles were detected. Seven samples were full or partial profiles corresponding to the drugs wrapper (C1), five samples were mixtures of C1 and C2. For three of these mixtures, C1 was the major contributor, whilst in the last two, the contributions were of equal proportions. Two samples were partial profiles with alleles corresponding to C2. The full dataset can be found in the Supplementary Material S2.

3.3. Shedder Status

The total *RFU* values (RFU_{tot}) from the direct PCR analysis varied from 0 to 458,705, variation was greater between individuals than within the samples from one individual (ANOVA, p = 0.04), Figure 4. However, some individuals, especially those that deposited low amounts of DNA, displayed lower variation. Individuals were classified as low, medium or high shedders based on the criteria defined by Johannessen et al. [15] with the following adjustments according to the observed values of the current dataset: high shedder class was assigned to participants that had two out of three samples above the average RFU_{tot} (62,520) and two out of three samples with 20 out of 24 full loci. Low shedder class was assigned to participants where all samples were below 8000 RFU_{tot} and two out of three with negative or partial profiles. The rest were classified as medium shedders. This resulted in 4 high, 11 medium and 5 low shedders (Figure 3). The full dataset can be found in the Supplementary Material S2.

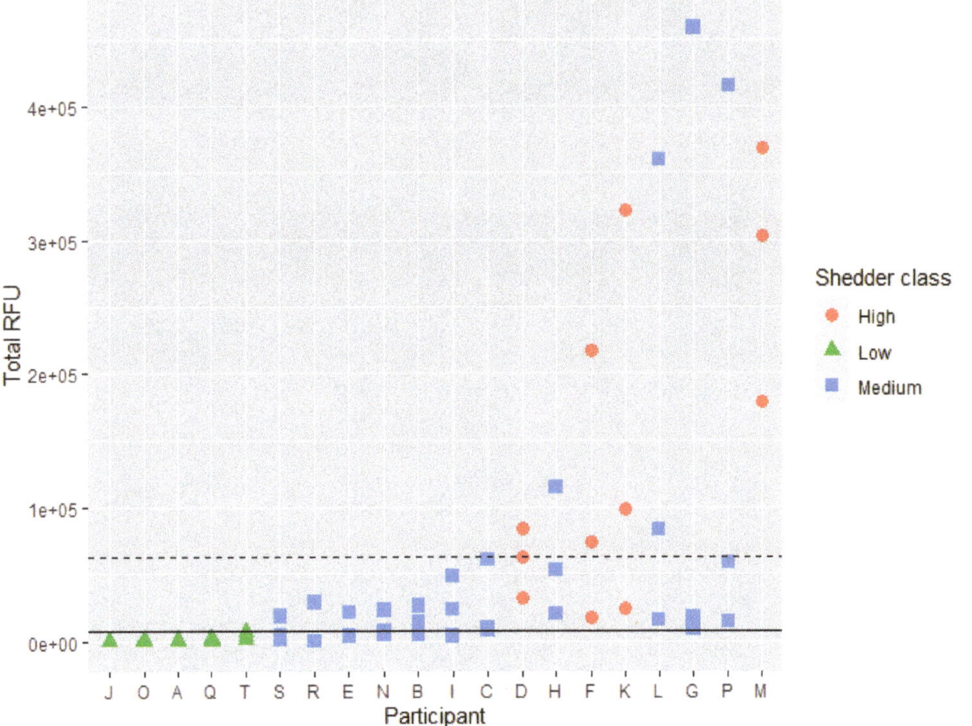

Figure 4. Scatter plot showing the total RFU_{tot} values (multiplied by M_x if sample was a mixture) for each sample collected from each participant and according to their shedder status, high (red circle), medium (blue square) low (green triangle). The average RFU_{tot} (6.25E+04) and low shedder limit of 8.00E+03 RFU_{tot} are represented with the dotted and straight lines, respectively.

DNA from unknown contributors was detected in 30/90 samples, the average M_x proportion from unknown contributors was highest for low shedders, Table 1.

Table 1. Detection of unknown alleles in the shedder samples and the proportion of unknown DNA detected for the three different shedder classes.

	Number of Samples	Average M_x Unknown Contrib.
High	4/12 (33%)	7.1
Medium	19/33 (58%)	8.5
Low	7/15 (47%)	52.0

3.4. Transfer in Relation to Shedder Status

Data from experiment 1 (direct transfer to zip-lock drugs bag) showed highest transfer rates with high shedders (Figure 5). More variation was observed in the medium shedder group, than for the low and high shedders. The trend is not as obvious for experiment 2 (indirect transfer from personal bag to zip-lock drugs bag). In fact, the best quality profile was detected in a sample from a low shedder participant. Based on the number of samples in each group, there were insufficient data to evaluate the effect using Bayesian networks described in Section 3.5.1.

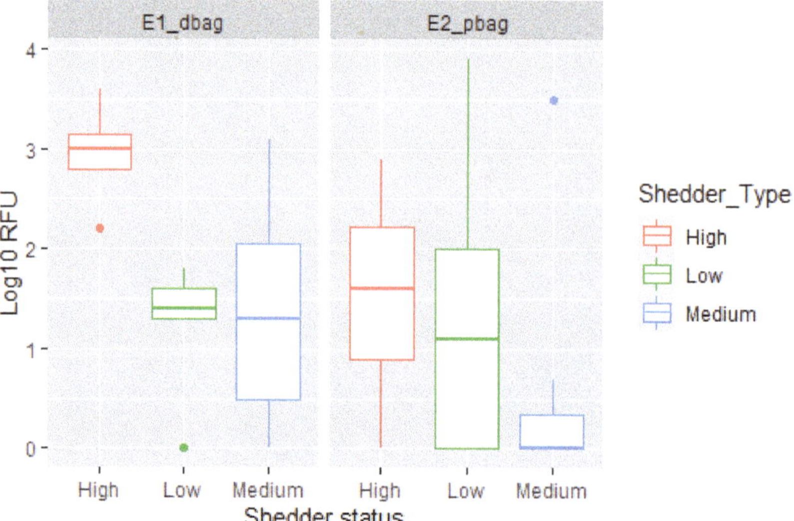

Figure 5. Boxplot displaying the log10 $\overline{RFU}$ detected in the direct transfer experiment ($E1_{dbag}$) and indirect transfer from personal bag ($E2_{pbag}$) according to the participants' shedder classification.

Data from persistence and detection of DNA from a previous user of a tape roll experiment showed that low shedders only provided low quality profiles and that higher quality profiles were provided by high shedders. Medium shedders provided both high and low quality results. (Figure 6).

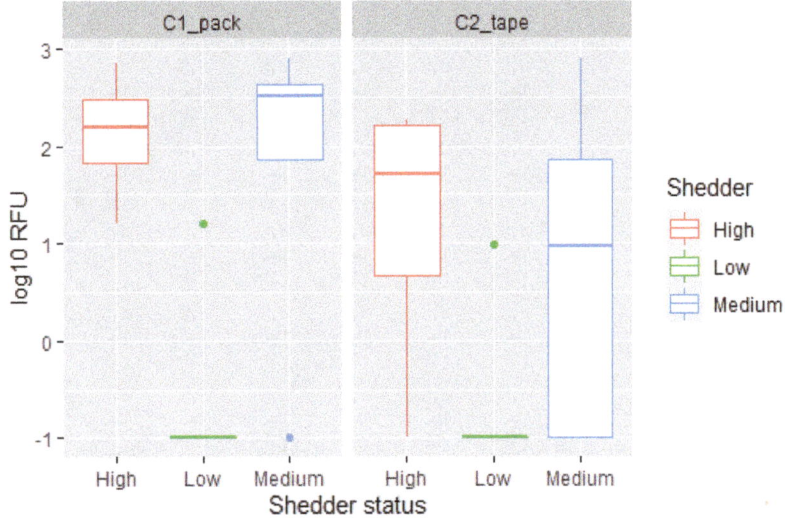

Figure 6. Boxplot displaying the log10 $\overline{RFU}$ for the drugs wrapper (C1$_{pack}$) and the previous handler (C2$_{tape}$) of the tape according to the shedder classification of the participants.

3.5. Case Examples

To demonstrate the potential use of the datasets obtained, we will use two fictive case examples that are based on actual experiences from case work, using a Bayesian network to evaluate the evidence.

3.5.1. Potential DNA Transfer from Storage in a Personal Bag

Case Circumstances

1. A large depot of drugs was found at a hideout;
2. The drugs were packed in zip-lock bags and placed in a black gym bag;
3. Upon questioning, person A claims to have no knowledge of the drugs. However, he recognizes a gym bag that the drugs had been stored in and claims that it used to belong to him but it was lost or stolen two weeks previously.

DNA Analysis

DNA samples were collected from the outside and opening of the zip-lock bag

4. Example 1: Result is a full DNA profile of a single individual. There is a candidate in the national DNA database who is identified as person A;
5. Example 2: Result is a mixture of two individuals. There is a candidate in the national DNA database who is identified as person A but there is no candidate for the second individual.

Propositions

Sub-source likelihood ratios were calculated for both contributors using EuroForMix [21], although this information was not used in any further analysis. To proceed with activity level analysis, it is assumed that the sub-source LR is sufficient for a court to agree the identity of a POI [2].

The alternative activity level propositions (for both examples) are as follows:

H_p: The suspect packed the drugs;

H_d: The suspect has no relation to the drugs but was the owner of the gym bag which was stolen two weeks previously. An unknown individual packed the drugs.

The BN used to instantiate probabilities is identical to that described by [6] (Supplement S1), except that the title of the nodes are changed to represent the case circumstances (Figure 7). Log-normal distributions were used to calculate drug bag (direct) and personal bag (indirect) TPR probabilities, conditioned upon values of $\overline{RFU}_A$ modelled with $\overline{RFU}_{E1dbag}$ and $\overline{RFU}_{E2pbag}$ distributions respectively. $\overline{RFU}_{unknown}$ was modelled with $\overline{RFU}_{E2pbag}$ distribution (Table 2), the assigned probabilities (Figure 8) were subsequently used in the BN (Figure 7) to calculate the results. To carry out sensitivity analysis, $1000\times$ bootstraps (with replacement) were taken of the $\overline{RFU}_{E1\_dbag}$ and $\overline{RFU}_{E2\_pbag}$ data (Supplementary Material S2) to provide 1000 new sets of data. For each bootstrap, a new set of log-normal parameters (mean log and SD log) were calculated using the *fitdistrplus* R package and the variation was represented by percentiles in Table 3.

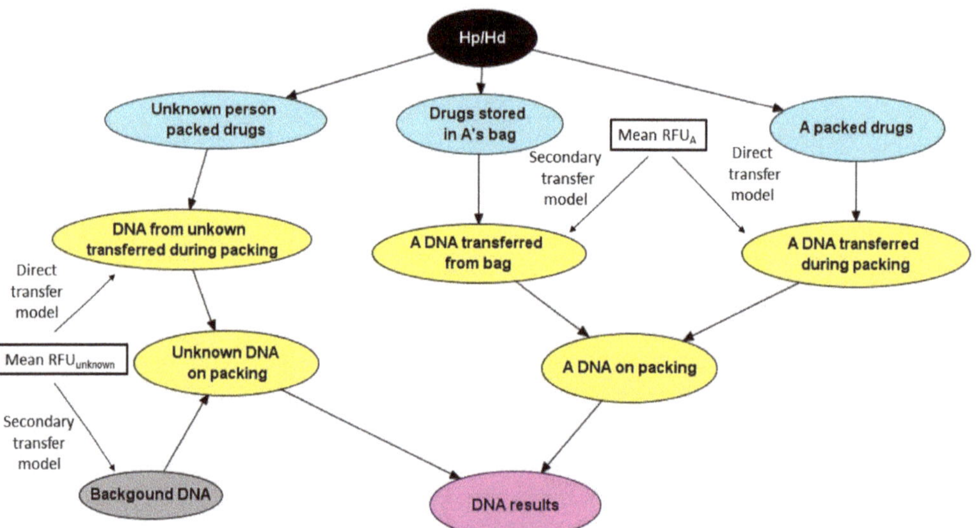

Figure 7. Bayesian network for the "drugs stored in gym bag" example showing data sets and models used to instantiate the nodes.

Table 2. Relationship of probabilities of DNA transfer from individuals A (POI) and U (unknown), showing the datasets that were used to calculate probability distributions, along with the BN nodes instantiated. See nomenclature Section 2.5.1 for definitions of probabilities.

Probability	Description	Contributor	Data used to Inform Probability Distribution	BN Nodes
t_A	Packing transfer	A	RFU_{E1dbag}	A DNA transferred during packing
t'	Packing transfer	U	RFU_{E1dbag}	DNA from unknown transferred during packing
s	Bag transfer	A	RFU_{E2pbag}	A DNA transferred from bag
b	Background	U	RFU_{E2pbag}	Background DNA

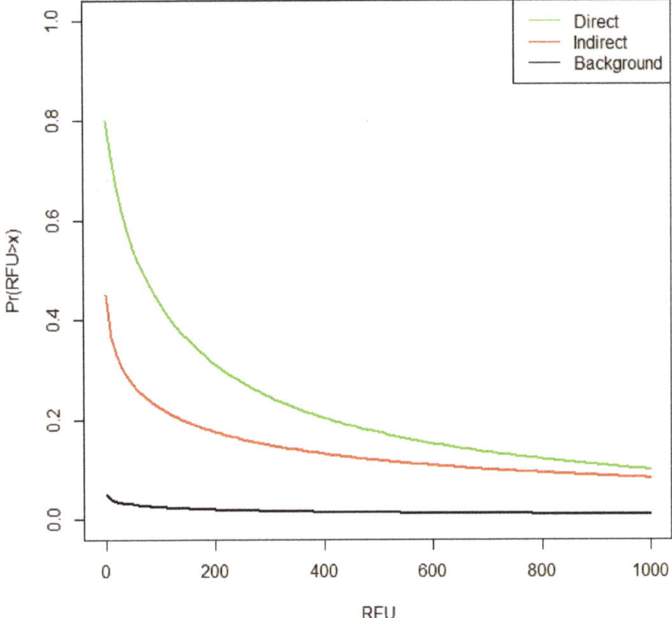

Figure 8. Comparison of probabilities of direct, indirect and background TPPR for the zip-lock drugs bag example. Direct transfer was modelled from $\overline{RFU}_{E1dbag}$; personal bag (indirect transfer) was modelled from $\overline{RFU}_{E2pbag}$ data and background was also modelled from $\overline{RFU}_{E2pbag}$ data, with adjusted $k = 0.95$ (the proportion of observations with no background) in order to scale results as described in Supplementary Material S1.

Table 3. Activity level likelihood ratios where only contributor A is recovered, with sensitivity analysis, showing 2.5–97.5 percentiles. The median (50 percentile) values are those that are reported. Results for the discrete model are shown in the top row; continuous models conditioned upon $\overline{RFU}_A > x$ are shown in remaining rows.

RFU$_A$ > x	2.50%	5%	10%	25%	50%	75%	90%	95%	97.50%
0	5	5	6	8	11	17	27	39	6×10^1
200	5	5	7	9	14	23	47	82	2×10^3
400	4	5	6	9	13	24	52	122	1×10^4
600	4	5	6	8	12	24	52	153	4×10^4
800	4	5	6	8	12	24	53	196	9×10^4
1000	4	4	5	8	12	24	54	218	2×10^5
2000	4	4	5	7	11	24	63	448	3×10^6
4000	3	4	4	6	10	23	77	1016	6×10^7
6000	3	4	4	6	9	21	87	1752	4×10^8

Derivation of the formulae used in the calculations are the same as those described in Supplementary Material S1 of Gill et al. [6]. Likelihood ratios were calculated as shown in Formulae 3–5 (nomenclature in Table 2):

(a)   Only the POI (A) is observed

$$LR = \frac{(s(1 - t_A) + t_A) \times (1 - b)}{s \times (1 - \Pr(U_d))} \tag{3}$$

(b) POI (A) and unknown is observed

$$LR_a = \frac{(s(1 - t_A) + t_A) \times b}{s \times \Pr(U_d)} \tag{4}$$

(c) Probability of recovery of DNA from an unknown contributor

$$\Pr(U_d) = t'b + t'(1 - b) + b(1 - t') = t' + b(1 - t') \tag{5}$$

There were only three observations of background (datasets $E1_{dbag}$ and $E2_{pbag}$). Background is from indeterminate (unknown) sources and can comprise both direct and indirect transfer. Here, it was modelled using $\overline{RFU}_{E1pbag} > x$ data (where x is a threshold value; first column in Table 3), except that the model was scaled relative to $k = 1 - \Pr(b)$ as described in the Supplementary Material S1; where k is the proportion of observations where no background was observed. From experimental observation $\Pr(b) = 0.05$ and $k = 0.95$.

Two possible outcomes of the DNA results were analysed in detail. Either a profile from the POI individual A is recovered, or A is recovered in combination with an unknown contributor which forms the basis of the proposition under H_d, else the unknown contributor is background under H_p.

Contributor A Recovered Alone

When contributor A is recovered alone, Table 3 shows that the median (50 percentile) LRs always favour the proposition that he/she packed the drugs; the evidence provides moderate support. If a discrete model is used where allele peak height is not considered, then LR = 11 (top row of Table 3). Taking peak height into account has little effect in this example. The sensitivity analysis shows the evidence always favours H_p at the 2.5 percentile.

Unknown and Contributor A Recovered

A different result is obtained when a mixture of unknown and contributor A is recovered. For the discrete model (top row of Table 4) the LR ≈ 0.1, favouring the proposition that an unknown contributor wrapped the drugs. When allele peak height is considered, similar results are obtained (Table 4).

Table 4. Activity level likelihood ratios where contributor A and an unknown are recovered, with sensitivity analysis, showing 2.5–97.5 percentiles. The median (50 percentile) values are those that are reported. Results for the discrete model are shown in the top row; continuous models conditioned upon $\overline{RFU}_A > x$ and $\overline{RFU}_{unknown} > x$ are shown in remaining rows.

$RFU_A > x$	$RFU_{Unknown} > x$	2.50%	5%	10%	25%	50%	75%	90%	95%	97.50%
0	0	0.1	0.1	0.1	0.1	0.1	0.1	0.2	0.2	0.2
100	2000	0.1	0.1	0.1	0.2	0.3	0.6	1.1	1.5	2
100	7000	0.1	0.2	0.2	0.3	0.6	1.1	1.8	2.4	4
2000	100	0.1	0.1	0.1	0.1	0.1	0.2	0.5	1.4	24
7000	100	0.1	0.1	0.1	0.1	0.1	0.1	0.6	3.6	307
1000	2000	0.1	0.1	0.2	0.2	0.3	0.5	0.9	1.5	20
1000	7000	0.2	0.2	0.2	0.3	0.5	0.9	1.3	2.7	35
2000	1000	0.1	0.1	0.1	0.1	0.2	0.3	0.7	1.8	45
7000	1000	0.1	0.1	0.1	0.1	0.2	0.3	1.0	4.2	717

3.5.2. Cardboard Drug Wrap Experiment

Case Circumstances

A large depot of drugs was detected by the police during a house search of A's house.

The drugs were wrapped in cardboard and covered by packing tape;

Person A admits that he packed the drugs and does not implicate anyone else;

Person B claims to have no knowledge of the drugs. However, he worked for a moving agency and often handles packing tape. Remains of packing tapes are often left behind and could be picked up and used by others.

DNA Analysis

DNA samples were collected from the wrappings. The results of the DNA analysis were a mixture of person A and an unknown contributor. A candidate was identified as person B from a national DNA database search.

Propositions

Sub-source likelihood ratios were calculated for both contributors using EuroForMix [20], although this information was not used in any further analysis. To proceed with activity level analysis, it is assumed that the sub-source LR is sufficient for a court to agree the identity of a POI [2].

The prosecution and defence activity level propositions are as follows:

H_p: A and B packed the drugs together and B did not previously handle the tape;

H_d: A packed the drugs alone; B had previously handled the tape

From the case information, a Bayesian network incorporating the relevant nodes was prepared (Figure 9). See Supplementary Materials S1 for details. Since both H_p and H_d agree that contributor A packed the drugs, his/her presence or absence of DNA has no effect upon the likelihood ratio. Only contributor B has an effect.

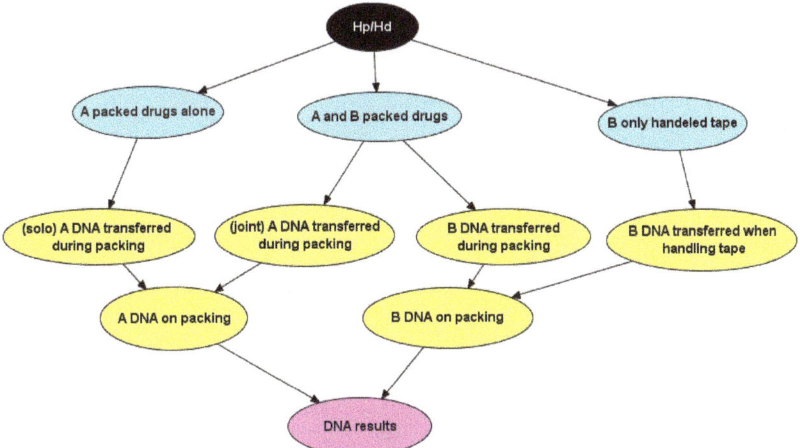

Figure 9. Bayesian network for the evaluation of evidence in the case where DNA evidence was collected from cardboard drug wrap.

Statistical Analysis

The data are provided in Supplementary Materials S2. In the experiment, contributor B previously handled the tape as described in Section 3.5.1, and contributor A packed the drugs. The mean $\overline{RFU}$ of the observed DNA profile was split per contributor ($\overline{RFU}_A$ and $\overline{RFU}_B$), based upon their respective mixture proportions (M_x): i.e., $\overline{RFU}_A = \overline{RFU}_{tot} \times M_{xA}$ and $\overline{RFU}_B = \overline{RFU}_{tot} \times M_{xB}$, where M_x was calculated using EuroForMix [20]. Log-normal distributions were fitted to each set of data using the *fitdistrplus* R package (Figure 10). Distributions for the BN node "B DNA transferred when handling tape" (Figure 9) were modelled from $\overline{RFU}_{C2tape}$; distributions for BN nodes" (solo) A DNA transferred during packing" and "(joint) B DNA transferred during the packing" were both modelled from $\overline{RFU}_{C1pack}$ (Table 5).

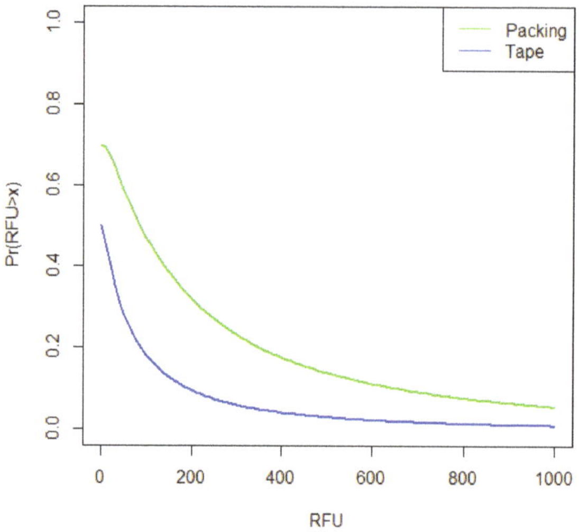

Figure 10. Lognormal distributions of $\overline{RFU}_{C1pack}$ and $\overline{RFU}_{C2tape}$.

Table 5. Relationship of probabilities of DNA transfer from individuals A and B, showing the datasets that were used to calculate probability distributions, along with the BN nodes instantiated. Nomenclature is described in Section 2.5.1.

Probability	Description	Contributor	Data Used to Inform Probability Distribution	BN Nodes
t_A	Packing transfer	A	RFU_{C1pack}	(solo) A DNA transferred during packing (joint) A DNA transferred during packing
t_B	Packing transfer	B	RFU_{C1pack}	(joint) B DNA transferred during packing
s	Tape transfer	B	RFU_{C2tape}	B DNA transferred when handling tape

Likelihood ratios were calculated as follows (see Table 5 for context):

(a) A DNA is recovered: $LR = \frac{(1-t_B)}{(1-s)}$

(b) B DNA is recovered: $LR = t_B/s$

(c) A and B DNA are recovered: $LR = t_B/s$

(d) no DNA is recovered: $LR = \frac{(1-t_B)}{(1-s)}$

The formulae are derived in Supplementary Material S1. Note that likelihood ratios of (a) and (d) are the same, as are (b) and (c). This is because both H_p and H_d condition upon contributor A, hence his/her presence is cancelled out. To carry out sensitivity analysis, 1000× bootstraps (with replacement) were taken of the $\overline{RFU}_A$ and $\overline{RFU}_B$ data (Supplementary Material S1). For each bootstrap, a new set of log-normal parameters (mean log and SD log) were calculated using the *fitdistrplus* R package.

Results of Analysis

Log-normal distributions were used to calculate the tape handling and drug packing TPR probabilities, conditioned upon values of $\overline{RFU}_B > x$ from simulated profiles and subsequently used in the BN (Figure 8) to calculate the results (Table 6).

Table 6. Activity level likelihood ratios, with sensitivity analysis, showing 1–99 percentiles. The median (50 percentile) values are those that are reported. Results for the discrete model are shown in the top row; continuous model conditioned upon $\overline{RFU}_B > x$ shown in remaining rows.

$RFU_B > x$	1%	2.50%	5%	10%	25%	50%	75%	90%	95%	97.50%	99%
0	0.8	0.8	0.9	1.0	1.2	1.4	1.7	2.0	2.3	2.6	3.0
100	1.2	1.4	1.5	1.7	2.1	2.7	3.9	5.6	7.3	10.0	16.2
200	1.3	1.5	1.7	2.0	2.6	3.7	6.6	12.9	20.5	34.0	90.5
300	1.3	1.5	1.7	2.1	2.8	4.5	10	23	43	93	282
400	1.3	1.5	1.7	2.0	3.0	5.1	13	39	78	190	953
500	1.2	1.4	1.6	2.0	3.1	5.5	17	65	147	371	2152
600	1.1	1.3	1.5	1.9	3.0	5.9	20	97	238	603	4441
700	1.0	1.2	1.4	1.8	3.0	6.1	24	133	360	1157	8454
800	0.8	1.1	1.3	1.7	3.0	6.4	29	179	563	1872	15,118
900	0.7	1.0	1.3	1.6	3.0	6.7	35	227	833	2951	27,012
1000	0.6	1.0	1.2	1.6	2.9	6.9	40	291	1176	5202	52,019

Likelihood ratios, along with sensitivity analyses are calculated against a range of $RFU_B > x$ values (Table 6). If a profile is obtained where only contributor A is present and there is no DNA present that can be attributed to contributor B, then the LR = 0.6, i.e., supports the proposition that suspect B did not package the drugs. If DNA is present that can be attributed to B, then the LR > 1, favouring the proposition that suspect B did package the drugs. The presence/absence of individual B as a contributor to the evidence can be described either as discrete: $\Pr(\overline{RFU}_B > 0)$ vs. absence, or as a continuous distribution where $\Pr(\overline{RFU}_B > x)$, where x is a threshold value. With a discrete model, LR=1.4 (first row of Table 6). Taking the value of $\overline{RFU}_B > x$, with the continuous model in subsequent rows of Table 6, a higher LR is achieved, reaching a maximum median LR=6.9 if $RFU_B > 1000$ (the limit of observations in Supplementary Materials S2), although the evidence can only be described as "weak" following the ENFSI verbal scale [22]. The sensitivity analysis shows the observed range between 1–99 percentiles from $1000\times$ bootstraps of the data. The variation increases greatly as $\overline{RFU}_B$ increases—a reflection of the small size of the datasets. In conclusion, the discrete model understates the value of the evidence, compared with the continuous model.

4. Discussion

4.1. Zip-Lock Drugs Bag Experiment

The DNA from the POI was detected more frequently on a zip-lock drugs bag if the bag was directly handled. However, the best quality profile observed in the study was collected from a zip-lock drugs bag stored in a personal bag (purse). From the literature, indirect transfer to a sleek surface such as the zip-lock drugs bag is expected to be low [8]. Most of the personal bags used in the experiments had previously been frequently used by the participants, although there are few observations in each class of bags, there is an indication that larger quantities of DNA can be detected on a zip-lock drugs bag after storage in purses. More DNA could be accumulated from the user on the inside of a purse as several personal items (e.g., phone, hairbrush, wallet) containing owner DNA are frequently stored there. In addition, the surface of the inside of the bag will influence accumulation and further transfer [8,23]. In the case example, it is shown that personal bags that are used to store everyday items, such as clothing or personal effects that are frequently handled, accumulate amounts of DNA that may be indirectly transferred to other objects. This resulted in low likelihood ratios (moderate evidence to support H_p) when DNA from only the POI was recovered. There was little difference between the discrete model and the continuous model, the latter takes the allele peak height into account. With mixtures, both discrete and continuous models favour H_d (LR $\approx$ 0.1; Table 4). In the experiment, only low amounts of background (DNA from unknown contributors) were detected. Combined with the relatively low difference between indirect and direct transfer probabilities (Figure 8), especially when $\overline{RFU} > 1000$, this has an impact of reducing the LR if the sample is in admixture with an unknown contributor, so that it always favours the defence proposition (H_d).

4.2. Cardboard Drug Wrap Experiment

In this study, the persistence of DNA from previous handlers of a roll of tape was investigated. As the top surface of the tape is hard and non-porous, the expectation is that low amounts of DNA would be transferred and detected after direct contact, in addition to a rapid removal of DNA from the previous user [8,12,13]. The findings of this study generally correlate with these expectations: a large proportion of samples produced no results or only a few alleles. The packer (last handler) was the only contributor or the one contributing a larger amount of DNA in most of the samples that gave results. Some exceptions were observed with two profiles showing results that only corresponded to the tape handler (person B). The sides of the tape have a rougher surface where more DNA is expected to be transferred upon initial contact [9,23]. In addition to DNA from the previous user persisting on the surface of the tape, it is possible that some of the DNA deposited on the side of tape could be transferred to the new user's hands and to the cardboard during the wrapping of the drugs. As no other items were touched in between handling the tape and performing the wrapping, there was no opportunity for the loss of person B's DNA to other surfaces. We did not monitor the wrapping procedure and recognise that the manner of contact during the procedure could influence the result. However, information regarding this will rarely be known in casework.

In the Bayesian network case example, we considered that an individual B claims that he/she handled tape which was later used to prepare drug wraps. Individual A has admitted the offence, hence, his/her presence of DNA on the drug wrap has no bearing on the value of the evidence. If contributor B's DNA is recovered, without taking account of $\overline{RFU}$ in the discrete model, the evidence is close to neutral LR = 1.4, whereas if $\overline{RFU}$ is taken into account, the value of the evidence increases with RFU, although it does not exceed LR = 7 where $\overline{RFU} > 1000$ (the upper limit of experimental observations), i.e., the evidence would be described as weak using the ENFSI scale [22]. However, if B's DNA is absent, then this favours the defence proposition LR = 0.6.

The experimental set up is similar to that used in [13] where the question was if the POI previously cut an aluminium foil or used this foil in lock picking. The activity LR in the lock-picking study, calculated with a discrete model (7.4) was greater than that observed in the current study (1.4). However, the LR was in the same range as the maximum (median) level of the continuous model employed (LR = 6.9). Some of the differences could be explained by the difference in transfer to and persistence on aluminium foil vs. tape.

4.3. Shedder Status and Transfer Probabilities

A person's shedder status has previously been shown to influence the probability of transfer, persistence, and detection of DNA [14,24]. Fonneløp et al. [14] demonstrated that DNA was more frequently detected in samples collected from the T-shirts of a victim if the attacker was a high shedder and that the probability of detection increased further if the victim was a low shedder. While Otten et al. [24] observed a correspondence between shedder stratus and DNA transfer to gloves. The correspondence between shedder status and the amount of DNA transferred is further demonstrated by our findings when it comes to direct transfer to zip-lock drugs bags (Figure 11), direct transfer during wrapping with a tape and transfer and persistence after touching a role of tape. On the other hand, when indirect transfer from the inside of a personal bag was considered, no clear association with shedder status was observed, and the best quality profile was detected after storage in a low shedder's personal bag. We hypothesised the amount of previous use and the surface of the inside of the bag could be of higher importance for this type of transfer. The low number of samples collected in each category is also a limitation and a clearer correspondence may be seen with a larger collection of data. Shedder status was not incorporated into the Bayesian networks because dividing the results into three categories would lead to too few data in each group to analyse. Secondly, it would also be important to properly characterise the effect of shedder status on indirect transfer before applying this variable to the model.

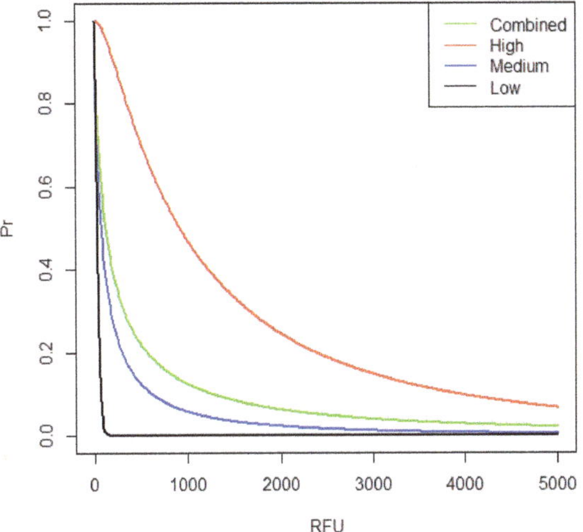

Figure 11. Effect of high/medium/low shedder status on direct transfer (E1) data.

The LRs calculated in this study are comparable to other studies where DNA transferred by hands is considered [6,13,25]. It is likely that including more information—especially shedder status, would, to some degree, change the LR calculations [14].

4.4. Detection of Unknown DNA

This experiment was performed during the COVID-19 pandemic where a general recommendation to keep a social distance of at least two meters and to wash hands frequently or use antibacterial liquid was given. It is likely that these measures could have had an impact on the detection of unknown DNA in the samples, which was low compared to previous studies [9,16,26].

5. Conclusions

We have created datasets on direct and indirect transfer to zip-lock bags and transfer and persistence to tape and further shown how the data can be used to inform Bayesian Networks. As the indirect and persistence scenarios tested are realistic under the circumstances utilised in this study, only moderate to low support for H_p was obtained. We have shown that applying a continuous model based on the profile quality can alter LRs compared to a discrete model and is preferable. There are challenges with limited datasets, and we were not able to implement shedder status into our models. More data on the influence of shedder status are required when indirect transfer is considered.

Supplementary Materials: The following are available online at https://www.mdpi.com/article/10.3390/genes13010018/s1, Supplementary Material S1: Derivation of formulae from experiment 2: Cardboard drug wraps, Supplementary Material S2: Supplementary table 2.1 Results from the direct and indirect transfer to zip-lock bags experiment; Supplementary table 2.2 Results from the persistence and detection of DNA from a previous user of a tape roll experiment; Supplementary table 2.3 The results of the shedder status experiment.

Author Contributions: Conceptualization, A.E.F. methodology, A.E.F. and P.G..; software, P.G.; formal analysis, A.E.F., S.F. and P.G.; investigation, S.F and G.S.; data curation, A.E.F. and S.F.; writing—original draft preparation, A.E.F., S.F. and P.G.; writing—review and editing, G.S.; supervision, A.E.F. and G.S.; project administration, A.E.F. All authors have read and agreed to the published version of the manuscript.

Funding: This research received no external funding.

Institutional Review Board Statement: This project was approved by the data protection officer at Oslo University Hospital (Approval Code: 20/22532, Approval Date: 21 October 2020).

Informed Consent Statement: Informed consent was obtained from all participants involved in the study.

Data Availability Statement: The data supporting the findings reported in this manuscript can be found in the supplementary material S2, Tables S1–S3.

Acknowledgments: We would like to thank Arne Roseth for his help with the direct PCR analysis and all the participants that contributed to the study.

Conflicts of Interest: The authors declare no conflict of interest.

References

1. Cook, R.; Evett, I.; Jackson, G.; Jones, P.; Lambert, J. A Hierarchy of Propositions: Deciding Which Level to Address in Casework. *Sci. Justice* **1998**, *38*, 231–239. [CrossRef]
2. Gill, P.; Hicks, T.; Butler, J.M.; Connolly, E.; Gusmão, L.; Kokshoorn, B.; Morling, N.; van Oorschot, R.A.; Parson, W.; Prinz, M.; et al. DNA commission of the International society for forensic genetics: Assessing the value of forensic biological evidence—Guidelines highlighting the importance of propositions. Part II: Evaluation of biological traces considering activity level propositions. *Forensic Sci. Int. Genet.* **2020**, *44*, 102186. [CrossRef]
3. Taylor, D.; Kokshoorn, B.; Biedermann, A. Evaluation of forensic genetics findings given activity level propositions: A review. *Forensic Sci. Int. Genet.* **2018**, *36*, 34–49. [CrossRef] [PubMed]
4. Biedermann, A.; Taroni, F. Bayesian networks for evaluating forensic DNA profiling evidence: A review and guide to literature. *Forensic Sci. Int. Genet.* **2012**, *6*, 147–157. [CrossRef] [PubMed]
5. Taylor, D.; Biedermann, A.; Hicks, T.; Champod, C. A template for constructing Bayesian networks in forensic biology cases when considering activity level propositions. *Forensic Sci. Int. Genet.* **2018**, *33*, 136–146. [CrossRef]
6. Gill, P.; Bleka, Ø.; Roseth, A.; Fonneløp, A.E. An LR framework incorporating sensitivity analysis to model multiple direct and secondary transfer events on skin surface. *Forensic Sci. Int. Genet.* **2021**, *53*, 102509. [CrossRef] [PubMed]
7. Van Oorschot, R.A.; Szkuta, B.; Meakin, G.E.; Kokshoorn, B.; Goray, M. DNA transfer in forensic science: A review. *Forensic Sci. Int. Genet.* **2019**, *38*, 140–166. [CrossRef]
8. Goray, M.; Mitchell, R.J.; van Oorschot, R.A. Investigation of secondary DNA transfer of skin cells under controlled test conditions. *Leg. Med.* **2010**, *12*, 117–120. [CrossRef]
9. Daly, D.J.; Murphy, C.; McDermott, S.D. The transfer of touch DNA from hands to glass, fabric and wood. *Forensic Sci. Int. Genet.* **2012**, *6*, 41–46. [CrossRef]
10. Fonneløp, A.; Johannessen, H.; Gill, P. Persistence and secondary transfer of DNA from previous users of equipment. *Forensic Sci. Int. Genet. Suppl. Ser.* **2015**, *5*, e191–e192. [CrossRef]
11. Raymond, J.; Van Oorschot, R.A.; Walsh, S.J.; Roux, C.; Gunn, P.R. Trace DNA and street robbery: A criminalistic approach to DNA evidence. *Forensic Sci. Int. Genet. Suppl. Ser.* **2009**, *2*, 544–546. [CrossRef]
12. Van Oorschot, R.A.; Glavich, G.; Mitchell, R.J. Persistence of DNA deposited by the original user on objects after subsequent use by a second person. *Forensic Sci. Int. Genet.* **2014**, *8*, 219–225. [CrossRef]
13. Mayuoni-Kirshenbaum, L.; Waiskopf, O.; Finkelstein, N.; Pasternak, Z. How did the DNA of a suspect get to the crime scene? A practical study in DNA transfer during lock-picking. *Aust. J. Forensic Sci.* **2020**, 1–11. [CrossRef]
14. Fonnelop, A.E.; Ramse, M.; Egeland, T.; Gill, P. The implications of shedder status and background DNA on direct and secondary transfer in an attack scenario. *Forensic Sci. Int. Genet.* **2017**, *29*, 48–60. [CrossRef] [PubMed]
15. Johannessen, H.; Gill, P.; Roseth, A.; Fonneløp, A.E. Determination of shedder status: A comparison of two methods involving cell counting in fingerprints and the DNA analysis of handheld tubes. *Forensic Sci. Int. Genet.* **2021**, *53*, 102541. [CrossRef]
16. Goray, M.; van Oorschot, R. Shedder status: Exploring means of determination. *Sci. Justice* **2021**, *61*, 391–400. [CrossRef]
17. Schmidt, M.; Bamberg, M.; Dierig, L.; Kunz, S.N.; Wiegand, P. The diversity of shedder tests and a novel factor that affects DNA transfer. *Int. J. Leg. Med.* **2021**, *135*, 1267–1280. [CrossRef]
18. Gill, P.; Bleka, Ø.; Fonneløp, A.E. RFU derived LRs for activity level assignments using Bayesian Networks. *Forensic Sci. Int. Genet.* **2021**, *56*, 102608. [CrossRef]

19. Gill, P.; Benschop, C.; Buckleton, J.; Bleka, Ø.; Taylor, D. A Review of Probabilistic Genotyping Systems: EuroForMix, DNAStatistX and STRmix. *Genes* **2021**, *12*, 1559. [CrossRef]
20. Butler, J.M. *Forensic DNA Typing: Biology, Technology, and Genetics of STR Markers*; Academic Press: Cambridge, MA, USA, 2005.
21. Bleka, Ø.; Storvik, G.O.; Gill, P. EuroForMix: An open source software based on a continuous model to evaluate STR DNA profiles from a mixture of contributors with artefacts. *Forensic Sci. Int. Genet.* **2016**, *21*, 35–44. [CrossRef]
22. European Network of Forensic Science Institutions "ENFSI" Guideline for Evaluative Reporting in Forensic Science [Online]. Available online: http://enfsi.eu/wp-content/uploads/2016/09/m1_guideline.pdf (accessed on 1 November 2021).
23. Fonneløp, A.E.; Egeland, T.; Gill, P. Secondary and subsequent DNA transfer during criminal investigation. *Forensic Sci. Int. Genet.* **2015**, *17*, 155–162. [CrossRef]
24. Otten, L.; Banken, S.; Schürenkamp, M.; Schulze-Johann, K.; Sibbing, U.; Pfeiffer, H.; Vennemann, M. Secondary DNA transfer by working gloves. *Forensic Sci. Int. Genet.* **2019**, *43*, 102126. [CrossRef] [PubMed]
25. Szkuta, B.; Ballantyne, K.N.; Kokshoorn, B.; van Oorschot, R.A. Transfer and persistence of non-self DNA on hands over time: Using empirical data to evaluate DNA evidence given activity level propositions. *Forensic Sci. Int. Genet.* **2018**, *33*, 84–97. [CrossRef] [PubMed]
26. Goray, M.; Fowler, S.; Szkuta, B.; van Oorschot, R. Shedder status—An analysis of self and non-self DNA in multiple handprints deposited by the same individuals over time. *Forensic Sci. Int. Genet.* **2016**, *23*, 190–196. [CrossRef] [PubMed]

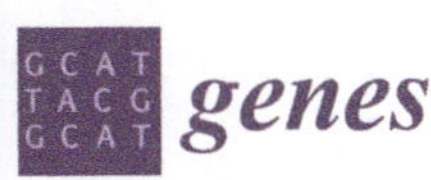

Article

Precision DNA Mixture Interpretation with Single-Cell Profiling

Jianye Ge [1,2,*], Jonathan L. King [1], Amy Smuts [1] and Bruce Budowle [1,2]

1   Center for Human Identification, University of North Texas Health Science Center,
    Fort Worth, TX 76107, USA; Jonathan.King@unthsc.edu (J.L.K.); Amy.Smuts@unthsc.edu (A.S.);
    Bruce.Budowle@unthsc.edu (B.B.)
2   Department of Microbiology, Immunology and Genetics, University of North Texas Health Science Center,
    Fort Worth, TX 76107, USA
*   Correspondence: Jianye.Ge@unthsc.edu; Tel.: +1-(817)-735-2477

Abstract: Wet-lab based studies have exploited emerging single-cell technologies to address the challenges of interpreting forensic mixture evidence. However, little effort has been dedicated to developing a systematic approach to interpreting the single-cell profiles derived from the mixtures. This study is the first attempt to develop a comprehensive interpretation workflow in which single-cell profiles from mixtures are interpreted individually and holistically. In this approach, the genotypes from each cell are assessed, the number of contributors (NOC) of the single-cell profiles is estimated, followed by developing a consensus profile of each contributor, and finally the consensus profile(s) can be used for a DNA database search or comparing with known profiles to determine their potential sources. The potential of this single-cell interpretation workflow was assessed by simulation with various mixture scenarios and empirical allele drop-out and drop-in rates, the accuracies of estimating the NOC, the accuracies of recovering the true alleles by consensus, and the capabilities of deconvolving mixtures with related contributors. The results support that the single-cell based mixture interpretation can provide a precision that cannot beachieved with current standard CE-STR analyses. A new paradigm for mixture interpretation is available to enhance the interpretation of forensic genetic casework.

Keywords: DNA forensics; DNA mixture; mixture interpretation; single-cell; clustering algorithm; number of contributors; consensus profile

Citation: Ge, J.; King, J.L.; Smuts, A.; Budowle, B. Precision DNA Mixture Interpretation with Single-Cell Profiling. *Genes* **2021**, *12*, 1649. https://doi.org/10.3390/genes12111649

Academic Editor: Niels Morling

Received: 29 September 2021
Accepted: 14 October 2021
Published: 20 October 2021

Publisher's Note: MDPI stays neutral with regard to jurisdictional claims in published maps and institutional affiliations.

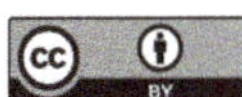

1. Introduction

Interpreting DNA mixtures is one of the most challenging problems in forensics genetics. The current standard workflow and mixture interpretation processes are used to extract DNA from a crime scene sample (e.g., swabs), quantify the extracted DNA (although in some protocols this step can be skipped), amplify targeted Short Tandem Repeat (STR) regions, detect DNA fragments through Capillary Electrophoresis (CE), call alleles with accompanying software, and interpret or deconvolve the contributors' DNA profiles as best as is possible from the collection of allelic peaks in an electropherogram primarily by a DNA analyst(s) based on training and experience with or without the assistance of probabilistic genotyping software programs (such as STRmix [1], LRmix [2], TrueAllele [3]). With this generalized CE-STR analysis process—although the DNA may still be contained in individual cells when collected—during extraction the cells, and thus the DNA, are pooled. If there is more than one contributor to the sample, a mixture is obtained. Subsequent to generating the mixture profile, an analyst(s) attempts to decipher the information to determine, for example, the number of contributors (NOC) in a mixture, the genotypes of individual contributors, if a particular individual is or is not a contributor of a mixture, and so forth. Given the available information generated through this standard process, the mixture profile is usually interpreted by indirect methods, such as inferring the NOC by counting the observed allelic peaks or evaluating the weight of the evidence assuming a person as being a contributor vs. an unknown person being a contributor by a likelihood ratio (LR) approach. The LR compares the likelihoods of observing the same evidence given two or more competing hypotheses (e.g., the mixture is composed of the victim and the suspect vs. the mixture is composed of the victim and a random person in a population). At times, the deconvolution of the contributing genotypes can be very challenging because of overlapping alleles, allele drop-out (ADO), allele drop-in (ADI), and uncertainty in the NOC. All forensic genetic methods to date, and likely for the foreseeable future, suffer from these phenomena. For example, it can be formidable with the current standard analysis to determine the NOC of a three-person mixture formed by two parents and their child, since both alleles of the child are shared with the parents. In addition, it is difficult to determine if a peak in a stutter position of a major contributor allele is composed of an allele from a minor contributor and stutter or solely a stutter product. Thus, some details of a mixture may not be able to be ascertained with a high degree of certainty.

To reduce the limitations of current standard mixture analyses, alternate methods have been proposed, such as enzymatic digestion differential extraction [4,5], reducing the allele overlap by using sequence-based alleles instead of traditional length-based alleles [6], employing probabilistic genotyping software [1–3], and so forth. While these alternate methods have added some value for mixture interpretation, the recent single-cell detection and analysis technologies may also reduce the challenges of DNA mixture interpretation. In theory, no mixture is generated as each cell is independently analyzed and thus the data from a single cell are derived from a single contributor. The DNA quantity of the contributors of a mixture can be more precisely determined by counting the isolated cells and cell types; the mixture ratio can be easily determined even though ratios may not be necessary anymore; and the alleles of each single cell can be called independently. The interpretation of these results is fundamentally different from the current interpretation approaches but should be much simpler. In other words, the computational intensive probabilistic genotyping methods, which are notably superior to previous manual methods, "guess", and often quite well, the possible genotypes of the contributors [1–3]; instead, single-cell profiles can be directly compared with the reference/known profiles to support whether or not an individual is a contributor of a mixture, if a good quality profile is obtained. However, due to technology limitations, a single-cell DNA profile usually contains ADO and/or ADI; in such scenarios, the consensus profiles from clustered cells can be used in single source profile comparisons or database searches. The consensus methods have been successfully used in single cell RNA studies [7,8] and forensic applications [9,10]. Therefore, this approach can reduce uncertainty regarding the profiles contributing to a mixture and thus provide stronger support for investigative leads and the judicial processes.

In a single-cell analysis workflow, cells are individually isolated from forensic samples. There are several methods developed that are capable of isolating single cells, such as manual micromanipulation [11–17], Laser Capture Microdissection (LCM) [18,19], Magnetic Activated Cell Sorting (MACS) flow cytometry [20], Fluorescent Activated Cell Sorting (FACS) flow cytometry [21–25], and a dielectrophoresis system (e.g., DEPArray) [26–28]. After isolation, the single cells can be individually amplified for the targeted regions (e.g., STRs) or subjected to Whole Genome Amplification (WGA) before amplification to enrich the DNA targets [17,29–33].

Li et al. [34] used the Identifiler kit (Thermo Fisher Scientific, South San Francisco, CA, USA) to amplify 15 autosomal STRs from 20 single sperm cells from one donor, and Han et al. [19] performed a similar study on 37 single sperm cells (from three donors) typing ten autosomal STRs with amplicon sizes <300 bp. In both studies, the consensus genotypes were consistent with the known donor genotypes. In Li et al. [34], the ADO rate was 25% and the ADI rate was 1.3%. In Han et al. [19] the ADO rate was lower (15%), possibly because the overall amplicon sizes were shorter, and the ADI rate was similar (1.4%). In these studies, the ADIs did not all reside at stutter positions of the true alleles. Some ADIs may have been due to DNA fragments from the other lysed cells which were co-amplified with a single cell and/or some ADIs might be due to genotype errors or low-level contamination. Anslinger et al. [27] collected 11 white blood cells with the DEPArray and genotyped 16 autosomal STRs using the PowerPlex ESXfast kit (Promega Corp., Madison, WI, USA). They found that 82% of alleles were obtained (i.e., 18% ADO rate), only one ADI was observed at a stutter position (i.e., 0.3% ADI rate), and the full profile was recovered by consensus. Even with ADO and ADI, full profiles of the donors were obtained by consensus of the single-cell profiles.

A recent study by Chen et al. [33] employed a WGA kit (Qiagen REPLI-g single cell kit, Hilden, Germany) and subsequently typed the products with both the GlobalFiler kit (Thermo Fisher Scientific, South San Francisco, CA, USA) on the CE platform and the ForenSeq DNA Signature Prep kit (Verogen, San Diego, CA, USA), on a Massive Parallel Sequencing (MPS) platform (i.e., MiSeq FGx, Verogen, San Diego, CA, USA). For the three single cells analyzed with the GlobalFiler kit only four STR alleles dropped out (i.e., 3.2% ADO rate), and no ADI was observed. For the three single cells amplified with the ForenSeq kit, all autosomal STR alleles were successfully recovered without any ADI. The better performance of the ForenSeq kit, compared with that of the GlobalFiler kit, may be due to the overall shorter amplicon sizes of the STR alleles and/or a different way noise is presented with MPS data. Deleye et al. [31] recently compared four commercial WGA kits, Ampli1 (Menarini Silicon Biosystems, Castel Maggiore, BO, Italy), DOPlify (PerkinElmer, Waltham, MA, USA), PicoPLEX (Takara Bio, Kusatsu, Japan), and REPLI-g (Hilden, Germany) with single B-lymphoblastoid cells and found that the REPLI-g had the lowest ADO rate for STR profiling (i.e., 8.33%), while the other kits had ADO rates varying from 35.71%–60.71%. According to Chen et al. [35], the major commercial WGA kits yield various genome coverages (41%–92%) and ADO rates (25%–65%). Thus, it is reasonable to assume that substantial ADO and ADI would be observed with single-cell WGA per cell if a larger number of single cells are sampled.

All these studies demonstrate that single-cell technologies can recover the STR alleles of single cells with a high success rate. However, to date, no study has provided a systematic approach to interpret the STR data from single-cells derived from mixtures. This study is the first attempt to develop and assess performance of interpretation methods for characterizing multiple donors from single-cell profiles of mixtures. The study herein evaluates these interpretation methods by a simulation approach with various mixture scenarios and reasonable ADO and ADI rates, and provides data in terms of the number of cells, NOC, and ADO and ADI rates. Through this study, the potential of the single-cell technology workflow was evaluated for the probabilities of not detecting a minor contributor during cell sampling, the accuracies of estimating the NOC with single cells and sampling, the accuracies of recovering the true alleles by single-cell profile consensus, and the capabilities of single-cell approach for deconvolving mixtures with related contributors. The results convey the high precision that a single cell workflow could achieve for mixture interpretation.

2. Methods

2.1. Simulation Methods

The autosomal STR genotypes of the single diploid cells (e.g., epithelial cells) were simulated using the method described in [36,37] for mixtures with unrelated and related contributors. In the simulation, the genotype of each marker of an individual was randomly simulated based on the allele frequencies and the population substructure correction (i.e., F_{st}) following Balding et al. [38]; the markers were assumed to be independent; the genotypes of related individuals were simulated assuming the parents transmit with equal probability a single allele at each locus to their children; the Two-Phase mutation model [39] was employed in the parent–child allelic transmissions; the mutation rates in the AABB report [40] were used. First, the genotype profile of each contributor in a mixture was simulated for the 21 autosomal STR loci in the GlobalFiler PCR amplification kit [41] using Caucasian population allele frequency data [42] and a F_{st} of 0.01. Second, based on the simulated genotype profiles of the contributors, ADO and ADI were incorporated to simulate the profiles of every single cell with a given number of cells of the contributors (e.g., 20 cells of contributor A and 20 cells of contributor B). Third, a mixture was formed by pooling the single-cell profiles of the contributors (e.g., a mixture with 40 cells in total from contributors A and B). Multiple mixtures with various mixture ratios were simulated, including mixtures with either unrelated (UR) or related contributors, namely, parent-child (PC), full-sibling (FS), and standard family trio (Table 1). Supplementary Table S1 gives an example of a simulated mixture with two unrelated contributors (20 cells each) in the ARFF format defined by WEKA [43], in which one attribute represents one allele of a locus (i.e., two attributes for a diploid genotype). The smaller allele was always assigned as the first allele for a heterozygous genotype, and alleles were listed in a defined attribute order.

Table 1. Accuracies of estimating the NOC with the EM algorithm and Silhouettes method for the various mixture scenarios. UR = unrelated, PC = parent-child, and FS = full-sibling. $D = 0.2$; $e = 0.01$; 10,000 simulations for each mixture scenario.

| No. of Cells | Mixture | 2-Person Mixture | | | | | | Mixture | 3-Person Mixture | | |
| | | Diploid | | | Haploid | | | | Diploid | | Haploid |
		UR	PC	FS	UR	PC	FS		UR	Trio	UR
160	80,80	100.00%	100.00%	99.90%	99.90%	98.04%	92.16%	53,53,53	99.96%	88.32%	96.55%
	106,54	100.00%	99.98%	99.74%	99.88%	96.53%	89.27%	32,32,96	99.69%	85.64%	81.79%
	128,32	100.00%	99.85%	98.87%	99.16%	91.35%	81.70%	16,48,96	98.60%	78.46%	52.55%
	144,16	99.97%	98.54%	94.86%	95.97%	87.64%	81.28%				
	152,8	99.55%	91.59%	86.12%	92.43%	87.98%	83.97%				
80	40,40	100.00%	99.93%	99.91%	99.93%	98.73%	96.32%	26,26,26	99.97%	87.94%	96.44%
	53,27	100.00%	99.94%	99.78%	99.87%	98.17%	94.40%	16,16,48	99.68%	86.51%	82.47%
	64,16	99.99%	99.96%	99.53%	99.71%	94.37%	87.68%	8,24,48	98.36%	80.54%	54.15%
	72,8	99.96%	98.99%	96.55%	95.56%	85.95%	81.09%				
	76,4	99.67%	93.47%	88.56%	88.91%	83.54%	79.10%				
40	20,20	100.00%	99.99%	99.93%	99.72%	95.25%	92.41%	13,13,13	99.96%	88.29%	91.81%
	26,14	100.00%	99.93%	99.87%	99.76%	94.56%	90.23%	8,8,24	99.79%	86.06%	76.22%
	32,8	100.00%	99.89%	99.22%	99.18%	89.52%	81.95%	4,12,24	98.44%	79.79%	46.55%
	36,4	99.90%	98.03%	95.37%	93.40%	76.58%	71.13%				
	38,2	95.49%	78.98%	74.69%	84.31%	68.47%	65.89%				
20	10,10	100.00%	99.54%	99.02%	97.21%	82.30%	79.50%	6,6,6	99.81%	85.59%	69.19%
	13,7	99.98%	99.48%	98.84%	97.30%	82.77%	79.09%	4,4,12	99.52%	82.22%	51.34%
	16,4	99.96%	99.62%	98.92%	95.34%	73.85%	70.30%	2,6,12	89.80%	72.16%	21.69%
	18,2	99.61%	97.00%	94.29%	81.92%	59.54%	58.65%				
	19,1	98.51%	86.74%	82.46%	60.82%	53.45%	53.40%				
10	5,5	99.95%	96.77%	94.02%	82.78%	56.59%	55.61%	3,3,3	97.16%	66.81%	33.58%
	6,4	99.84%	96.65%	93.90%	80.38%	55.79%	53.41%	2,2,6	99.05%	76.26%	38.63%
	8,2	99.68%	94.61%	91.60%	78.59%	49.60%	48.24%	1,3,6	59.31%	37.65%	12.44%
	9,1	98.91%	89.19%	85.09%	65.71%	41.74%	42.05%				

The ADO model described in Balding et al. [44] was used in the simulation, in which D represents the probability of drop-out of one allele at a heterozygous locus, and D_2 represents the probability of drop-out at a homozygous locus, with $D_2 \approx \frac{1}{2}D^2$. The rare scenarios that a locus of a diploid cell or a haploid cell presents more than two alleles or more than one allele, respectively, were ignored in this study (i.e., only up to two alleles or one allele with strongest signal(s) for diploid and haploid cells, respectively, would be called), allele size dependent degradation was ignored, and somatic mutations (i.e., the genotypes of the diploid cells from the same contributor may be different) were also ignored. The ADI was incorporated as a random genotyping error (with an ADI rate of e); namely, one allele may be randomly called as any other allele at this locus in the population data with equal chance. For example, changes to genotypes 10,10 → 10,15 or 10,11 → 10,15 for a homozygous and heterozygous locus, respectively, for diploid cells were produced to approximate ADI. Thus, a heterozygous locus with ADI has to have one ADO involved. However, the ADO and ADI events in general were assumed to be independent for the purposes of this study. When the ADO and ADI rates are 0, the genotype profiles of single diploid cells from the same contributor should be identical.

For the profiles of the single haploid cells the interpretation is slightly different because only one allele out of two at each autosomal locus is randomly distributed in the haploid cells. Therefore, the interpretation of haploid single-cell mixture profiles may be more complicated than that of diploid cells, even without ADO or ADI. In the haploid profile simulations, the alleles were generated by randomly selecting one allele of the two simulated diploid alleles at each locus and assuming independence among the loci. The same population data, parameters, ADO model, and ADI model as in the diploid simulations were used in simulating the haploid single-cell profiles.

2.2. Clustering Single Cells

To estimate the NOC of a mixture and allele consensus of each contributor, the single cells need to be grouped into clusters (or contributors). There is a large number of clustering algorithms that may serve this purpose. This study tested two classic clustering algorithms, Expectation–Maximization (EM) [45,46] and K-Means [47]. The EM algorithm assigns a probability distribution for the latent variables to each instance in the dataset (i.e., each single cell), which indicates the probability of it belonging to each of the clusters (i.e., each contributor in a mixture), computes parameters to optimize the likelihood of the model, and then repeats these two steps until convergence [43,45]. The EM algorithm implemented in WEKA uses multivariate Gaussians with diagonal covariance matrices as mixture components [46]. The EM algorithm does not explicitly require a distance measure between the instances. The K-Means algorithm randomly chooses an initial centroid for each cluster, each instance is assigned to its nearest centroid to form clusters, the centroids are updated with the instances in the same clusters, and these two steps are repeated until convergence [47]. The K-Means algorithm requires a distance measure between instances, which is Euclidean distance by default. The EM and SimpleKMeans algorithm implementations with default setting in the WEKA software package [43] were used in this study.

The clustering algorithms usually require a predefined number of clusters. To determine the best number of clusters, the Silhouettes method [48] implemented in Cluster-Maker [49] was used. For a given number of clusters, the Silhouettes coefficient measures how similar an instance is to its own cluster compared to other clusters. The maximum value of the Silhouettes coefficient indicates the most likely number of clusters for a given range of the number of clusters [50]. For the mixtures in Table 1, the Silhouettes coefficients of two to six clusters were calculated and compared, and the number of clusters with the highest Silhouettes coefficient was determined as the NOC.

2.3. Single-Cell Profile Visualization

Multidimensional Scaling (MDS) was used to visualize the clustering of single-cell profiles. The three-dimensional (3D) MDS coordinates of every single-cell profile of a mixture were calculated using MDSJ [51], in which the distance between two profiles was measured as the number of mismatched alleles normalized by the total number of alleles. Then, the 3D coordinates were visualized by JTableSaw [52].

2.4. Consensus Method

For the single-cell profiles clustered into the same cluster, the genotype profiles of these single cells were determined by consensus and then compared with the true genotypes to assess the accuracies of recovering the true alleles by the clustering approach. For both diploid and haploid cells, the consensus of each allele was determined independently (i.e., alleles at the same position defined in the order as described in Section 2.1 and Supplementary Table S1). The consensus allele at a position (e.g., the first allele of the vWA locus in a diploid cell, or the only allele of the vWA locus in a haploid cell) in a cluster was defined as the most frequent allele at this position among the single-cell profiles in this cluster. The missing data due to ADO were ignored during consensus.

3. Results

3.1. The Probability of Not Detecting a Contributor during Sampling

The current standard CE-STR mixture analysis process may not be able to provide a precise estimate of the DNA input quantities of the contributors, nor the probability that a minor contributor is not observed in a mixture. The limitations are due in part to only the contributors with sufficient input quantities showing allele peaks above a detection threshold, and allele sharing may mask a minor contributor; these phenomena become more exacerbating as the number of contributors increases. Thus, a minor contributor may not be detected through this process. With the single-cell analysis, however, the quantity of a sample can be directly determined by counting the cells in a sample, although sampling error can occur during cell isolation. Therefore, the probability of not detecting a minor contributor can be estimated with the single-cell profiling.

Assuming a large number of cells are available in a forensic sample (i.e., the sampling process follows a binomial distribution) and each cell has an equal chance to be sampled, the probability that none of the cells from a contributor with a mixture proportion of p is sampled in the total sampled n cells is $(1-p^n)$. Table 2 estimates these probabilities for various mixture proportions of a contributor(s) and different total numbers of sampled cells, either diploid or haploid cells, with 6.6 pg DNA for a diploid cell and 3.3 pg DNA for a haploid cell [53]. The mixtures containing both diploid and haploid cells (e.g., a mixture of epithelial cells and sperm cells) were not considered (but can be readily determined if desired); these cellular mixtures can be separated either by counting the number of alleles across the loci or by technologies (e.g., DEPArray) to select cells from different tissues.

Table 2. The probability of not detecting a minor contributor in a set of single-cell samplings.

No. of Cells	DNA Quantity (pg)		The Mixture Proportion of a Contributor				
	Diploid	Haploid	1%	5%	10%	20%	50%
1	6.6	3.3	99.00%	95.00%	90.00%	80.00%	50.00%
5	33	16.5	95.10%	77.38%	59.05%	32.77%	3.13%
10	66	33	90.44%	59.87%	34.87%	10.74%	0.10%
15	99	49.5	86.01%	46.33%	20.59%	3.52%	0.00%
20	132	66	81.79%	35.85%	12.16%	1.15%	0.00%
40	264	132	66.90%	12.85%	1.48%	0.01%	0.00%
80	528	264	44.75%	1.65%	0.02%	0.00%	0.00%
160	1056	528	20.03%	0.03%	0.00%	0.00%	0.00%
500	3300	1650	0.66%	0.00%	0.00%	0.00%	0.00%

In general, as more cells are sampled the chance of not detecting a contributor decreases. For example, if 80 diploid cells are sampled (~528 pg DNA in total, close to the recommended DNA input of some commercial CE-STR kits, that is, 500 pg), there is a 44.75% chance that none of the cells from a 1% minor contributor is sampled; however, for a 5% minor contributor there is only a 1.65% chance of not detecting the minor contributor. For a low quantity DNA sample with only 15 cells (~99 pg), there is a 46.33% chance that a 5% minor contributor would not be detected. To obtain a high confidence of detecting a minor contributor with 1% or lower proportion, ≥500 single cells may need to be sampled.

3.2. The Accuracies of NOC Estimation

3.2.1. NOC Estimation by Clustering

The two-person and three-person mixtures were simulated with various numbers of cells, various mixture ratios, unrelated or related contributors, and both diploid and haploid cells (Table 1). In the simulation, the ADO and ADI rates were set as 0.2 and 0.01, respectively, which were similar to the estimations of several studies [19,27,34] and reflected the current performance of single-cell studies. For each mixture scenario, 10,000 cases were simulated, and the NOC for each case was estimated by the EM and K-Means clustering algorithms, together with the Silhouettes method. Table 1 shows the accuracies of estimating the NOC for the simulated mixture scenarios with the EM algorithm, which provides higher accuracies compared with the K-Means algorithm. The NOC accuracies estimated by K-Means are listed in Supplementary Table S2.

For diploid cells, in general, higher accuracies were achieved with more cells and/or more balanced mixture ratios. If contributors were unrelated, almost all scenarios had >98% accuracy, except for three-person mixtures with a very few number of cells sampled and severely imbalanced mixture ratios (e.g., 2,6,12 and 1,3,6). Almost 100% accuracies were obtained if the contributors were unrelated, and there were more than 20 cells in total sampled. For PC and FS pairs, most of the estimated accuracies were higher than 98%, although, as expected, lower than those of UR pairs. Estimating the NOC for a mixture composed of a family trio can be particularly challenging with CE-STR analyses as well as with MPS; however, the accuracies with single cell analyses and the EM algorithm together with Silhouettes method were mostly >80%, except for scenarios with an extremely low number of sampled cells (e.g., ten cells) or highly imbalanced mixture ratios (e.g., 1:3:6).

The NOC accuracies with haploid cells were lower than those of diploid cells, because the same contributor may have many different haploid profiles due to meiosis, and the ADO and ADI would add more variants making the clustering of haploid cells more challenging. However, even with these limitations, high accuracies were achieved when the mixture ratios were relatively balanced and the number of sampled cells was high (e.g., 98.17% accuracy with a (53,27) Parent-Child mixture). Even for highly imbalanced mixtures (for example, 72,8), NOC accuracies were 95.56% and 85.95% for UR and PC contributors, respectively, which were still reasonably high.

3.2.2. Impact of ADO and ADI on NOC Estimation by Clustering

The accuracies of estimating the NOC can be impacted by the ADO and ADI rates. To investigate the impact of ADO and ADI, the same simulations as above were conducted for three mixture examples (Figure 1) with the same number of contributor cells (two, six, and 12 cells) for a three-person mixture, with different relationships among the contributors, different cell types, and various ADO and ADI rates.

For diploid unrelated cells (Figure 1a), the accuracies with lower ADO rates are higher and decrease with increasing ADO rates (e.g., 99.16% with $D = 0.05$ and $e = 0.01$, compared with 89.88% with $D = 0.2$ and $e = 0.01$). The ADI had less impact with the NOC accuracies due to the relatively low ADI rates (i.e., at the level of 0.01) compared with relatively high ADO rates (i.e., at the level of 0.1). The accuracies dropped more so with family trio mixtures (Figure 1b), likely because the related contributors share at least half of their alleles (assuming no mutation), and ADO and ADI could contribute to some cells from a different contributor sharing more alleles than expected, and eventually blur the boundaries between contributors (see Figure 2a as an example). The haploid mixtures, as expected, had a lower estimation of NOC accuracies. Even with no ADO or ADI, the accuracy was low (i.e., 41.38%), which is mostly due to the varied haploid profiles from each cell of the same contributor, a small number of sampled cells, and poor performance of the EM algorithm for imbalanced mixtures. Sampling more cells, as well as algorithms better designed specifically for imbalanced single-cell genotype data, should improve the accuracies.

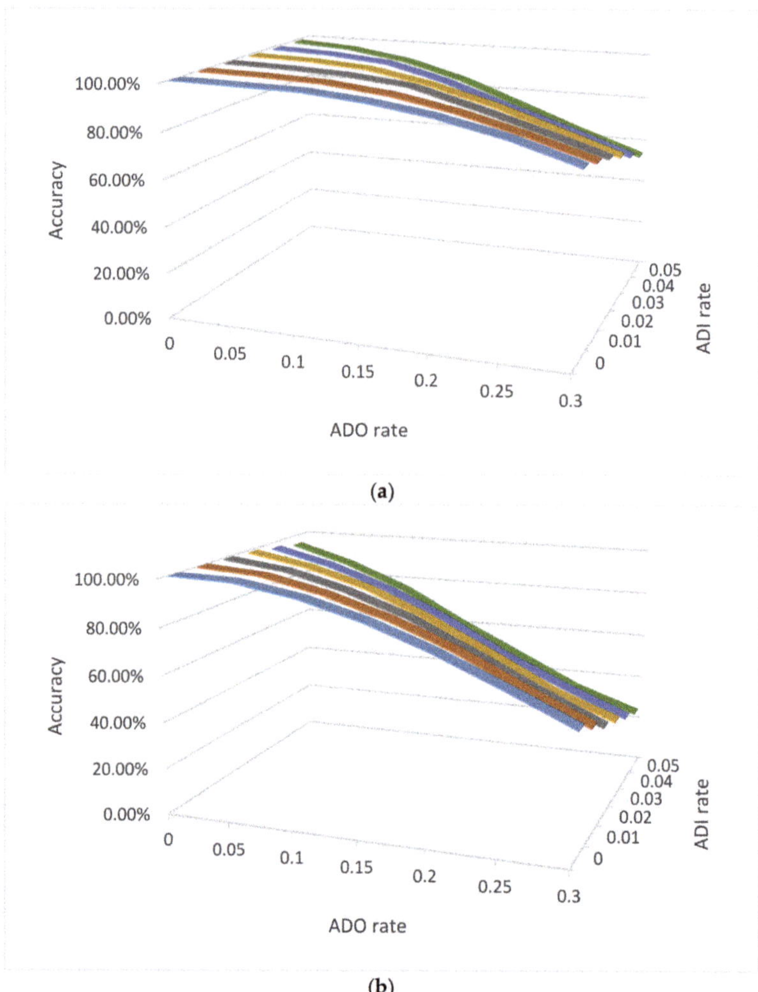

Figure 1. *Cont.*

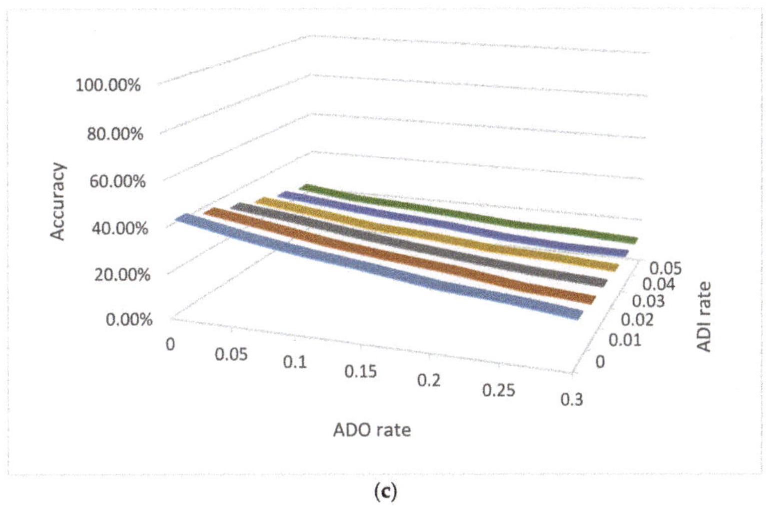

(**c**)

Figure 1. The accuracies of NOC estimation for 3-person mixtures with 2, 6, and 12 single cells with various ADO and ADI rates in three scenarios: (**a**) Diploid cells with three unrelated contributors, (**b**) Diploid cells with three family trio contributors (father, mother, and child), and (**c**) Haploid cells with three unrelated contributors. $D = 0.2$; $e = 0.01$; 10,000 simulations for each mixture scenario.

3.2.3. NOC Estimation by Visualization

Among these tested mixtures, the accuracies dropped substantially when the mixture ratios were extremely imbalanced (i.e., 9:1 and 19:1), which is mostly because the classic clustering algorithms do not perform well with imbalanced data (i.e., large sample size differences between or among clusters) [54]. The related contributors (i.e., the data points are closer to each other), haploid data (i.e., genotype uncertainty), and small numbers of cells (i.e., clustering with sparse data) can further reduce the accuracies. In such scenarios, particularly when the number of sampled cells is small, visualization of the distance between and among single-cell profiles may facilitate human judgement on the NOC. Visualization has been shown to be an effective way to estimate the NOC and differentiate cell types in single-cell applications [55,56].

Figure 2 displays several examples of 3D MDS plots. In Figure 2a, the EM algorithm and Silhouettes method together incorrectly determined a family trio mixture as a two-person mixture, because many cells of two specific contributors (i.e., one of the parents and the child) were very close to each other and the algorithm considered them as one contributor. However, with visualization, the NOC most likely could be determined as three. Figure 2b is an example with a correct NOC estimation, in which all contributors were clearly separated. In Figure 2c, two contributors (2 and 12) were incorrectly clustered into a single contributor, but with the MDS plot they appear separated. In Figure 2d, a three-person mixture was incorrectly determined as a four-person mixture. In one of the minor contributors, one single-cell profile was distant from the other three single-cells, which led to an incorrect NOC estimation. Even with MDS plot, it was challenging to determine the NOC, as both three and four clusters appeared possible.

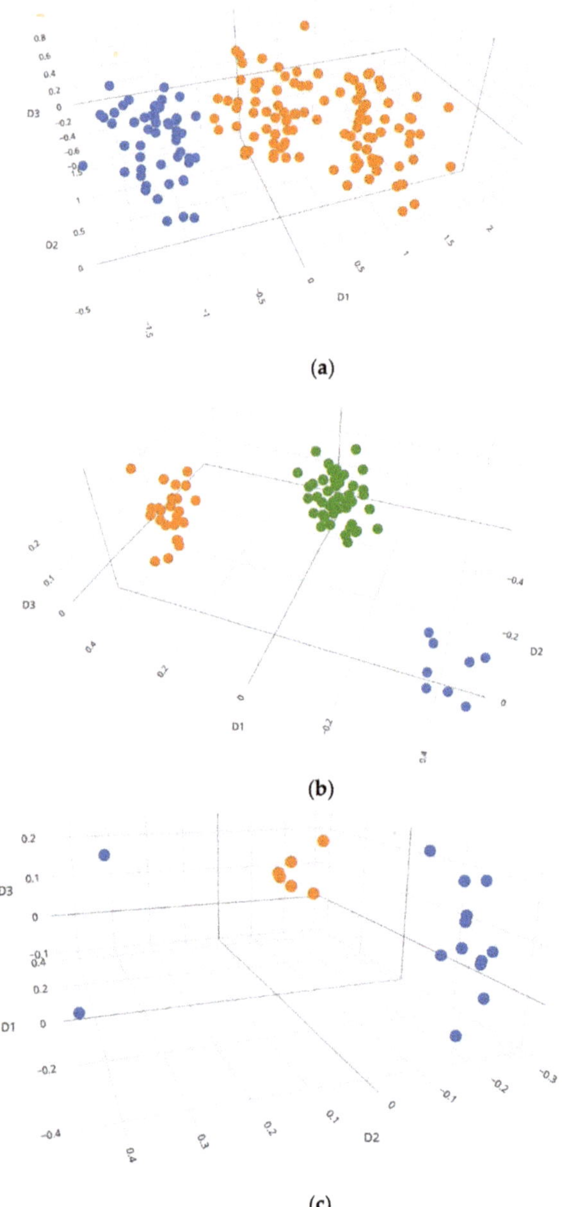

(a)

(b)

(c)

Figure 2. *Cont.*

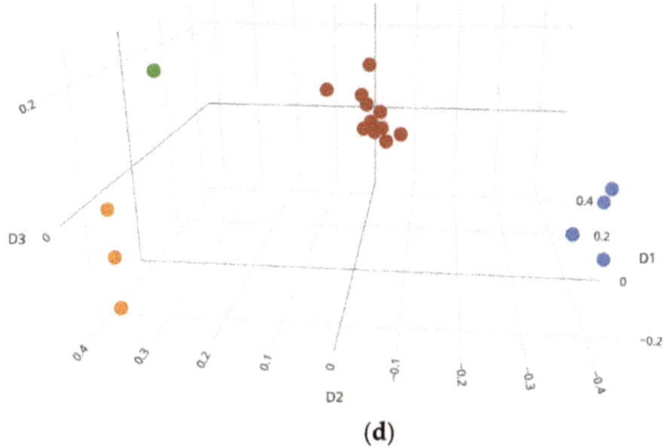

(d)

Figure 2. Mixture visualization examples with 3D MDS plots: (**a**) A family trio diploid cell mixture (53, 53, 53) incorrectly clustered with the EM algorithm and Silhouettes method as two contributors. (**b**) A family trio diploid cell mixture (8,24,48) correctly clustered with the EM algorithm and Silhouettes method as three contributors. (**c**) A 3-person haploid cell mixture (2,6,12) incorrectly clustered with the EM algorithm and Silhouettes method as two contributors. (**d**) A 3-person diploid cell mixture (4, 4, 12) incorrectly clustered with the EM algorithm and Silhouettes method as four contributors. Each color represents each cluster. Rotatable plots of these figures can be found in Supplementary Figure S1.

3.2.4. NOC Estimation by Identity-by-State (IBS) Distance Measure

Another way to estimate the NOC is to measure the distances between single-cell profiles using predefined IBS thresholds. Figure 3 shows the IBS distributions of unrelated and related pairs of individuals (UR, PC, and FS) and pairs of the known alleles of a contributor versus the consensus alleles with a given number of sampled cells, assuming the clustered profiles were from the same contributor. Apparently, there was no overlap between the IBS distribution of the unrelated and one cell with diploid cells, which means two unrelated diploid cells can be clearly separated simply by a reasonable IBS threshold (e.g., IBS $\leq$ 24 for the scenario of $D = 0.2$ and $e = 0.01$). This simple approach can readily determine if a group of single cells is from one contributor or multiple unrelated contributors (i.e., single source or mixture), as well as if a cell profile and a known profile from an unrelated individual may be from the same source. Thus, the NOC can be precisely determined by measuring the IBS distance between every pair of diploid cell profiles and a predefined maximum IBS distance for cells within the same cluster (e.g., IBS $\leq$ 24), assuming all contributors are unrelated. However, this approach may not work well for haploid cell profiles, because the consensus diploid profile relying on a single haploid cell would be homozygous across the loci. There would be a good proportion of the IBS distributions of UR and 1 haploid cell profile that would overlap. For example, 9.6% of unrelated pairs had IBS $\geq$ 16, and 9.7% of the consensus profiles from one haploid cell had IBS $\leq$ 17 (Figure 3b).

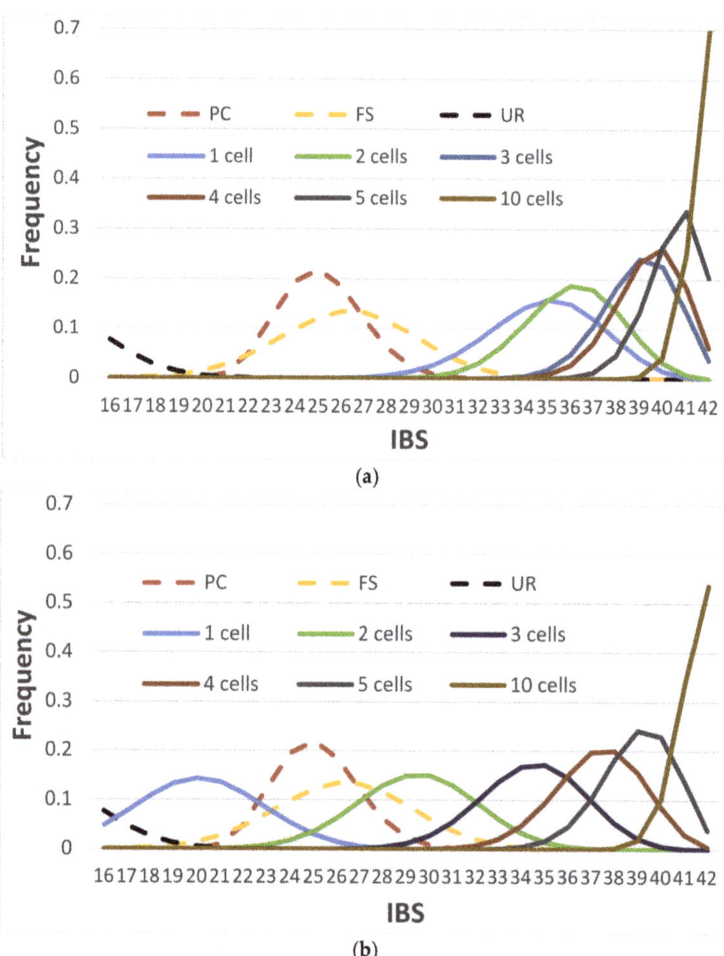

Figure 3. IBS distributions of unrelated and related pairs (UR, PC, and FS, in dotted lines) and pairs of the true profile versus the consensus profile with a given number of cells (in solid lines) based on (**a**) diploid cells and (**b**) haploid cells. $D = 0.2$; $e = 0.01$; 1,000,000 simulations for each distribution. The IBS of "n cell(s)" is the IBS between true genotypes and the consensus genotypes from n cell(s). These distributions are based on 21 GlobalFiler markers and thus the maximum IBS is 42. The consensus profile might contain missing alleles, and these missing alleles were excluded in counting IBS.

If the contributors are related, the IBS measure may not reach 100% accuracy to differentiate two unrelated cells from two related single cells (i.e., there were overlaps between the "one cell" distribution and the FS or PC distributions (Figure 3)). However, if multiple cells could be associated by either clustering, measured distances, or visualization, the consensus profile could differentiate a profile from his/her parent or full-siblings simply by IBS counting (e.g., a false rate less than 0.05% with a consensus profile from five cells for both PC and FS, and almost no error with ten cells (Figure 3)), which was similar to haploid cells (Figure 3b).

3.3. Accuracies of Consensus

3.3.1. IBS Distributions with Consensus

Once the NOC is estimated for a mixture, the consensus profile of each contributor can be generated by common alleles of the clustered single cells. As shown in Figure 3a, one single diploid cell as a single contributor mostly shared at least 28 alleles (with an average of 35 alleles) with the true profile, and the mismatches were mostly due to the high ADO rate (i.e., 0.2). Thus, there is sufficient precision to differentiate one single-cell profile from a random person profile (~0.03% average error rate with a threshold of IBS $\leq$ 24; the average error rate was the average of the false positive rate of determining a consensus profile and an unrelated profile as from the same source, and the false negative rate of determining the two profiles as being from different sources).With more cell profiles clustering in the same contributor, more shared alleles are found between the consensus profile and the true profile.

The consensus of haploid cell profiles would be more challenging, but would have more success than the current standard process. It is unlikely to determine the source of a single haploid cell profile (Figure 3b). However, the consensus profile of two haploid cells in a cluster, if they truly belong to the contributor, could be differentiated from a random person (<0.13% average error rate with a threshold of IBS $\leq$ 21), even though, on average, ~30% of the consensus alleles might not be correct (i.e., different from the true alleles or missing). For a contributor with $\geq$1 haploid cells, the consensus profile most likely would have $\leq$3 inconsistent alleles compared with the true profile. In general, these results were consistent with the simulation study by Lucy et al. [57], although ADO and ADI were not included in their study.

In addition, the results in Figure 3 indicated that the mixture ratio estimation of the sperm samples with the current CE-STR analysis might not be accurate for the extremely low quantity DNA samples, even if there is no ADO, ADI, or degradation. Each sperm cell has only one allele at a locus, and a contributor with a few sperm cells may have highly imbalanced allele sampling. For example, three out of four sampled sperm cells may share one particular allele of a heterozygote and the other sperm could have a different allele, which could make this contributor appear as a 3:1 mixture with two homozygotes. The mixture ratio at different loci may randomly vary when the number of sampled haploid cells is small, which likely could lead to an incorrect interpretation or more alternate genotypes to consider with the CE-STR mixture analysis.

3.3.2. A Suspect or His/Her Close Relatives as Contributors

In certain cases, it may be necessary to determine if a suspect or one of the suspect's close relatives is a potential contributor to a mixture. Based on the IBS distributions in Figure 3a, with only a few diploid cell profiles, an IBS threshold of $\leq$34 can precisely differentiate the related individuals if a consensus profile is from a known profile or a full-sibling of this known profile. With only three diploid cell profiles, 0.68% of the consensus profiles would have an IBS $\leq$ 34 (i.e., false negatives), 0.18% of the FS pairs would have IBS $\geq$ 35 (i.e., false positives or more appropriately adventitious associations). Sampling more cells can reduce the false rates. For haploid mixtures, if the same threshold is used (i.e., IBS $\leq$ 34), five haploid cell profiles would be needed to achieve high accuracy (i.e., 0.64% false negative rate). Thus, it only requires a consensus accuracy as low as 83.3% (35/42) to precisely differentiate if a consensus profile is from a known individual (e.g., suspect) or this individual's first-degree relative(s).

The average accuracies of consensus for all diploid mixtures and most haploid mixtures with balanced contributors were higher than 83.3% (Table 3). Therefore, except for minor contributors with $\leq$2 diploid cells or $\leq$4 haploid cells sampled, the consensus profiles of each contributor in the mixtures should be able to determine the source of the profile with very high accuracies (Table 3). Again, more cells sampled would increase these accuracies.

Table 3. The average of the average accuracies of consensus alleles compared with the true alleles of the contributors. Only the mixtures with the correct NOC estimation were included. The NOC was determined using the EM algorithm and Silhouettes method. $D = 0.2$; $e = 0.01$; 10,000 simulations for each mixture scenario.

No. of Cells.	2-Person Mixture							3-Person Mixture			
	Mixture	Diploid			Haploid			Mixture	Diploid		Haploid
		UR	PC	FS	UR	PC	FS		UR	Trio	UR
160	80,80	100.00%	100.00%	100.00%	100.00%	99.93%	99.28%	53,53,53	100.00%	100.00%	100.00%
	106,54	100.00%	100.00%	99.99%	100.00%	99.80%	98.83%	32,32,96	100.00%	100.00%	99.94%
	128,32	100.00%	99.98%	99.90%	99.55%	98.64%	97.17%	16,48,96	99.96%	99.95%	99.47%
	144,16	99.85%	98.91%	97.91%	94.96%	93.92%	91.86%				
	152,8	98.01%	90.16%	89.05%	81.77%	85.70%	84.88%				
80	40,40	100.00%	100.00%	100.00%	100.00%	99.96%	99.73%	26,26,26	99.99%	99.99%	99.97%
	53,27	100.00%	100.00%	99.99%	99.99%	99.90%	99.49%	16,16,48	99.91%	99.91%	99.73%
	64,16	99.94%	99.93%	99.89%	99.75%	99.09%	97.90%	8,24,48	99.47%	99.45%	98.53%
	72,8	99.19%	98.65%	98.01%	95.15%	92.18%	90.78%				
	76,4	96.40%	93.09%	91.63%	81.77%	83.45%	83.02%				
40	20,20	99.96%	99.96%	99.96%	99.93%	99.80%	99.52%	13,13,13	99.69%	99.68%	99.00%
	26,14	99.88%	99.87%	99.87%	99.67%	99.41%	98.90%	8,8,24	98.94%	98.95%	97.56%
	32,8	99.21%	99.18%	99.08%	98.37%	96.61%	95.43%	4,12,24	97.79%	97.78%	94.55%
	36,4	96.79%	96.17%	95.85%	91.16%	87.64%	86.57%				
	38,2	85.79%	81.23%	81.22%	76.48%	78.91%	78.88%				
20	10,10	99.16%	99.17%	99.13%	98.20%	96.75%	95.68%	6,6,6	96.98%	96.97%	92.68%
	13,7	98.90%	98.87%	98.85%	97.53%	95.57%	94.51%	4,4,12	95.72%	95.71%	89.05%
	16,4	96.83%	96.80%	96.71%	93.02%	89.51%	88.51%	2,6,12	94.02%	94.02%	84.83%
	18,2	92.78%	92.31%	92.01%	81.99%	77.81%	78.35%				
	19,1	90.85%	88.80%	87.86%	69.30%	68.57%	69.78%				
10	5,5	96.33%	96.34%	96.30%	91.56%	87.57%	86.61%	3,3,3	92.68%	92.74%	78.80%
	6,4	95.37%	95.33%	95.33%	90.70%	86.72%	85.95%	2,2,6	89.45%	89.47%	75.58%
	8,2	92.11%	91.99%	91.97%	82.58%	78.46%	77.78%	1,3,6	90.86%	90.42%	66.12%
	9,1	90.81%	90.36%	90.17%	71.50%	67.26%	67.31%				

3.3.3. Accuracies of Consensus by Clustering

The distributions in Figure 3 assumed the cells clustered into contributors were truly the cells from this contributor. In fact, cells may be clustered to an incorrect contributor. However, the incorrectly clustered cells should be overwhelmed (assuming a sufficient number) by the cells correctly belonging to a contributor and the incorrect alleles should be filtered out by consensus, if a good clustering algorithm is used and there are enough cells clustered to this contributor.

To test this hypothesis, the consensus accuracies of clustering results were estimated using the same simulations conducted as in Table 1, and the average accuracies of consensus alleles were calculated for each simulated mixture. For example, a mixture with two contributors may have consensus accuracies of 0.8 and 0.9, respectively, and the average accuracy would be 0.85. For mixtures with an imbalanced mixture ratio (e.g., 1:3:6), the minor contributor(s) usually had lower consensus accuracies, mostly due to the small numbers of sampled cells. Table 3 shows the average of 10,000 simulations for the average accuracies of the consensus profile. Only the cases with the correct NOC estimation were included in these calculations.

As expected, given the correct NOC estimation, mixtures with a relatively high number of cells have very high consensus accuracies. Full profiles can be precisely obtained by consensus of the cells in the same clusters, if there are enough sampled diploid cells for a mixture with relatively balanced contributor ratios. The mixtures with relatively low consensus accuracies were mainly due to the low accuracies of the minor contributors with really low numbers of sampled cells. For example, the mixtures with (152,8) had an average accuracy of 98.01%, but the average consensus accuracy of the major contributor (i.e., 152) was 100%, but the minor contributor (i.e., eight) had a lower accuracy (i.e., ~96%).

Even with imbalanced contributors, all mixtures with at least five diploid cell profiles for the minor contributors achieved >96% average consensus accuracy, mostly greater than 97.6% (i.e., one allele mismatch or missing, 41/42). Particularly, the individual profiles of the family trio mixtures could be recovered even with only 40 sampled cells and imbalanced contributors, if one allele mismatch or missing was allowed. These observations were consistent with those in Figure 3, which indicates that consensus was able to filter out most incorrect alleles, if not all, caused by either ADO and ADI or incorrect clustering. These consensus profiles with just a few mismatched or missing alleles should be precise enough to generate reasonable partial matches (or hits) in a forensic DNA database (e.g., CODIS) search and support the potential identities of the contributors.

The consensus accuracies of the haploid cell mixtures, in line with expectations, were lower than those of diploid cell mixtures. However, the accuracies were still high for mixtures with enough sampled cells (e.g., $\geq$20 cells) and relatively balanced contributors, even with related contributors (e.g., 94.51% for FS mixtures of 13:7). Similar to the NOC estimation with haploid cell profiles, the accuracy dropped substantially for extremely imbalanced contributors. This observation is most likely because the EM algorithm does not perform well for imbalanced data. When the number of cells of a cluster is few (e.g., $\leq$4), together with ADI and relatively high ADO, 1 or 2 incorrectly clustered cells may dramatically change the consensus alleles. Better clustering algorithms specifically designed for imbalanced data may be able to improve the consensus accuracies.

Moreover, the relationships between the contributors appear to have little impact on the consensus accuracies when the number of cell profiles of each contributor is high (e.g., $\geq$16) or the contributors are relatively balanced; the consensus accuracies of unrelated and related contributors of the mixtures were almost identical for diploid cells (Table 3). In other words, the relationships between the contributors could impact the NOC estimation, but once NOC was correctly estimated, the consensus within each cluster solely relied on the profiles in the same cluster. However, when the number of cells from a contributor is small, the consensus accuracies vary more so, since a few incorrectly clustered cells may change the consensus alleles.

In addition, the two-person mixtures with 1:1 ratio were used as examples to investigate the consensus accuracy as a function of the number of cells in the cluster (Figure 4), for both diploid and haploid cells. The accuracies increase fastly with more cells added into the same clusters when the number of cells in a cluster is relatively small. With these balanced mixtures, a cluster with $\geq$5 diploid cells or $\geq$7 haploid cells had $\geq$97.6% accuracy (i.e., one allele mismatched or missing), which was consistent with the results in Table 3. For the extremely imbalanced mixtures, the consensus accuracy of the minor contributor can fluctuate more due to the EM algorithm's poor performance with imbalanced mixture ratios.

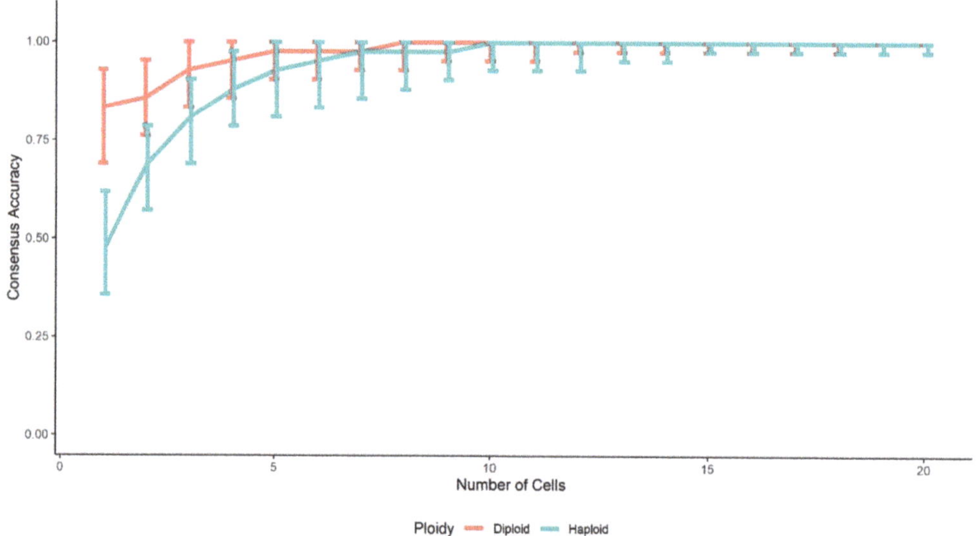

Figure 4. Consensus accuracy as a function of the number of cells in the cluster, with 1:1 ratio mixtures. $D = 0.2$; $e = 0.01$; 10,000 simulations for each mixture. The bars represent the 95% confidence intervals.

3.3.4. Impact of ADO and ADI on Consensus Accuracies

The above analysis used the typical ADO and ADI rates as an example ($D = 0.2$ and $e = 0.01$) to investigate the performance of consensus. The consensus accuracies are expected to be higher with lower ADO and ADI rates. Figure 5 shows the IBS distributions of the consensus profiles from one diploid cell (Figure 5a) and four haploid cells (Figure 5b), as examples, compared with the IBS distributions of UR, PC and FS. The IBS distribution of two diploid cell profiles was only slightly higher than that of one diploid cell profile, particularly when the ADO and ADI rates were low. Therefore, only one diploid cell profile scenario was used here to assess whether one diploid cell profile can provide high accuracies of determining the sources of contributors. If $D = 0$ and $e = 0$, the IBS should always be 42 for diploid cells. Thus, this scenario is not included in Figure 5a.

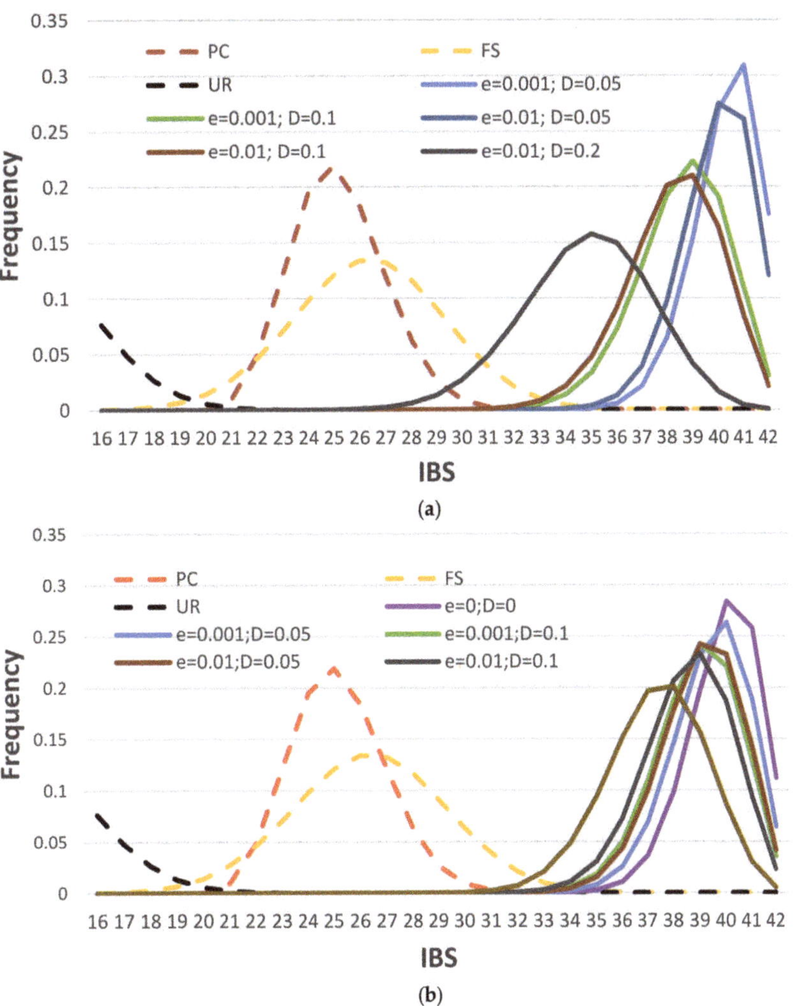

Figure 5. IBS distributions of unrelated and related pairs (UR, PC, and FS, in dotted lines) and pairs of the true profile versus the consensus profile with a given number of cells (in solid lines) for (**a**) 1 diploid cell and (**b**) 4 haploid cells. 1,000,000 simulations for each distribution. Missing alleles are excluded in counting IBS.

As expected, lower ADO and ADI rates provided higher IBS values on average. ADO had a larger impact on the distributions, mostly because the ADO rates were much larger than ADI rates in the simulated scenarios. Same as shown in Figure 3a, with $D = 0.2$ and $e = 0.01$, one diploid cell profile would be good enough to differentiate if it is from a known reference person or an unrelated person. If contributors are related, $D \leq 0.05$ may be required to precisely differentiate a known individual from his/her full-siblings (i.e., ~0.15% average error rate with a threshold of IBS ≤ 34), although $D = 0.1$ may also be acceptable (i.e., ~0.8% average error rate with a threshold of IBS ≤ 32). With more cells sampled and clustered, the consensus accuracies are expected to be higher, which would tolerate higher ADO and ADI rates to obtain similar accuracies.

With four haploid cells, even without ADO and ADI, the full profile may not be able to be recovered in most cases. However, the consensus profile, even partial, can be differentiated from an unrelated person, even with an ADO rate of 0.2. To differentiate a known individual from his/her full-siblings, with four haploid cells in a single cluster, it would be desirable to have an ADO ≤ 0.05 (i.e., ~0.35% average error rate with a threshold of IBS ≤ 34).

Additionally, the same examples as in Figure 1 were simulated to assess the consensus accuracies with potential incorrectly clustered cells even with correct NOC estimations (Figure 6). The accuracies decrease with either increasing ADO or ADI rates. As expected, the accuracies of diploid cell mixtures decrease slower than those of haploid cell mixtures, because haploid cells have half the alleles of diploid cells. The ADI seems to have a bigger impact on haploid mixtures compared with diploid mixtures. Therefore, for genotyping mixture samples comprised of sperm, it would be better to have a low ADI rate, while a relatively high ADO rate may be acceptable.

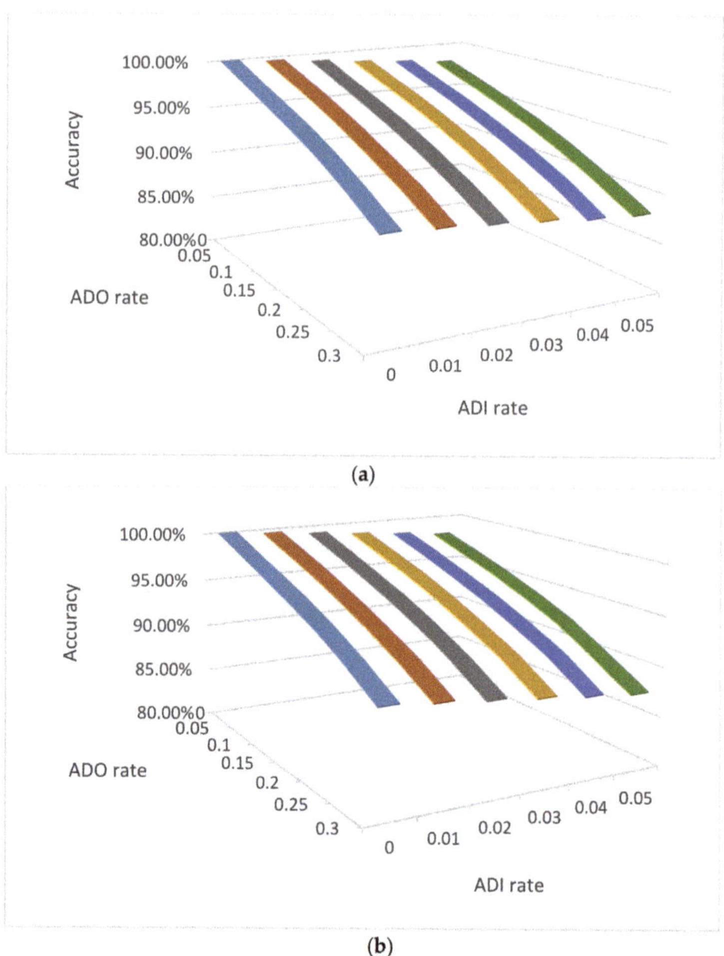

Figure 6. *Cont.*

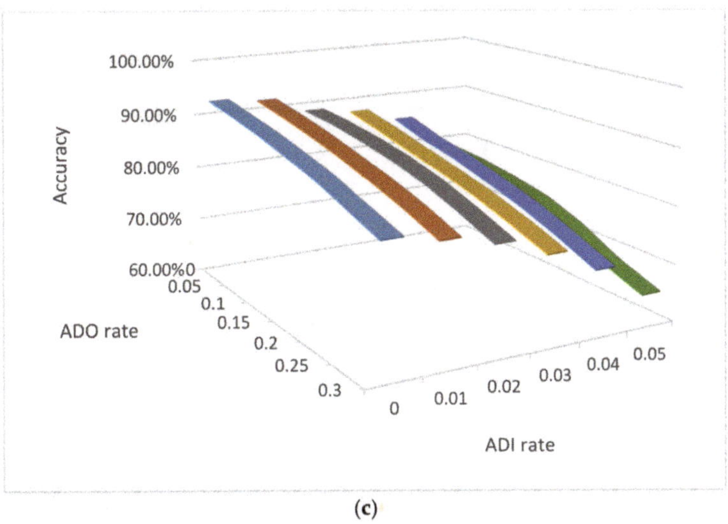

(**c**)

Figure 6. The accuracies of consensus for 3-person mixtures with 2, 6, and 12 single cells with various ADO and ADI rates in three scenarios: (**a**) diploid cells with three unrelated contributors, (**b**) diploid cells with three family trio contributors (father, mother, and child), and (**c**) haploid cells with three unrelated contributors.

In addition, similar to the data in Table 3, the unrelated and family trio diploid mixtures had almost identical consensus accuracies for diploid cells. In other words, although clustering may provide better NOC estimations for mixtures with unrelated contributors than family trio mixtures (i.e., 89.80% vs. 72.16%, respectively), if the NOC is correctly estimated, clustering performs similarly for the unrelated and family trio contributor mixtures.

4. Discussion

4.1. A Paradigm Shift of Mixture Interpretation

With the emergence of single-cell technologies, a number of studies have employed these technologies for forensic applications, mostly on the wet-lab work to generate genotype profiles from single cells. The simulation studies herein are the first one to provide guidance on a comprehensive interpretation workflow for single-cell mixture profiles, evaluate the capabilities of single-cell profiles for mixture interpretation, and support that the single-cell based mixture interpretation can provide a precision that cannot be achieved by manual or the probabilistic genotyping interpretation approaches with DNA profiles generated by standard CE-STR analyses.

Figure 7 illustrates the general mixture interpretation workflow with the single-cell mixture profiles. First, with the single-cell profiles generated from a mixture, the NOC of the single-cell profiles is estimated, either by clustering (e.g., EM algorithm and Silhouettes method), distance measure (e.g., IBS), or visualization. Second, the consensus profile of each cluster/contributor is generated from the single-cell profiles in each cluster. Then, the consensus profile(s) would be either directly searched against a DNA database(s) for partial or full matches (or hits), or compared with known profiles (e.g., suspect's profile) to determine if these profiles, or these profiles' relatives, potentially could be the contributor(s) of the mixture. In cases in which a full, or close to full profile, is obtained from a single cell(s), the profile may be directly compared with a known reference profile(s) or searched in a DNA database(s).

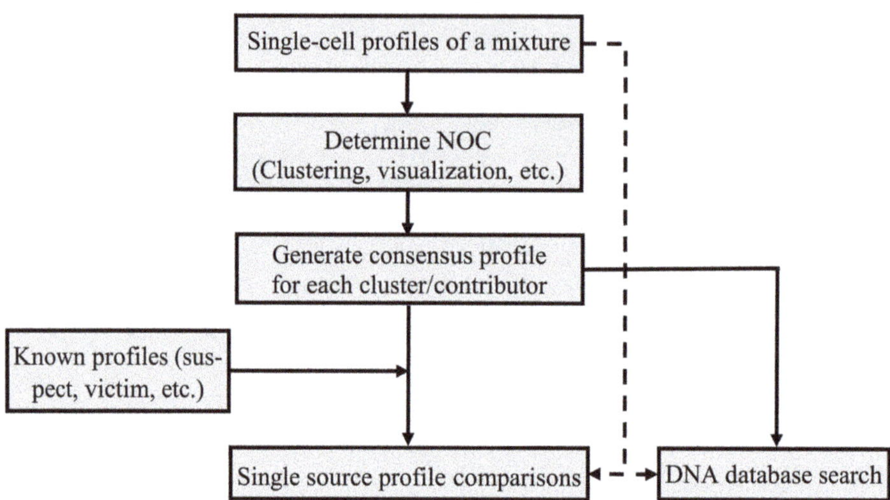

Figure 7. The interpretation workflow of single-cell profiles generated from a mixture.

With single-cell technologies, a DNA mixture is not formed during the DNA extraction process. Thus, the interpretation is simplified and based on single source profile comparisons. Therefore, the need for methods, such as probabilistic genotyping, that indirectly determine the genotypes of the contributors, may not be required in some cases. Instead, the single-cell based approach can directly determine the profiles of the contributors from single-cell profile clusters or from the single source profiles of the individual cells.

For the single source comparisons to confirm or exclude individuals, IBS counting can be employed to determine the potential source or relationship between a consensus profile from single cells and a reference profile to be compared by a predefined IBS threshold as shown in Figures 3 and 4. A LR based approach still can apply in these comparisons [58]. Let A be the consensus profile and B be a reference profile (e.g., a suspect's profile). The hypotheses can be framed, for example, as A and B are from the same source or from different and unrelated sources. Then, the following equation can be used to calculate an LR, with ADO and ADI incorporated to explain the allele difference between A and B, if there are any. However, the ADO and ADI rates of the consensus profile are different from the rates for single cell profiles. These rates should be calculated by consensus similar to the methods of estimating quality scores in MPS [59].

$$LR = \frac{Pr(A, B | A \& B \text{ are from same source})}{Pr(A, B | A \& B \text{ are unrelated})}. \tag{1}$$

In Equation (1), the numerator is the product of the transition probabilities in Table 1 of [60] and the genotype frequency of B, and the denominator is simply the product of the genotype frequencies of A and B. When all alleles of A and B are identical and there is no ADO and ADI, this equation reduces to the inverse of the traditional Random Match Probability (RMP) of A or B.

In cases when a relative of, for example, the suspect is hypothesized as the contributor, both IBS and LR approaches can still apply. For the IBS approach, a different threshold can be used, as shown in Figures 3 and 4. For the LR approach, the denominator hypothesis would be different (Equation (2)). The numerator can be calculated by expanding Table 1 in [61] with the incorporation of ADO and ADI, using a similar model to that described in [60].

$$LR = \frac{Pr(A, B | A \& B \text{ are related as a specific relationship})}{Pr(A, B | A \& B \text{ are unrelated})}. \tag{2}$$

If there is no known profile to compare, the consensus profile (full or partial) may be searched against a forensic DNA database(s) (e.g., CODIS). If a consensus profile is generated from a cluster with a good number of sampled cells (e.g., ≥10), the partial matches (or hits) highly likely belong to family members of the sample donor or the sample donor.

4.2. The Capabilities and Limitations

This study supports that, based on the single-cell technologies, the DNA mixtures can be precisely deconvoluted with proper interpretation methods. With the single-cell profiles of any DNA mixture, the chance of missing a minor contributor can be quantified, and the proportion of each contributor in the mixture can be determined at the level of single cells or chromosomes through the single-cell profile clusters. These proportions may not reflect the true proportions in the whole mixture sample before cell isolation, particularly when the proportion is small or the number of sampled cells is small, because of cell extraction efficiency and sampling error, as only a small percentage of the cells may be isolated for genotype profiling. However, depending on the case scenario, mixture proportions may not be important or relevant compared with just identifying the cells that are present.

The probabilities of not detecting a minor contributor estimated in Table 2 assume a large number of cells are available for analysis. For low-quantity DNA samples, which may contain a few cells, hypergeometric distribution may be a better model to estimate these probabilities. However, the hypergeometric distribution requires knowing the total number of cells in a forensic sample, which may not be possible or precisely determined. In contrast, binomial distribution does not require the total number of cells in the estimation, and thus it may still be a good option in low-quantity DNA samples.

NOC estimation is the key component in this interpretation workflow. If the NOC is overestimated (e.g., a two-person mixture is determined as a three-person mixture), most likely the single cells of a contributor(s) are separated into two or more clusters, and the consensus profile of each cluster may still be valid. However, if the NOC is underestimated, cells from multiple contributors would be merged into one cluster, which could lead to an incorrect consensus profile. Nevertheless, by the clustering approach, the NOC of a mixture can be precisely determined for the mixtures with a high number of cells and relatively balanced mixture ratios, even for mixtures with related contributors.

In this study, for the tested classic clustering algorithms, EM performed better than K-Means in general, but K-Means performed better in some mixtures, such as the (5,5) mixture with unrelated contributors. Both of these classic algorithms do not perform well with imbalanced mixture ratios [54]. The EM algorithm does not explicitly require a distance measure, and the Euclidean distance was used in the K-Means algorithm. While the Euclidean distance measure may not be the best distance for this application, it was used herein as a proof of concept. Specifically designed distances for STR alleles, such as counting the number of step differences between STR alleles, only counting the heterozygous loci to mitigate the impact of ADO, or allele or genotype matching based measures (e.g., IBS), could be better choices for algorithms which require a distance measure. The Silhouettes method was used in this study to determine the number of clusters, but it does not work for the scenarios when NOC = 1 and is not necessarily the best method for single-cell STR data. Other methods, such as the Davies–Bouldin index, the Dunn index, and the Akaike information criterion (AIC), may help determine the number of clusters and may be tested in the future. Overall, better clustering algorithms (such as t-SNE clustering [62], semi-supervised and self-supervised learning [63,64]) and better methods of determining the number of clusters should be pursued for the single-cell profiles with imbalanced mixtures. In addition, similar to that of other single-cell applications, visualization can be helpful to estimate the NOC, as human judgment may do better deciding the NOC when the number of instances is small (e.g., few to hundreds), which is the case for many forensic mixture samples. However, human judgment can be subjective; different individuals may reach different conclusions. Thus, visualization is more of a tool to assist the users to decide NOC or limit the range of possible NOCs.

With a correct NOC, a high precision consensus profile can be obtained through the clustered cell profiles. The sources of these consensus profiles can be precisely determined by comparing them with the known profiles or considering the untyped relatives. The accuracy relies on the number of cell profiles in the clusters, as well as the ADO and ADI rates. But even with $D = 0.2$ and $e = 0.01$, the consensus accuracies of all contributors approach 100% for mixtures with ≥ 40 cells and relatively balanced mixture ratios. Particularly, the family trio mixtures can be deconvoluted to recover the genotypes of the individual contributors, even though related, which in theory is more challenging with CE-STR analysis without conditioning on one of the contributors [65]. This study did not investigate the consensus accuracies when the estimated NOC was incorrect. It was mainly because, if the number of the true profiles (e.g., two) and the number of consensus profiles (e.g., three) are different, it is not easy to decide which consensus profiles should compare with which true profiles. The accuracies with NOC overestimation and underestimation will be investigated in future studies.

The success of the single-cell mixture interpretations was based on the assumption that a reasonable number of intact single cells can be isolated from a DNA sample, there are no doublets or triplets of cells during cell isolation, and most of the alleles of these isolated single cells can be successfully genotyped or sequenced. Although these assumptions may not be held, low quality data per call could be filtered out using a threshold or with algorithms. For example, doublets can be detected by an outlier detection algorithms [66] or simply counting the number of alleles (i.e., triplet and/or quadruplet allele genotypes per locus) or heterozygotes. Regardless, the interpretation methods developed in this study allowed for imperfect data, such as small sample sizes, ADO, and ADI.

For some degraded forensic samples, many of the cells may be lysed, and thus isolating intact cells may be difficult. Additionally, if extracellular DNA is present, the DNA fragments released from the lysed cells may be isolated with an intact cell(s), which could cause extra alleles to appear for some of the single-cell profiles. Validation studies should be able to determine the impact of such events occurring. However, the impact may be small because the extracellular fragments are a small subset of the genome; forensic applications currently target only a very small percentage of the human genome (i.e., ~10k bp out of 3 billion bp). In addition, if the NOC is estimated correctly and the consensus works well, the drop-in alleles still may be able to be filtered out.

Even if a good number of cells are isolated, genotype profiling of the single copy alleles in each single cell can be challenging, depending on the ADO and ADI rates. The ADO and ADI rates can have a substantial impact on the analysis, such as NOC estimation and allele consensus. The current ADO and ADI rates observed in various studies [19,27,34] may still be high for each single-cell profile compared with the profiles generated from bulk cells. However, WGA could help enrich targets [31,33] for higher accuracies of genotype profiling, and single-cell isolation and amplification technologies are likely to become more robust.

Generating consensus profiles from multiple single cells that are clustered can mitigate the effects of high ADO and ADI rates, as described in Section 3.3. If there are ≥ 10 cell profiles in a cluster, with $D = 0.2$ and $e = 0.01$, a full consensus profile can be generated with no mismatched alleles or only one mismatched allele on average, with up to three mismatched alleles, in ~99.96% of the diploid mixtures and ~99.7% of the haploid mixtures. The process is also highly successful for developing the consensus profile among related profiles.

In addition, the NOC estimation and allele consensus with single-cell profiles do not need to assume independence among the tested alleles and markers, since the machine learning algorithms by nature are able to accommodate dependent variants. Therefore, in contrast to the complexity of current practices to incorporate dependence among the markers, the single-cell based mixture interpretation can directly use the genetically linked markers and markers in Linkage-Disequilibrium (LD) together, as well as the dependence among the alleles at the same locus, without any statistical corrections. This feature makes the single-cell based interpretation readily able to include as many markers as possible to increase the discriminating power and better identify individual contributors. However, current methods, including the current probabilistic genotyping approach, do not readily address dependent markers.

4.3. Future Improvements

As a proof-of-concept, this study only simulated the 21 STR loci in the GlobalFiler kit by simplified but reasonable ADO and ADI models to demonstrate the capabilities of using single-cell profiles to deconvolve mixtures. The same principles should apply for other autosomal markers as well, either more STRs, Single Nucleotide Polymorphisms (SNPs), or Insertion-Deletions (InDels). With more markers typed, the accuracy of NOC estimation should increase. ADO may have a higher impact on performance using SNPs than using STRs, since most of the SNPs have only two alleles at a locus and three possible genotypes at each locus. But the huge numbers of SNPs in the human genome should be able to overcome this limitation quite well. Indeed, whole genome sequencing (WGS) of single cells has been described for other applications [67].

The lineage markers on mitochondrial DNA (mtDNA) and the Y chromosome can be very useful for NOC estimation and allele consensus due to their unique features. The diploid cells from the same contributor should have the same Y chromosome markers (if a male contributor) and mtDNA haplotype (except for heteroplasmy or somatic mutations). Use of Y markers in the haploid cells is more complicated. Half of all sperm from a male contributor should have the same Y chromosome barring mutation, and the other half of the sperm should carry the same X chromosome barring mutation. Therefore, an interpretation process could be designed that first clusters profiles based on Y chromosome markers, followed by autosomal or X chromosome markers. X chromosome markers have been useful in certain cases, such as incest cases. However, mixture interpretation using X chromosome markers with CE-STR analysis has been problematic. With single-cell profiling, X chromosome markers could be used routinely for mixture deconvolution, especially when combined with Y markers.

The ADO model employed in this study did not consider degradation due to different allele and locus sizes. Accuracies could increase if degradation was included in the ADO model, such as including the pattern of the ADO rates for different sizes of alleles could improve the modeling of ADO rates for different alleles. A detection threshold still needs to be determined to differentiate alleles from noise. The ADI model used in this study assumed a random genotyping error while a large proportion of the ADIs are likely exaggerated stutters for specific STR alleles. It would be desirable to incorporate a stutter model, which should increase the accuracies of NOC estimation and allele consensus; less distinctly different alleles would be observed in each cluster with a stutter model allowing the profiles to cluster more effectively. However, not all wet-lab technologies would generate stutters. For SNPs and Indels, there is no stutter. For STRs, the stutters may be minimized by the recently developed Unique Molecular Index (UMI) technology [68]. There are many factors that may impact ADO and ADI, such as types of markers, sequencing platforms, library preparation kits, amplification kits, sequencing kits, protocols, software programs to call alleles, detection thresholds, and so forth. Thus, technology and marker specific ADO and ADI models may be the better options. In addition, the independence of the ADO and/or ADI events among the cells may not be assumed with real samples [69]. Therefore, more sophisticated ADO and ADI models that incorporate the underlying dependence between the cells may be better refracting the actual scenarios. Furthermore, this study used all single cells in analysis. In real casework, a filter should be implemented to remove the single cells with the number of missing alleles or loci beyond a certain threshold, and thus, only good quality data would be used in clustering and profile comparisons, which in general should improve interpretation accuracies.

Another improvement in accuracy could be to use clustering algorithms with a better performance on imbalanced data [70]. Particularly, when a minor contributor is represented with an extremely small number of sampled cells (e.g., one or two), outlier detection algorithms (e.g., Isolation Forest [71]) or self-supervised learning [72], instead of the classic clustering algorithms, may be used to select the single cell(s) of the minor contributor(s). Improving accuracies of determining the number of clusters, other NOC methods, such as Davies–Bouldin index, Dunn index, Akaike information criterion (AIC), and so forth, may also be considered. The current allele consensus method treats two alleles at the same locus independently. Performance may be improved if consensus is performed at the genotype level. With such improvements, it is reasonable to expect that this single-cell interpretation workflow should be able to interpret mixtures with a higher number of contributors (i.e., NOC $\geq$ 4).

In addition, the measures of several different NOCs may be very close to each other, and multiple alleles may be close likely being the consensus allele in the consensus profile. Picking one among multiple similarly likely NOCs or alleles could lead to error. Thus, the interpretation methods may allow multiple possible scenarios with estimated weights, similar to the continuous probabilistic genotyping approaches. These scenarios may be evaluated, compared, and combined in a Bayesian or LR fashion.

4.4. Costs

The whole mixture interpretation workflow with the current routine methods includes wet-lab work, data interpretation, judicial proceedings, law enforcement investigation, and so forth, and a cost benefit analysis should be considered in a systems fashion as opposed to solely the laboratory cost. The cost of the wet-lab workflow may be $50–100 per sample currently (including sample collection, DNA extraction, quantification, amplification, genotyping, but not including the labor), depending on the costs of the reagents and local infrastructure. There are more costs that tend to occur after the DNA mixture profile is generated, such as DNA interpretation (including software and hours of work interpreting mixture profiles), evidence presentation in the court, and so forth. Additional costs may also occur, including the law enforcement investigation, reanalyzing samples/aliquots, hiring external reviewers for complex mixture interpretation, and so forth.

Compared with the current routine methods, the single-cell based mixture interpretation methods will add more costs to the wet-lab workflow, depending on the number of cells to be analyzed and the reagents used in the workflow. In general, the more cells that are analyzed, the higher are the costs. However, the cost increase may not be linear to the number of cells to be tested, as the volume of reagents may be reduced in many steps (such as amplification), and some steps of the workflow will not be needed (such as extraction and quantification). More importantly, the single-cell based methods provide a much more simplified interpretation with higher precision. Thus, the costs of the subsequent work (such as data interpretation, additional wet-lab analysis, law enforcement investigation, external review, judicial proceedings, etc.) may be substantially reduced, and the overall costs of mixture cases, at a systems level, may be reduced.

Thus, while sampling multiple single cells will be more costly for the wet lab work than analyzing one mixture (i.e., pooled cell) sample, costs of analyses, such as MPS, continue to drop, and more facile single-cell technologies are likely to be developed. However, more importantly, the cost of analysis should be weighed against the value of reducing uncertainty in mixture interpretation, saving time and resource for law enforcement investigations and saving costs of judicial proceedings, which in turn would save the overall costs of an investigation by the government.

5. Conclusions

Overall, this study has demonstrated that the single-cell based mixture interpretation can provide a precision that cannot be achieved with current standard CE-STR analyses. A new paradigm for mixture interpretation is available to enhance the success of forensic genetic casework. More effort should be dedicated to improving the details of the interpretation methods, as well as the single-cell isolation and genotype profiling methods. In addition, as we see with other recent advances (such as familial searching or investigative genetic genealogy), this single-cell profiling approach could also be used after other approaches have not been able to achieve a desired outcome, assuming a sufficient sample for additional testing or by preserving part of the biological evidence to repeat the analyses with a different approach.

Supplementary Materials: The following are available online at https://www.mdpi.com/article/10.3390/genes12111649/s1, Supplementary Table S1. A simulated mixture example with two unrelated contributors (20 diploid cells each) in the ARFF format defined by WEKA. "?" = missing or dropout allele. Supplementary Table S2. Accuracies of NOC with K-Means algorithm and Silhouettes method for various mixture scenarios. UR = unrelated, PC = parent-child, and FS = full-sibling. Supplementary Figure S1, which includes the rotatable plots of Figure 2.

Author Contributions: Conceptualization, J.G.; Methodology, J.G.; Software, J.G.; Data Analysis, J.G.; Visualization J.G. and J.L.K.; writing—original draft preparation, J.G.; writing—review and editing, J.G., J.L.K., A.S. and B.B. All authors have read and agreed to the published version of the manuscript.

Funding: Internal funds from Center for Human Identification.

Institutional Review Board Statement: Not applicable, as this study used simulation data.

Informed Consent Statement: Not applicable.

Data Availability Statement: No data to report.

Conflicts of Interest: A patent application in pending.

References

1. Bright, J.-A.; Taylor, D.; McGovern, C.; Cooper, S.; Russell, L.; Abarno, D.; Buckleton, J. Developmental validation of STRmix™, expert software for the interpretation of forensic DNA profiles. *Forensic Sci. Int. Genet.* **2016**, *23*, 226–239. [CrossRef] [PubMed]
2. Gill, P.; Haned, H.; Eduardoff, M.; Santos, C.; Phillips, C.; Parson, W. The open-source software LRmix can be used to analyse SNP mixtures. *Forensic Sci. Int. Genet. Suppl. Ser.* **2015**, *5*, e50–e51. [CrossRef]
3. Perlin, M.W.; Legler, M.M.; Spencer, C.E.; Smith, J.L.; Allan, W.P.; Belrose, J.L.; Duceman, B.W. Validating TrueAllele DNA mixture interpretation. *J. Forensic Sci.* **2011**, *56*, 1430–1447. [CrossRef]
4. Gill, P.; Jeffreys, A.J.; Werrett, D.J. Forensic application of DNA 'fingerprints'. *Nature* **1985**, *318*, 577–579. [CrossRef] [PubMed]
5. Voorhees, J.C.; Ferrance, J.P.; Landers, J.P. Enhanced elution of sperm from cotton swabs via. enzymatic digestion for rape kit analysis. *J. Forensic Sci.* **2006**, *51*, 574–579. [CrossRef] [PubMed]
6. Novroski, N.M.; King, J.L.; Churchill, J.D.; Seah, L.H.; Budowle, B. Characterization of genetic sequence variation of 58 STR loci in four major population groups. *Forensic Sci. Int. Genet.* **2016**, *25*, 214–226. [CrossRef] [PubMed]
7. Gan, Y.; Li, N.; Zou, G.; Xin, Y.; Guan, J. Identification of cancer subtypes from single-cell RNA-seq data using a consensus clustering method. *BMC Med. Genom.* **2018**, *11*, 117. [CrossRef]
8. Cui, Y.; Zhang, S.; Liang, Y.; Wang, X.; Ferraro, T.N.; Chen, Y. Consensus clustering of single-cell RNA-seq data by enhancing network affinity. *Brief. Bioinform.* **2021**, bbab236. [CrossRef]
9. Kling, D.; Tillmar, A.O.; Egeland, T. Familias 3-extensions and new functionality. *Forensic Sci. Int. Genet.* **2014**, *13*, 121–127. [CrossRef] [PubMed]
10. Vullo, C.M.; Catelli, L.; Rodriguez, A.A.I.; Papaioannou, A.; Merino, J.C.Á.; Lopez-Parra, A.; Gaviria, A.; Baeza-Richer, C.; Romanini, C.; González-Moya, E. Second GHEP-ISFG exercise for DVI: "DNA-led" victims' identification in a simulated air crash. *Forensic Sci. Int. Genet.* **2021**, *53*, 102527. [CrossRef]
11. Budowle, B.; Eisenberg, A.J.; Van Daal, A. Validity of low copy number typing and applications to forensic science. *Croat. Med. J.* **2009**, *50*, 207–217. [CrossRef]
12. Li, C.; Qi, B.; Ji, A.; Xu, X.; Hu, L. The combination of single cell micromanipulation with LV-PCR system and its application in forensic science. *Forensic Sci. Int. Genet. Suppl. Ser.* **2009**, *2*, 516–517. [CrossRef]
13. Huffman, K.; Hanson, E.; Ballantyne, J. Recovery of single source DNA profiles from mixtures by direct single cell subsampling and simplified micromanipulation. *Sci. Justice* **2021**, *61*, 13–25. [CrossRef] [PubMed]
14. Xu, C.; Feng, L.; Yang, F.; Jia, J.; Ji, A.-Q.; Hu, L.; Li, C.-X. Mucosal cell isolation and analysis from cellular mixtures of three contributors. *J. Forensic Sci.* **2015**, *60*, 783–786. [CrossRef] [PubMed]
15. Brück, S.; Evers, H.; Heidorn, F.; Müller, U.; Kilper, R.; Verhoff, M.A. Single cells for forensic DNA analysis-from evidence material to test tube. *J. Forensic Sci.* **2010**, *56*, 176–180. [CrossRef] [PubMed]

16. Schneider, C.; Müller, U.; Kilper, R.; Siebertz, B. Low copy number DNA profiling from isolated sperm using the aureka®-micromanipulation system. *Forensic Sci. Int. Genet.* **2012**, *6*, 461–465. [CrossRef] [PubMed]

17. Theunissen, G.M.; Rolf, B.; Gibb, A.; Jäger, R. DNA profiling of sperm cells by using micromanipulation and whole genome amplification. *Forensic Sci. Int. Genet. Suppl. Ser.* **2017**, *6*, e497–e499. [CrossRef]

18. Vandewoestyne, M.; Deforce, D. Laser capture microdissection in forensic research: A review. *Int. J. Leg. Med.* **2010**, *124*, 513–521. [CrossRef] [PubMed]

19. Han, J.-P.; Yang, F.; Xu, C.; Wei, Y.-L.; Zhao, X.-C.; Hu, L.; Ye, J.; Li, C.-X. A new strategy for sperm isolation and STR typing from multi-donor sperm mixtures. *Forensic Sci. Int. Genet.* **2014**, *13*, 239–246. [CrossRef]

20. Xu, Y.; Xie, J.; Chen, R.; Cao, Y.; Ping, Y.; Xu, Q.; Hu, W.; Wu, D.; Gu, L.; Zhou, H.; et al. Fluorescence- and magnetic-activated cell sorting strategies to separate spermatozoa involving plural contributors from biological mixtures for human identification. *Sci. Rep.* **2016**, *6*, 36515. [CrossRef] [PubMed]

21. Schoell, W.M. Separation of sperm and vaginal cells with flow cytometry for DNA typing after sexual assault. *Obstet. Gynecol.* **1999**, *94*, 623–627. [CrossRef]

22. Verdon, T.J.; Mitchell, R.J.; Chen, W.; Xiao, K.; van Oorschot, R.A. FACS separation of non-compromised forensically relevant biological mixtures. *Forensic Sci. Int. Genet.* **2015**, *14*, 194–200. [CrossRef]

23. Miller, J.M.; Brocato, E.R.; Yadavalli, V.K.; Greenspoon, S.A.; Ehrhardt, C.J. Testing hormone-specific antibody probes for presumptive detection and separation of contributor cell populations in trace DNA mixtures. *bioRxiv* **2019**. [CrossRef]

24. Stokes, N.A.; Stanciu, C.E.; Brocato, E.R.; Ehrhardt, C.J.; Greenspoon, S.A. Simplification of complex DNA profiles using front end cell separation and probabilistic modeling. *Forensic Sci. Int. Genet.* **2018**, *36*, 205–212. [CrossRef]

25. Dean, L.; Kwon, Y.J.; Philpott, M.K.; Stanciu, C.E.; Seashols-Williams, S.J.; Cruz, T.D.; Sturgill, J.; Ehrhardt, C.J. Separation of uncompromised whole blood mixtures for single source STR profiling using fluorescently-labeled human leukocyte antigen (HLA) probes and fluorescence activated cell sorting (FACS). *Forensic Sci. Int. Genet.* **2015**, *17*, 8–16. [CrossRef] [PubMed]

26. Williamson, V.R.; Laris, T.M.; Romano, R.; Marciano, M.A. Enhanced DNA mixture deconvolution of sexual offense samples using the DEPArray™ system. *Forensic Sci. Int. Genet.* **2018**, *34*, 265–276. [CrossRef]

27. Anslinger, K.; Graw, M.; Bayer, B. Deconvolution of blood-blood mixtures using DEPArrayTM separated single cell STR profiling. *Rechtsmedizin* **2019**, *29*, 30–40. [CrossRef]

28. Fontana, F.; Rapone, C.; Bregola, G.; Aversa, R.; de Meo, A.; Signorini, G.; Sergio, M.; Ferrarini, A.; Lanzellotto, R.; Medoro, G.; et al. Isolation and genetic analysis of pure cells from forensic biological mixtures: The precision of a digital approach. *Forensic Sci. Int. Genet.* **2017**, *29*, 225–241. [CrossRef] [PubMed]

29. England, R.; Nancollis, G.; Stacey, J.; Sarman, A.; Min, J.; Harbison, S. Compatibility of the ForenSeq™ DNA signature prep kit with laser microdissected cells: An exploration of issues that arise with samples containing low cell numbers. *Forensic Sci. Int. Genet.* **2020**, *47*, 102278. [CrossRef]

30. Lim, H.H.; Srisiri, K.; Rerkamnuaychoke, B.; Bandhaya, A. A comparative study of whole genome amplification and low-template DNA profiling. *Forensic Sci. Int. Genet. Suppl. Ser.* **2019**, *7*, 509–511. [CrossRef]

31. Deleye, L.; Plaetsen, A.-S.V.; Weymaere, J.; Deforce, D.; Van Nieuwerburgh, F. Short tandem repeat analysis after whole genome amplification of single B-lymphoblastoid cells. *Sci. Rep.* **2018**, *8*, 1–6. [CrossRef]

32. Schneider, P.; Balogh, K.; Naveran, N.; Bogus, M.; Bender, K.; Lareu, M.; Carracedo, A. Whole genome amplification—the solution for a common problem in forensic casework? *Int. Congr. Ser.* **2004**, *1261*, 24–26. [CrossRef]

33. Chen, M.; Zhang, J.; Zhao, J.; Chen, T.; Liu, Z.; Cheng, F.; Fan, Q.; Yan, J. Comparison of CE- and MPS-based analyses of forensic markers in a single cell after whole genome amplification. *Forensic Sci. Int. Genet.* **2020**, *45*, 102211. [CrossRef]

34. Li, C.-X.; Han, J.-P.; Ren, W.-Y.; Ji, A.-Q.; Xu, X.-L.; Hu, L. DNA profiling of spermatozoa by laser capture microdissection and low volume-PCR. *PLoS ONE* **2011**, *6*, e22316. [CrossRef] [PubMed]

35. Chen, C.; Xing, D.; Tan, L.; Li, H.; Zhou, G.; Huang, L.; Xie, X.S. Single-cell whole-genome analyses by linear amplification via transposon insertion (LIANTI). *Science* **2017**, *356*, 189–194. [CrossRef] [PubMed]

36. Ge, J.; Budowle, B.; Chakraborty, R. Choosing relatives for DNA identification of missing persons. *J. Forensic Sci.* **2011**, *56*, S23–S28. [CrossRef] [PubMed]

37. Ge, J.; Budowle, B. Kinship index variations among populations and thresholds for familial searching. *PLoS ONE* **2012**, *7*, e37474. [CrossRef] [PubMed]

38. Balding, D.J.; Nichols, R.A. DNA profile match probability calculation: How to allow for population stratification, relatedness, database selection and single bands. *Forensic Sci. Int.* **1994**, *64*, 125–140. [CrossRef]

39. Ge, J.; Budowle, B.; Chakraborty, R. DNA identification by pedigree likelihood ratio accommodating population substructure and mutations. *Investig. Genet.* **2010**, *1*, 8. [CrossRef]

40. AABB. *Relationship Testing Annual Reports*; AABB: Bethesda, MD, USA, 2008.

41. Wang, D.Y.; Gopinath, S.; Lagacé, R.E.; Norona, W.; Hennessy, L.K.; Short, M.L.; Mulero, J.J. Developmental validation of the GlobalFiler® express PCR amplification kit: A 6-dye multiplex assay for the direct amplification of reference samples. *Forensic Sci. Int. Genet.* **2015**, *19*, 148–155. [CrossRef]

42. Moretti, T.R.; Moreno, L.I.; Smerick, J.B.; Pignone, M.L.; Hizon, R.; Buckleton, J.S.; Bright, J.-A.; Onorato, A.J. Population data on the expanded CODIS core STR loci for eleven populations of significance for forensic DNA analyses in the United States. *Forensic Sci. Int. Genet.* **2016**, *25*, 175–181. [CrossRef]

43. Eibe, F.; Hall, M.A.; Witten, I.H. *Online Appendix for Data Mining: Practical Machine Learning Tools and Techniques*; The WEKA Workbench; Morgan Kaufmann: Burlington, MA, USA, 2016.

44. Balding, D.J.; Buckleton, J. Interpreting low template DNA profiles. *Forensic Sci. Int. Genet.* **2009**, *4*, 1–10. [CrossRef]

45. Dempster, A.P.; Laird, N.M.; Rubin, D.B. Maximum likelihood from incomplete data via the EM algorithm. *J. R. Stat. Soc. Ser. B* **1977**, *39*, 1–22.

46. Witten, I.H.; Frank, E.; Hall, M.A. *Data Mining: Practical Machine Learning Tools and Techniques*, 3rd ed.; Elsevier/Morgan Kaufmann: San Francisco, CA, USA, 2011. [CrossRef]

47. Kanungo, T.; Mount, D.; Netanyahu, N.; Piatko, C.; Silverman, R.; Wu, A. An efficient k-means clustering algorithm: Analysis and implementation. *IEEE Trans. Pattern Anal. Mach. Intell.* **2002**, *24*, 881–892. [CrossRef]

48. Rousseeuw, P.J. Silhouettes: A graphical aid to the interpretation and validation of cluster analysis. *J. Comput. Appl. Math.* **1987**, *20*, 53–65. [CrossRef]

49. Morris, J.H.; Apeltsin, L.; Newman, A.M.; Baumbach, J.; Wittkop, T.; Su, G.; Bader, G.D.; Ferrin, T.E. ClusterMaker: A multi-algorithm clustering plugin for cytoscape. *BMC Bioinform.* **2011**, *12*, 436. [CrossRef]

50. Kaufman, L.; Rousseeuw, P.J. *Finding Groups in Data: An Introduction to Cluster Analysis*; John Wiley and Sons: Hoboken, NJ, USA, 2009.

51. Pich, C. MDSJ: Java Library for Multidimensional Scaling (Version 0.2). 2009. Available online: http://www.inf.uni-konstanz.de/algo/software/mdsj (accessed on 21 October 2020).

52. Java Data Frame and Visualization Library. Available online: https://jtablesaw.github.io/tablesaw/ (accessed on 21 October 2020).

53. Cairns, P. Gene methylation and early detection of genitourinary cancer: The road ahead. *Nat. Rev. Cancer* **2007**, *7*, 531–543. [CrossRef] [PubMed]

54. Xuan, L.; Zhigang, C.; Fan, Y. Exploring of clustering algorithm on class-imbalanced data. In Proceedings of the 2013 8th International Conference on Computer Science & Education, Colombo, Sri Lanka, 26–28 April 2013; pp. 89–93.

55. Wang, B.; Zhu, J.; Pierson, E.; Ramazzotti, D.; Batzoglou, S. Visualization and analysis of single-cell RNA-seq data by kernel-based similarity learning. *Nat. Methods* **2017**, *14*, 414–416. [CrossRef]

56. Amir, E.-A.D.; Davis, K.L.; Tadmor, M.D.; Simonds, E.; Levine, J.H.; Bendall, S.C.; Shenfeld, D.K.; Krishnaswamy, S.; Nolan, G.P.; Pe'Er, D. ViSNE enables visualization of high dimensional single-cell data and reveals phenotypic heterogeneity of leukemia. *Nat. Biotechnol.* **2013**, *31*, 545–552. [CrossRef] [PubMed]

57. Lucy, D.; Curran, J.; Pirie, A.; Gill, P. The probability of achieving full allelic representation for LCN-STR profiling of haploid cells. *Sci. Justice* **2007**, *47*, 168–171. [CrossRef] [PubMed]

58. Council, N.R. *An Update: The Evaluation of Forensic DNA Evidence*; National Academies Press: Washington, DC, USA, 1996.

59. Wall, J.D.; Tang, L.F.; Zerbe, B.; Kvale, M.N.; Kwok, P.-Y.; Schaefer, C.; Risch, N. Estimating genotype error rates from high-coverage next-generation sequence data. *Genome Res.* **2014**, *24*, 1734–1739. [CrossRef] [PubMed]

60. Ge, J.; Budowle, B. Modeling one complete versus triplicate analyses in low template DNA typing. *Int. J. Leg. Med.* **2013**, *128*, 259–267. [CrossRef] [PubMed]

61. Ge, J.; Chakraborty, R.; Eisenberg, A.; Budowle, B. Comparisons of familial DNA database searching strategies. *J. Forensic Sci.* **2011**, *56*, 1448–1456. [CrossRef] [PubMed]

62. Kobak, D.; Berens, P. The art of using t-SNE for single-cell transcriptomics. *Nat. Commun.* **2019**, *10*, 1–14. [CrossRef]

63. Chen, L.; He, Q.; Zhai, Y.; Deng, M. Single-cell RNA-seq data semi-supervised clustering and annotation via. structural regularized domain adaptation. *Bioinformatics* **2021**, *37*, 775–784. [CrossRef]

64. Chen, L.; Zhai, Y.; He, Q.; Wang, W.; Deng, M. Integrating deep supervised, self-supervised and unsupervised learning for single-cell RNA-seq clustering and annotation. *Genes* **2020**, *11*, 792. [CrossRef]

65. Lin, M.-H.; Bright, J.-A.; Pugh, S.N.; Buckleton, J.S. The interpretation of mixed DNA profiles from a mother, father, and child trio. *Forensic Sci. Int. Genet.* **2020**, *44*, 102175. [CrossRef]

66. Stoeckius, M.; Zheng, S.; Houck-Loomis, B.; Hao, S.; Yeung, B.Z.; Mauck, W.M.; Smibert, P.; Satija, R. Cell hashing with barcoded antibodies enables multiplexing and doublet detection for single cell genomics. *Genome Biol.* **2018**, *19*, 1–12. [CrossRef]

67. Zhang, L.; Dong, X.; Lee, M.; Maslov, A.Y.; Wang, T.; Vijg, J. Single-cell whole-genome sequencing reveals the functional landscape of somatic mutations in B lymphocytes across the human lifespan. *Proc. Natl. Acad. Sci. USA* **2019**, *116*, 9014–9019. [CrossRef]

68. Woerner, A.E.; Mandape, S.; King, J.L.; Muenzler, M.; Crysup, B.; Budowle, B. Reducing noise and stutter in short tandem repeat loci with unique molecular identifiers. *Forensic Sci. Int. Genet.* **2021**, *51*, 102459. [CrossRef]

69. Sheth, N.; Swaminathan, H.; Gonzalez, A.J.; Duffy, K.R.; Grgicak, C.M. Towards developing forensically relevant single-cell pipelines by incorporating direct-to-PCR extraction: Compatibility, signal quality, and allele detection. *Int. J. Leg. Med.* **2021**, *135*, 727–738. [CrossRef] [PubMed]

70. Lin, W.-C.; Tsai, C.-F.; Hu, Y.-H.; Jhang, J.-S. Clustering-based undersampling in class-imbalanced data. *Inf. Sci.* **2017**, *409–410*, 17–26. [CrossRef]

71. Liu, F.T.; Ting, K.M.; Zhou, Z.-H. Isolation forest. In Proceedings of the 2008 Eighth IEEE International Conference on Data Mining, Washington, DC, USA, 15–19 December 2008; pp. 413–422.

72. Yang, Y.; Xu, Z. Rethinking the value of labels for improving class-imbalanced learning. *arXiv* **2006**, arXiv:2006.07529 2020.

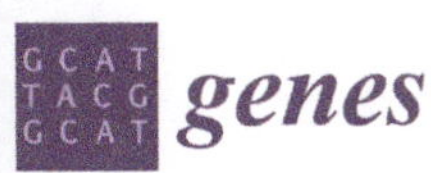

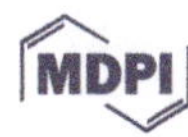

Article

Cross-Amplification in Strigiformes: A New STR Panel for Forensic Purposes

Patrizia Giangregorio [1,*], Lorenzo Naldi [1,2], Chiara Mengoni [1], Claudia Greco [1], Anna Padula [1], Marco Zaccaroni [3], Renato Fani [3], Giovanni Argenti [2] and Nadia Mucci [1]

1. Conservation Genetics Area, Institute for Environmental Protection and Research, Via Ca' Fornacetta 9, Ozzano dell'Emilia, 40064 Bologna, Italy; lorenzonaldi95@gmail.com (L.N.); chiara.mengoni@isprambiente.it (C.M.); claudia.greco@isprambiente.it (C.G.); anna.padula@isprambiente.it (A.P.); nadia.mucci@isprambiente.it (N.M.)
2. Department of Agriculture, Food, Environment and Forestry (DAGRI), University of Florence, Piazzale delle Cascine 18, 50144 Florence, Italy; giovanni.argenti@unifi.it
3. Department of Biology, University of Florence, Via Madonna del Piano 6, Sesto Fiorentino, 50019 Florence, Italy; marco.zaccaroni@unifi.it (M.Z.); renato.fani@unifi.it (R.F.)
* Correspondence: patrizia.giangregorio@isprambiente.it

Abstract: Strigiformes are affected by a substantial decline mainly caused by habitat loss and destruction, poaching, and trapping. Moreover, the increasing trend in bird trade and the growing interest in wild-caught rather than captive-bred birds are expected to encourage illegal trade. The biomolecular investigation represents a valuable tool to track illegal trade and to explore the genetic variability to preserving biodiversity. Microsatellite loci (STRs) are the most used markers to study genetic variability. Despite the availability of species-specific microsatellite loci in Strigiformes, a unique panel permitting the description of the genetic variability across species has not been identified yet. We tested 32 highly polymorphic microsatellite markers to evaluate the reliability of a unique microsatellite panel in different species of Strigiformes and its use for conservation and forensic purposes. We included in the study 84 individuals belonging to 28 parental groups and 11 species of Strigiformes. After screening polymorphic microsatellite loci, the description of genetic variability, and the kinship assessment, we characterized a final panel of 12 microsatellite loci able to identify individuals in 9 Strigiformes species. This STR panel might support the authorities in the forensic investigation for suspected smugglers and false parental claims; moreover, it can be useful to evaluate relatedness among individuals in captive-bred populations and to implement research projects finalized to the description of the genetic variability in wild populations.

Keywords: cross-amplification; microsatellites; Strigiformes; forensic; illegal trade; kinship; nocturnal raptors

Citation: Giangregorio, P.; Naldi, L.; Mengoni, C.; Greco, C.; Padula, A.; Zaccaroni, M.; Fani, R.; Argenti, G.; Mucci, N. Cross-Amplification in Strigiformes: A New STR Panel for Forensic Purposes. *Genes* **2021**, *12*, 1721. https://doi.org/10.3390/genes12111721

Academic Editor: Niels Morling

Received: 5 October 2021
Accepted: 25 October 2021
Published: 28 October 2021

Publisher's Note: MDPI stays neutral with regard to jurisdictional claims in published maps and institutional affiliations.

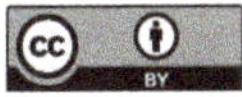

1. Introduction

Habitat loss and fragmentation represent the main threats to the survival of wildlife species. Several studies have well documented their effect on biodiversity loss [1]. Moreover, also international wildlife trade contributes to the depletion of natural resources; hence, the over-exploitation of natural populations, such as the withdrawal of individuals from the wild, is considered one of the leading causes driving the species into extinction [2–4]. It is known that seafood, furniture, and fashion are the main categories requested from the international trade; in addition to this, the commerce of pets affects many individuals. At least 5% of the import/export requests regards parrots and bird of prey (raptors and owls), a quote that equals the sum of all other commercialized birds [1].

Baker and colleagues [5] calculated that animals' demand for pets and entertainment purposes contributed to at least one-fifth of the wildlife trade [6–8], and they showed that the removal of wild individuals from native populations was accounted in migrating species for the second threat that pushes species into extinction, lower only to the habitat loss [9].

Species over-exploitation increases the negative effects produced by habitat unsuitability, causing the reduction of individuals in wild populations that, in turn, can produce a fast loss of genetic variability in a short timescale. Domínguez et al. [10] showed that decreasing populations and pet trade could have generated a bottleneck, reducing genetic variability in the yellow cardinal, *Gubernatrix cristata*, an endangered passerine from the southern region of South America. Harris et al. [11] found that 14 species routinely traded in Indonesian wildlife markets had undergone population decline differently from the other 22 untraded species, which did not suffer any number reduction. Evans and Sheldon [12] found a correlation between the decline of mean heterozygosity with an increasing extinction risk and identified the smaller population sizes as the main cause of this correlation.

Valuable tools to rule or forbid the trade of threatened species to save them from extinction have been provided since the application in 1976 of the Washington Convention. All the countries belonging to the European Community joined the convention that has been applied through several Council (EU) Regulations. Species subjected to maximum protection are listed in Annex A that includes most of the species listed in Appendix I and several species of Appendix II recorded as critically endangered in the European Community.

One of the orders suffering a strong decline in Europe is Strigiformes, which includes two main families: Tytonidae and Strigidae. While the first family is split into two subfamilies, each of which including one genus (*Tyto* and *Phodilus*), the taxonomy of Strigidae is quite controversial [13]. Differently from traditional systematics, Wink et al. [14] recognized the existence of three subfamilies (Ninoxinae, Striginae, Surninae) with several tribes in the last two through a molecular phylogenetic approach. Concerning the substantial decline of Strigiformes in Europe, it is caused mainly by pesticides, changing agricultural techniques with the loss of the structures for nesting and lower rodent availability than in traditional farming, and caught of individuals from the wild. Several main factors threatening owl survival in the Gaza Strip were identified by Abdel Rabou [15], including habitat loss and destruction, poaching and trapping, myths and superstitions, secondary poisoning, road kills, and fence agricultural lands. Wan et al. [16] found a negative influence of fragmentation on the population size and genetic diversity. Despite their inclusion in CITES Appendix II, they enjoy the greatest protection and are listed in Annex A. As for other species included in the CITES Appendix II, only individuals imported into the EU before the Convention of Washington entered into force can be traded. This permission is also applicable to these individuals' descendants, but only if their birth in captivity is proved.

The demand for pets among birds gradually increased in the past decades [17]. Panter, Atkinson and White [7] recorded a wild-caught export of 18,948 individuals belonging to 86 owl species from 1975 to 2015. In 2019, Ribeiro and colleagues [18] denounced a future trend in legal bird trade driven by sociocultural motivations with an increased demand that will interest wild-caught rather than captive-bred birds. This preference is expected to drive towards an increase in the illegal trade of the rarest or more popular species. Also, the reduced number of wild individuals increases their commercial value, encouraging, even more, their illegal trade. Remarkably, the illicit traffic involves the smuggling of eggs and the laundering through captive breeding facilities of wild-caught animals [7].

Owls trade increased in the last decades and has also been influenced by a change in habits; for example, Nijman and Nekaris [19] recorded an increased owl trade, from <0.06% before 2002 to >0.43% post 2008, in wildlife markets in Java and Bali and suggested a delayed "Harry Potter effect". Siriwat and colleagues [20] identified the same increasing trade in Thailand without finding a correlation with the "Harry Potter effect"; nevertheless, they found an association between the increasing owl request, the novel online market and more popularity of owls as a pet. Moreover, they related the higher market price of some species to lower individual availability.

Even though the main actions aim to prevent and hamper over-exploitation and illegal trade represent the first steps in preserving biodiversity, a biomolecular investigation can give valuable hints for either verifying the depletion of genetic variability or tracking illegal trade. This can be carried out through individual identification using molecular techniques and kinship analyses. One of the most used genetic markers to study genetic variability is microsatellite loci (i.e., short tandem repeats or STRs). They are multiallelic and PCR multiplexable, allowing the description of genetic variability with reduced costs. Although the comparability between different laboratories has often proved to represent a limit for their use, this hampering can be easily resolved by using an allelic ladder for each marker—that identifies the position of all the alleles—and by sharing reference samples.

Despite the availability of species-specific panels of microsatellite loci in Strigiformes [21–26] and the cross-amplification of some markers in species lacking their markers [27], a unique panel permitting the description of the genetic variability across species has not been found yet. Such a protocol would permit the recording of comparable variability indices among different species and speed the process, reducing molecular analyses costs; it could also be informative in detecting illegal trade of individuals collected from the wild.

Thus, we tested 32 highly polymorphic microsatellite markers available from literature in 11 species of Strigiformes with the following aims:

- To evaluate the reliability of a unique panel of microsatellite loci for several species of Strigiformes;
- To test its use for conservation and forensic purposes;
- To assess the use of the panel in confirming phylogenetic relationships among species.

2. Materials and Methods

The overall experimental strategy used in this work was based on the following steps:

(i) Thirty-two microsatellite markers selected from the literature were tested on two unrelated individuals of a restricted panel of three species (*Athene noctua, Strix aluco, Bubo bubo*) (Table 1).

Table 1. List of species and individuals used in each step: family groups from 1 to 9 were tested in the first and second screening; additional species and family groups (from 10 to 28) were tested in the third step.

Family	Subfamily	Tribe	Species	ID	Gender	Relationships	Family Group
				S_al 1	Male	Father	1
				S_al 2	Female	Mother	
				S_al 3	unknown	Offspring	
				S_al 4	Male	Father	2
		Strigini	*Strix aluco*	S_al 5	Female	Mother	
				S_al 6	unknown	Offspring	
				S_al 7	Male	Father	3
				S_al 8	Female	Mother	
Strigidae	Striginae			S_al 9	unknown	Offspring	
				B_bu 1	Male	Father	4
				B_bu 2	Female	Mother	
				B_bu 3	unknown	Offspring	
				B_bu 4	Male	Father	5
		Bubonini	*Bubo bubo*	B_bu 5	Female	Mother	
				B_bu 6	unknown	Offspring	
				B_bu 7	Male	Father	6
				B_bu 8	Female	Mother	
				B_bu 9	unknown	Offspring	

Table 1. *Cont.*

Family	Subfamily	Tribe	Species	ID	Gender	Relationships	Family Group
				A_no 1	Male	Father	7
				A_no 2	Female	Mother	
				A_no 3	unknown	Offspring	
				A_no 4	Male	Father	8
	Surninae	Athenini	*Athene noctua*	A_no 5	Female	Mother	
				A_no 6	unknown	Offspring	
				A_no 7	Male	Father	9
				A_no 8	Female	Mother	
				A_no 9	unknown	Offspring	
				S_ne 1	Male	Father	
				S_ne 2	Female	Mother	10
				S_ne 3	unknown	Offspring	
				S_ne 4	Male	Father	
			Strix nebulosa	S_ne 5	Female	Mother	11
				S_ne 6	unknown	Offspring	
		Strigini		S_ne 7	Male	Father	
Strigidae				S_ne 8	Female	Mother	12
				S_ne 9	unknown	Offspring	
				S_ur 1	Male	Father	
				S_ur 2	Female	Mother	13
			Strix uralensis	S_ur 3	unknown	Offspring	
	Striginae			S_ur 4	Male	Father	
				S_ur 5	Female	Mother	14
				S_ur 6	unknown	Offspring	
				B_sc 1	Male	Father	
				B_sc 2	Female	Mother	15
				B_sc 3	unknown	Offspring	
				B_sc 4	Male	Father	
		Bubonini	*Bubo scandiacus*	B_sc 5	Female	Mother	16
				B_sc 6	unknown	Offspring	
				B_sc 7	Male	Father	
				B_sc 8	Female	Mother	17
				B_sc 9	unknown	Offspring	

Table 1. *Cont.*

Family	Subfamily	Tribe	Species	ID	Gender	Relationships	Family Group
Strigidae	Striginae	Otini	*Otus scops*	O_sc 1	Male	Father	18
				O_sc 2	Female	Mother	
				O_sc 3	unknown	Offspring	
				O_sc 4	Male	Father	19
				O_sc 5	Female	Mother	
				O_sc 6	unknown	Offspring	
				O_sc 7	Male	Father	20
				O_sc 8	Female	Mother	
				O_sc 9	unknown	Offspring	
		Asionini	*Asio otus*	A_ot 1	Male	Father	21
				A_ot 2	Female	Mother	
				A_ot 3	unknown	Offspring	
				A_ot 4	Male	Father	22
				A_ot 5	Female	Mother	
				A_ot 6	unknown	Offspring	
	Surninae	Surnini	*Surnia ulula*	S_ul 1	Male	Father	23
				S_ul 2	Female	Mother	
				S_ul 3	unknown	Offspring	
				S_ul 4	Male	Father	24
				S_ul 5	Female	Mother	
				S_ul 6	unknown	Offspring	
				S_ul 7	Male	Father	25
				S_ul 8	Female	Mother	
				S_ul 9	unknown	Offspring	
			Glaucidium passerinum	G_pa 1	Male	Father	26
				G_pa 2	Female	Mother	
				G_pa 3	unknown	Offspring	
				G_pa 4	Male	Father	27
				G_pa 5	Female	Mother	
				G_pa 6	unknown	Offspring	
Tytonidae	Tytoninae		*Tyto alba*	T_al 1	Male	Father	28
				T_al 2	Female	Mother	
				T_al 3	unknown	Offspring	

(ii) Microsatellite markers giving polymorphic profiles in all the species tested at step (i) were used for genotyping three family groups per species (Table 1).

(iii) Microsatellite primers giving polymorphic amplification patterns at step (ii) were then used to evaluate the STR panel for forensic purposes on a larger panel of family groups, comprising different subfamilies, tribes and species, aiming at identifying a unique shared panel of polymorphic loci (Table 1). The selected species are the most commonly traded in the Italian market.

According to the manufacturer's instructions, DNA was isolated from feathers using DNeasy Blood and Tissue Kit (Qiagen, Hilden, Germany). After digestion in 180 µL ATL buffer, 20 µL proteinase K and 20 µL DTT and incubation overnight at 56 °C, the lysate was loaded in a QIAcube HT robotic station (Qiagen, Hilden, Germany) for further purification steps.

DNA was amplified in an 8 µL final volume reaction. The PCR reactions were carried out as follows: in 8 µL of the final volume, we added 1x reaction buffer, 0.02% BSA, 1.5 mM $MgCl_2$, 0.125 mM of dNTPs, Hot Start Taq Polymerase 0.025 U (Qiagen, Hilden, Germany), 0.125 mM primer (forward and reverse), 1 µL DNA template and nuclease-free water to reach the final volume.

Twenty-five out of 32PCR primers used in this work were originally isolated from five species of Strigidae *(Bubo bubo, Otus elegans, Strix occidentalis, Strix nebulosa, Glaucidium brasilianum)*, one from the goshawk *(Accipiter gentilis)*. Six were previously designed to and/or shown to display high cross utility throughout many genetically distant passerine and shorebirds and were found polymorphic in *Tyto alba*. (Table 2); each forward primer was labelled with fluorescent ABI dyes. Amplification reactions were performed in simplex to test for the right allelic range and no specific amplification. According to melting temperature and reference bibliography, we chose the following thermal profile: 94 °C for 15′, followed by 35 cycles at 94 °C for 40″, 60 °C for 40″, ending with a final extension at 72 °C for 10′.

Table 2. Loci chosen from literature and tested for the cross-species amplification study.

Primer ID	Forward Primer Sequence	Reverse Primer Sequence	Original Species	References
54f2	GAGAGATGTTGGGCTCTTGTG	TGTTAATTGCATTGAATGTCAGC	Passerine and shorebird species	[25]
BOOW19	GGAAACTTACTAGAAAATAAATGACTGG	CTTTCTAACTTTCCCATGCAAC	Passerine and shorebird species	[25]
Calex05	TCCAGCTGAAGTCTTCCGTGAAT	TCCACACCTGTTCGACAGTTCAATA	Passerine and shorebird species	[25]
HvoB1	AAGCAAGGACTTTCCTTCCAG	TCTCAAATTGGAACAGAGAAAGG	Passerine and shorebird species	[25]
Tgu06	CGAGTAGCGTATTTGTAGCGA	AGGAGCGGTGATTGTTCAGT	Passerine and shorebird species	[25]
TG04-061	GACAATGGCTATGAAATAAATTAGGC	AGAAGGGCATTGAAGCACAC	Passerine and shorebird species	[25]
BbuS027	TCATGAGGAACTTTCAGTGCTC	GAAGAAAGGCAGCTCTCACC	*Bubo bubo*	[28]
BbuS102	AACTGATTTGGAAACCACCATC	CTGGAACACCCAGTGTTTGTC	*Bubo bubo*	[28]
Bbus116	GTTTCTGCAGCTGGGTCAG	AAACAGTTTCCATGCCTTACG	*Bubo bubo*	[28]
BbuS132	TCATTGTAGGTCCCATCCAAC	CCATATCTATCAAGCAACCTTGG	*Bubo bubo*	[28]
Oe050	AGAGTTGTCCTTGGTTGG	TTCTAGTAACCTCATCTGC	*Otus elegans*	[29]
Oe054	TCAGAAAGAAAACTTCAGCAACC	CATATATGTATACACAGGCACATGC	*Otus elegans*	[29]
15A6	ACCTCAGAAGCAGACAGAACC	CCTTTGCGATTGCTGTAAC	*Strix occidentalis*	[30]
Age5	ACGTTACAGACACCGATTACTTCC	AGCCACGCGTCTGATACTTT	*Accipiter gentilis*	[31]
Bb101	AATAACCCCAATAGAAGC	ACCAGAAGGAGATGAGACC	*Bubo bubo*	[21]
Bb126	TCTCCAGAAGGGTTGTCATC	TGCTAAAACCTTACAGAATAACAG	*Bubo bubo*	[21]
Oe142	TGAATCAGCAAACCTGTGCCTG	AGCTAACCTAGAGTCAGCCAGC	*Otus elegans*	[29]

Table 2. *Cont.*

Primer ID	Forward Primer Sequence	Reverse Primer Sequence	Original Species	References
Oe171	TTTTACAAACTACTAGTGCATGTCTCC	AGATGTTGTATTTCAGTGTCAG	*Otus elegans*	[29]
Oe3-21	GATTAGAGACCCGATTCCACA	TTATCTGAGTGGAAGGGTAGTGC	*Otus elegans*	[29]
Oe3-7	GTGGGTTTATTGCCCCCTCG	CAGATGAATGAATGGATAGATGG	*Otus elegans*	[22]
Oe149	CACACATCCATTTTGGGGTGC	GGATGCTGGAACTGACCTGC	*Otus elegans*	[22]
Oe081	GTAAGGGAAGTAGACGTCTGTTGG	CAACTTTGTGTCATCTGAAAGG	*Otus elegans*	[22]
Oe084	GGGCATAGTTAGACCTTTGCAG	CACATCTGTTGTTCTCCGTGTTACC	*Otus elegans*	[22]
SneD105	AGCCTTGGGAGGTTAAGTCCT	ACACGCAATCACTGAAGCAGT	*Strix nebulosa*	[24]
SneD113	AGCTCTTTCCCGACAGTGTCTA	GCCAAAAAACCCCATATCCTAG	*Strix nebulosa*	[24]
SneD202	GCTGGGCTTAGAAATTACATGG	CTCTGCCCTAATCAGGAACACT	*Strix nebulosa*	[24]
SneD211	TAGCCCTGTGGATTTGCATTAG	TCACCAGAAGTTCAAAGCAGGTAG	*Strix nebulosa*	[24]
SneD218	GGGTGTGAGAATGACCTACCTG	AGCAGACAGGAGATGGCTTTTA	*Strix nebulosa*	[24]
Fepo42	CGTATACATCGAAATAAATACC	CGAATAAAACATCCCTAACC	*Glaucidium brasilianum*	[23]
Oe053	CTCTGCATCTTAACGCACAGGAC	CCTCCAAGTGGACAGGAAAAGC	*Otus elegans*	[29]
Oe128	CGTTGTAAATGATGAATCGCCTAGTGC	ATGCATGTATACATACAAACCTGG	*Otus elegans*	[29]
Oe129	GTCACCTCTTGACATCCGAGTAGC	GCTAAGAGTCCATTTGCCCATCTG	*Otus elegans*	[29]

Amplicons were separated through capillary electrophoresis in an ABI 3130xl genetic analyzer (Thermo Fisher Scientific); alleles were scored in GeneMapper 4.0 using GeneScan 500 ROX size standard (Thermo Fisher Scientific, Waltham, MA, USA). An allelic ladder was constructed in Genemapper, merging the sample electropherograms at each locus. Scoring has been reported for each peak, allowing the data comparison among laboratories (Supplementary Material Figure S1: allelic ladders).

Genotypes resulting from the screening were analyzed for the selected loci. Allele number (NA), effective allele number (NE), number of private alleles, observed and expected heterozygosities (Ho, He) were computed using GenAlEx 6.41 [32]. Gimlet 1.3.3 [33] was used to evaluate the probability of identity (PID) among individuals of each cluster species, to calculate the minimum number of markers necessary to achieve a reliable individual genotyping for unrelated (PID) and related samples (PID$_{sib}$, sibling).

A factorial correspondence analysis (FCA) was carried out in Genetix 4.05 [34] to check the genetic distances between species, tribes and subfamilies.

Parentage relationships among individuals within the family cluster were reconstructed in Colony 2.0 [35]. This analysis allows to check if an individual that is claimed to be bred in captivity truly descends from the declared parents. A single analysis was performed including all genotypes of all species together. We used non-inbreeding data and monogamy models, and set the genotyping error rate value 0.0001. The same analysis was conducted in Cervus [36,37] and the LOD score was computed using a proportion of loci typed = 0.60 and mistyped = 0.01. An additional computation with the same parameters was performed using the Delta score defined as the difference in LOD scores between the most and the second most likely candidate parents. The confidence levels were set to 80% (relaxed) and 95% (strict) in both analyses.

3. Results

3.1. Preliminary Screening of STR Polymorphic Loci

Thirty-two microsatellite markers were chosen to evaluate their cross-species amplification potential on three species (*Athene noctua, Strix aluco, Bubo bubo*) (Table 1), belonging to two different sub-families, Striginae and Surninae, and three tribes (Strigini, Bubonini, Athenini) respectively [14].

Two unrelated individuals per species were selected from the CITES sample database (managed since 1995 by the Italian Institute of Environmental Protection and Research

–ISPRA-on behalf of the Italian Environmental Ministry). Data obtained revealed that twenty-one out of 32 markers used (15a6, Age5, Bb101, Bb126, BbuS027, Bbus116, Calex05, Fepo42, Oe054, Oe128, Oe129, Oe142, Oe149, Oe321, Oe53, Oe81, Oe84, SneD113, SneD202, SneD218, Tgu06) gave amplicons in *A. noctua*, *S. aluco* and *B. bubo* DNA samples. The remaining 11 microsatellites were discarded because they either did not give any amplification product or led to unreliable PCR amplicons.

3.2. Evaluation of the STR Potential in Family Groups

Three family groups (father, mother and one offspring) for each species ($n = 9$, Table 1) were chosen from the CITES database and analyzed at the twenty-one loci selected in the previous section.

Data obtained revealed that 12 of them resulted polymorphic in at least 2 species (15a6, Fepo42, Oe053, Oe054, Oe128, Oe129, Oe142, Oe149, Oe321, SneD113, SneD218, Tgu06) and were retained for further analyses. Fepo42 and Oe054 resulted monomorphic in *S. aluco*, and Oe129 did not give any amplification product in *B. bubo* but were retained.

3.3. Evaluation of the STR Potential in Other Subfamilies of Strigidae

In order to evaluate the potential application of the STR panel for forensic purposes, the 12 microsatellites were used on a larger panel of samples (Table 1), which included:

1. Additional species belonging to the already analyzed tribes of Bubonini and Strigini (*Bubo scandiacus, Strix uralensis, Strix nebulosa*);

2. Two species belonging to the tribes of Asionini (*Asio otus*) and Otini (*Otus scops*);

3. Two species belonging to the Surninae subfamily, Tribes Surnini (*Surnia ulula, Glaucidium passerinum*).

4. *Tyto alba*, belonging to the Tytonidae family, subfamily Tytoninae.

Three family groups were chosen for each species except for *A. otus*, *S. uralensis* and *G. passerinum* because only two confirmed parental nuclei were available in the database. The final dataset consisted of 81 individuals belonging to 27 families.

The DNA of each of the 81 individuals was amplified using the twelve primer sets. Data obtained revealed that the DNA from the additional species included in the analysis (*O. scops, A. otus, B. scandiacus, S. ulula, S. uralensis, S. nebulosa, G. passerinum, T. alba*) was amplified at the examined loci with the following exceptions:

1. *S. ulula* showed fixed genotypes at four loci (Oe054, Oe129, Oe053, Oe321);

2. Ten loci were amplified in *G. passerinum*. However, only four loci were polymorphic. Because of lack of variable loci, *G. passerinum* was removed from the further analysis;

3. *S. uralensis* and *S. nebulosa* showed no polymorphisms at Oe321 and Oe054 loci;

4. In *A. otus*, a unique fixed allele was recorded at locus Oe142;

5. Six loci were amplified in *T. alba* (FePo42, Oe54, Oe128, Oe129, Oe321, Tgu06), but only 2 were variable (FePo42, Tgu06). Thus, this species was discarded from further analyses because two loci are too few to be able to distinguish individuals reliably.

All the percentage values of polymorphic loci per species varied between 100% ($n = 12$ in *A. noctua* and *O. scops*) and 66.67% ($n = 8$ in *S. ulula*), if we do not take into account the value in *G. passerinum* and *T. alba* (Table 3).

Table 3. Variability indices: Allele number (NA), effective allele number (NE); observed heterozygosity (HO), expected heterozygosity (HE), unbalanced expected heterozygosity (uHE), percentage of polymorphic loci (P%). Standard errors are shown in brackets.

Species	NA	NE	HO	HE	uHE	P%
Strix aluco	3.6 (±0.5)	2.8 (±0.4)	0.528 (±0.091)	0.525 (±0.083)	0.556 (±0.087)	83.33%
Strix nebulosa	3.0 (±0.3)	2.2 (±0.2)	0.565 (±0.096)	0.471 (±0.074)	0.499 (±0.079)	83.33%
Strix uralensis	3.0 (±0.5)	2.3 (±0.4)	0.528 (±0.119)	0.429 (±0.092	0.468 (±0.100)	75.00%
Bubo bubo	4.2 (±0.6)	2.6 (±0.4)	0.539 (±0.090)	0.545 (±0.068)	0.578 (±0.072)	91.67%
Bubo scandiacus	3.3 (±0.4)	2.6 (±0.3)	0.515 (±0.092)	0.550 (±0.061)	0.584 (±0.065)	91.67%
Otus scops	6.3 (±0.6)	4.6 (±0.5)	0.733 (±0.049)	0.750 (±0.027)	0.798 (±0.030)	100.00%
Athene noctua	4.1 (±0.5)	3.3 (±0.5)	0.620 (±0.061)	0.604 (±0.060)	0.641 (±0.064)	100.00%
Asio otus	3.2 (±0.4)	2.5 (±0.3)	0.681 (±0.097)	0.529 (±0.062)	0.590 (±0.070)	91.67%
Surnia ulula	2.2 (±0.3)	1.70 (±0.21)	0.356 (±0.088)	0.318 (±0.074)	0.338 (±0.079)	66.67%
Mean	3.7 (±0.2)	2.8 (±0.14)	0.566 (±0.030)	0.525 (±0.025)	0.561 (±0.026)	87.04 (±3.70)%

3.4. Genetic Variability between and within Species

Statistical analysis was carried out on 9 species at 12 loci (Table 3). The mean allele number (NA) was 3.7 (±0.2), with the highest values recorded respectively in *O. scops* (6.3 ± 0.6) and the lowest one in *S. ulula* (2.2 ± 0.3). Mean expected and observed heterozygosity (He and Ho) ranged from 0.750 ± 0.027 and 0.733 ± 0.049 in *O. scops* to 0.318 ± 0.074 and 0.356 ± 0.088 in *S. ulula* with an average value of 0.525 ± 0.025 and 0.566 ± 0.030, respectively. The probability of identity resulted in different thresholds depending on the species and if it was estimated for unrelated or related individuals (Figure 1). A PID value lower than 0.001 was reached in all the species using an average of 3.9 markers, while the same value was achieved with PID$_{sib}$ using at least an average of 9.2 loci. *S. ulula*, *S. nebulosa* and *S. uralensis* were not included in this last computation because their threshold resulted higher using all the loci (minimum values respectively of 0.0155, 0.00162 and 0.00246) (Table 4).

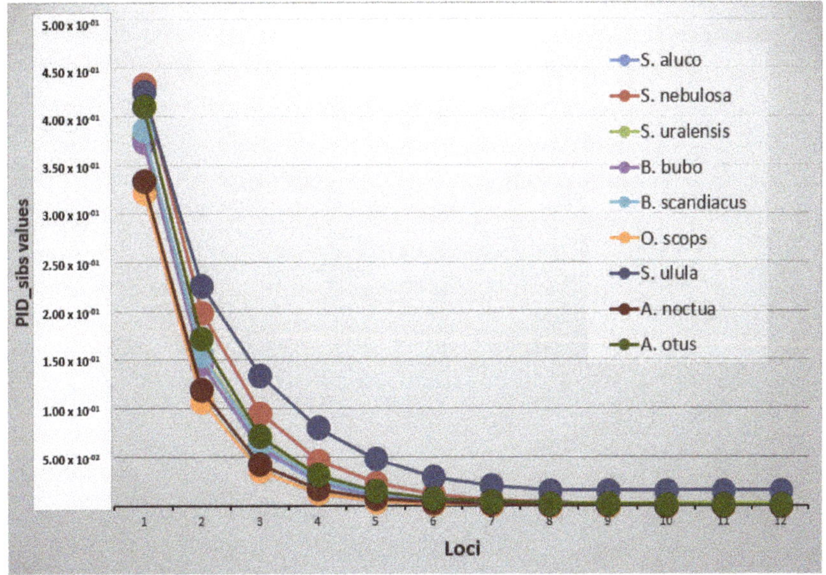

Figure 1. Graph of the PID$_{sib}$ trend in the species.

Table 4. PID and PID_sib values: In the table, values lower than 0.001 were bold-evidenced. In the PID_sib columns, this threshold wasindicated with (*). The PID_sib never reached this value in *Surnia ulula* (0.0155), *Strix nebulosa* (0.00162) and *Strix uralensis* (0.0246). When PID or PID_sib values stop decreasing it means that the markers are not variable and informative (underlined).

	Strix aluco			*Strix nebulosa*			*Strix uralensis*	
locus	PID	PID_sib	locus	PID		locus	PID	PID_sib
Oe149	8.16×10^{-02}	3.78×10^{-01}	15a6	1.40×10^{-01}	4.33×10^{-01}	Oe128	8.16×10^{-02}	3.82×10^{-01}
15a6	6.98×10^{-03}	1.46×10^{-01}	Oe53	2.38×10^{-02}	1.99×10^{-01}	Oe53	9.28×10^{-03}	1.57×10^{-01}
SneD218	$\mathbf{7.10 \times 10^{-04}}$	5.87×10^{-02}	SneD218	4.82×10^{-03}	9.54×10^{-02}	Oe142	1.25×10^{-03}	6.72×10^{-02}
Oe53	7.22×10^{-05}	2.36×10^{-02}	Oe149	1.01×10^{-03}	4.68×10^{-02}	Oe149	$\mathbf{1.86 \times 10^{-04}}$	2.96×10^{-02}
Oe142	7.77×10^{-06}	9.59×10^{-03}	Fepo42	$\mathbf{2.28 \times 10^{-04}}$	2.35×10^{-02}	SneD218	3.23×10^{-05}	1.38×10^{-02}
Oe128	1.45×10^{-06}	4.56×10^{-03}	Oe142	5.18×10^{-05}	1.18×10^{-02}	15a6	7.33×10^{-06}	6.93×10^{-03}
Oe129	3.52×10^{-07}	2.42×10^{-03}	SneD113	1.24×10^{-05}	6.07×10^{-03}	Oe129	2.14×10^{-06}	3.82×10^{-03}
SneD113	9.97×10^{-08}	1.33×10^{-03}	Oe129	3.17×10^{-06}	3.20×10^{-03}	Fepo42	1.20×10^{-06}	2.87×10^{-03}
Oe321	3.77×10^{-08}	7.97×10^{-04} *	Oe128	1.14×10^{-06}	1.99×10^{-03}	Tgu06	$\underline{8.74 \times 10^{-07}}$	$\underline{2.46 \times 10^{-03}}$
Tgu06	$\underline{2.11 \times 10^{-08}}$	$\underline{5.99 \times 10^{-04}}$	Tgu06	$\underline{7.53 \times 10^{-07}}$	$\underline{1.62 \times 10^{-03}}$	Oe054	$\underline{8.74 \times 10^{-07}}$	$\underline{2.46 \times 10^{-03}}$
Fepo42	$\underline{2.11 \times 10^{-08}}$	$\underline{5.99 \times 10^{-04}}$	Oe054	$\underline{7.53 \times 10^{-07}}$	$\underline{1.62 \times 10^{-03}}$	Oe321	$\underline{8.74 \times 10^{-07}}$	$\underline{2.46 \times 10^{-03}}$
Oe054	$\underline{2.11 \times 10^{-08}}$	$\underline{5.99 \times 10^{-04}}$	Oe321	$\underline{7.53 \times 10^{-07}}$	$\underline{1.62 \times 10^{-03}}$	SneD113	$\underline{8.74 \times 10^{-07}}$	$\underline{2.46 \times 10^{-03}}$

	Bubo bubo			*Bubo scandiacus*			*Otus scops*	
locus	PID	PID_sib	locus	PID	PID_sib	locus	PID	PID_sib
SneD218	7.65×10^{-02}	3.74×10^{-01}	Oe53	8.79×10^{-02}	3.86×10^{-01}	Oe054	2.99×10^{-02}	3.22×10^{-01}
Oe53	7.26×10^{-03}	1.46×10^{-01}	SneD218	8.94×10^{-03}	1.55×10^{-01}	Oe149	1.18×10^{-03}	1.08×10^{-01}
15a6	$\mathbf{8.09 \times 10^{-04}}$	6.01×10^{-02}	SneD113	1.01×10^{-03}	6.48×10^{-02}	SneD113	$\mathbf{4.70 \times 10^{-05}}$	3.60×10^{-02}
Oe142	9.11×10^{-05}	2.56×10^{-02}	Oe142	$\mathbf{1.36 \times 10^{-04}}$	2.76×10^{-02}	15a6	2.73×10^{-06}	1.28×10^{-02}
Fepo42	1.48×10^{-05}	1.16×10^{-02}	Oe128	2.52×10^{-05}	1.31×10^{-02}	Fepo42	1.85×10^{-07}	4.70×10^{-03}
SneD113	2.70×10^{-06}	5.77×10^{-03}	Oe054	5.84×10^{-06}	6.70×10^{-03}	Oe142	1.48×10^{-08}	1.79×10^{-03}
Oe128	8.03×10^{-07}	3.16×10^{-03}	Tgu06	1.50×10^{-06}	3.49×10^{-03}	SneD218	1.47×10^{-09}	7.19×10^{-04} *
Oe149	2.23×10^{-07}	1.78×10^{-03}	Oe149	4.68×10^{-07}	2.03×10^{-03}	Oe128	1.48×10^{-10}	2.93×10^{-04}
Oe054	6.17×10^{-08}	1.00×10^{-03}	Fepo42	1.68×10^{-07}	1.26×10^{-03}	Oe53	2.49×10^{-11}	1.34×10^{-04}
Tgu06	2.33×10^{-08}	5.98×10^{-04} *	15a6	6.83×10^{-08}	7.92×10^{-04} *	Oe321	4.46×10^{-12}	6.45×10^{-05}
Oe321	1.55×10^{-08}	4.89×10^{-04}	Oe129	$\underline{2.78 \times 10^{-08}}$	$\underline{4.99 \times 10^{-04}}$	Tgu06	8.29×10^{-13}	3.13×10^{-05}
Oe129	\\	\\	Oe321	$\underline{2.78 \times 10^{-08}}$	$\underline{4.99 \times 10^{-04}}$	Oe129	1.76×10^{-13}	1.54×10^{-05}

	Surnia ulula			*Athene noctua*			*Asio otus*	
locus	PID	PID_sib	locus	PID	PID_sib	locus	PID	PID_sib
SneD218	1.34×10^{-01}	4.26×10^{-01}	SneD113	3.94×10^{-02}	3.34×10^{-01}	Tgu06	1.14×10^{-01}	4.10×10^{-01}
Oe142	3.56×10^{-02}	2.27×10^{-01}	Oe149	2.42×10^{-03}	1.20×10^{-01}	SneD218	1.36×10^{-02}	1.72×10^{-01}
15a6	1.34×10^{-02}	1.35×10^{-01}	Oe129	$\mathbf{1.51 \times 10^{-04}}$	4.30×10^{-02}	Fepo42	1.62×10^{-03}	7.20×10^{-02}
Fepo42	4.63×10^{-03}	8.06×10^{-02}	SneD218	1.46×10^{-05}	1.71×10^{-02}	Oe129	$\mathbf{2.41 \times 10^{-04}}$	3.17×10^{-02}
Oe128	1.77×10^{-03}	4.86×10^{-02}	Oe142	1.96×10^{-06}	7.27×10^{-03}	Oe128	4.70×10^{-05}	1.50×10^{-02}
SneD113	$\mathbf{5.87 \times 10^{-04}}$	2.95×10^{-02}	15a6	3.66×10^{-07}	3.38×10^{-03}	15a6	9.91×10^{-06}	7.33×10^{-03}
Tgu06	2.86×10^{-04}	2.06×10^{-02}	Fepo42	6.59×10^{-08}	1.59×10^{-03}	Oe149	3.24×10^{-06}	4.31×10^{-03}
Oe149	$\underline{1.60 \times 10^{-04}}$	$\underline{1.55 \times 10^{-02}}$	Oe321	1.34×10^{-08}	7.88×10^{-04} *	SneD113	1.24×10^{-06}	2.60×10^{-03}
Oe054	$\underline{1.60 \times 10^{-04}}$	$\underline{1.55 \times 10^{-02}}$	Oe054	5.22×10^{-09}	4.80×10^{-04}	Oe321	5.04×10^{-07}	1.64×10^{-03}
Oe129	$\underline{1.60 \times 10^{-04}}$	$\underline{1.55 \times 10^{-02}}$	Oe128	2.59×10^{-09}	3.39×10^{-04}	Oe054	2.00×10^{-07}	1.06×10^{-03}
Oe321	$\underline{1.60 \times 10^{-04}}$	$\underline{1.55 \times 10^{-02}}$	Tgu06	1.36×10^{-09}	2.50×10^{-04}	Oe53	$\underline{9.20 \times 10^{-08}}$	$\underline{7.18 \times 10^{-04}}$ *
Oe53	$\underline{1.60 \times 10^{-04}}$	$\underline{1.55 \times 10^{-02}}$	Oe53	7.63×10^{-10}	1.87×10^{-04}	Oe142	$\underline{9.20 \times 10^{-08}}$	$\underline{7.18 \times 10^{-04}}$

A principal component analysis was then carried out, revealing that, as expected, the three species of the genus *Strix* (*S. uralensis, S. nebulosa, S. aluco*) overlapped in the PCA graphic (Figure 2). *A. otus* and *O. scops* showed a low distance from each other and resulted not very distant from the *Strix* species. *S. ulula* exhibited the greatest genetic distance from the other species while *A. noctua* was in a mid-range position (Figure 2). *B. scandiacus* and *B. bubo* did not overlap, but the genetic distance of the two species is low.

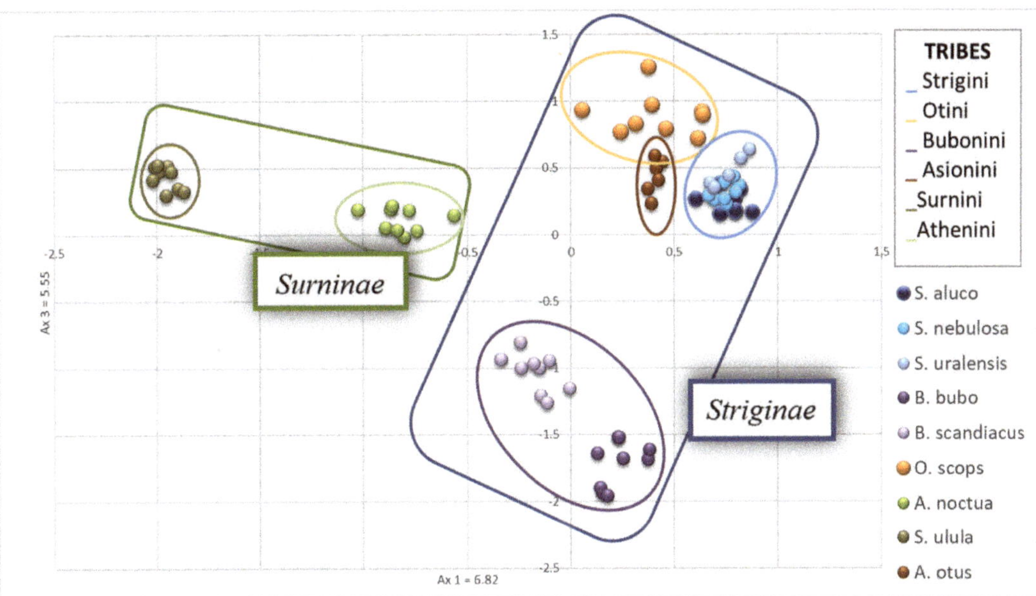

Figure 2. Principal Component Analysis plot obtained using Genetix and visualized in Excel. *Strix* sp. overlapped while *Bubo bubo* and *Bubo scandiacus* plotted very closed each other. *Surnia ulula* individuals diverged consistently from other species. Ovals in different colors represent the distribution of individuals belonging to six tribes of Striginae and Surninae, in the blue and green squares, respectively.

3.5. Evaluation of the STR Potential Panel for Parentage Analysis in Family Groups

The paternity test yielded inconsistent results and different reliability values depending on the species (Tables 5 and 6). In Colony, the correct parent pair was assigned with the maximum probability value (1.00) but decreased in *S. nebulosa* (0.992 and 0.907), *S. uralensis* (0.997), and *S. ulula* (0.983 and 0.753) when the computation has been limited to association with putative mother or father. In two individuals, respectively, of *S. uralensis* (S_ur6) and *S. ulula* (S_ul3), the probability of assignment to the right parent is reduced to 0.500.

In Cervus, using the LOD computation, all the individuals have been correctly associated with the right parents with trio confidence values higher than 95%, except for S_ul3 that has been associated with the wrong father (S_ul5 instead of S_ul2). In *S. uralensis* (S_ur6), the assignment to the right mother did not reach a significant value. Using the Delta calculation, the probability values decreased in *S. nebulosa*, *S. uralensis* and *S. ulula* (see Table 6 for more details). Again, S_ul3 was associated with the wrong father.

Table 5. Parental assignment values from Colony: the lowest values were recovered when the one-parent assignment was tested. In the table, misallocation or low assignment probabilities are highlighted in bold.

	Parent Pair Probability			Single Parent Probability		
Offspring	Father	Mother	Probability Value	Main Probability		Second Probability
S_al 3	S_al 1	S_al 2	1.00			
S_al 6	S_al 4	S_al 5	1.00			
S_al 9	S_al 7	S_al 8	1.00			
S_ne 3	S_ne 1	S_ne 2	1.00	S_ne 2	0.907	S_ne 8
S_ne 6	S_ne 4	S_ne 5	1.00	S_ne 4	0.992	S_ne 1
S_ne 9	S_ne 7	S_ne 8	1.00			
S_ur 3	S_ur 1	S_ur 2	1.00	S_ur 2	0.997	S_ur 5
S_ur 6	S_ur 4	S_ur 5	1.00	S_ur 5	**0.500**	S_ur 2
B_bu 3	B_bu 1	B_bu 2	1.00			
B_bu 6	B_bu 4	B_bu 5	1.00			
B_bu 9	B_bu 7	B_bu 8	1.00			
B_sc 3	B_sc 1	B_sc 2	1,00			
B_sc 6	B_sc 4	B_sc 5	1.00	B_sc 6	0.999	
B_sc 9	B_sc 7	B_sc 8	1,00			
O_sc 3	O_sc 1	O_sc 2	1.00			
O_sc 6	O_sc 4	O_sc 5	1.00			
O_sc 9	O_sc 7	O_sc 8	1.00			
A_no 3	A_no 1	A_no 2	1.00			
A_no 6	A_no 4	A_no 5	1.00			
A_no 9	A_no 7	A_no 8	1.00			
S_ul 3	S_ul 1	S_ul 2	1.00	S_ul 1	**0.500**	S_ul 4
S_ul 6	S_ul 4	S_ul 5	1.00	S_ul 4	0.983	S_ul 7
				S_ul 5	**0.753**	S_ul 2
S_ul 9	S_ul 7	S_ul 8	1.00			
A_ot 3	A_ot 1	A_ot 2	1.00			
A_ot 6	A_ot 7	A_ot 8	1.00			

Table 6. Parentage analysis in Cervus using the LOD and Delta computation. The different confidence values are indicated by the following codes: * = confidence level higher than 95%. In the table, misallocation or low assignment probabilities are highlighted in bold.

	LOD						Delta			
Offspring	Candidate Mother	Pair Confidence	Candidate Father	Pair Confidence	Trio Confidence	Offspring	Candidate Mother	Pair Confidence	Candidate Father	Pair Confidence
S_al 3	S_al 1	*	S_al 2	*	*	S_al 3	S_al 1	*	S_al 2	*
S_al 6	S_al 3	*	S_al 4	*	*	S_al 6	S_al 3	*	S_al 4	*
S_al 9	S_al 7	*	S_al 8	*	*	S_al 9	S_al 7	*	S_al 8	*
S_ne 3	S_ne 1	*	S_ne 2	*	*	S_ne 3	S_ne 1	*	S_ne 2	*
S_ne 6	S_ne 4	*	S_ne 5	*	*	S_ne 6	S_ne 4	*	S_ne 5	*
S_ne 9	S_ne 7	*	S_ne 8	*	*	S_ne 9	S_ne 7	*	S_ne 8	*
S_ur 3	S_ur 1	*	S_ur 2	*	*	S_ur 3	S_ur 1	*	S_ur 2	*
S_ur 6	S_ur 4		S_ur 5	*	*	S_ur 6	S_ur 4		S_ur 5	*
B_bu 3	B_bu 1	*	B_bu 2	*	*	B_bu 3	B_bu 1	*	B_bu 2	*

Table 6. *Cont.*

	LOD						Delta			
Offspring	Candidate Mother	Pair Confidence	Candidate Father	Pair Confidence	Trio Confidence	Offspring	Candidate Mother	Pair Confidence	Candidate Father	Pair Confidence
B_bu 6	B_bu 4	*	B_bu 5	*	*	B_bu 6	B_bu 4	*	B_bu 5	*
B_bu 9	B_bu 7	*	B_bu 8	*	*	B_bu 9	B_bu 7	*	B_bu 8	*
B_sc 3	B_sc 1	*	B_sc 2	*	*	B_sc 3	B_sc 1	*	B_sc 2	*
B_sc 6	B_sc 4	*	B_sc 5	*	*	B_sc 6	B_sc 4	*	B_sc 5	*
B_sc 9	B_sc 7	*	B_sc 8	*	*	B_sc 9	B_sc 7	*	B_sc 8	*
O_sc 3	O_sc 1	*	O_sc 2	*	*	O_sc 3	O_sc 1	*	O_sc 2	*
O_sc 6	O_sc 4	*	O_sc 5	*	*	O_sc 6	O_sc 4	*	O_sc 5	*
O_sc 9	O_sc 7	*	O_sc 8	*	*	O_sc 9	O_sc 7	*	O_sc 8	*
A_no 3	A_no 1	*	A_no 2	*	*	A_no 3	A_no 1	*	A_no 2	*
A_no 6	A_no 4	*	A_no 5	*	*	A_no 6	A_no 4	*	A_no 5	*
A_no 9	A_no 7	*	A_no 8	*	*	A_no 9	A_no 7	*	A_no 8	*
S_ul 3	S_ul 1	*	S_ul 5	*	*	S_ul 3	S_ul 1	*	**S_ul 5**	*
S_ul 6	S_ul 4	*	**S_ul 5**	*	*	S_ul 6	S_ul 4	*	S_ul 5	*
S_ul 9	S_ul 7	*	S_ul 8	*	*	S_ul 9	S_ul 7	*	S_ul 8	*
A_ot 3	A_ot 1	*	A_ot 2	*	*	A_ot 3	A_ot 1	*	A_ot 2	*
A_ot 6	A_ot 7	*	A_ot 8	*	*	A_ot 6	A_ot 7	*	A_ot 8	*

4. Discussion

International wildlife trafficking today is recognized as one of the largest organized transnational crimes [38], which equals the trafficking of drugs, arms and humans (World Wildlife Report, United Nations: Office on Drugs and Crime).

Genotyping assays through microsatellites are a quick, informative and low-cost approach for linking items of evidence to crimes in forensic investigations [39]. Since microsatellites have high mutation rates, they are used within the context of monitoring illegal wildlife trade primarily to identify individuals, assign individuals to specific populations or for relatedness testing. Oklander et al. [39] generated a multilocus microsatellite genotype reference database of the black and gold howler monkey (*Alouatta caraya*), a neotropical primate threatened by habitat loss and capture for illegal trade in Argentina, to assign confiscated individuals to localities of origin, illustrating the applicability of genotype databases for inferring hotspots of illegal capture. Potoczniak et al. [39] developed a STR genotyping assay able to associate a biological sample to Asian elephant (*Elephas maximus*) or African elephant (*Loxodonta africana*). Fitzsimmons et al. [40] designed a panel of 26 microsatellite loci for *Crocodylus* spp. to answer questions regarding population assignment, mating system and geneflow. Jan and Fumagalli [41] isolated DNA microsatellite markers in seven parrot species threatened with extinction and subjected to illegal trafficking, characterized a total of 106 polymorphic microsatellite markers and tested them for individual identification and parental analyses. Mucci and colleagues [42] developed a panel of 16 de novo sequenced microsatellites (STRs) for *Testudo graeca* and tested its effectiveness for parentage analysis in two other species of endangered tortoises, *T. hermanni* and *T. marginata*.

Given the utility of STR-based approaches to answer questions related to wildlife crime investigations as forensic genetics, efforts should be devoted to the characterization of microsatellite primers for species threatened by illegal trafficking. However, while in human forensics, the selection of around 20 core STR loci allowed the standardization around the globe for human identity testing [43,44], accomplishing this same achievement is more challenging for the hyper-diverse animal assemblage encountered in wildlife forensics [38].

The lack of species-specific molecular markers or their inadequate representation in genetic databases is major limitation in wildlife forensics [45].

Cross-amplification is a widely used approach permitting to avoid investing time and money in the development of new markers, and many studies have proven the efficiency of microsatellite loci developed in closely related species [42,46–49].

The first aim of this study was to test for the presence of a minimum number of microsatellite loci reliable for individual identification and parentage analysis for forensic purposes in 11 species of Strigiformes listed in the CITES Appendix II and regularly traded in the Italian national market.

Literature data show that cross-species transferability is unevenly distributed across taxa. Barbará et al. [50] reviewed 64 primer notes and found more than 40% transfer success in mammals, more than 25% in fishes and more than 10% in birds. Our results permitted to define a unique panel of 12 out of 32 highly polymorphic microsatellites (37%), able to identify individuals in nine species of two subfamilies of Strigiformes (Striginae and Surninae) belonging to Family Strigidae (*A. otus, A. noctua, B. bubo, B. scandiacus, O. scops, S. aluco, S. nebulosa, S. uralensis, S. ulula*).

The test was non-efficient in individuals of *T. alba* in which only six markers yield a positive result but four of them resulted monomorphic. Such results could rely on the fact that *T. alba* is the only species of this study belonging to a different family [51]. The two monophyletic families of Strigiformes, Tytonidae and Strigidae, diverged in the middle of the Eocene [52]. The phylogenetic divergence of Tytonidae from Strigidae could be justified by the retrieved inefficiency of markers panel tested on species. Since only two subfamilies represent Tytonidae family with a single genus each [53]—Tytoninae with *Tyto* and Phodilinae with *Phodilus*—it is not possible to verify the discriminant power of tested markers on other species of the same taxon.

The common barn owl *T. alba* is one of the most cosmopolitan species and represents a taxon-rich species complex with several subspecies [54]. The interest in its conservation status clears the need for integrating this set with more polymorphic loci for this species. Twenty-one microsatellite loci already isolated and characterized in *T. alba* [26] could be tested for cross-amplification in CITES species to implement this panel.

The principal component analysis results reflect the most recent knowledge about taxonomy and systematics of Strigiformes [53].

A slightly better but similar result was obtained for *G. passerinum*, for which only 4 markers were polymorphic. The high number of monomorphic loci in this species could be due to several cumulative factors: the low number of related individuals analyzed, the high inbreeding of captive-bred individuals, or the inefficiency of the selected markers for this species. Unlike *T. alba*, microsatellites were developed only for a species of the same genera: *Glaucidium brasilianum* [23].

Evaluating the STR panel potential in identifying family groups, we found that in two out of the nine species analyzed (*S. uralensis* and *S. ulula*), the probability value associated with parent pairs was reduced. The PID_{sib} almost reached the 0.001 threshold value in *S. ulula, S. nebulosa* and *S. uralensis* (see Table 4: Probability of identity values, PID and PID_{sibs}). However, PID and PID_{sib} values are subjected to bias due to the low number of tested individuals per species and bottleneck in captive breeding facilities. For these three species, it could be helpful to increase the number of samples and markers to obtain a more confident individual identification and association to parent pairs.

Besides reducing time and costs when adopting a cross-amplification approach, another advantage of using a shared panel among several species is the possibility of comparing genetic variability values among species. Nevertheless, even if microsatellites loci are very useful genetic markers in studying the mating system, population genetics, and conservation of owls, many studies focus on species belonging to the same genus. Dial et al. [55] screened many markers developed in strigids but found only four polymorphic pairs in the great horned owl (*Bubo virginianus*), short-eared owl (*Asio flammeus*) and the snowy owl (*Bubo scandiacus*). In addition, another eight reliably amplified polymorphic fragments only in the great horned owl, eleven in the short-eared owl, and ten in the snowy owl.

Hsu et al. [22] developed six new microsatellite markers containing tetranucleotide repeat motifs (GATA/CTAT) for Lanyu scops owl (*Otus elegans botelensis*). They tested them, and additional further microsatellite primer pairs previously developed from *O. elegans* on four other species of owls (*O. lettia, O. spilocephalus, O. scops* and *Ninox scutulata*). Data obtained showed a reduced degree of polymorphism with most of the loci resulting polymorphic in the three *Otus* owls but only five in *N. scutulata*.

Our study gives a valuable tool to implement research involving most Strigidae threatened by illegal trafficking, habitat loss and fragmentation in Italy and other countries.

Delport et al. [56] tested 19 loci originally developed for Vidua and Geospiza for cross-amplification in Nesospiza buntings. They detected a degree of polymorphism and heterozygosity lower in loci developed for Vidua than those explicitly developed for Nesospiza. These data demonstrate that microsatellite markers isolated in the reference species are frequently less variable in related species. Moreover, cross-species amplification is usually limited to the loci that were found polymorphic in the referent species. In this study, we selected from the literature the most variable loci in each reference species: most polymorphic loci were discarded only when they were found monomorphic or did not give amplification products in all the target species, with only three exceptions as mentioned in Results (Paragraph ii), because of their utility in other species. We are aware that this a priori selection can cause an ascertainment bias, as suggested by Delport et al. [56]; however, we found high levels of polymorphisms in nine out 11 analyzed species.

Variability indices found in different species using this panel were not discordant from the ones found in the natural populations with different markers: Pellegrino et al. [57] found in the *A. noctua* European populations an average and an effective number of alleles = 5.6 and 3.5, respectively, and observed and expected heterozygosities equal to 0.59 and 0.61, respectively. Pertoldi et al. [58] found lower alleles in the Danish population (effective number of alleles = 2.8; Ho = 0.51 and He = 0.60), probably caused by a population bottleneck in the last decades.

Microsatellite loci represent reliable molecular markers to describe genetic variability or its drastic reduction, as demonstrated by Macías-Duarte et al. [59] that found different values in three different populations of *Athene cunicularia*, with the average number of alleles varying from 2.7 in Clarion Islands to 5.1 in Florida and 22.5 in Western North America.

Though their high polymorphism makes them adequate for conservation and forensic genetics purposes, the main difficulties are represented by comparing samples between laboratories.

This problem that has been resolved through the exchange of reference samples has been recently fixed by the set-up of an allelic ladder [60]. According to these authors, we constructed an allelic ladder for each locus to standardize a protocol between laboratories for conservation and forensic purposes.

Comparability between laboratories is now also possible thanks to high-throughput sequencing (HTS) technologies [61]. This application that has been developed and used in human forensics [62–64] has been already applied also in conservation genetics [65–68]. This method permits the sequencing of STRs, allowing the identification of the correct number of repeats. The possibility of multiplexing several dozen of markers from a single individual will allow cost and time reduction. De Barba et al. [69] used this protocol in the study of a brown bear population yielded reliable results of parentage analysis also from low quality DNA, confirming a broader application in conservation genetics and forensics.

5. Conclusions

The newly optimized 12 loci can provide the authorities with the ability to investigate suspected smugglers and false parental claims or establish a link between evidence and an individual (e.g., identifying when a bird is illegally transferred between different breeding facilities). In addition to this, the selected markers can be used to assess relatedness among captive-bred individuals, which can be crucial in designing optimal breeding protocols to avoid genetic variability loss and minimize inbreeding. Moreover, these markers are useful for applications in research projects on wild populations where individual genotype identification allows to describe the mating system, genetic variability, population structure and geneflow among nine different species of Strigiformes with conservation concern.

Supplementary Materials: The following are available online at https://www.mdpi.com/article/10.3390/genes12111721/s1, Figure S1: allelic ladders; Figure S2: individual genotypes.

Author Contributions: Conceptualization, N.M., G.A., R.F., M.Z.; methodology: N.M., C.M., C.G., P.G.; Validation: P.G., N.M., C.G.; formal analysis, P.G., L.N., A.P.; writing—original draft preparation, N.M., P.G.; writing—review and editing, P.G., C.M., A.P., C.G., M.Z., R.F., G.A.; supervision, N.M., R.F.; project administration, N.M., C.M. All authors have read and agreed to the published version of the manuscript.

Funding: This research received no external funding.

Institutional Review Board Statement: Ethical review and approval were waived for this study since they are not officially required by national regulations. In any case, the study abided by local policies and regulations. The methods applied in this study were carried out in strict accordance with the Nature and Sea Protection Directorate (DPNM, which belongs to the Ministry for the Ecological Transition) and the Italian Institute for Environmental Protection and Research (ISPRA). The breeders authorized the feather's sampling of their own animals. The handling of animals and feather's samplings were carried out by qualified veterinary personnel in accordance with animal welfare procedures and in the presence and under the jurisdiction of the Italian forest police units (Carabinieri Command). The Carabinieri Command exercises management, coordination and control functions of the CITES operational units, in charge for the application of CITES directives. The CITES units checked that the breeders fulfilled requirements of the art. 54 of Reg. (CE) n. 865/2006 for investigations of birth in captivity.

Informed Consent Statement: Not applicable.

Acknowledgments: The authors gratefully acknowledge the Italian Ministry for Ecological Transition (MITE), particularly the Italian CITES Management Authority, which since 1997 granted support to the Unit for Conservation Genetics (BIO-CGE) at ISPRA, and allowed us to develop molecular procedures for improving wildlife forensics.

Conflicts of Interest: The authors declare no conflict of interest.

References

1. Anderson, S.C.; Elsen, P.R.; Hughes, B.B.; Tonietto, R.K.; Bletz, M.C.; Gill, D.A.; Holgerson, M.A.; Kuebbing, S.E.; McDonough MacKenzie, C.; Meek, M.H.; et al. Trends in ecology and conservation over eight decades. *Front. Ecol. Environ.* **2021**, *19*, 274–282. [CrossRef]
2. Bishop, J.M.; Leslie, A.J.; Bourquin, S.L.; O'Ryan, C. Reduced effective population size in an overexploited population of the Nile crocodile (*Crocodylus niloticus*). *Biol. Conserv.* **2009**, *142*, 2335–2341. [CrossRef]
3. Betancourth-Cundar, M.; Palacios-Rodríguez, P.; Mejía-Vargas, D.; Paz, A.; Amézquita, A. Genetic differentiation and overexploitation history of the critically endangered Lehmann's Poison Frog: Oophaga lehmanni. *Conserv. Genet.* **2020**, *21*, 453–465. [CrossRef]
4. Righi, T.; Splendiani, A.; Fioravanti, T.; Casoni, E.; Gioacchini, G.; Carnevali, O.; Barucchi, V.C. Loss of mitochondrial genetic diversity in overexploited mediterranean swordfish (*Xiphias gladius*, 1759) population. *Diversity* **2020**, *12*, 170. [CrossRef]
5. Baker, S.E.; Cain, R.; Kesteren, F.V.; Zommers, Z.A.; D'Cruze, N.; MacDonald, D.W. Rough trade: Animal welfare in the global wildlife trade. *BioScience* **2013**, *63*, 928–938. [CrossRef]
6. Tingley, M.W.; Harris, J.B.C.; Hua, F.; Wilcove, D.S. The pet trade's role in defaunation. *Science* **2017**, *356*, 1–916. [CrossRef] [PubMed]
7. Panter, C.T.; Atkinson, E.D.; White, R.L. Retraction: Quantifying the global legal trade in live CITES-listed raptors and owls for commercial purposes over a 40-year period. *Avocetta* **2019**, *43*, 23–36. [CrossRef]
8. Vall-Llosera, M.; Su, S. Trends and characteristics of imports of live CITES-listed bird species into Japan. *Ibis* **2019**, *161*, 590–604. [CrossRef]
9. Brochet, A.L.; Van Den Bossche, W.; Jbour, S.; Ndang'Ang'A, P.K.; Jones, V.R.; Abdou, W.A.L.I.; Al-Hmoud, A.R.; Asswad, N.G.; Atienza, J.C.; Atrash, I.; et al. Preliminary assessment of the scope and scale of illegal killing and taking of birds in the Mediterranean. *Bird Conserv. Int.* **2016**, *26*, 1–28. [CrossRef]

10. Domínguez, M.; Tiedemann, R.; Reboreda, J.C.; Segura, L.; Tittarelli, F.; Mahler, B. Genetic structure reveals management units for the yellow cardinal (*Gubernatrix cristata*), endangered by habitat loss and illegal trapping. *Conserv. Genet.* **2017**, *18*, 1131–1140. [CrossRef]

11. Harris, J.B.C.; Green, J.M.H.; Prawiradilaga, D.M.; Giam, X.; Giyanto; Hikmatullah, D.; Putra, C.A.; Wilcove, D.S. Using market data and expert opinion to identify overexploited species in the wild bird trade. *Biol. Conserv.* **2015**, *187*, 51–60. [CrossRef]

12. Evans, S.R.; Sheldon, B.C. Interspecific patterns of genetic diversity in birds: Correlations with extinction risk. *Conserv. Biol.* **2008**, *22*, 1016–1025. [CrossRef] [PubMed]

13. Enríquez, P.L.; Eisermann, K.; Mikkola, H.; Motta-Junior, J.C. A review of the systematics of Neotropical owls (Strigiformes). *Neotrop. Owls Divers. Conserv.* **2017**, 1–670. [CrossRef]

14. Wink, M.; El-Sayed, A.A.; Sauer-Gürth, H.; Gonzalez, J. Molecular phylogeny of owls (Strigiformes) inferred from DNA sequences of the mitochondrial cytochrome b and the nuclear RAG-1 gene. *Ardea* **2009**, *97*, 581–591. [CrossRef]

15. Abdel Rabou, A.F.N. On the Owls (Order Strigiformes) Inhabiting the Gaza Strip—Palestine. *JOJ Wildl. Biodivers.* **2020**, *3*, 1–11. [CrossRef]

16. Wan, H.Y.; Ganey, J.L.; Vojta, C.D.; Cushman, S.A. Managing emerging threats to spotted owls. *J. Wildl. Manag.* **2018**, *82*, 682–697. [CrossRef]

17. Li, L.; Jiang, Z. International trade of CITES listed bird species in China. *PLoS ONE* **2014**, *9*, e85012. [CrossRef]

18. Ribeiro, J.; Reino, L.; Schindler, S.; Strubbe, D.; Vall-llosera, M.; Araújo, M.B.; Capinha, C.; Carrete, M.; Mazzoni, S.; Monteiro, M.; et al. Trends in legal and illegal trade of wild birds: A global assessment based on expert knowledge. *Biodivers. Conserv.* **2019**, *28*, 3343–3369. [CrossRef]

19. Nijman, V.; Nekaris, K.A.I. The Harry Potter effect: The rise in trade of owls as pets in Java and Bali, Indonesia. *Glob. Ecol. Conserv.* **2017**, *11*, 84–94. [CrossRef]

20. Siriwat, P.; Nekaris, K.A.I.; Nijman, V. Digital media and the modern-day pet trade: A test of the 'Harry Potter effect' and the owl trade in Thailand. *Endanger. Species Res.* **2020**, *41*, 7–16. [CrossRef]

21. Isaksson, M.; Tegelström, H. Characterization of polymorphic microsatellite markers in a captive population of the eagle owl (*Bubo bubo*) used for supportive breeding. *Mol. Ecol. Notes* **2002**, *2*, 91–93. [CrossRef]

22. Hsu, Y.C.; Li, S.H.; Lin, Y.S.; Severinghaus, L.L. Microsatellite loci from Lanyu scops owl (*Otus elegans botelensis*) and their cross-species application in four species of strigidae. *Conserv. Genet.* **2006**, *7*, 161–165. [CrossRef]

23. Proudfoot, G.; Honeycutt, R.; Douglas Slack, R. Development and characterization of microsatellite DNA primers for ferruginous pygmy-owls (*Glaucidium brasilianum*). *Mol. Ecol. Notes* **2005**, *5*, 90–92. [CrossRef]

24. Hull, J.M.; Keane, J.J.; Tell, L.A.; Ernest, H.B. Development of 37 microsatellite loci for the great gray owl (*Strix nebulosa*) and other *Strix* spp. owls. *Conserv. Genet.* **2008**, *9*, 1357–1361. [CrossRef]

25. Klein, A.; Horsburgh, G.J.; Kupper, C.; Major, A.; Lee, P.L.M.; Hoffmann, G.; Matics, R.; Dawson, D.A. Microsatellite markers characterized in the barn owl (*Tyto alba*) and high utility in the other owls (Strigiformes: AVES). *Mol. Ecol. Resour.* **2009**, *9*, 1513–1519. [CrossRef]

26. Burri, R.; Antoniazza, S.; Siverio, F.; Klein, Á.; Roulin, A.; Fumagalli, L. Isolation and characterization of 21 microsatellite markers in the barn owl (*Tyto alba*). *Mol. Ecol. Resour.* **2008**, *8*, 977–979. [CrossRef] [PubMed]

27. Hogan, F.E.; Cooke, R.; Norman, J.A. Reverse ascertainment bias in microsatellite allelic diversity in owls (Aves, Strigiformes). *Conserv. Genet.* **2009**, *10*, 635–638. [CrossRef]

28. Kleven, O.; Dawson, D.A.; Gjershaug, J.O.; Horsburgh, G.J.; Jacobsen, K.O.; Wabakken, P. Isolation, characterization and predicted genome locations of Eurasian eagle-owl (*Bubo bubo*) microsatellite loci. *Conserv. Genet. Resour.* **2013**, *5*, 723–727. [CrossRef]

29. Hsu, Y.C.; Severinghaus, L.L.; Lin, Y.S.; Li, S.H. Isolation and characterization of microsatellite DNA markers from the Lanyu scops owl (*Otus elegans botelensis*). *Mol. Ecol. Notes* **2003**, *3*, 595–597. [CrossRef]

30. Thode, A.B.; Maltbie, M.; Hansen, L.A.; Green, L.D.; Longmire, J.L. Microsatellite markers for the Mexican spotted owl (*Strix occidentalis* lucida). *Mol. Ecol. Notes* **2002**, *2*, 446–448. [CrossRef]

31. Topinka, J.R.; May, B. Development of polymorphic microsatellite loci in the northern goshawk (*Accipiter gentilis*) and cross-amplification in other raptor species. *Conserv. Genet.* **2004**, *5*, 861–864. [CrossRef]

32. Peakall, R.; Smouse, P.E. GenAlEx 6.5: Genetic analysis in Excel. Population genetic software for teaching and research–an update. *Bioinformatics* **2012**, *28*, 2537–2539. [CrossRef] [PubMed]

33. Valière, N. GIMLET: A computer program for analysing genetic individual identification data. *Mol. Ecol. Notes* **2002**, *2*, 377–379. [CrossRef]

34. Jones, O.R.; Wang, J. COLONY: A program for parentage and sibship inference from multilocus genotype data. *Mol. Ecol. Resour.* **2010**, *10*, 551–555. [CrossRef]

35. Marshall, T.C.; Slate, J.; Kruuk, L.E.B.; Pemberton, J.M. Statistical confidence for likelihood-based paternity inference in natural populations. *Mol. Ecol.* **1998**, *7*, 639–655. [CrossRef]

36. Kalinowski, S.T.; Taper, M.L.; Marshall, T.C. Revising how the computer program CERVUS accommodates genotyping error increases success in paternity assignment. *Mol. Ecol.* **2007**, *16*, 1099–1106. [CrossRef] [PubMed]

37. Belkhir, K.; Borsa, P.; Chikhi, L.; Raufaste, N.; Bonhomme, F. *Genetix 4.05, Logiciel Sous Windows Tm Pour La Génétique Des Populations*; Laboratoire Genome, Populations, Interactions, CNRS UMR 5000, Universite de Montpellier II: Montpellier, France, 1996–2004.

38. Smart, U.; Cihlar, J.C.; Budowle, B. International Wildlife Trafficking: A perspective on the challenges and potential forensic genetics solutions. *Forensic Sci. Int. Genet.* **2021**, *54*, 102551. [CrossRef] [PubMed]

39. Potoczniak, M.J.; Chermak, M.; Quarino, L.; Tobe, S.S.; Conte, J. Development of a multiplex, PCR-based genotyping assay for African and Asian elephants for forensic purposes. *Int. J. Leg. Med.* **2020**, *134*, 55–62. [CrossRef]

40. Fitzsimmons, N.N.; Tanksley, S.; Forstner, M.R.J.; Louis, E.E.; Daglish, R.; Gratten, J.; Davis, S. Microsatellite markers for Crocodylus: New genetic tools for population genetics, mating system studies and forensics. *Crocodilian Biol. Evol.* **2001**, 51–57.

41. Jan, C.; Fumagalli, L. Polymorphic DNA microsatellite markers for forensic individual identification and parentage analyses of seven threatened species of parrots (family Psittacidae). *PeerJ* **2016**, *2016*, 1–7. [CrossRef]

42. Mucci, N.; Giangregorio, P.; Cirasella, L.; Isani, G.; Mengoni, C. A new STR panel for parentage analysis in endangered tortoises. *Conserv. Genet. Resour.* **2020**, *12*, 67–75. [CrossRef]

43. Zhou, Z.; Shao, C.; Xie, J.; Xu, H.; Liu, Y.; Zhou, Y.; Liu, Z.; Zhao, Z.; Tang, Q.; Sun, K. Genetic polymorphism and phylogenetic analyses of 21 non-CODIS STR loci in a Chinese Han population from Shanghai. *Mol. Genet. Genom. Med.* **2020**, *8*, 1–8. [CrossRef] [PubMed]

44. Kumar, A.; Kumar, R.; Kumawat, R.K.; Shrivastava, P.; Chaubey, G. Genomic diversity at 22 STR loci (extended CODIS STR) in the population of Rajasthan, India. *Gene Rep.* **2021**, *23*, 101150. [CrossRef]

45. Rocco, F.D.; Anello, M. The Use of Forensic DNA on the Conservation of Neotropical Mammals. In *Molecular Ecology and Conservation Genetics of Neotropical Mammals*; Springer Nature Switzerland AG: Cham, Switzerland, 2021; pp. 85–98.

46. Gebhardt, K.J.; Waits, L.P. Cross-species amplification and optimization of microsatellite markers for use in six Neotropical parrots. *Mol. Ecol. Resour.* **2008**, *8*, 835–839. [CrossRef] [PubMed]

47. Dawson, D.A.; Horsburgh, G.J.; Küpper, C.; Stewart, I.R.K.; Ball, A.D.; Durrant, K.L.; Hansson, B.; Bacon, I.; Bird, S.; Klein, Á.; et al. New methods to identify conserved microsatellite loci and develop primer sets of high cross-species utility—As demonstrated for birds. *Mol. Ecol. Resour.* **2010**, *10*, 475–494. [CrossRef] [PubMed]

48. Maulidi, A.; Fatchiyah, F.; Hamidy, A.; Kurniawan, N. Microsatellite Marker for Cross-Species Amplification: Study Case for Indonesian Sundaland Python (Serpentes: Pythonidae). *J. Exp. Life Sci.* **2018**, *8*, 61–65. [CrossRef]

49. Du Toit, Z.; Dalton, D.L.; du Plessis, M.; Jansen, R.; Grobler, J.P.; Kotzé, A. Isolation and characterization of 30 STRs in Temminck's ground pangolin (*Smutsia temminckii*) and potential for cross amplification in other African species. *J. Genet.* **2020**, *99*. [CrossRef]

50. Barbará, T.; Palma-Silva, C.; Paggi, G.M.; Bered, F.; Fay, M.F.; Lexer, C. Cross-species transfer of nuclear microsatellite markers: Potential and limitations. *Mol. Ecol.* **2007**, *16*, 3759–3767. [CrossRef]

51. König, C.; Weick, F. *Owls of the World*; AandC Black Publishers Ltd.: London, UK, 2008.

52. Prum, R.O.; Berv, J.S.; Dornburg, A.; Field, D.J.; Townsend, J.P.; Lemmon, E.M.; Lemmon, A.R. A comprehensive phylogeny of birds (Aves) using targeted next-generation DNA sequencing. *Nature* **2015**, *526*, 569–573. [CrossRef] [PubMed]

53. Wink, M.; Sauer-Gurth, H. Molecular taxonomy and systematics of owls (Strigiformes)—An update. *Airo* **2021**, *29*, 487–500.

54. Aliabadian, M.; Alaei-Kakhki, N.; Mirshamsi, O.; Nijman, V.; Roulin, A. Phylogeny, biogeography, and diversification of barn owls (Aves: Strigiformes). *Biol. J. Linn. Soc.* **2016**, *119*, 904–918. [CrossRef]

55. Dial, C.R.; Talbot, S.L.; Sage, G.K.; Seidensticker, M.T.; Holt, D.W. Cross-species Amplification of Microsatellite Markers in the Great Horned Owl *Bubo virginianus*, Short-eared Owl *Asio flammeus* and Snowy Owl *B. scandiacus* for Use in Population Genetics, Individual Identification and Parentage Studies. *J. Yamashina Inst. Ornithol.* **2012**, *44*, 1–12. [CrossRef]

56. Delport, W.; Grant, T.J.; Ryan, P.G.; Bloomer, P. Ten microsatellite loci for evolutionary research on Nesospiza buntings. *Mol. Ecol. Notes* **2006**, *6*, 1180–1183. [CrossRef]

57. Pellegrino, I.; Negri, A.; Boano, G.; Cucco, M.; Kristensen, T.N.; Pertoldi, C.; Randi, E.; Šálek, M.; Mucci, N. Evidence for strong genetic structure in European populations of the little owl Athene noctua. *J. Avian Biol.* **2015**, *46*, 462–475. [CrossRef]

58. Pertoldi, C.; Pellegrino, I.; Cucco, M.; Mucci, N.; Randi, E.; Laursen, J.T.; Sunde, P.; Loeschcke, V.; Kristensen, T.N.; du Toit, Z.; et al. Genetic consequences of population decline in the Danish population of the little owl (*Athene noctua*). *Mol. Ecol.* **2020**, *14*, 358–367. [CrossRef]

59. Macías-Duarte, A.; Conway, C.J.; Holroyd, G.L.; Valdez-Gómez, H.E.; Culver, M. Genetic Variation among Island and Continental Populations of Burrowing Owl (*Athene cunicularia*) Subspecies in North America. *J. Raptor Res.* **2019**, *53*, 127–133. [CrossRef]

60. Biello, R.; Zampiglia, M.; Corti, C.; Deli, G.; Biaggini, M.; Crestanello, B.; Delaugerre, M.; Di Tizio, L.; Leonetti Francesco, L.; Stefano, C.; et al. Mapping the geographic origin of captive and confiscated Hermann's tortoises: A genetic toolkit for conservation and forensic analyses. *Forensic Sci. Int. Genet.* **2021**, *51*, 102447. [CrossRef] [PubMed]

61. Glenn, T.C. Field guide to next-generation DNA sequencers. *Mol. Ecol. Resour.* **2011**, *11*, 759–769. [CrossRef]

62. Fordyce, S.L.; Ávila-Arcos, M.C.; Rockenbauer, E.; Børsting, C.; Frank-Hansen, R.; Petersen, F.T.; Willerslev, E.; Hansen, A.J.; Morling, N.; Gilbert, T.P. High-throughput sequencing of core STR loci for forensic genetic investigations using the Roche Genome Sequencer FLX platform. *BioTechniques* **2011**, *51*, 127–133. [CrossRef] [PubMed]

63. Bornman, D.M.; Hester, M.E.; Schuetter, J.M.; Kasoji, M.D.; Minard-Smith, A.; Barden, C.A.; Faith, S.A. Short-read, high-throughput sequencing technology for STR genotyping. *BioTechniques. Rapid Dispatches* **2012**, *23*, 1–7. [CrossRef]

64. Van Neste, C.; Van Nieuwerburgh, F.; Van Hoofstat, D.; Deforce, D. Forensic STR analysis using massive parallel sequencing. *Forensic Sci. Int. Genet.* **2012**, *6*, 810–818. [CrossRef]

65. Stoeckle, B.C.; Theuerkauf, J.; Rouys, S.; Gula, R.; Lorenzo, A.; Lambert, C.; Kaeser, T.; Kuehn, R. Identification of polymorphic microsatellite loci for the endangered Kagu (*Rhynochetos jubatus*) by high-throughput sequencing. *J. Ornithol.* **2012**, *153*, 249–253. [CrossRef]

66. Pimentel, J.S.M.; Carmo, A.O.; Rosse, I.C.; Martins, A.P.V.; Ludwig, S.; Facchin, S.; Pereira, A.H.; Brandão-Dias, P.F.P.; Abreu, N.L.; Kalapothakis, E. High-throughput sequencing strategy for microsatellite genotyping using neotropical fish as a model. *Front. Genet.* **2018**, *9*, 1–8. [CrossRef]

67. Qi, W.H.; Lu, T.; Zheng, C.L.; Jiang, X.M.; Jie, H.; Zhang, X.Y.; Yue, B.S.; Zhao, G.J. Distribution patterns of microsatellites and development of its marker in different genomic regions of forest musk deer genome based on high throughput sequencing. *Aging* **2020**, *12*, 4445–4462. [CrossRef] [PubMed]

68. Song, C.; Feng, Z.; Li, C.; Sun, Z.; Gao, T.; Song, N.; Liu, L. Profile and development of microsatellite primers for Acanthogobius ommaturus based on high-throughput sequencing technology. *J. Oceanol. Limnol.* **2020**, *38*, 1880–1890. [CrossRef]

69. De Barba, M.; Miquel, C.; Lobréaux, S.; Quenette, P.Y.; Swenson, J.E.; Taberlet, P. High-throughput microsatellite genotyping in ecology: Improved accuracy, efficiency, standardization and success with low-quantity and degraded DNA. *Mol. Ecol. Resour.* **2017**, *17*, 492–507. [CrossRef] [PubMed]

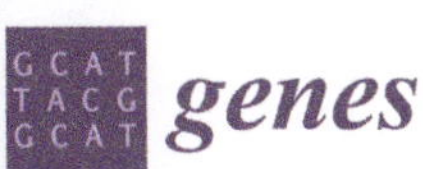

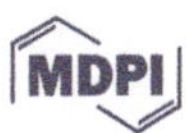

Article

Individual Identification with Short Tandem Repeat Analysis and Collection of Secondary Information Using Microbiome Analysis

Solip Lee [1], Heesang You [1], Songhee Lee [2], Yeongju Lee [2], Hee-Gyoo Kang [3], Ho-Joong Sung [3], Jiwon Choi [4] and Sunghee Hyun [1,2,*]

[1] Department of Senior Healthcare, Graduate School, Eulji University, Uijeongbu-si 11759, Korea; zhdndl@naver.com (S.L.); yhs1532@nate.com (H.Y.)

[2] Department of Biomedical Laboratory Science, Graduate School, Eulji University, Uijeongbu-si 11759, Korea; song-1107@naver.com (S.L.); dlddwn1@gmail.com (Y.L.)

[3] Department of Biomedical Laboratory Science, College of Health Sciences, Eulji University, Seongnam 13135, Korea; kanghg@eulji.ac.kr (H.-G.K.); hjsung@eulji.ac.kr (H.-J.S.)

[4] Forensic DNA Analysis Division, National Forensic Service, Seoul 08636, Korea; ridnf@paran.com

* Correspondence: hyunsh@eulji.ac.kr; Tel.: +82-10-9412-8853

Abstract: Forensic investigation is important to analyze evidence and facilitate the search for key individuals, such as suspects and victims in a criminal case. The forensic use of genomic DNA has increased with the development of DNA sequencing technology, thereby enabling additional analysis during criminal investigations when additional legal evidence is required. In this study, we used next-generation sequencing to facilitate the generation of complementary data in order to analyze human evidence obtained through short tandem repeat (STR) analysis. We examined the applicability and potential of analyzing microbial genome communities. Microbiological supplementation information was confirmed for two of four failed STR samples. Additionally, the accuracy of the gargle sample was confirmed to be as high as 100% and was highly likely to be classified as a body fluid sample. Our experimental method confirmed that anthropological and microbiological evidence can be obtained by performing two experiments with one extraction. We discuss the advantages and disadvantages of using these techniques, explore prospects in the forensic field, and highlight suggestions for future research.

Keywords: next-generation sequencing; short tandem repeat; forensic microbiology; identification; microbiome

Citation: Lee, S.; You, H.; Lee, S.; Lee, Y.; Kang, H.-G.; Sung, H.-J.; Choi, J.; Hyun, S. Individual Identification with Short Tandem Repeat Analysis and Collection of Secondary Information Using Microbiome Analysis. *Genes* **2022**, *13*, 85. https://doi.org/10.3390/genes13010085

Academic Editor: Niels Morling

Received: 15 December 2021
Accepted: 27 December 2021
Published: 29 December 2021

Publisher's Note: MDPI stays neutral with regard to jurisdictional claims in published maps and institutional affiliations.

1. Introduction

Evidence analysis helps to support the alibis of individuals involved in legal cases and is crucial in the courtroom for scene reconstruction and suspect tracking. Evidence obtained regarding the victim or suspect is important in an investigation. Finding traces of a person who meets certain conditions at the scene is critical to forensic investigation because this evidence makes a connection with the perpetrator or victim and helps solve the case. There are various properties of important trace evidence, and the most prominent is evidence of human origin. Most of this evidence contains human DNA, which is useful for forensic judgment. Additionally, other types of evidence, such as unidentified and post-mortem traces, body hair, and behavior traces on the body of the victim or human-derived materials, can be collected. Based on the analysis, the results can be used to identify the crime scene and as proof of alibi. Such DNA evidence connects the case, victim, and suspect [1].

Short tandem repeat (STR) analysis is effective when there is clear evidence of human DNA. Human genetic material can be identified through DNA typing, thus providing proofs regarding individuals involved in the case [2,3]. Securing human DNA and analyzing STRs are important to identify comparable suspects and victims. Therefore, laboratories worldwide are studying the most efficient and effective way to acquire DNA evidence. Additionally, studies on evidence generated from low-level DNA profiles from trace DNA suggest that trace DNA can lead to successful case resolution [4,5]. However, some laboratories do not analyze trace DNA evidence because of low biomass of trace DNA or touch DNA samples [6].

STR analysis cannot guarantee a 100% success rate, and the assay success varies with the sample quantity and quality. Human DNA is considerably affected by environmental factors. The STR analysis may not be possible because DNA is damaged by high temperature, humidity, UV light, and microbial activation [7]. Therefore, low copy number (LCN) samples subjected to STR analysis sometimes render uninterpretable or inconclusive results [8]. Additionally, other results cannot be inferred from the results of LCN samples alone. Even if a sample contains non-existent or non-identifiable human DNA, it is likely that other substances or genes are present, as samples are collected from various sites and situations. Thus, other analytical methods may supplement information from low-quality STR results.

The human body hosts numerous microorganisms, and the human microbiome is influenced by the human body. For example, the microbiome is affected by various factors such as living environment [9], eating habits [10], age, sex [11,12], race [13], and the existence of a distinct microbiome field [14]. Thus, studies investigating whether individuals can be identified using microbiome characteristics that differ from one individual to another are being actively conducted [15–17]. Analysis of the microbiome has progressed to the point that the microbiome can be traced using biodiversity analysis. Furthermore, the microbiome is unique to an individual or a group and can reveal characteristic features known as the "microbial fingerprint." Individual microorganisms are used in the forensic field and in research related to individual identification during the progression of a case. Studies have included object and owner tracking [17,18], environmental tracking using soil microbes [19], bloodstain tracking [20], post-mortem interval tracking [14], and oral saliva identification [21–23]. By examining the characteristics of microorganisms (bacteria, fungi, and viruses) and linking them to individuals and case evidence, forensic microbiology can help obtain clues that can help resolve the case. Additionally, analyzing the microbiome makes it possible to montage trace DNA from suspects or victims and provides information on background tracing and scene reconstruction. Microorganisms are ubiquitous, and their quantity is considerably greater than that of human DNA. Proofs found at the scene may include those that do not have visible features, such as blood. The discovery of human DNA at crime scenes alone may not lead to prosecution based on genetic evidence. In fact, the prosecution of a case in Korea was canceled, despite the fact that the suspect was identified using Y-STR (STR on the Y chromosome) analysis [24]. Therefore, additional analysis is needed to supplement human genetic information and reveal the case background, proof of alibi, and connection of evidence.

Herein, we propose a human bacterial profiling method using next-generation sequencing to collect secondary information. In this study, using bacterial profiling, we investigated whether additional information can be obtained from samples of failed STR assays (Figure 1). Furthermore, we devised a method to classify and identify samples of unknown origin.

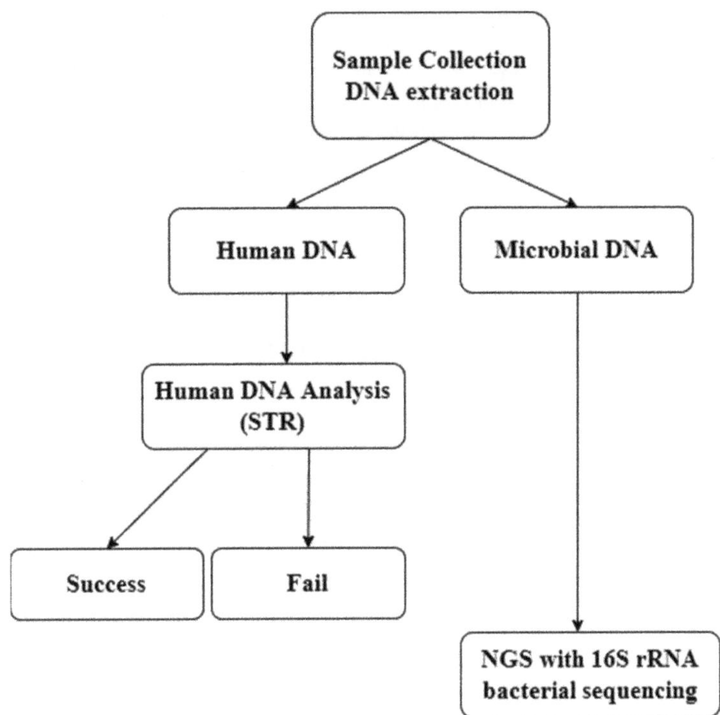

Figure 1. Schematic of the application of Bacterial profiling. Human DNA analysis and microbial DNA analysis are possible simultaneously through one DNA extraction.

2. Materials and Methods

2.1. Sample Collection and DNA Extraction

Samples were collected from student volunteers of Eulji University (Republic of Korea, Daejeon). The study protocol was approved by the internal review board of Eulji University (IRB No. EUIRB 2020-13). All volunteers were healthy adults in their 20s, with one male and nine female university students, and samples were collected from each individual during the same visit. A questionnaire was used to determine if the participant was under treatment with antibiotics or if there was environmental contamination, such as alcoholic disinfection of the hand or mobile phone. If a volunteer was administered antibiotics or had disinfected the hand or mobile phone within 2 h before sampling, sampling was discontinued (Table S1).

We used sterile, DNA-free cotton-tipped applicators (Puritan Medical Products Co., Guilford, ME, USA) to swab individual mobile phones and surface skin of the fingertip of the ventral joint. The tip of the applicator was then cut with sterile pair of scissors and collected in a 1.5 mL collection tube. Oral gargle and urine samples were collected in sterile 8 mL collection tubes. To obtain gargle samples, the volunteers were provided drinking water to swirl the floor of their mouths 10 times. The samples were stored at −80 °C until DNA extraction. Each sample swab was mixed with 700 μL of phosphate-buffered saline and 12 glass beads (2 mm) in a 1.5 mL Eppendorf (Ep) tube. The mixture was vortexed for 15 min and centrifuged at 8000 rpm for 5 min. The supernatant was removed, and the pellet was mixed with 20 μL of egg white lysozyme (Amresco, Solon, OH, USA) and incubated at 37 °C for 1 h. Subsequently, the total DNA was extracted using a QIAamp® DNA Mini Kit (Qiagen, Hilden, Germany). The DNA was eluted with 80 μL of elution buffer. The extracted DNA samples were stored at -80 °C until library preparation and sequencing.

2.2. STR Analysis

The extracted DNA samples were quantified using a Quantifiler Trio Quantification kit (Thermo Fisher Scientific, Waltham, MA, USA) and an Applied Biosystems 7500 Real-Time Polymerase Chain Reaction (PCR) System (Thermo Fisher Scientific, Waltham, MA, USA). The cycling parameters were set and data analysis was performed in accordance with the recommendations of the manufacturer. The samples were amplified in triplicate. The DNA concentration was adjusted to 1.0 ng/µL in a final PCR mixture volume of 25 µL. The samples with higher DNA concentrations were diluted to 1 ng/µL.

The PCR product (1 µL) was added to 8.5 µL of highly deionized (Hi-Di) formamide (Applied Biosystems, Zug, Switzerland) and 0.5 µL of 600 LIZ (20–600 nucleotide range, Applied Biosystems) Size Standard (Applied Biosystems). STR amplification was performed using 1 ng of template DNA and an AmpFLSTR Identifiler PCR Amplification Kit (Thermo Fisher Scientific). Amplification was performed using an ABI Prism 310 Genetic Analyzer, and the data were analyzed with GeneMapper ID software v3.2.1 (Thermo Fisher Scientific, MA, USA).

2.3. Library Preparation of 16S rRNA Amplicons

Forty samples were analyzed by high-throughput 16S rRNA gene amplicon sequencing on an Ion GeneStudio S5 platform (Thermo Fisher Scientific). The V3–V4 regions of the 16S rRNA gene from each sample were amplified using the following primers: 341F (5′-CCTACGGGNGGCWGCAG-3′), which contained a sample-specific 6–8-base pair tag sequence, and 805R (5′-GACTACHVGGGTATCTAATCC-3′). PCR amplification was performed using Platinum PCR SuperMix High Fidelity master mix (Invitrogen, Carlsbad, CA, USA) with 2.5 ng of template DNA and 50 nmol of each primer in a 27-µL reaction mixture volume. The PCR conditions were as follows: 94 °C for 3 min, followed by 30 cycles at 94 °C for 30 s, 50 °C for 30 s, and 72 °C for 30 s. To remove residual primer dimers and contaminants, the amplicon libraries were purified using an Agencourt AMPure XP DNA purification kit (Beckman Coulter Life Sciences, Indianapolis, IN, USA). The samples were eluted with 15 µL of low Tris-EDTA (TE) buffer. The DNA concentration and quality were assessed using the dsDNA High Sensitivity Assay Kit on a Qubit 4 Fluorometer (Thermo Fisher Scientific, Waltham, MA, USA). The fragment size and quality of the pooled DNA were assessed using an Agilent 2100 Bioanalyzer (Agilent Technologies, Palo Alto, CA, USA). The enriched particles were loaded on to an Ion 530 chip (Thermo Fisher Scientific) and sequenced using an Ion GeneStudio S5 instrument [25].

2.4. Analysis of 16S rRNA Amplicon Sequences

Reads were excluded from the analysis if they were shorter than 500 bp or were inappropriately paired. The sequence data were analyzed using EzBioCloud 16S rRNA gene-based microbiome taxonomic profiling (MTP) and the PICRUST algorithm (ChunLab, Seoul, Korea) with "Bacteria" as a target taxon in the prokaryotic 16S rRNA gene database PKSSU4.0. Sequences processed using the EzBio Cloud 16S rRNA gene-based MTP pipeline were clustered into operational taxonomic units (OTUs) using a 97%-similarity cut-off and identified using QIIME-MOTHUR algorithms.

2.5. Statistical Analysis

To examine differences in the bacterial community diversity, Microbiome Analyst software (www.microbiomeanalyst.ca, accessed on 25 January 2021,) [26] was used to evaluate α and β diversities and to conduct group comparison and classification. The Shannon index was used to evaluate α diversity. Principal coordinate analysis (PCoA) was conducted using Jensen–Shannon divergence and evaluated using the permutational multivariate analysis of variance (PERMANOVA). The microbial composition among groups was compared using linear discriminant analysis (LDA) effect size (LEfSe), and the relative abundance of the core microbiome taxa was assessed at the genus level. Kruskal–

Wallis H test correction was performed using SPSS ver. 20.0 to evaluate the inter-group significance at the genus and species levels.

3. Results

3.1. STR Analysis

The samples were subjected to STR analysis. The concentration of DNA isolated from the gargle, urine, finger, and mobile phone samples was 16.67, 2.16, 0.85, and 0.42 ng/µL, respectively. In the case of fingertip and mobile phone samples, four undetected concentrations of DNA (under 0 ng/µL low concentration) were analyzed.

The STR analysis results are shown in Table 1. For actual individual identification, statistical analysis should be performed for each gene peak. However, in this study, the number of samples to be confirmed was not large enough for a statistical approach, and the general approach of simply counting the number of matching loci was able to distinguish them from each other [27]. The urine and gargle fluid samples provided a full profile that could identify individuals. For both fingertip and mobile phone samples, 8 of the 10 samples were confirmed identifiable full profiles. Two fingertip and two mobile phone samples from two subjects could not be used to identify individuals.

Table 1. Results of STR analysis.

	Sample (n = 40)	Full Profile (Loci = 24)	Partial Profile			Mixed	Full + Minor
			1~10	11~19	20~23		
Fingertip	10	4	1	1	1	1	2
Mobile phone	10	7	1	1	0	0	1
Urine	10	9	0	0	0	0	1
Gargle	10	9	0	0	0	0	1

Mixed = although mixed with other genes, the degree to which an individual profile can be identified.

3.2. Microbiome Analysis

3.2.1. Overview of Taxonomic Diversity

The samples were classified into gargle, urine, mobile phone, and fingertip according to the collection site. Among the 40 samples, 5 were discarded during quality control processing. Thus, 35 samples were used in the study. We obtained 660,095 valid 16S rRNA reads after quality filtering. For each group, 340,525 (gargle), 103,510 (urine), 112,877 (fingers), and 103,183 (mobile phone) reads were obtained.

The composition of the bacterial community of each sample was examined for relative abundance at the genus level. The genera that accounted for the highest proportion in the gargle samples were *Streptococcus*, *Rothia*, *Gemella*, *Heamophillus*, *Neisseria*, and *Granulicatella*. The genera that accounted for the highest proportion in the urine samples were *Lactobacillus*, *Gardnerella*, *Streptococcus*, and *Prevotella*. The genera with the highest proportion in the fingertip samples were *Streptococcus*, *Rothia*, *Cutibacterium*, and *Staphylococcus*. Finally, the genera that accounted for the highest proportion in the mobile phone samples were *Streptococcus*, *Rothia*, *Porphyromonas*, and *Neisseria*. The average number of OTUs in each sample was 643 for gargle, 229 for urine, 520 for finger, and 400 for mobile phone.

3.2.2. α and β Diversities

α-Diversity analysis was performed to determine the abundance of each species (Figure 2). The analysis was performed at the species level and tested using the Kruskal–Wallis method. The overall p-value was less than 0.05, which indicated significant diversity of all species. In the α-diversity analysis, the samples with high abundance, diversity, and uniformity were the gargle, fingertip, and mobile phone samples. Urine had lower diversity than the other three sample types.

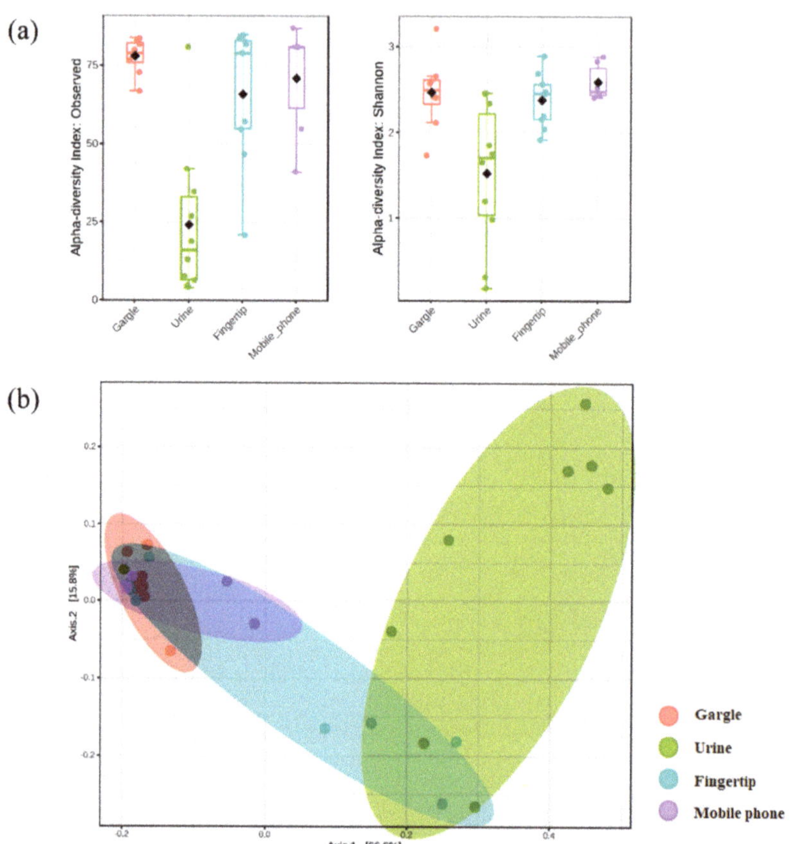

Figure 2. Results of α and β diversity, which reveal the total strain abundance and type (**a**) α diversity with Observed (left) and Shannon (right) index and (**b**) β diversity with Jensen-Shannon divergence index.

β-Diversity analysis using Jensen–Shannon divergence demonstrated bacterial community clustering for each sample type. Urine samples had a few overlapping parts with the other sample types, indicating differences in the bacterial community composition from other sample types. Several communities in the fingertip samples were similar to the bacterial communities from the gargle and mobile phone samples, suggesting that the fingers share bacterial species through contact with other body parts.

3.2.3. Creation of a List of Strains and Matching Assessment

Next, a list was prepared using the representative markers reported for each site and the sample analysis method used in the study (Table 2). This list was prepared at the genus level using LEfSe, the core microbiome, and the reported general microbiome from previous studies (see Table S2 and references therein). LEfSe was used to analyze gargle, urine, and finger metagenomics data. The linear discriminant analysis (LDA) score was derived using a Kruskal–Wallis rank sum test, where the significant LDA scores were more than 2.0. The false discovery rate (FDR) was set to 0.05. In the core microbiomes, the relative abundance of the bacteria in each group was determined using a relative abundance cut-off value of 0.01. The LEfSe and core microbiome data were analyzed by selecting the most abundant strain present in each body part and a representative species present in the urine and gargle samples. The detailed strain-selection methods are included in Table S2.

Table 2. Ten representative strains at the Genus level for each region, constructed using the microbiome or indicative bacteria reported in previous studies and sample analysis conducted within the study.

Gargle	Urine	Fingertip
Streptococcus	*Escherichia*	*Corynebacterium*
Veillonella	*Staphylococcus*	*Streptococcus*
Prevotella	*Finegoldia*	*Staphylococcus*
Neisseria	*Atopobium*	*Micrococcus*
Haemophilus	*Lactobacillus*	*Veillonella*
Porphyromonas	*Corynebacterium*	*Dermacoccus*
Rothia	*Gardnerella*	*Cutibacterium*
Actinomyces	*Campylobacter*	*Enhydrobacter*
Campylobacter	*Peptoniphilus*	*Sphingomonas*
Tannerella	*Anaerococcus*	*Lawsonella*

Table S3 shows the results of verification of the presence or absence of microbial species in each sample compared to the reference list. For the mobile phone samples, the classification was based on the fingertip panel, as contact with the hand was common.

We observed that gargle samples had the highest probability of confirming the microbiome composition, followed by the fingertip and mobile phone samples. For the urine samples, the average agreement rate was 66%, which was lower than that of the gargle and finger samples. Unlike the microbiome of other body parts, the number of bacteria present in urine is small and is classified using strains originating from the genital tract according to sex [28]. Identification of the strains from mobile phones was confirmed using the list of fingertip strains. The average coincidence rate was approximately 60%. Among the eight target samples, six matched the fingertip strain by more than 60%. Thus, it was inferred that the corresponding sample is related to the skin.

By confirming 10 genera in the gargle samples, significant differences were observed in the gargle and urine samples compared, thereby making it possible to discriminate body fluids ($p < 0.05$). However, for *Streptococcus* and *Prevotella*, there was no significant difference because these strains are commonly found in urine and the mouth [28,29]. Among the remaining eight strains, *Tannerella* was the most different compared with the other strains. There was no significant difference in the gargle samples compared to the finger and mobile phone samples, which is consistent with the findings of a previous study, showing that a large number of oral bacteria are introduced via exposure to external environments such as fingers and mobile phones or by personal habits and behaviors [30].

In urine samples, *Staphylococcus*, *Finegoldia*, *Corynebacterium*, and *Campylobacter* showed significant differences compared with those in the other groups. For the fingertip samples, no significant differences were observed compared to the mobile phone samples. Similarly, no significant differences were found when compared with the gargle samples. However, there were strains with significant differences between the urine and gargle samples and the mobile phone samples. *Staphylococcus*, *Dermacoccus*, *Cutibacterium*, and *Enhydrobacter* were specifically identified on mobile phones. *Sphingomonas* was the most frequent in urine.

The possibility of final classification was investigated by applying our classification method to the selected sample using the strain reported as the major microbiome component at the species level. The strains observed in the gargle samples were *Streptococcus salivarius*, *S. sanguinis*, and *Neisseria subflava* [31], whereas those in the urine samples were *Lactobacillus* spp. and *Gardnerella vaginalis* [32]. There are three strains in the fingertip samples: *Cutibacterium acnes*, *Corynebacterium tuberculostearicum*, and *Micrococcus lutes* [33]. Using our classification method, three strains were identified in all gargle samples and *Lactobacillus* species were found in all urine samples. Among them, *G. vaginalis* was found in only 5 of 10 samples. *Gardnerella vaginalis* is found in females and is increased in the presence of bacterial vaginosis [21]. In fingertip and mobile phone samples, *C. acnes* was found in all samples on the fingers, *C. tuberculostearicum* was found in eight out of nine samples, and *M. luteus* was detected in six out of nine samples. In the mobile phone samples, *C. acnes* was found in all individuals, whereas the other two bacterial species were not detected in mobile phone samples. Thus, by identifying skin-related microorganisms, it can be inferred whether the sample is directly related to humans or was obtained from a surface where primary or secondary transfer occurred.

3.3. Personal Feature Tracking and Unique Bacterial Features

The bacterial strains present in each sample type were as follows. First, numerous strains derived from microorganisms in the human upper respiratory tract, oral cavity, feces, and intestines were found in the gargle samples [22,29]. Additionally, microorganisms related to the environment, such as plant roots, sea water, and soil were observed. *Avibacterium*, which is found in chicken beaks, and *Bombiscardovia*, which is found in the digestive tract of bees, were also detected [23,34]. Among environmental microorganisms, *Skermanella*, which is found in Korean aerial environments, was observed [34]. In the case of urine, microbes associated with the intestines, urethra, vagina, and cervix, as well as oral bacteria, were found [21,31]. By matching samples with female subjects, we confirmed that the sex-related information was consistent.

3.4. Bacterial Analysis of Failed STR an Analysis Samples

We performed 16S rRNA bacterial profiling by NGS on samples of failed STR analysis (Figure 3). All samples of failed STR analysis showed valid results in bacterial sequencing. The bacterial profiles were different between mobile phone and finger samples. Therefore, the bacterial sequencing results were compared with the results of an earlier study in which the mobile phone and hand of individuals shared a similar microorganism profile [16]. Sample No. 12, 25, 34, and 44 from finger tips and mobile phones, which had failed STR analysis, were combined and subjected to bacterial profiling. These samples were analyzed using Jensen–Shannon divergence to determine the degree of similarity between samples. We confirmed that the samples that failed STR analysis could be distinguished from each other at different sample locations.

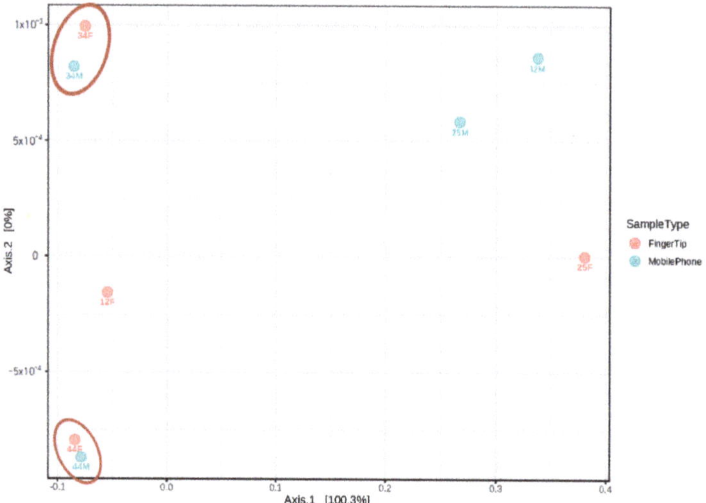

Figure 3. β diversity and relationship of failed STR samples with fingertip-mobile phone (Jensen-Shannon divergence). The correlation is confirmed by measuring the similar distance between each sample using a two-dimensional distance measurement expression. The red circle means nearest sample).

4. Discussion

DNA extracted for forensic analysis is often contaminated with non-human DNA. The study objective was to confirm that additional microbiome analysis can be performed when STR analysis fails. We also showed that sample classification and tracking of individual characteristics are possible using microbiome analysis. The origin of the sample could be determined based on the bacterial composition of each sample. In experimental samples that do not return valid results in the STR analysis, additional NGS analysis can supplement information on the relationship between the samples. Additionally, by analyzing bacterial strains in each sample according to partial microbial characteristics, it is possible to obtain information regarding the sex, environment, or physical condition of the source of the sample.

Owing to the wide distribution of microorganisms, complete individual results were not obtained through microbial profiling, although tracked information could be obtained about the surrounding environment, sex, or physical condition of the subject using survey and subject information matching. In gargle samples, we observed strains derived from various communities such as those from feces and intestines, in addition to human oral microbes. Furthermore, the observed environmental microorganisms were derived from various environments, such as plant roots, sea water, soil, and deep mineral water. Therefore, we were able to observe whether bacteria were included because of respiration through the mouth. However, unlike oral bacteria, periodontal and upper respiratory tract bacteria were present in small proportions and excluded from the oral microbiome composition. Using these strains, environmental tracking was possible. Of the bacteria found in the oral cavity, *Skermanella* is found in the air of Korea [35], suggesting that individuals with this species in the gargle samples currently reside in Korea.

In urine, bacteria related to the intestines, urethra, cervix, vagina, soil or water environment, and outdoor air were found to be similarly diverse. Urine is particularly likely to be contaminated by contact with the hand of the subject at the time of collection, and the distribution of bacteria may vary depending on the collection environment and method. Additionally, urine is a body fluid that is linked to health status and sex-related information. In females, the perineum is shorter than that in men, and intestinal microbes found in the anus or large intestine are found in the female genitalia. Thus, not only urinary-tract-related bacteria but also anal-, fecal-, and intestinal-related bacteria are found in urine-related samples with high abundance. Thus, sex can be predicted using this method. Females may suffer from bacterial vaginosis, and the associated bacteria may be detected in large amounts [36]. In this study, many *Lactobacillus* species were found in the urinary tract. Additionally, *G. vaginalis*, the causative agent of bacterial vaginosis, was frequently observed. However, the volunteers were not questioned regarding vaginitis. Our results indicate that the biological environment or sex of the volunteers can be inferred by analyzing the bacterial profile.

Generally, specific strains were found related to the sample collection site, such as the mouth and urinary tract, although this was not the case for skin sites. The existence of skin microbes related to the genus *Cutibacterium*, as reported in other studies, was confirmed in this study [19]. However, as the fingers are most exposed to the external environment and often come into contact with other surfaces, the bacterial community composition is complicated by various environments [37]. Thus, it is possible to find a characteristic bacterial community related to the contact environment, although contrarily, it is appropriate to interpret skin microbiome analysis results with the possibility of contamination in mind. At the time of sample collection, it was recommended not to wash hands for 3 h before sample collection, although no specific precautions were taken. Thus, the volunteers may have been in contact with each other or other college students, for example, by touching or unconscious contact. DNA transfer can occur by two routes: primary and secondary; it has been reported that human DNA as well as bacterial DNA can be transferred [38]. These external factors may have attributed to the difficulty in identifying tracing microorganisms using skin samples.

Owing to the outbreak of COVID-19 at the time of sample collection, the Korean government recommended the regular use of disinfectants. Hence, hand sanitizers were actively used. Any subjects who disinfected and washed their hands more than a certain number of times a day were excluded. As bacteria are vulnerable to alcohol-mediated degradation, if disinfection is carried out several times a day there is a high possibility that characteristic bacteria will be killed [39]. As these habits are related to social changes, it may be helpful to consider the variables for changes according to social aspects when conducting skin microbiome studies of the hand. Additionally, although there are microbes on surfaces such as the skin and mobile phones, they do not necessarily share all strains because of different biological and nutritional conditions [38]. Therefore, when performing a microbiome-wide analysis, it is necessary to confirm the characteristics of the possession identified from the owner. The method by which information of the object surface is analyzed can also help the investigation.

In the case of sample information derived from a single person, profiling can be integrated with information of other samples. In the case of volunteer 7, *Mobiluncus*, a bacterium found in the male partner of a woman with bacterial vaginosis, was found in the gargle sample [40]. Additionally, numerous *Lactobacillus* species were found in the urine of volunteer 7, and it was confirmed through the questionnaire that the subject was a man with a girlfriend. In the case of volunteer 21, *Neiserria sicca* was found in all collection sites. This bacterium is found in patients with weakened immunity or atopy [41]. Volunteer 21 was confirmed to have atopic skin disease using the questionnaire. In the case of volunteer 2, *Massilia aerilata* and *Corynebacterium kreppenstedtii*, which are commonly found on the hands, mobile phones, plant-related substances, or plant roots, were observed [42,43]. Volunteer 2 confirmed the presence of companion plants at home in the survey. Volunteer 20 had *Lactobacillus iners*, *Gardnella vaginalis*, and *Atopobium vaginae* on the mobile phone. These bacteria are found in the vagina and urinary tract of females, suggesting that the owner of the mobile phone was a woman [16]. Additionally, as volunteer 20 did not disinfect the mobile phone, there is a high probability that the microbiological composition is associated with the owner. Our results suggest that individual profiles can be obtained by microbial analysis through information matching between multiple samples and confirmation using questionnaires.

Microbiome analysis of samples from human sources has potential for forensic applications by providing information on the identification of individuals at crime scenes. However, the analysis range of the microbiome is wide and there are many variables, such as the distribution and composition of bacteria, environment, and differences among individuals. Considering that the above results showed a concordance rate of approximately 80% or more, the STR analysis is the best test for human-derived samples. However, only human genetic information can be obtained, and additional environmental or circumstantial information cannot be completely obtained [27]. As with human DNA, there are no specific marker loci such as STR. Hence, it is difficult to perform specific tests. However, this study suggests that sample-derived tracking and sample-related information tracking are possible using NGS, by preparing a panel list using specific bacteria in a manner similar to the STR analysis. As the bacterial abundance is different for each sample type, it is better to determine the abundance for each cluster rather than use a specific marker for feature tracking. The use of a single strain is risky as the strain may exist extensively in other sites [16]. Accordingly, we prepared lists using various microbiomes and presented a proposal to selectively select strains using these lists. Using this approach, additional analyses can be employed for samples of unknown origin. Furthermore, samples that fail STR analysis can be analyzed using a secondary method.

An era has arrived when human DNA alone cannot be used as valid evidence in court. In an actual case, although DNA of the suspect was found and the Y-STR was matched, the evidence used in the case did not contain the suspect's fingerprint. Furthermore, the DNA of the police personnel involved in the case at the time matched the Y-STR of the suspect, thus invalidating the sentence of the perpetrator [14]. This indicates that oral descriptions of the victim and the human DNA profile applicable to suspects are not valid in court, and additional evidence must be presented. Therefore, for a clear trial and fair judgment, not only the main body of evidence but also additional evidence supporting and/or linking the suspect or victim to the case is inevitable. For example, supplemental information can be provided by identifying oral bacteria in bite marks that occur in sexual assault cases. In this regard, we would like to emphasize that information of forensic microorganisms that can identify human traces is also necessary for creating secondary profiles and collecting additional evidence. In addition, the method used for DNA extraction is important. Since analyzing traces of microbial genes and human genes via a single sample collection can be applied in a forensic approach, it has the advantage of securing more evidence in case resolution.

In this study, only the V3–V4 region was analyzed using 16S rRNA sequencing. Analysis of other V regions could identify more microbial communities and individual strains. The classification of the V region compared to the actual analyzed region is also different. In addition, if the sample itself is not of acceptable quality, the number of bacteria that can be analyzed is small, and complete information according to individual tracking may not be available. Moreover, high-quality DNA can be obtained using various tools and swabbing solutions in the DNA collection method [44,45].

5. Conclusions

In forensic analysis, samples collected are often of variable quality. Evidence not belonging to humans is also found, and even if clear human evidence such as blood is detected, human DNA can be destroyed or can be difficult to recover and extract. Our findings indicate that by creating a list of microbial classifications according to each site, site tracking can be achieved. Moreover, through microbiome analysis, a selective experimental method could be performed even with a single extraction step; secondary analysis of samples that failed STR analysis can be performed as well. We believe that the findings of this study lay a foundation for the development of methodologies in forensic microbiology for analyzing low-quality evidence.

Supplementary Materials: The following supporting information can be downloaded at: https://www.mdpi.com/article/10.3390/genes13010085/s1. Table S1: Survey and results, Table S2: Listing of major strains by site using LEfSe, Core Microbiome and reported studies, Table S3: Sample discrimination result using a random microbial panel.

Author Contributions: Conceptualization, methodology, software, formal analysis, writing—original draft preparation, and writing—review and editing, S.L. (Solip Lee); validation, investigation, and resources, S.L. (Songhee Lee) and H.Y.; data curation and visualization, Y.L.; supervision and project administration, H.-G.K., H.-J.S., J.C. and S.H. All authors have read and agreed to the published version of the manuscript.

Funding: This research received no external funding.

Institutional Review Board Statement: The study was conducted according to the guidelines of the Declaration of Helsinki and approved by the Institutional Review Board of Eulji University Institutional Bioethics Committee (IRB No. EUIRB 2020-13).

Informed Consent Statement: Informed consent was obtained from all subjects involved in the study.

Data Availability Statement: The data presented in this study are available in the article and Supplementary Materials. The raw data are available on reasonable request from the corresponding author.

Acknowledgments: This research was supported and funded by the Korean National Police Agency [Project Name: Development of bloodstain analysis system for scene reconstruction/Project Number: POLICE_I_00001_01_101].

Conflicts of Interest: The authors declare no conflict of interest.

References

1. Reid, C.A.; Howes, L.M. Communicating forensic scientific expertise: An analysis of expert reports and corresponding testimony in Tasmanian courts. *Sci. Justice* **2020**, *60*, 108–119. [CrossRef] [PubMed]
2. Dumache, R.; Ciocan, V.; Muresan, C.; Enache, A. Molecular DNA Analysis in Forensic Identification. *Clin. Lab.* **2016**, *62*, 245–248. [CrossRef] [PubMed]
3. Silva, N.M.; Pereira, L.; Poloni, E.S.; Currat, M. Human neutral genetic variation and forensic STR data. *PLoS ONE* **2012**, *7*, e49666. [CrossRef] [PubMed]
4. Dziak, R.; Peneder, A.; Buetter, A.; Hageman, C. Trace DNA Sampling Success from Evidence Items Commonly Encountered in Forensic Casework. *J. Forensic Sci.* **2018**, *63*, 835–841. [CrossRef] [PubMed]
5. Raymond, J.J.; van Oorschot, R.A.; Walsh, S.J.; Roux, C. Trace DNA analysis: Do you know what your neighbour is doing? A multi-jurisdictional survey. *Forensic Sci. Int. Genet.* **2008**, *2*, 19–28. [CrossRef]
6. Harbison, S.; Fallow, M.; Bushell, D. An analysis of the success rate of 908 trace DNA samples submitted to the Crime Sample Database Unit in New Zealand. *Aust. J. Forensic Sci.* **2008**, *40*, 49–53. [CrossRef]
7. Alaeddini, R.; Walsh, S.J.; Abbas, A. Forensic implications of genetic analyses from degraded DNA—A review. *Forensic Sci. Int. Genet.* **2010**, *4*, 148–157. [CrossRef]
8. Kloosterman, A.; Kersbergen, P. Efficacy and limits of genotyping low copy number DNA samples by multiplex PCR of STR loci. *Int. Congr. Ser.* **2003**, *1239*, 795–798. [CrossRef]
9. Meadow, J.F.; Altrichter, A.E.; Bateman, A.C.; Stenson, J.; Brown, G.Z.; Green, J.L.; Bohannan, B.J. Humans differ in their personal microbial cloud. *PeerJ* **2015**, *3*, e1258. [CrossRef]
10. Eetemadi, A.; Rai, N.; Pereira, B.M.P.; Kim, M.; Schmitz, H.; Tagkopoulos, I. The Computational Diet: A Review of Computational Methods Across Diet, Microbiome, and Health. *Front. Microbiol.* **2020**, *11*, 393. [CrossRef]
11. Pasolli, E.; Asnicar, F.; Manara, S.; Zolfo, M.; Karcher, N.; Armanini, F.; Beghini, F.; Manghi, P.; Tett, A.; Ghensi, P.; et al. Extensive Unexplored Human Microbiome Diversity Revealed by over 150,000 Genomes from Metagenomes Spanning Age, Geography, and Lifestyle. *Cell* **2019**, *176*, 649–662.e20. [CrossRef] [PubMed]
12. De la Cuesta-Zuluaga, J.; Kelley, S.T.; Chen, Y.; Escobar, J.S.; Mueller, N.T.; Ley, R.E.; McDonald, D.; Huang, S.; Swafford, A.D.; Knight, R.; et al. Age- and Sex-Dependent Patterns of Gut Microbial Diversity in Human Adults. *mSystems* **2019**, *4*, e00261-19. [CrossRef] [PubMed]
13. Huttenhower, C.; Gevers, D.; Knight, R.; Abubucker, S.; Badger, J.; Chinwalla, A.; Giglio, M.G. Structure, function and diversity of the healthy human microbiome. *Nature* **2012**, *486*, 207.
14. Metcalf, J.L. Estimating the postmortem interval using microbes: Knowledge gaps and a path to technology adoption. *Forensic Sci. Int. Genet.* **2019**, *38*, 211–218. [CrossRef]
15. Schmedes, S.E.; Woerner, A.E.; Novroski, N.M.M.; Wendt, F.R.; King, J.L.; Stephens, K.M.; Budowle, B. Targeted sequencing of clade-specific markers from skin microbiomes for forensic human identification. *Forensic Sci. Int. Genet.* **2018**, *32*, 50–61. [CrossRef]
16. Fierer, N.; Lauber, C.L.; Zhou, N.; McDonald, D.; Costello, E.K.; Knight, R. Forensic identification using skin bacterial communities. *Proc. Natl. Acad. Sci. USA* **2010**, *107*, 6477–6481. [CrossRef]
17. Goga, H. Comparison of bacterial DNA profiles of footwear insoles and soles of feet for the forensic discrimination of footwear owners. *Int. J. Legal Med.* **2012**, *126*, 815–823. [CrossRef]
18. Yang, J.; Tsukimi, T.; Yoshikawa, M.; Suzuki, K.; Takeda, T.; Tomita, M.; Fukuda, S. *Cutibacterium acnes* (*Propionibacterium acnes*) 16S rRNA genotyping of microbial samples from possessions contributes to owner identification. *mSystems* **2019**, *4*, e00594-19. [CrossRef]
19. Concheri, G.; Bertoldi, D.; Polone, E.; Otto, S.; Larcher, R.; Squartini, A. Chemical elemental distribution and soil DNA fingerprints provide the critical evidence in murder case investigation. *PLoS ONE* **2011**, *6*, e20222. [CrossRef]
20. López, C.D.; González, D.M.; Haas, C.; Vidaki, A.; Kayser, M. Microbiome-based body site of origin classification of forensically relevant blood traces. *Forensic Sci. Int. Genet.* **2020**, *47*, 102280. [CrossRef] [PubMed]
21. Aroutcheva, A.A.; Simoes, J.A.; Behbakht, K.; Faro, S. *Gardnerella vaginalis* isolated from patients with bacterial vaginosis and from patients with healthy vaginal ecosystems. *Clin. Infect. Dis.* **2001**, *33*, 1022–1027. [CrossRef]
22. Alcaraz, L.D.; Belda-Ferre, P.; Cabrera-Rubio, R.; Romero, H.; Simón-Soro, A.; Pignatelli, M.; Mira, A. Identifying a healthy oral microbiome through metagenomics. *Clin. Microbiol. Infect.* **2012**, *18* (Suppl. 4), 54–57. [CrossRef]
23. Bisgaard, M.; Nørskov-Lauritsen, N.; De Wit, S.; Hess, C.; Christensen, H. Multilocus sequence phylogenetic analysis of *Avibacterium*. *Microbiology* **2012**, *158*, 993–1004. [CrossRef]
24. Ho, W. What's the Y-STR Gene? Determined for a 12-Year Sentence of Not Guilty. NEWSIS. 2020. Available online: https://news.v.daum.net/v/20200529142012559 (accessed on 29 May 2020).
25. Lee, S.H.; You, H.S.; Kang, H.G.; Kang, S.S.; Hyun, S.H. Association between Altered Blood Parameters and Gut Microbiota after Synbiotic Intake in Healthy, Elderly Korean Women. *Nutrients* **2020**, *12*, 3112. [CrossRef] [PubMed]
26. Dhariwal, A.; Chong, J.; Habib, S.; King, I.L.; Agellon, L.B.; Xia, J. MicrobiomeAnalyst: A web-based tool for comprehensive statistical, visual and meta-analysis of microbiome data. *Nucleic Acids Res.* **2017**, *45*, W180–W188. [CrossRef] [PubMed]
27. Romsos, E.L.; French, J.L.; Smith, M.; Figarelli, V.; Harran, F.; Vandegrift, G.; Moreno, L.I.; Callaghan, T.F.; Brocato, J.; Vaidyanathan, J. Results of the 2018 rapid DNA maturity assessment. *J. Forensic Sci.* **2020**, *65*, 953–959. [CrossRef]

28. Abelson, B.; Sun, D.; Que, L.; Nebel, R.A.; Baker, D.; Popiel, P.; Amundsen, C.L.; Chai, T.; Close, C.; DiSanto, M. Sex differences in lower urinary tract biology and physiology. *Biol. Sex Differ.* **2018**, *9*, 45. [CrossRef]
29. Willis, J.R.; Gabaldón, T. The human oral microbiome in health and disease: From sequences to ecosystems. *Microorganisms* **2020**, *8*, 308. [CrossRef] [PubMed]
30. Edmonds-Wilson, S.L.; Nurinova, N.I.; Zapka, C.A.; Fierer, N.; Wilson, M. Review of human hand microbiome research. *J. Dermatol. Sci.* **2015**, *80*, 3–12. [CrossRef]
31. Ohta, J.; Sakurada, K. Oral gram-positive bacterial DNA-based identification of saliva from highly degraded samples. *Forensic Sci. Int. Genet.* **2019**, *42*, 103–112. [CrossRef]
32. Petrova, M.I.; Lievens, E.; Malik, S.; Imholz, N.; Lebeer, S. *Lactobacillus* species as biomarkers and agents that can promote various aspects of vaginal health. *Front. Physiol.* **2015**, *6*, 81. [CrossRef] [PubMed]
33. Li, Z.; Xia, J.; Jiang, L.; Tan, Y.; An, Y.; Zhu, X.; Ruan, J.; Chen, Z.; Zhen, H.; Ma, Y. Characterization of the human skin resistome and identification of two microbiota cutotypes. *Microbiome* **2021**, *9*, 47. [CrossRef]
34. Killer, J.; Kopečný, J.; Mrázek, J.; Havlík, J.; Koppová, I.; Benada, O.; Rada, V.; Kofroňová, O. *Bombiscardovia coagulans* gen. nov., sp. nov., a new member of the family Bifidobacteriaceae isolated from the digestive tract of bumblebees. *Syst. Appl. Microbiol.* **2010**, *33*, 359–366. [CrossRef] [PubMed]
35. Weon, H.-Y.; Kim, B.-Y.; Hong, S.-B.; Joa, J.-H.; Nam, S.-S.; Lee, K.H.; Kwon, S.-W. *Skermanella aerolata* sp. nov., isolated from air, and emended description of the genus *Skermanella*. *Int. J. Syst. Evol. Microbiol.* **2007**, *57*, 1539–1542. [CrossRef]
36. Mitra, A.; MacIntyre, D.A.; Mahajan, V.; Lee, Y.S.; Smith, A.; Marchesi, J.R.; Lyons, D.; Bennett, P.R.; Kyrgiou, M. Comparison of vaginal microbiota sampling techniques: Cytobrush versus swab. *Sci. Rep.* **2017**, *7*, 9802. [CrossRef] [PubMed]
37. Tozzo, P.; D'Angiolella, G.; Brun, P.; Castagliuolo, I.; Gino, S.; Caenazzo, L. Skin Microbiome analysis for forensic human identification: What do we know so far? *Microorganisms* **2020**, *8*, 873. [CrossRef]
38. Thornbury, D.; Goray, M.; van Oorschot, R.A. Indirect DNA transfer without contact from dried biological materials on various surfaces. *Forensic Sci. Int. Genet.* **2021**, *51*, 102457. [CrossRef]
39. Bondurant, S.W.; Duley, C.M.; Harbell, J.W. Demonstrating the persistent antibacterial efficacy of a hand sanitizer containing benzalkonium chloride on human skin at 1, 2, and 4 hours after application. *Am. J. Infect. Control.* **2019**, *47*, 928–932. [CrossRef]
40. Tuzil, J.; Filkova, B.; Malina, J.; Kerestes, J.; Doležal, T. Smoking in women with chronic vaginal discomfort is not associated with decreased abundance of Lactobacillus spp. but promotes *Mobiluncus* and *Gardnerella* spp. overgrowth: Secondary analysis of trial data including microbiome analysis. *Ceska Gynekol.* **2021**, *86*, 22–29. [CrossRef]
41. Dzidic, M.; Abrahamsson, T.R.; Artacho, A.; Collado, M.C.; Mira, A.; Jenmalm, M. Oral microbiota maturation during the first 7 years of life in relation to allergy development. *Allergy* **2018**, *73*, 2000–2011. [CrossRef]
42. Du, Y.; Yu, X.; Wang, G. *Massilia tieshanensis* sp. nov., isolated from mining soil. *Int. J. Syst. Evol. Microbiol.* **2012**, *62*, 2356–2362. [CrossRef] [PubMed]
43. Barka, E.A.; Vatsa, P.; Sanchez, L.; Gaveau-Vaillant, N.; Jacquard, C.; Klenk, H.-P.; Clément, C.; Ouhdouch, Y.; van Wezel, G.P. Taxonomy, physiology, and natural products of *Actinobacteria*. *Microbiol. Mol. Biol. Rev.* **2016**, *80*, 1–43. [CrossRef] [PubMed]
44. Hedman, J.; Jansson, L.; Akel, Y.; Wallmark, N.; Liljestrand, R.G.; Forsberg, C.; Ansell, R. The double-swab technique versus single swabs for human DNA recovery from various surfaces. *Forensic Sci. Int. Genet.* **2020**, *46*, 102253. [CrossRef] [PubMed]
45. You, H.S.; Lee, S.H.; Ok, Y.J.; Kang, H.-G.; Sung, H.J.; Lee, J.Y.; Kang, S.S.; Hyun, S.H. Influence of swabbing solution and swab type on DNA recovery from rigid environmental surfaces. *J. Microbiol. Methods* **2019**, *161*, 12–17. [CrossRef]

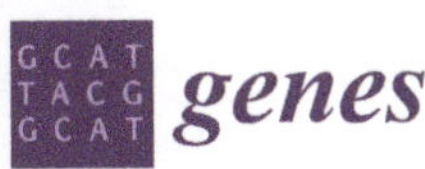 *genes*

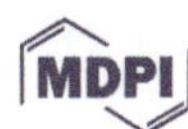

Article

Improved DNA Extraction and Illumina Sequencing of DNA Recovered from Aged Rootless Hair Shafts Found in Relics Associated with the Romanov Family

Odile Loreille [1,*], **Andreas Tillmar** [2,3], **Michael D. Brandhagen** [1], **Linda Otterstatter** [4] and **Jodi A. Irwin** [1]

1   Federal Bureau of Investigation Laboratory, DNA Support Unit, Quantico, VA 22135, USA; mdbrandhagen@fbi.gov (M.D.B.); jairwin@fbi.gov (J.A.I.)
2   Department of Forensic Genetics and Forensic Toxicology, National Board of Forensic Medicine, SE-587 58 Linkoping, Sweden; andreas.tillmar@rmv.se
3   Department of Biomedical and Clinical Sciences, Faculty of Medicine and Health Sciences, Linköping University, SE-582 25 Linkoping, Sweden
4   Federal Bureau of Investigation Laboratory, Trace Evidence Unit, Quantico, VA 22135, USA; lmotterstatter@fbi.gov
*   Correspondence: oploreille@fbi.gov

Citation: Loreille, O.; Tillmar, A.; Brandhagen, M.D.; Otterstatter, L.; Irwin, J.A. Improved DNA Extraction and Illumina Sequencing of DNA Recovered from Aged Rootless Hair Shafts Found in Relics Associated with the Romanov Family. *Genes* **2022**, *13*, 202. https://doi.org/10.3390/genes13020202

Academic Editor: Niels Morling

Received: 29 November 2021
Accepted: 20 January 2022
Published: 23 January 2022

Publisher's Note: MDPI stays neutral with regard to jurisdictional claims in published maps and institutional affiliations.

Abstract: This study describes an optimized DNA extraction protocol targeting ultrashort DNA molecules from single rootless hairs. It was applied to the oldest samples available to us: locks of hairs that were found in relics associated with the Romanov family. Published mitochondrial DNA genome sequences of Tsar Nicholas II and his wife, Tsarina Alexandra, made these samples ideal to assess this DNA extraction protocol and evaluate the types of genetic information that can be recovered by sequencing ultrashort fragments. Using this method, the mtGenome of the Tsarina's lineage was identified in hairs that were concealed in a pendant made by Karl Fabergé for Alexandra Feodorovna Romanov. In addition, to determine if the lock originated from more than one individual, two hairs from the locket were extracted independently and converted into Illumina libraries for shotgun sequencing on a NextSeq 500 platform. From these data, autosomal SNPs were analyzed to assess relatedness. The results indicated that the two hairs came from a single individual. Genetic testing of hairs that were found in the second artifact, a framed photograph of Louise of Hesse-Kassel, Queen of Denmark and maternal grandmother of Tsar Nicholas II, revealed that the hair belonged to a woman who shared Tsar Nicholas' maternal lineage, including the well-known point heteroplasmy at position 16169.

Keywords: Romanov family; next generation sequencing (NGS); hybridization capture; mitochondrial DNA; heteroplasmy; single nucleotide polymorphism (SNP); kinship analyses; biological sexing; ancient DNA

1. Introduction

The fate of the Romanov family was considered one of the greatest mysteries of the 20th century and generates interest and speculation to this day. While official written records are scarce, reports indicate that Tsar Nicholas and his family were held prisoner and shot in July 1918 by a Bolshevik firing squad in the Ipatiev House (Ekaterinburg, Russia). According to accounts, the bodies were then buried in a superficial, hastily dug pit [1,2].

In 1991, nine skeletons were recovered from a shallow grave in Ekaterinburg and tentatively identified by Russian authorities as the Tsar, the Tsarina, three of their five children, and four family retainers. Subsequent DNA testing confirmed the identification of the five Romanovs [3]. The testing included mitochondrial DNA (mtDNA) analysis of the purported Tsarina and three of her daughters. Their mtDNA profile was compared to the profile of one of the Tsarina's living grandnephews, Prince Philip, Duke of Edinburgh, who belonged to the same maternal lineage. Testing also included biological sex determination and autosomal short tandem repeats (STR) analyses and all the DNA results established the presence of a family group consistent with the Romanovs. Additionally, mtDNA testing of the putative remains of the Tsar yielded a sequence that was consistent with the mtDNA profiles of two living maternal relatives of the Tsar as well as the mtDNA profile of the exhumed remains of the Tsar's brother, Grand Duke George Romanov [3,4]. After 16 years following the discovery of the first grave, the missing son and daughter were accounted for when a few small bone fragments were discovered close to the site of the previous recoveries. Anthropological as well as mitochondrial and nuclear DNA analyses of these bone fragments confirmed the presence of the two Romanov children that were missing from the first grave [5,6].

Recently, the DNA Support Unit (DSU) of the FBI laboratory was made aware of two artifacts containing biological material believed to be associated with the Romanov family. The items are part of a collection owned by Mr. Nikolai Bachmakov, an expert restorer in Fabergé collectibles. The first item was a pre-1899 locket purchased by Mr. Bachmakov from another dealer. The locket, a Karl Fabergé pendant, was decorated with three precious stones (Figure 1A). Inside and under glass, was an old black and white photograph of Empress Alexandra Feodorovna Romanov (Figure 1B). On the other side, also under glass, was a lock of light-colored hairs.

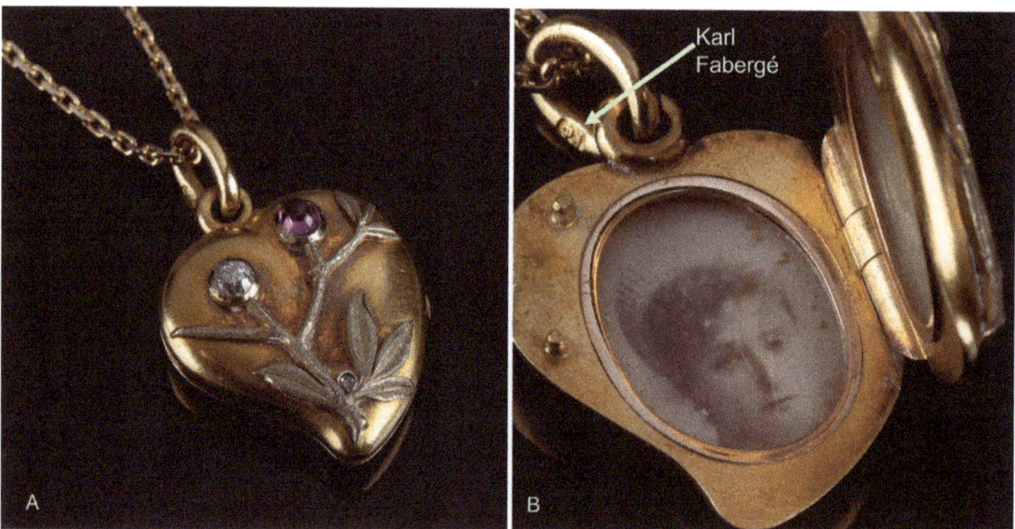

Figure 1. (**A**) Closed Fabergé locket showing precious stones. (**B**) The open locket showing a picture of Tsarina Alexandra Feodorovna Romanov. The stamped initials from Karl Fabergé can be seen on the jump ring. Photographed by Richard Walker. Courtesy of the Russian History Museum.

Shortly after, Mr. Bachmakov informed the DSU that he was also in possession of a framed photograph of Queen Louise of Hesse-Kassel (1817–1898), wife of King Christian IX of Denmark and maternal grandmother of Tsar Nicholas II (Figure 2). Positioned between the glass of the frame and the photograph was a large lock of light hairs that were presumed to belong to Queen Louise.

Although genetic characterization seemed to be the only way to confirm the provenance of the hairs, it was well understood that DNA recovery from such aged and degraded hairs would be challenging. MtDNA, which is sometimes targeted in forensic casework, is increasingly difficult to recover with increasing sample age. In 2005, Melton et al. [7] showed that the likelihood of obtaining a full hypervariable region I/hypervariable region II (HVI/HVII) mtDNA profile decreased from 90% in single shed hairs 0–5 years old to ~60% in hairs greater than 20 years old. Similarly, in a 2017 study, mtDNA averaged only

61 bp in human hairs that had been collected 50 to 100 years ago [8]. For older samples, next generation sequencing (NGS) techniques that do not rely on predefined amplicons have proven necessary for DNA recovery [9–11]. In these particular cases, it is likely that the quantities of hair that were used (between 20 mg and 2 g), the beneficial conditions of preservation, and/or the presence of some hair roots contributed to successful DNA typing.

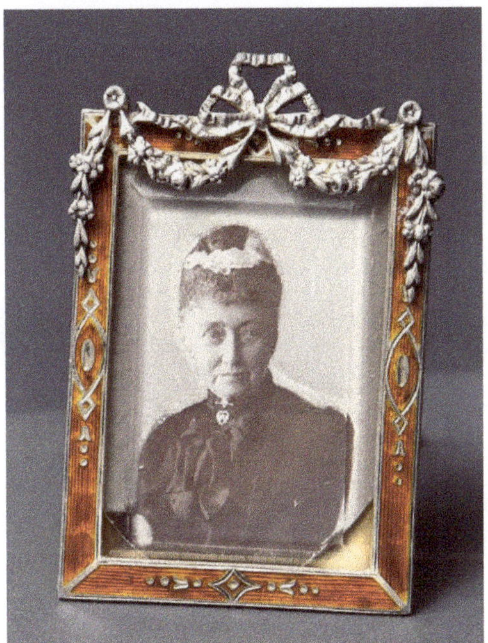

Figure 2. Picture frame containing a picture of Queen Louise of Hesse-Kassel after restoration. Courtesy of M. Perekrestov, from the Russian History Foundation.

We recently employed NGS to develop DNA data from the types of hair samples that are routinely encountered in forensic casework: single shed hairs that are generally comprised of less than 1 mg of biological material [12]. Here, we extended this work by testing even older (i.e., more degraded) rootless hairs that were believed to be associated with Russian royalty. We first assessed the feasibility of recovering DNA from hairs believed to be over a century old. Multiple hairs were pooled together for DNA extraction to improve the likelihood of DNA recovery and to optimize DNA recovery methodologies. We then applied these optimized protocols to the analysis of the types of single hair shafts that are routinely encountered in forensic DNA casework. Overall, the results not only shed light on the hypothesis that the hairs may have originated from members of the Russian Royal family, but also demonstrate the potential value of low coverage sequence data in resolving investigative questions from single decades-old-shed hairs.

2. Material

2.1. The Fabergé Locket

The Fabergé pendant is shown in Figure 1A,B. It is a 14 karat yellow gold heart locket that weighs 8.7 g and measures 24.75 mm × 19.84 mm × 7.15 mm. On the front side, a floral pattern is entwined over the heart and is embellished with three stones: one old-cut round diamond stone of ~0.10 carat (ct), one Cabochon-shaped ruby stone of ~0.12 ct, and a small rose-cut diamond of 0.001 ct (Figure 1A).

On the back, the Russian monogram AΘ (Θ being an old Cyrillic equivalent to the letter F) is engraved as well as the great Imperial crown of Russia (Supplementary Figure S1C). The initials of the locket's maker, stamped on the loose jump ring, are KΦ, as in Karl Fabergé (Figure 1B). The interior of the locket is fitted with two oval-shaped glazed picture frames and on the right side, the scratched inventory number 15,650 means that the locket was made between late 1897 and early 1898. One side contained a black and white portrait of the Empress Alexandra Feodorovna (1872–1918) and on the other side was a lock of light brown/dark blond hairs (Supplementary Figure S1A–E).

2.2. The Picture Frame

The frame, made of silver 925 standard, is covered with red enamel, and decorated with silver ribbons. The size of the black and white cabinet card of Queen Louise is 6.7 cm by 4.3 cm (Figure 2).

A picture of the pre-restored frame containing the lock of hair can be found in Supplementary Figure S2A.

2.3. Hair Samples

The hair samples tested from both the locket and the frame are described in Table 1. In addition to DNA testing, three hairs from the locket and one hair from the frame were examined microscopically by an FBI trace analyst examiner. These hairs were mounted on slides and permanently stored in the FBI hair reference collection.

Table 1. Description of the hair shaft samples that were used in this study and purification methods that were used during DNA extraction.

Associated Item	Hair Shafts Tested	Experiment	Purification Protocol
	Single hair of ~5 cm (light brown). **Lo1a**	Microscopic examination	
	Single hair of ~2.5 cm (light brown). **Lo1b**	Microscopic examination	NA
	Single hair of ~3.8 cm (light brown). **Lo1c**	Microscopic examination	
Fabergé Locket	5 hairs for a total of ~16 cm. **Lo5h**	DNA	MinElute column
	Single hair of 4 cm (light brown). **Lo2**	DNA	Magnetic silica beads
	Single hair of 3.2 cm (light brown). **Lo3**	DNA	Magnetic silica beads
	Single hair of 6 cm (white). **Q3**	Microscopic examination	NA
Frame	6 hairs for a total of ~27 cm. **Q6h**	DNA	MinElute column
	Single hair of 5.5 cm (white). **Q1**	DNA	Magnetic silica beads
	Single hair of 7 cm (brown). **Q2**	DNA	Magnetic silica beads

To maximize the chances of DNA recovery, initial experiments were performed with multiple hairs. From the locket, and under the assumption that all the hairs shared the same mtDNA lineage, five hairs totaling ~16 cm were extracted (Locket 5 hairs: Lo5h). Similarly for the frame, six hairs totaling ~27 cm were tested (Queen 6 hairs: Q6h). Following extraction protocol optimization involving the replacement of MinElute columns with silica coated magnetic beads, and successful results when co-extracting multiple hairs at once, DNA extraction from single hair shafts was attempted for both historical items.

3. Methods

3.1. Microscopic Examination

A total of four hairs were prepared on glass microscope slides using Permount mounting media (Table 1; hairs Lo1a, Lo1b, Lo1c, and Q3). The hairs were examined using a high magnification transmitted light microscope (Leica DM4000B with a Leica FS4000 optical bridge) and photographed with a Leica MC190 HD.

3.2. DNA Extraction Protocols

DNA extraction and library preparation were performed in a laboratory dedicated to low-quantity and low-quality DNA samples with limited personnel access. Personal protective equipment to minimize the risk of contamination included Tyvek® IsoClean® single-use garments (frocks, sleeves, masks from DuPont™, Wilmington, DE, USA), goggles, and double gloving. The reagents were aliquoted and irradiated before the samples were introduced and all plastic consumables were irradiated in a cross-linker prior to use.

A total of three DNA extracts were generated from both the locket hairs and the frame hairs, for a total of six extracts. Of these six extracts, two were developed from multiple hairs (Lo5h and Q6h), and four were developed from single hair shafts (Lo2, Lo3, Q1, and Q2).

Two different purification methods were used. Protocol B from Brandhagen et al. [12] was applied first for the extractions of multiple hairs samples (Lo5h and Q6h). In brief, DNA was extracted using a lysis buffer optimized for hair digestion and then purified with MinElute silica columns from the Qiagen PCR purification kit (Qiagen, Germantown, MD, USA) using large volumes of binding buffer. To accommodate the large volumes of solution, the MinElute columns were fitted with Qiagen extension columns and placed on a vacuum manifold (VacConnector, Qiagen).

DNA from single strands of hair was extracted using the same optimized digestion buffer and volumes as in protocol B, but instead of using MinElute columns, DNA was purified with magnetic beads coated with silica (cat#: 786–915, G-Bioscience, Maryland Heights, MO, USA) as recommended by Rohland et al. [13]. A detailed description of the new protocol can be found in Supplementary Material #1.

DNA quantification via qPCR was not performed on the extracts, as previous experiments had demonstrated that DNA fragments present in hair samples of considerable age are generally too small to yield a 105 bp amplicon with the mtDNA qPCR assay routinely used in DSU [12,14]. Although fluorometric quantification was attempted using a Qubit™ Fluorometer and a dsDNA High Sensitivity Assay Kit (Invitrogen, Waltham, MA, USA), no dsDNA could be detected. The final concentration of the adapters was arbitrarily set at 300 nM.

3.3. Library Preparation

A total of 50 µL from all six DNA extracts (Lo5h, Lo2, Lo3, Q6h, Q1, Q2) and four reagent controls (RB1 to RB4) were converted into double stranded DNA Illumina libraries using the NEBNext® Ultra™ II DNA Library Prep Kit for Illumina® (NEB, Ipswich, MA, USA) and looped adapters from the NEBNext® Multiplex Oligos for Illumina® kit (NEB). Illumina libraries were prepared according to the manufacturer's instructions except for ligation which used highly diluted adapters and was performed overnight at 7 °C. Following ligation, the ligated looped adapters were converted into Y-shaped adapters with the USER® Enzyme kit (NEB). The libraries were then purified with 1.8× AMPure XP beads (Beckman Coulter, Sykesville, MD, USA). All the libraries were dual indexed with primers from the NEBNext® Multiplex Oligos for Illumina® kit and subsequently amplified for 25 cycles with the NEBNext® Q5® Hot Start HiFi PCR Master Mix (NEB). Purification of the amplified libraries was performed using 1.5× AMPure XP beads. The libraries were then shotgun sequenced on an MiSeq Forensic Genomics System (FGx™) instrument (Illumina Inc., San Diego, CA, USA) with a v2 cartridge and 2 × 151 cycles and/or on a NextSeq 500/550 (Illumina) with a High Output kit v2.5 and 2 × 75 cycles in order to obtain additional data.

3.4. Hybridization Capture

Mitochondrial DNA enrichment via hybridization capture was performed on all RBs and on four libraries, one from the locket (Lo5h) and three from the frame (Q6h, Q1, and Q2), using biotinylated RNA baits (myBaits Mito Human, Modern Global, Daicel Arbor Biosciences, Ann Arbor, MI, USA). Each hybridization capture was performed at 62 °C for 24 h using 100 ng of 80 bp long RNA baits. The captured product was then amplified for 16 to 19 cycles and purified with AMPure XP beads. DNA from the purified enriched libraries was successfully quantified using a Qubit™ Fluorometer and the Qubit™ dsDNA Broad Range Assay Kit (Invitrogen), then diluted and analyzed on a 2100 Bioanalyzer with the High Sensitivity DNA Kit (Agilent, Santa Clara, CA, USA). Following quantification, libraries were pooled and sequenced on a MiSeq FGx^{TM} instrument with a v2 cartridge and 2 × 151 cycles. The very first capture library that was sequenced, Lo5h-mt, was also sequenced on the NextSeq 500 with 2 × 75 cycles. The comparison of the data from both instruments showed that a MiSeq run was sufficient to accurately sequence the small mtGenome. As a result, all the subsequent capture libraries were only sequenced on the MiSeq FGx^{TM}.

3.5. Data Analyses

Raw Fastq reads were first imported as paired-end reads, quality trimmed, and the overlapping pairs were merged in the CLC Genomics Workbench, version 12.0 (CLC Bio/Qiagen, Aarhus, Denmark). Merged reads were then mapped to the human genome by a supercomputer using the Burrows-Wheeler Aligner (BWA aln, v0.7.17–r1188) with seed disabled [15] and SAMTools v.1.11 [16]. BWA aln was chosen over CLC because this algorithm is more efficient at mapping very short reads (i.e., reads under 50 bp). Reads with mapping quality below 30 were removed and, to circumvent the fact that BWA can't map reads to a circular reference, a chimeric mtDNA reference was created to allow reads that overlap the mtGenome origin to map. The 33,152 bp sequence was developed by combining the sequence of the standard revised Cambridge reference (rCRS) 16,569 bp genome, followed by 14 N and a second mtGenome sequence starting at position 8284 and ending at position 8283. This chimeric mtDNA reference also replaced the mtDNA reference ChrM in the human genome reference hg19 (a.k.a GRCh37). Duplicate reads were removed using Picard v.2.23.8 [17]. Mappings were imported back into CLC as bam files and the mtDNA reads were extracted and re-mapped to the standard 16,569 bp circular rCRS reference. Duplicate mtDNA reads were removed and CLC was used to develop variant calls, DNA size distribution, and read depth. The shotgun data from single hair extracts were used to assess biological sex using the R_X method published by Mittnik et al. [18]. This method compares the number of sequences originating from the X chromosome to the number of sequences originating from the 22 autosomes. A male assignment is made if the upper bound of the 95% CI is less than 0.60, while a female assignment is made if the lower bound is greater than 0.80.

Next, the shotgun data were used to analyze ~1.3 million nuclear SNPs that were covered by at least one read. From the SNP results, a "forced haploid" approach was used to assess relatedness between the two locket hairs, Lo2 and Lo3 (Figure 3).

In brief, relatedness was assessed by comparing allele mismatch proportions between the two locket hairs to expected allele mismatch proportions for unrelated, parent-child, sibling, and same individual relationships. Specifically, the shotgun datasets from Lo2 and Lo3 were first reduced to 1.3 million SNPs that include the SNPs generally typed by genetic genealogy companies and used in GEDmatch [19,20]. The number of SNPs was then further reduced to SNPs that overlapped between the two hair samples. Next, using a custom R script, the datasets were forced into pseudo-haploid genomes for which the allele mismatch proportion was calculated. The resulting SNP marker set (i.e., SNPs with allele calls in both samples) was used as the input in the mismatch proportion simulation method. To obtain expected mismatch proportion distributions, pseudo-haploid datasets for various degrees of relatedness (i.e., same individual, parent/child, full siblings, or unrelated individuals) were simulated using the European allele frequencies of the Genomes Project Consortium [21] and SNP-nexus [22,23] for the specific set of SNPs that were included in the sample comparison. In addition, a simplistic error model was included to account for the possibility of different genotype errors such as deamination, depurination, PCR error, sequencing error, and mapping error, that may occur for low-quality and low-quantity DNA samples. An error rate of 0 to 2% was used in our simulations. As controls, shotgun data from two 50 year-old-sourced hair samples, completely unconnected to this project and that were known to originate from the same individual (189A and 189B) were analyzed and compared. In addition, data from hair samples 189A and Lo2, which were known to originate from two unrelated individuals, were compared (a more detailed description of the method can be found in Supplementary Material #2).

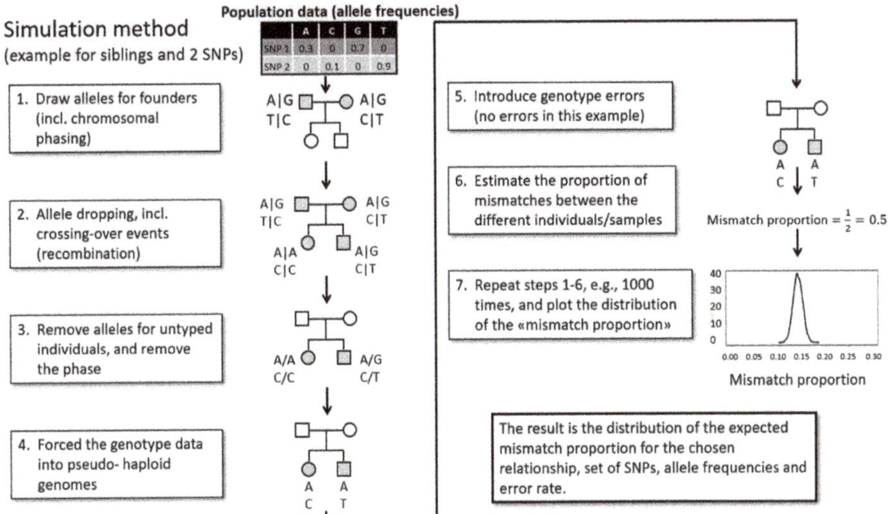

Figure 3. Simulation approach applied to infer the degree of relatedness between low coverage DNA datasets based on allele mismatch proportions.

Finally, some of the unmapped reads were analyzed using the Metagenomics RAST (MG-RAST) server [24] in an effort to identify the source of the non-human reads.

4. Results

4.1. Histology Examination

The four microscopically-examined hairs were very well preserved overall (Figures 4A–C and 5) as characteristics of decomposition, insect damage, or fungal damage were not observed. Nor was there any indication of artificial treatment, such as dyeing or bleaching. Based on pigment arrangement, pigment density, overall diameter, cross-sectional shape of the hair shaft and the cuticle thickness, the examiner determined that all four hairs were most likely human head hairs of European ancestry.

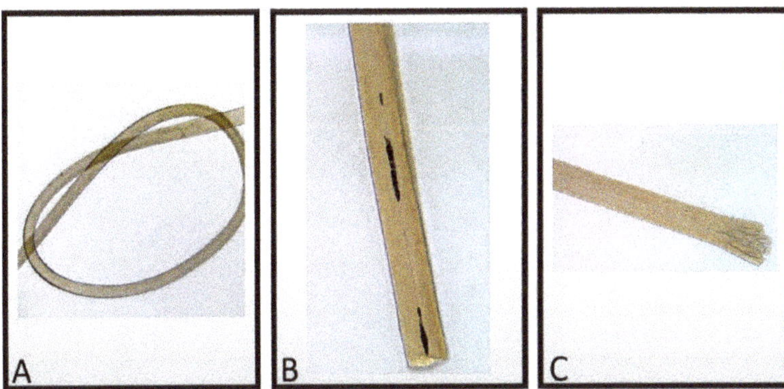

Figure 4. Photographs taken from three different hairs that were found in the Fabergé locket. (**A**) Magnification 100×. (**B**) Magnification 200× shows that the proximal end of the hair appears cut. (**C**) Magnification 200× shows that the proximal end of the hair appears broken.

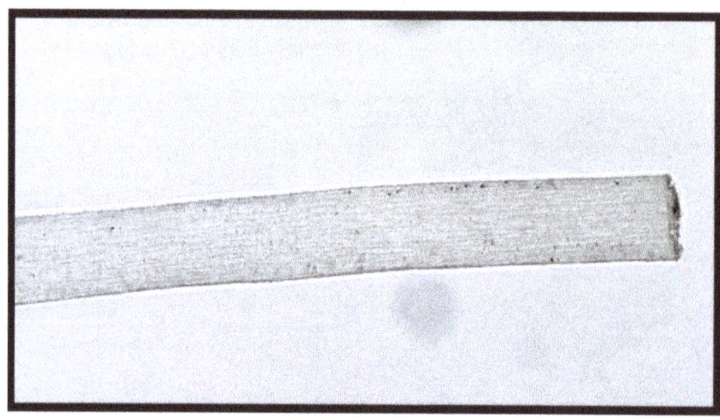

Figure 5. Magnification: 200×. Photograph taken from a white hair that was found in the picture frame. The proximal end of the hair appears cut.

Based on microscopic examination, it was established that no root was present on any of the samples examined.

4.2. Illumina Sequencing Results from the Fabergé Locket Hairs

Three libraries were produced with the locket samples. From sample Lo5h (extract/library from five hairs), a shotgun DNA library (Lo5h-sh, a library not enriched for any marker) as well as a mtDNA-enriched library (Lo5h-mt) were sequenced on a MiSeq FGx™. The mtDNA-enriched library Lo5h-mt was also sequenced on a NextSeq 500 to compare the data that were obtained from both instruments. For single hair extracts/library Lo2 and Lo3, shotgun libraries were only sequenced on a NextSeq 500 and no hybridization capture was performed. Sequencing statistics for the hair samples that were found in the locket are presented in Table 2 and more detailed information can be found in Supplementary Table S1. Shotgun library Lo5h-sh was only sequenced on a MiSeq FGx™ since our focus for the multi-hair extracts was to establish that DNA could be recovered from hairs of this age, and that is best addressed by targeting the mtGenome. In addition, since the locket had a picture of Tsarina Alexandra, it was conceivable that it contained hairs from herself and/or from some of her children. As a result, all the individuals would share the same mtGenome and data analysis would not be compromised by mixtures. Analysis of nuclear DNA, however, would have presented a challenge. Consequently, high throughput sequencing of Lo5h-sh for nuclear DNA analysis was not attempted on the NextSeq 500 platform.

Table 2. Sequencing statistics from the Fabergé locket hairs.

Shotgun Libraries	Platforms Used	Number of Mapped Reads	Percentage of Mapped Reads	Number of Unique Reads
Lo5h-sh (5 hairs)	MiSeq FGx™	6,229,985	48%	5,500,712
Lo2-sh (1 hair)	NextSeq 500	199,948,284	66.54%	38,036,020
Lo3-sh (1 hair)	NextSeq 500	151,630,120	78.91%	33,388,550

mtDNA-Enriched Library	Platforms Used	Number of Mapped Reads	Percentage of Mapped Reads	Number of Unique mtDNA Reads
Lo5h-mt (5 hairs)	NextSeq 500	21,109,044	97.50%	35,188

The percentage of endogenous human reads in the Lo5h-sh library was 48%. This percentage was a bit lower than expected considering that all hairs had been thoroughly decontaminated via Terg-a-zyme sonication before digestion. When unmapped reads of

75 bp or longer were analyzed with MG-RAST, close to 63% of the sequences remained unknown and most of the sequences that matched a sequence in GenBank belonged to the Proteobacteria phylum (Supplementary Material #2).

The percentage of endogenous human DNA was, however, higher when single hairs were extracted with the optimized protocol (66.54% for Lo2-sh and 78.91% for Lo3-sh). Additionally, as a precaution, purification reagents remained stored at 4°C between use to avoid potential mold growth. In this case, since both Lo2 and Lo3 were single source samples, high throughput sequencing of the libraries was carried out on the NextSeq 500 platform to collect as many DNA sequences as possible.

4.2.1. Mitochondrial DNA Results

MtDNA-enriched library Lo5h-mt produced 35,188 unique mtDNA reads representing >3.2 million bases. The entire mtGenome was successfully sequenced at an average depth of 198× (range: 159–273×; standard deviation (SD): 11.38). Shotgun sequencing of the Lo5h-sh produced 29,879 mtDNA reads representing >1.9 million bases. Once again, the complete mtGenome was sequenced at an average depth of 119× (range: 5–173×; SD: 17.77). The DNA length distributions of Lo5h-sh and Lo5h-mt are presented in Figure 6A.

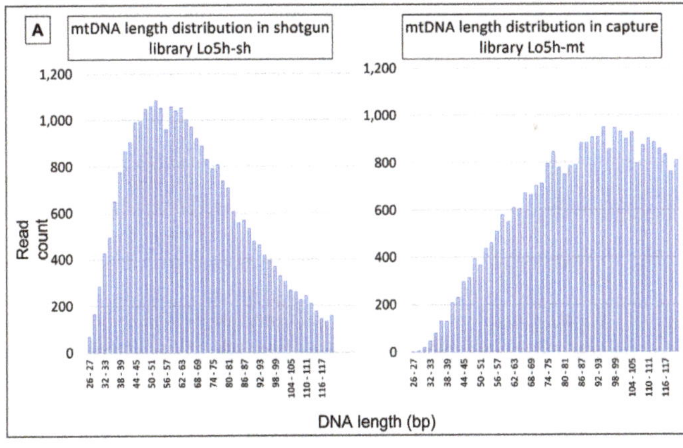

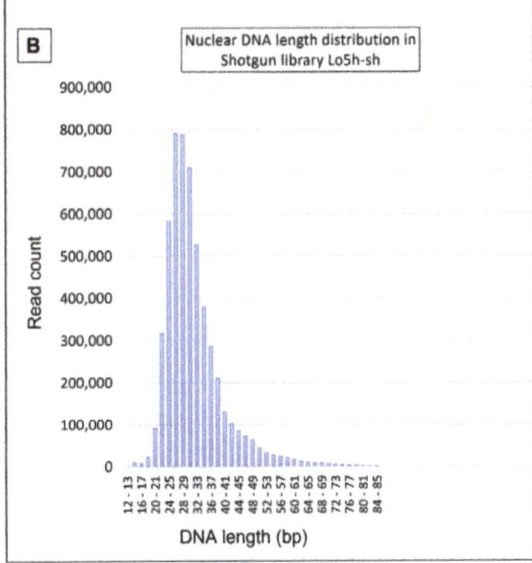

Figure 6. Length distribution of (**A**) mtDNA reads in Lo5h-sh and Lo5h-mt, and (**B**) nuclear DNA reads in Lo5h-sh.

Shotgun libraries Lo2-sh and Lo3-sh yielded 27,058 and 32,099 unique mtDNA sequences with an average depth of 111× (range: 22–148×; SD:13.08) and 164× (range: 26–219×; SD:12.06) respectively. MtDNA enrichment of the Lo2 and Lo3 libraries via hybridization capture was deemed unnecessary since there was sufficient coverage of the mtGenome in the shotgun data that were produced by the NextSeq.

The average mtDNA fragment length varied between 66.04 bp and 93.46 bp, depending on the library and the reference used for mapping (Tables 3 and S5). Interestingly, the hybridization capture library that was developed from Lo5h (Lo5h-mt) yielded an average mtDNA fragment size that was much larger than the one that was observed in the Lo5h shotgun library (Lo5h-sh).

Table 3. Average length of the mtDNA molecules in the locket libraries when mapped to hg19 (left) or to rCRS (right).

Library	Mapped mtDNA Reads Average Length (bp)
Lo2-sh	67.82/67.89
Lo3-sh	84.99/85.17
Lo5h-sh	66.04/69.16
Lo5h-mt	93.46

At 93.46 bp, the mean length of the mtDNA reads in the enriched Lo5h-mt library was substantially higher than the mean mtDNA length that were observed in the shotgun libraries (Table 3). This pattern between the shotgun and enriched libraries has been observed in several other studies involving ancient DNA [25–27]. Our hypothesis that the noticeable disparity in average length could be caused by a preferential binding of larger mtDNA molecules during hybridization capture was confirmed by Krasnenko et al. [28] who stated that "[…] insert size crucially impact(s) enrichment results" and that "the maximum efficiency of enrichment (>90%) is achieved with 250–330 bp insertion length". Of note, average DNA length estimates should be viewed with the following caveats in mind: they can be greatly influenced by factors such as DNA extraction protocol, library preparation protocol, number of sequencing cycles, and bioinformatics pipelines (trimming in particular).

Shotgun libraries Lo2-sh and Lo3-sh also showed substantial variation in mean mtDNA fragment length (67.82 versus 84.99 bp). These differences could be the result of a number of factors, including sample variability between individual hairs or variability resulting from the distance between the tested section and the root [12].

All the locket hair libraries produced the same mtGenome profile: 263G, 315.1C, 524.1A, 524.2C, 750G, 1438G, 3010A, 4137T, 4769G, 8860G, 15326G, 16111T, 16357C, and 16519C. The sequence belongs to haplogroup H1af2 and is identical to the mtGenome of Empress Alexandra's maternal lineage published as "Queen Victoria's profile" by Rogaev et al. [6], (GenBank # FJ656214). Detailed variant tables can be found in Supplementary Table S2.

4.2.2. Nuclear DNA Results

Sequencing of the shotgun libraries produced 38,008,962 (Lo2-sh), 33,328,275 (Lo3-sh), and 5,470,833 (Lo5h-sh) unique human nuclear sequences representing 1,256,322,853 (Lo2-sh), 1,104,095,334 (Lo3-sh), and 174,843,798 (Lo5h-sh) nucleotides, respectively. The average read depth was 0.40× (Lo2-sh), 0.35× (Lo3-sh) and 0.06× (Lo5h-sh), and the average nuclear DNA fragment length was 33.05 (Lo2-sh), 33.13 (Lo3-sh) and 31.96 bp (Lo5h-sh) (Table 4). In every library, at least 98.9% of the human DNA that was sequenced belonged to the nuclear genome.

Table 4. Average length of the nuclear DNA molecules in the locket libraries.

Library	Mapped Nuclear DNA Reads Average Length (bp)
Lo2-sh	33.05
Lo3-sh	33.13
Lo5h-sh	31.96

As has been previously observed in Brandhagen et al. [12], the average length of nuclear DNA fragments tends to be smaller than the average length of mtDNA fragments.

4.2.3. Biological Sex

The two single hairs that were shotgun sequenced (Lo2-sh and Lo3-sh) were assessed for biological sex. In both cases, the lower bound of the Rx confidence interval was >0.8, resulting in a biological sex of female (Table 5). This result excludes the Romanov's son, Tsarevich Alexis, as a possible source of these two hairs.

Table 5. Determination of the biological sex of the donor of the hairs that were found in the Fabergé locket using Rx as described in [18]. SD: standard deviation. CI: Confidence interval. The values indicating a biological sex of female are in bold.

Library	Rx	SD	CI	CI Low	CI Sup
Lo2-sh	0.965	0.231	0.097	**0.869**	1.062
Lo3-sh	0.935	0.229	0.097	**0.838**	1.031

4.2.4. Relatedness Estimates

In addition to being assessed for biological sex, hairs Lo2 and Lo3 were tested for relatedness. Only reads >35 bp were used for this analysis to avoid spurious mapping of bacterial sequences, as recommended by Meyer et al. [29]. Out of 1.3 million SNPs, 15,331 and 33,591 were covered by at least one read for Lo2-sh and Lo3-sh, respectively, and 1196 of these SNPs were covered in both samples. The proportion of allele mismatches was calculated to 0.11 after forcing the Lo2-sh and Lo3-sh datasets into pseudo-haploid genomes. Assuming a non-zero genotype error rate, such a proportion is expected among samples originating from the same individual and is, at the same time, unexpected for parent/child, siblings, and unrelated individuals (Figure 7). As controls for the forced haploid simulation approach, the mismatch proportions for the two known samples originating from the same individual as well as two samples originating from two known unrelated individuals were determined. The observed mismatch proportions for those comparisons fit well with the expected mismatch distributions for same individual and unrelated individuals, respectively (Supplementary Material #2). Based on the observed forced haploid mismatch proportion as evaluated against the simulated data and considering the error rate that is most appropriate for the given comparison, the data indicate that Lo2 and Lo3 originate from the same individual.

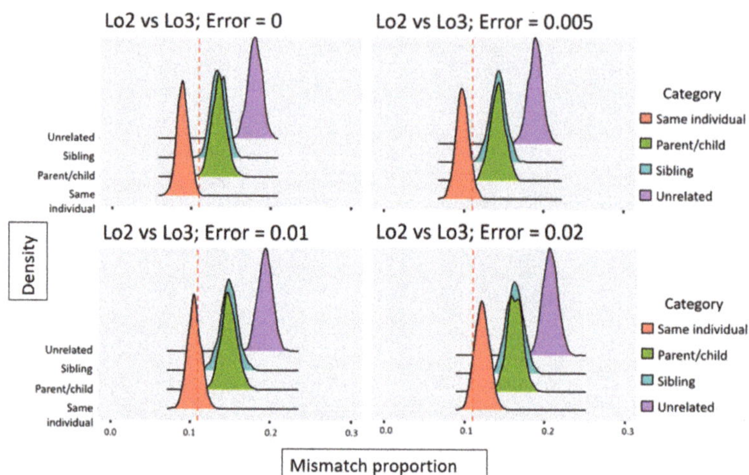

Figure 7. Observed mismatch proportion for the Lo2 vs. Lo3 comparison (red dashed line) in relation to the expected mismatch proportions for various degrees of relatedness and different genotype error rates.

4.3. Illumina Sequencing Results from the Picture Frame Hairs

Sequencing statistics for the hair samples that were found in the frame are shown in Table 6. The low percentage of endogenous human DNA in the library derived from six hairs (Q6h-sh) (21.17%) is even lower than the 48% that was observed with the library from five locket hairs (Lo5h-sh). However, as with the locket hairs, the percentage of human DNA improved substantially in the libraries that were derived from single hair shafts. Sample Q1-sh produced 70.12% human DNA, while Q2-sh produced 89%. The three hybridization capture libraries, not surprisingly, yielded the highest percentages of target DNA. In all three cases, ≥88% of the human reads were mtDNA sequences. Further details can be found in Supplementary Table S1.

Table 6. Sequencing data from libraries made with DNA extracted from hair shafts found in the picture frame.

Shotgun Libraries	Platforms Used	Number of Mapped Raw Reads	Percentage of Raw Mapped Reads	Number of Unique Human Reads
Q6h-sh (6 hairs)	MiSeq FGx	2,072,278	21.17%	1,817,968
Q1-sh (1 hair)	MiSeq FGx	267,392	70.12%	239,692
Q2-sh (1 hair)	NextSeq 500	278,531,240	89%	56,390,706
mtDNA-Enriched Libraries	**Platforms Used**	**Number of Mapped Raw Reads**	**Percentage of Raw Mapped mtDNA Reads**	**Number of Unique mtDNA Reads**
Q6h-mt (6 hairs)	MiSeq FGx	7,059,775	90.68%	26,038
Q1-mt (1 hair)	MiSeq FGx	3,586,989	96.69%	14,514
Q2-mt (1 hair)	MiSeq FGx	8,104,414	88%	24,636

Among the shotgun libraries, the number of endogenous molecules in Q1-sh was noticeably lower than in the other samples (Table 6). The high quantity of damage in this sample, exacerbated by an over- amplification of the DNA, resulted in a high percentage of noise in the data. As a result, the Q1-sh library was not sequenced on the NextSeq 500 instrument and fewer unique human reads were, therefore, recovered.

4.3.1. Mitochondrial DNA Results

Since the frame hairs seemed more degraded than the locket hairs, every Q library was enriched for mtDNA to produce the highest possible data quality.

For Q6h-mt, 26,038 unique mtDNA reads were obtained (>1.2 million bp) and the entire mtGenome was sequenced at an average depth of 74× (range: 27–117×; SD:11.45). At 47.26 bp, the average length of the DNA fragments was significantly shorter than the 93.08 bp average mtDNA size that was observed with Lo5h-mt.

For Q1-mt, a total of 14,514 unique mtDNA reads, spanning 563,192 bp were sequenced. In this case, the average read depth was 34× (range: 1–100×; SD: 14.98) and the average mtDNA length was 38.80 bp.

Finally, for Q2-mt, 24,636 unique reads totaling >1.1 million bp were recovered. Reads spanned the entire mtGenome, with an average read depth of 67× (range: 13–125×; SD: 15.49) and an average fragment length of 45.33 bp.

Mitochondrial DNA was also analyzed from the shotgun sequence data of Q6h-sh and Q2-sh (Table 7).

Table 7. Number of unique mitochondrial DNA reads and mean mtDNA lengths in the shotgun and capture libraries.

Sequencing Platform	Library	Number of Unique mtDNA Reads	Average mtDNA Size (bp). hg19/rCRS
MiSeq FGx™	Q6h-sh	11,052	45.78/45.56
MiSeq FGx™	Q6h-mt	26,038	47.26
MiSeq FGx™	Q1-sh	1281	NA
MiSeq FGx™	Q1-mt	14,514	38.80
NextSeq 500	Q2-sh	15,267	42.32/43.9
MiSeq FGx™	Q2-mt	24,636	45.33

The 1281 mtDNA reads obtained with Q1-sh were insufficient to produce reliable variant calls. Similar to what was observed with the locket hairs, the average mtDNA fragment size in the capture libraries was larger, although the magnitude of the difference was relatively small (Figure 8). This is likely due to the fact that the range of the average lengths for the mtDNA fragments in the frame hairs was smaller than the range that was observed with the locket hairs. Capture library Q6h-mt and shotgun library Q6h-sh both produced the following mtDNA profile: 73G, 263G, 315.1C, 709A, 750G, 1438G, 1842G, 1888A, 2706G, 2850C, 4216C, 4769G, 4917G, 6257A, 7022C, 7028T, 8697A, 8860G, 10463C, 11251G, 11719A, 11812G, 13368A, 13965C, 14233G, 14687G, 14766T, 14905A, 15326G, 15452A, 15607G, 15928A, 16126C, 16169Y, 16294T, 16296T, 16519C. The profile belongs to haplogroup T2a1a and is identical to the published sequence of Tsar Nicholas Romanov, including position 16169 which is characterized by a point heteroplasmy in the Tsar and his brother's mtGenome [3–6], (GenBank # FJ656215). Position 16169 had a read depth of 75× with 57 Ts and 18 Cs (76% T). In the shotgun data, the percentage of T versus C varies between 80% and 81% depending on the reference used for mapping. The reference can cause bias as a result of pseudogenes in the human genome. If data are mapped against hg19, which includes both the nuclear and the mitochondrial genome, unspecific sequences will be randomly mapped to one genome or the other, and true mtDNA sequences may be erroneously mapped to nuclear pseudogenes. On the other hand, if the data are mapped only to the rCRS, pseudogene sequences (although rare in these types of degraded samples) could erroneously map to the mtGenome. For this reason, the shotgun data were mapped to both references.

Since the Q6h library was prepared using six hairs, it is not possible to determine whether individual hairs were heteroplasmic or homoplasmic. That is, the mixed position at 16169 in both the shotgun and capture libraries could be the result of individual hairs being homoplasmic for the two variants.

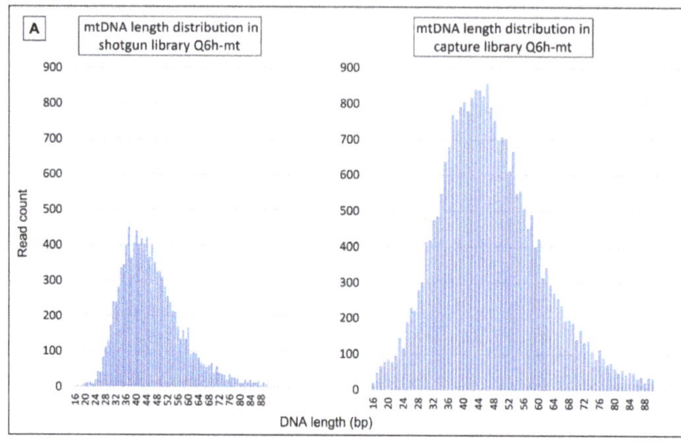

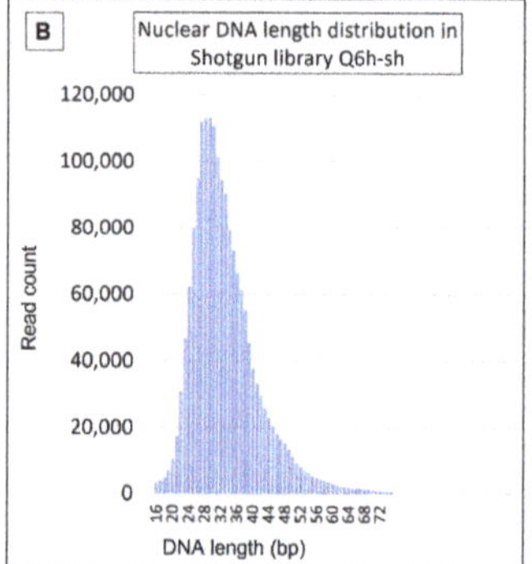

Figure 8. Length distribution of (**A**) mtDNA reads in Q6h-sh and Q6h-mt, and (**B**) nuclear DNA reads in Q6h-sh.

The mtGenome profile that was produced by Q1-mt is similar to the Q6h-mt profile with one exception: position 16169 appeared homoplasmic for thymine, with 27 out of 27 reads exhibiting a T.

In contrast to Q1-mt, position 16169 in library Q2-mt reflected primarily cytosine bases, with 53 C and 1 T. Since hydrolytic deamination is one of the most abundant forms of damage in ancient molecules, it is possible that the thymine base that was detected in the data was a deaminated cytosine [30,31]. In fact, in the shotgun library, all 25 reads have a C which supports 16169 being homoplasmic for cytosine.

4.3.2. Nuclear DNA Results

Sequencing of the library Q6h-sh produced 1,806,916 nuclear reads representing close to 60 million bases, an average read depth of $0.02\times$ (range: $1–109\times$; SD: 1.04), and a mean nuclear DNA length of 33.18 bp. Sequencing of library Q1-sh on a MiSeq FGx^{TM} produced 238,411 unique human nuclear sequences for a total of 8.4 million bases. The average read depth was $<0.01\times$ and the mean DNA length was 35.51 bp.

Finally, sequencing of library Q2-sh on a NextSeq 500 platform produced 56,375,439 unique human nuclear reads representing a total of 1.8 billion nucleotides. The average read depth was $0.58\times$ (range: 1–184; SD: 4.65) and the median nuclear read length was 32.06 bp.

Unfortunately, the number of quality reads that were recovered from Q1-sh was insufficient to perform a relatedness analysis between Q1 and Q2. However, the biological sex could be assessed.

For both hairs, the lower bound of the confidence interval was >0.8 (Table 8), resulting in a biological sex of female, the expected result if the hairs belonged to Queen Louise.

Table 8. Determination of the biological sex of the donor of two hairs that were found in the frame using Rx as described in [18]. SD: standard deviation. CI: Confidence interval. The values indicating a biological sex of female are in bold.

Library	Rx	SD	CI	CI Low	CI Sup
Q1-sh	0.903	0.201	0.084	**0.819**	0.987
Q2-sh	0.964	0.228	0.095	**0.868**	1.059

5. Discussion

The primary goal of this study was to explore the origin of the hairs in the locket and the frame using techniques and, more importantly, sample sizes that are relevant to forensic casework. By using these historical samples as a proxy for evidentiary material, protocols for extremely limited and compromised samples could be further optimized for routine casework. Overall, the results demonstrate that this method can successfully recover both full mitochondrial genomes and nuclear DNA data from the types of single, aged, and degraded hair samples that are routinely encountered in forensic casework. Furthermore, the results illustrate that limited genetic information can be useful for answering questions that are relevant to DNA identification. Specifically, the comparison between the single strands of hair that were tested from the locket indicate that despite partial SNP information for any given hair sample and limited overlapping data between any two hair samples, valuable information can be acquired. Typical forensic samples rarely, if ever, meet or exceed the suspected age and degradation states of the hairs tested here, yet the integrity of DNA in older cases with hairs recovered from less optimal storage conditions or that were originally collected from harsher environmental settings than those that were encountered here may make these studies directly applicable to some casework scenarios. Hence, the development of protocols for samples that challenge or exceed the lower detection limits of the currently employed methods demonstrates potential for the utility of the protocols in even the worst, or at least the vast majority of casework scenarios.

5.1. DNA Extraction Modifications

To maximize DNA recovery from the hair shafts, modifications were made to the purification step of the DNA extraction. Previous work has shown that both mtDNA and nuclear DNA can be obtained from single shed hairs up to 60 years old with a DNA extraction protocol that employed the MinElute PCR purification kit [12]. This particular protocol/purification method was used as a starting point to assess the feasibility of recovering DNA from hair this old, and extractions were performed with five (Lo5h) and six (Q6h) hairs to maximize the chances of detecting DNA.

When these two libraries were evaluated with the 2100 Bioanalyzer, the electropherograms of the reagent blanks showed a large curve that was similar to the ones that were observed with the hair libraries (Figure 9A).

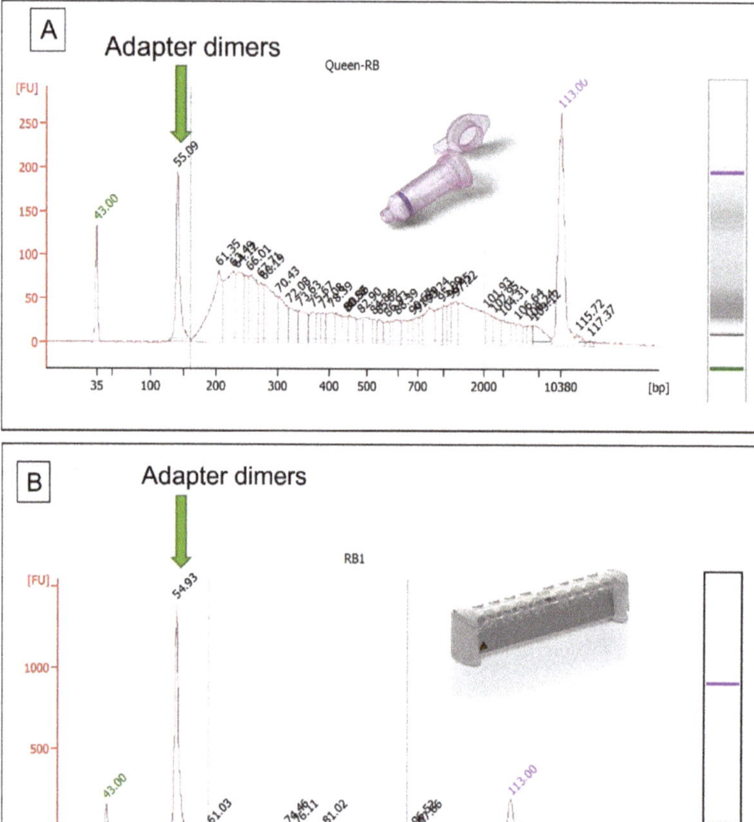

Figure 9. Bioanalyzer electropherograms of reagent blank libraries when DNA purification was performed using (**A**) MinElute columns, or (**B**) magnetic beads from G-Biosciences.

The sequencing of these reagent blank libraries produced data but the reads did not map to the human genome reference. These results suggest that the MinElute columns are contaminated with trace amounts of non-human DNA. For most human DNA identification applications, this type of very low-level contamination would have little impact on the final sequence data. Given that the contaminant is non-human and present only in trace quantities, the ratio of target human DNA to contaminant DNA would be high enough for the contaminant to go undetected. However, when the number of PCR cycles is high and when only a few target molecules are present in the extract, such as in the aged and degraded single hair shaft extracts that were tested here, the ratio of endogenous DNA to non-human contaminant DNA drops substantially. The MinElute columns were, therefore, replaced first with the Ultraclean Production (UCP) MinElute columns (cat # 56204, Qiagen). Though Bioanalyzer profiles of hair libraries that were purified with the UCP columns did not reflect the presence of any DNA, the columns were not used on the samples that were presented in this study for two reasons: (1) the use of a vacuum and extender columns was cumbersome and contamination-prone and (2) use of the columns resulted in a near doubling of library purification costs from ~$6 USD per sample to over $11 USD per sample. The columns were thus replaced with silica beads from G-Biosciences. These beads produced the same library purity as the UCP columns, but at a cost of ~$5 USD per sample. In addition, experiments that were performed on other aged hairs showed that the average size of DNA molecules that were collected by silica beads was slightly smaller than the DNA that was purified with MinElute and UCP MinElute columns. As a result, the columns were replaced by the more practical and cost-efficient DNA-free silica magnetic beads for all subsequent experiments.

The sequencing results of the bead-purified hair extracts demonstrated a substantial increase in the percentage of human DNA that was recovered (Tables 2 and 6). For the locket hairs, the recovery of human DNA improved from 48% in the MinElute-purified library (Lo5h-sh) to 66.54% (Lo2-sh) and 78.91% (Lo3-sh) in the two bead-purified shotgun libraries. Similarly, for the frame hairs, human DNA recovery increased from 21.17% (Q6h-sh) to 70.12% and 89% in Q1-sh and Q2-sh, respectively. Finally, unlike the Bioanalyzer electropherograms from the MinElute-purified libraries, the bead-purified RB library electropherograms exhibited only a single 140 bp peak of adapter dimers (Figure 9B).

In Brandhagen et al. [12], the previous version of our protocol had been tested as a way to save ultrashort DNA fragments that were lost during a wash step from the PrepFiler Kit protocol (Applied Biosystems, Waltham, MA, USA). We confirmed that the optimized silica beads protocol works equally well, or better, than the previous one in small fragment retention.

5.2. Authenticity of the Items

DNA testing is often employed to authenticate items of historical significance [32]. However, successful DNA testing is dictated by the type of item, its age and condition, how it has been stored, whether it has been handled/contaminated, etc. Items that can be decontaminated, such as hairs and calcified tissues, generally offer the best chance of success. Yet, even in cases for which the target DNA can often be recovered, authentication can still prove difficult, particularly when the direct or familial references that are required for identification are not straightforward to establish or acquire [33]. Fortunately, for historical items that are believed to be associated with the Romanov family, sufficient DNA reference information exists. Thus, on top of the historical evidence tying the locket and frame artifacts to the Romanov family, the DNA data that were recovered from the hairs may also prove useful.

5.2.1. Fabergé Locket
Historical Evidence of Authenticity

The photograph of Princess Alexandra displayed in the locket comes from a cabinet card, a type of photography mounted on a piece of cardboard that was very popular in the 1860s. It could be confidently identified as a copy of a photograph that was made in St Petersburg in 1895 by Alexander Pasetti, the photographer of the Imperial Russian court (see the original photograph in Supplementary Figure S4).

The pendant was crafted by the famous Russian jeweler and goldsmith, Karl Gustavovich Fabergé (also known as Peter Carl Fabergé; 1846–1920). Karl was the son of Gustav Fabergé, a German jeweler who moved to St. Petersburg in 1842 and opened the House of Fabergé. The association between Karl Fabergé and the Russian Imperial family is well documented. On Orthodox Easter of 1885, Tsar Alexander III Romanov offered his wife, Empress Maria Feodorovna, a jeweled Eastern Hen egg that was made by Fabergé [34]. The Empress liked it so much that Alexander named Fabergé goldsmith by special appointment to the Imperial crown and commissioned an Easter egg every following year. After Alexander's death in 1894, his son, Tsar Nicholas II, took over the tradition and asked Fabergé to create two unique eggs each year, one for his mother, the Dowager Empress Maria, and one for his wife Alexandra Feodorovna [35]. While Easter eggs made the House of Fabergé famous, they only represent a fraction of the Fabergé creations that were made for the Tsars and their families [34].

Genetic Evidence

The Tsarina's mtGenome was characterized in 2009 [6]. Hence, it was possible to directly compare the mtGenome haplotype that was developed from the locket hairs to the reference haplotype for the Tsarina; the two sequences are identical. The haplotype belongs to haplogroup H1af2 [36], which is characterized by a C4137T transition. To understand the rarity of the haplotype, three different mtDNA datasets were searched: the public FamilyTreeDNA© mitochondrial DNA Haplotree database [37], GenBank, and the European DNA Profiling Group mtDNA Population database (EMPOP, [38]). Sequence level data could not be compared in the FamilyTreeDNA© dataset. However, only ten of 170,000 complete mtGenome sequences were reported to belong to the H1af2 haplogroup. When the complete mtGenome sequence is compared to the GenBank database, no match is returned besides the profiles of the Tsarina, Alexei, and Maria, that were published by Rogaev et al. [6]. In fact, of more than 52,000 mtGenome profiles present in GenBank, only 38 sequences have a C4137T, and only five of those (including the three profiles mentioned above) belongs to haplogroup H [39]. H1af2 sequences are not currently present in EMPOP. While it is not possible to establish the identity based on mtDNA, the rarity of this profile increases the odds that the hairs that were found in the locket belonged to the Tsarina or a member of her maternal lineage.

To gain further insight into the source of the hairs and, in more general terms, explore the potential probative value of the nuclear DNA data that were recovered, autosomal SNPs were also analyzed. Autosomal SNP reference data was not available for the Tsarina or her relatives, so our goal with the SNP analysis was not source identity. Instead, the SNP results were used to assess if the strands of hair in the locket originated from the same individual or from multiple individuals from the same maternal lineage. Assuming the hairs belong to the Tsarina or one of her immediate maternal relatives (i.e., her children), the hairs would be over 100 years old. If this is indeed the case, the presence of mtDNA fragments that were larger than 90 bp in both the shotgun and the enriched library of Lo5h suggests that at least a portion of the molecules was well preserved.

In previous studies, hairs of somewhat similar age have yielded average mtDNA fragment sizes of approximately 60 bp [8], while younger hairs (between 40 and 60 years old) were shown to harbor mtDNA fragments averaging 70–80 bp [12]. There could be at least two explanations for the great preservation of the locket hair DNA. First, according to the locket owner, Mr. Bachmakov, the locket was extremely difficult to open and required specialized tools to do so. In Mr. Bachmakov's expert opinion, the locket had not been opened for years, perhaps even decades, and it is likely that the hairs remained safely sealed and protected from oxygen, light, and humidity. Second, saw dust that was found inside the locket may have acted as a desiccant. In the 19th and 20th centuries, jewels that were made of gold were treated with acid to enrich the proportion of gold on the surface and to change the color from a pink to a yellow gold [40]. After being rinsed with water, the objects were dried and saw dust was used to absorb moisture. In some cases, as in the case of this Fabergé locket, small amounts of saw dust remained inside the jewels. Unbeknown to the maker of the pendant, the desiccant properties of the saw dust may have played a key role in preserving the hairs and their genetic material.

5.2.2. Picture Frame
Historical Evidence

The origin of the framed picture of Queen Louise of Hesse Kassel is supported by documents that were provided to Mr. Bachmakov when the object was purchased. The paperwork indicates that the framed photograph had originally belonged to Maria Feodorovna (known as Princess Dagmar of Denmark prior to her marriage), one of Louise's daughters. It was passed down to one of Maria Feodorovna's daughters, Grand Duchess Xenia (1875–1960), and then again through various family members to a living descendant who kept it in his/her possession until 2017 when it was purchased by Mr. Bachmakov. The picture also comes from a cabinet card and the initials on the back show that the photograph was taken by Mary Steen, a famous Danish photographer who, in 1896, was appointed court photographer to Alexandra, Princess of Wales (1844–1925), later Queen Alexandra (Supplementary Figure S5).

Given the picture of Queen Louise and the fact that the strands of hair were white, it is presumed that they came from the Queen and were collected from her in her senior years. If these assumptions are correct, the hairs would be at least 120 years old.

Genetic Evidence and mtDNA Heteroplasmy

Mitochondrial DNA sequencing was performed to test the hypothesis that the frame hairs are from Tsar Nicholas' maternal grandmother, Queen Louise of Hesse-Kassel. Fortunately, the mtDNA sequence of the Tsar's maternal lineage is well documented. His control region (CR) haplotype was first reported in a study on the DNA analysis of skeletal remains that were discovered in Russia in 1991 and attributed to Nicholas II. The profile was compared to the CR of two living relatives who served as maternal references: James George Alexander Bannerman Carnegie, 3rd Duke of Fife (1929–2015), the Tsar's first cousin twice removed and Countess Xenia Cheremeteva Sfiris (b. 1942), his great grandniece [3] (Figure 10). The profile of Tsar Nicholas revealed a C/T point heteroplasmy at position 16169 that was not present in the two references CR profiles that only had the 16169T variant. Since little was known about the occurrence of mitochondrial DNA heteroplasmy variants in the early 1990s, the mixed C/T position was originally viewed by skeptics as a "mismatch" between the tsar's remains and his living relatives. However, two studies, both published in 1996, settled the debate. Ivanov et al. [4] analyzed the skeletal remains of the Tsar's brother, Grand Duke George (1871–1899) and the study revealed once more, the presence of a point heteroplasmy at position 16169, albeit with opposite ratios. While C was the predominant base in Nicholas' DNA, T was the dominant allele that was observed in his brother's profile. Concurrently, the CR from Tikhon Nikolaevich Kulikovsky-Romanov (1917–1993), one of Tsar Nicholas nephews, was also Sanger sequenced and, in this case, only cytosines were observed at position 16169, adding credence to the presence of an heteroplasmic variant in the Tsar's DNA [41].

The point heteroplasmy in the Tsar's lineage was again confirmed in 2009, following the discovery of skeletal remains that were believed to be the two missing Romanov children. Additional genetic analyses of all the skeletal remains that were found in 1991 not only confirmed that the two sets of newly discovered skeletal remains were the two missing Romanov children [5], but also re-established the presence of point heteroplasmy in the Tsar's remains [6].

In this study, the 16169 point heteroplasmy was not observed in skeletal remains, but in hair shafts. The occurrence of mtDNA heteroplasmy in human hairs has been extensively characterized [42,43]. Studies show that different levels of heteroplasmy can be observed in hairs from a single individual, as was seen in [44–47] and even along the length of a single hair shaft [48]. Our study followed the transmission of heteroplasmy through six generations. Interestingly, while it endured between the two generations that separate the Tsar from his grandmother, it seems to have rapidly evolved towards homoplasmy in the three different branches of the family that were studied. The perfect match between the sequence of the Tsar's mtGenome and the sequence from the frame hairs, as well as the presence of a point heteroplasmy at position 16169 are consistent with the hairs coming from Louise of Hesse-Kassel, Queen of Denmark or another individual that is maternally related to Tsar Nicholas II.

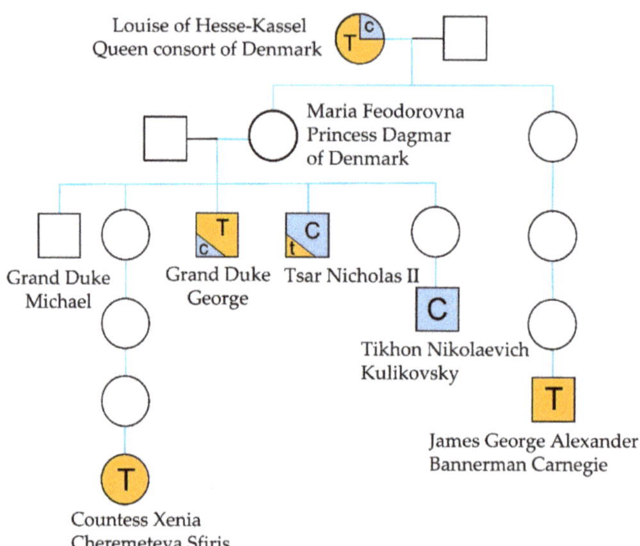

Figure 10. Family tree of the Romanov family showing the major allele (T or C) at heteroplasmic position 16169.

6. Conclusions

We have previously shown that nuclear DNA can be recovered from single rootless hair shafts [12]. Here, we extend that work by demonstrating that both mitochondrial and nuclear DNA can be recovered from single rootless hairs of substantial age when an extraction protocol that is designed for highly fragmented DNA is employed. Further, by optimizing the extraction protocol to eliminate/reduce low level contaminating DNA from the reagents and supplies, we improved both DNA yields and downstream sequencing results.

Given that traditional nuclear and mitochondrial DNA typing assays generally target DNA fragments larger than 100–150 bp, extraction protocols optimized for the retention of smaller fragments may often be unnecessary. For the most compromised specimens, however, this type of specialized extraction coupled with shotgun sequencing, may offer the best and perhaps only chance of recovering probative DNA data. With an average mtDNA and nuclear DNA fragment sizes of approximately 40–85 bp and 33 bp, respectively, the hair samples tested here would have failed to produce DNA results with even the smallest mtDNA amplicons routinely used in operational casework. In addition, standard extraction protocols would likely have discarded much or most of the endogenous target DNA. By combining an optimized extraction protocol and next generation shotgun sequencing, it was possible to recover complete mtGenomes from hair samples that are most likely older than any evidence or reference hair sample that is generally submitted to a crime laboratory. These very old samples not only produced 14-times more mtDNA sequencing data than the control region would, they also produced enough nuclear DNA to assess the biological sex and, in one case, relatedness among samples.

Our results further demonstrate that probative nuclear DNA can likely be recovered from the types of single rootless hair shafts encountered in casework and generally tested for mtDNA only. By extension, the results suggest that aged hair from keepsake lockets, hairbrushes, and other aged sources may serve as alternative direct or familial reference material for missing persons cases that are requiring nuclear DNA and for which hair samples are the only available material. Finally, it is likely that this or similar extraction protocol(s) can be useful on any type of highly degraded sample. Indeed, we have also used this protocol for samples that were not hairs and can confirm that it can be extremely successful with any sample type that contains highly degraded DNA molecules.

Supplementary Materials: The following supporting information can be downloaded at: https://www.mdpi.com/article/10.3390/genes13020202/s1. Supplementary Material #1: Description of the optimized DNA extraction protocol for hair shafts; Supplementary Material #2: Description of the forced haploid and simulation method; Table S1: Sequencing statistics for all the hairs that were analyzed in this study. Table S2: Variant calls for the hairs found in the Fabergé locket. Table S3: Variant calls for the hairs found in the picture frame. Table S4: Data from reagent blanks. Table S5: Nuclear and mitochondrial DNA length observed in all the libraries. Figure S1: Pictures of the Fabergé locket. A. Locket and items that were recovered inside the right side of the jewel. B. Open locket showing the engraved number 15,650. C. Back of the locket showing the Tsarina's initials and the imperial crown of Russia. D. Jump ring from the locket showing the stamped initials of Karl Fabergé. E. Lock of hairs that were found in the locket; Figure S2: Picture frame A. before and B. after restoration by Mr. Bachmakov; Figure S3: RAST results for Lo5h-sh. Figure S4: A. Cabinet card showing a photograph of Tsarina Alexandra made by Alexander Pasetti. B. Close up view of the Tsarina's face. C. Picture that was found in the locket; Figure S5: Picture of Queen Louise of Hesse-Kassel taken in 1863 (source: Wikipedia). B. Back of the cabinet card found in the picture frame partially showing the name of Danish photographer Mary Steen. C. Front of the picture found in the picture frame.

Author Contributions: O.L. conceived the experiments. O.L., M.D.B. and L.O. performed the experiments. O.L. and A.T. performed data analyses. O.L., J.A.I. and A.T., wrote the manuscript. All authors have read and agreed to the published version of the manuscript.

Funding: This research received no external funding.

Data Availability Statement: The mtDNA data can be found in GenBank under project number PRJNA782999. For GenBank Biosample numbers, see Tables S2 and S3.

Acknowledgments: Above all, we would like to express our deep gratitude to Nikolai Bachmakov and Peter Sarandinaki who entrusted us with very precious samples and for patiently responding to all our questions. We are also extremely grateful to have been allowed to use a supercomputer for our bioinformatics analyses. Jeroen van der Perk, Thomas Lehman, Brian D. Osmond, and Steven Jaslar, thank you. The authors would also like to acknowledge Michael Perekrestov from the Russian History Foundation for allowing us to use the Museum's photographs. Finally, we would like to thank our internal reviewers: Kyleen Elwick, Michelle Galusha, Jade Gray, Thomas Callaghan, Antony Onorato, and Lara Adams for their critical review of the manuscript.

Conflicts of Interest: Names of commercial manufacturers are provided for identification purposes only and inclusion does not imply endorsement of the manufacturer, or its products or services by the FBI. The views expressed are those of the authors and do not necessarily reflect the official policy or position of the FBI. This is FBI Laboratory publication #22–08.

References

1. Massie, R.K. *The Romanovs: The Final Chapter*; Random House: New York, NY, USA, 1995.
2. Byard, R.W. The execution of the Romanov family at Yekatarinberg. *Forensic Sci. Med. Pathol.* **2020**, *16*, 552–556. [CrossRef] [PubMed]
3. Gill, P.; Ivanov, P.L.; Kimpton, C.P.; Piercy, R.; Benson, N.; Tully, G.; Evett, I.; Hagelberg, E.; Sullivan, K. Identification of the remains of the Romanov family by DNA analysis. *Nat. Genet.* **1994**, *6*, 130–135. [CrossRef] [PubMed]
4. Ivanov, P.L.; Wadhams, M.J.; Roby, R.K.; Holland, M.M.; Weedn, V.W.; Parsons, T.J. Mitochondrial DNA sequence heteroplasmy in the Grand Duke of Russia Georgij Romanov establishes the authenticity of the remains of Tsar Nicholas II. *Nat. Genet.* **1996**, *12*, 417–420. [CrossRef] [PubMed]
5. Coble, M.; Loreille, O.; Wadhams, M.J.; Edson, S.; Maynard, K.; Meyer, C.E.; Niederstätter, H.; Berger, C.; Berger, B.; Falsetti, A.B.; et al. Mystery Solved: The Identification of the Two Missing Romanov Children Using DNA Analysis. *PLoS ONE* **2009**, *4*, e4838. [CrossRef]
6. Rogaev, E.I.; Grigorenko, A.P.; Moliaka, Y.K.; Faskhutdinova, G.; Goltsov, A.; Lahti, A.; Hildebrandt, C.; Kittler, E.L.W.; Morozova, I. Genomic identification in the historical case of the Nicholas II royal family. *Proc. Natl. Acad. Sci. USA* **2009**, *106*, 5258–5263. [CrossRef]

7. Melton, T.; Dimick, G.; Higgins, B.; Lindstrom, L.; Nelson, K. Forensic Mitochondrial DNA Analysis of 691 Casework Hairs. *J. Forensic Sci.* **2005**, *50*, 73–80. [CrossRef]
8. Tobler, R.; Rohrlach, A.; Soubrier, J.; Bover, P.; Llamas, B.; Tuke, J.; Bean, N.; Abdullah-Highfold, A.; Agius, S.; O'Donoghue, A.; et al. Aboriginal mitogenomes reveal 50,000 years of regionalism in Australia. *Nature* **2017**, *544*, 180–184. [CrossRef]
9. Rasmussen, M.; Li, Y.; Lindgreen, S.; Pedersen, J.S.; Albrechtsen, A.; Moltke, I.; Metspalu, M.; Metspalu, E.; Kivisild, T.; Gupta, R.; et al. Ancient human genome sequence of an extinct Palaeo-Eskimo. *Nature* **2010**, *463*, 757–762. [CrossRef]
10. Rasmussen, M.; Guo, X.; Wang, Y.; Lohmueller, K.E.; Rasmussen, S.; Albrechtsen, A.; Skotte, L.; Lindgreen, S.; Metspalu, M.; Jombart, T.; et al. An Aboriginal Australian Genome Reveals Separate Human Dispersals into Asia. *Science* **2011**, *334*, 94–98. [CrossRef]
11. Moltke, I.; Korneliussen, T.S.; Seguin-Orlando, A.; Moreno-Mayar, J.V.; LaPointe, E.; Billeck, W.; Willerslev, E. Identifying a living great-grandson of the Lakota Sioux leader Tatanka Iyotake (Sitting Bull). *Sci. Adv.* **2021**, *7*, 2013. [CrossRef]
12. Brandhagen, M.D.; Loreille, O.; Irwin, J.A. Fragmented Nuclear DNA Is the Predominant Genetic Material in Human Hair Shafts. *Genes* **2018**, *9*, 640. [CrossRef] [PubMed]
13. Rohland, N.; Glocke, I.; Aximu-Petri, A.; Meyer, M. Extraction of highly degraded DNA from ancient bones, teeth and sediments for high-throughput sequencing. *Nat. Protoc.* **2018**, *13*, 2447–2461. [CrossRef] [PubMed]
14. Kavlick, M.F. Development of a triplex mtDNA qPCR assay to assess quantification, degradation, inhibition, and amplification target copy numbers. *Mitochondrion* **2019**, *46*, 41–50. [CrossRef] [PubMed]
15. Li, H.; Durbin, R. Fast and accurate short read alignment with Burrows–Wheeler transform. *Bioinformatics* **2009**, *25*, 1754–1760. [CrossRef] [PubMed]
16. Li, H.; Handsaker, B.; Wysoker, A.; Fennell, T.; Ruan, J.; Homer, N.; Marth, G.; Abecasis, G.; Durbin, R.; 1000 Genome Project Data Processing Subgroup. The Sequence Alignment/Map format and SAMtools. *Bioinformatics* **2009**, *25*, 2078–2079. [CrossRef] [PubMed]
17. Picard. Available online: http://broadinstitute.github.io/picard (accessed on 15 September 2021).
18. Mittnik, A.; Wang, C.C.; Svoboda, J.; Krause, J. A Molecular Approach to the Sexing of the Triple Burial at the Upper Paleolithic Site of Dolni Vestonice. *PLoS ONE* **2016**, *11*, e0163019. [CrossRef] [PubMed]
19. Tillmar, A.; Sjölund, P.; Lundqvist, B.; Klippmark, T.; Älgenäs, C.; Green, H. Whole-genome sequencing of human remains to enable genealogy DNA database searches–A case report. *Forensic Sci. Int. Genet.* **2020**, *46*, 102233. [CrossRef] [PubMed]
20. Tillmar, A.; Fagerholm, S.A.; Staaf, J.; Sjölund, P.; Ansell, R. Getting the conclusive lead with investigative genetic genealogy –A successful case study of a 16 year old double murder in Sweden. *Forensic Sci. Int. Genet.* **2021**, *53*, 102525. [CrossRef]
21. 1000 Genomes Project Consortium; Auton, A.; Brooks, L.D.; Durbin, R.M.; Garrison, E.P.; Kang, H.M.; Korbel, J.O.; Marchini, J.L.; McCarthy, S.; McVean, G.A.; et al. A global reference for human genetic variation. *Nature* **2015**, *526*, 68–74.
22. Nexus. Available online: https://www.snp-nexus.org (accessed on 15 December 2020).
23. Oscanoa, J.; Sivapalan, L.; Gadaleta, E.; Ullah, A.Z.D.; Lemoine, N.R.; Chelala, C. SNPnexus: A web server for functional annotation of human genome sequence variation (2020 update). *Nucleic Acids Res.* **2020**, *48*, W185–W192. [CrossRef]
24. Meyer, F.; Paarmann, D.; Souza, M.D.; Olson, R.; Glass, E.M.; Kubal, M.; Paczian, T.; Rodriguez, A.; Stevens, R.; Wilke, A.; et al. The metagenomics RAST server—A public resource for the automatic phylogenetic and functional analysis of metagenomes. *BMC Bioinform.* **2008**, *9*, 386. [CrossRef] [PubMed]
25. Carpenter, M.; Buenrostro, J.D.; Valdiosera, C.; Schroeder, H.; Allentoft, M.; Sikora, M.; Rasmussen, M.; Gravel, S.; Guillén, S.; Nekhrizov, G.; et al. Pulling out the 1%: Whole-Genome Capture for the Targeted Enrichment of Ancient DNA Sequencing Libraries. *Am. J. Hum. Genet.* **2013**, *93*, 852–864. [CrossRef] [PubMed]
26. Enk, J.M.; Devault, A.M.; Kuch, M.; Murgha, Y.E.; Rouillard, J.M.; Poinar, H.N. Ancient whole genome enrichment using baits built from modern DNA. *Mol. Biol. Evol.* **2014**, *31*, 1292–1294. [CrossRef] [PubMed]
27. Ávila-Arcos, M.C.; Sandoval-Velasco, M.; Schroeder, H.; Carpenter, M.; Malaspinas, A.-S.; Wales, N.; Peñaloza, F.; Bustamante, C.D.; Gilbert, M.T.P. Comparative performance of two whole-genome capture methodologies on ancient DNA Illumina libraries. *Methods Ecol. Evol.* **2015**, *6*, 725–734. [CrossRef]
28. Krasnenko, A.; Tsukanov, K.; Stetsenko, I.; Klimchuk, O.; Plotnikov, N.; Surkova, E.; Ilinsky, V. Effect of DNA insert length on whole-exome sequencing enrichment efficiency: An observational study. *Adv. Genom. Genet.* **2018**, *8*, 13–15. [CrossRef]
29. Meyer, M.; Arsuaga, J.L.; de Filippo, C.; Nagel, S.; Aximu-Petri, A.; Nickel, B.; Martinez, I.; Gracia, A.; de Castro, J.M.B.; Carbonell, E.; et al. Nuclear DNA sequences from the Middle Pleistocene Sima de los Huesos hominins. *Nature* **2016**, *531*, 504–507. [CrossRef]
30. Hofreiter, M.; Jaenicke, V.; Serre, D.; von Haeseler, A.; Pääbo, S. DNA sequences from multiple amplifications reveal artifacts induced by cytosine deamination in ancient DNA. *Nucleic Acids Res.* **2001**, *29*, 4793–4799. [CrossRef]
31. Rathbun, M.M.; McElhoe, J.A.; Parson, W.; Holland, M.M. Considering DNA damage when interpreting mtDNA heteroplasmy in deep sequencing data. *Forensic Sci. Int. Genet.* **2017**, *26*, 1–11. [CrossRef]
32. King, T.E.; Fortes, G.G.; Balaresque, P.; Thomas, M.G.; Balding, D.; Delser, P.M.; Neumann, R.; Parson, W.; Knapp, M.; Walsh, S.; et al. Identification of the remains of King Richard III. *Nat. Commun.* **2014**, *5*, 5631. [CrossRef]
33. Parson, W.; Loreille, O.; Niederstätter, H.; Parsons, T.J.; Scheithauer, R. DNA Investigations of the putative Mozart cranium. In Proceedings of the 17th International Symposium on Human Identification, Nashville, TN, USA, 10 October 2006.
34. Bainbridge, C.; Peter, C.F. *Goldsmith and Jeweller to the Russian Imperial Court and the Principal Crowned Heads of Europe*; Batsford: London, UK, 1 January 1949.

35. Available online: https://www.christies.com/features/Faberge-15-things-a-collector-needs-to-know-8353-1.aspx (accessed on 15 September 2021).
36. van Oven, M.; Kayser, M. Updated comprehensive phylogenetic tree of global human mitochondrial DNA variation. *Hum. Mutat.* **2009**, *30*, e386–e394. [CrossRef]
37. FamilyTree DNA. Available online: https://www.familytreedna.com/public/mt-dna-haplotree/H (accessed on 20 December 2021).
38. EMPOP. Available online: https://www.empop.org (accessed on 20 December 2021).
39. MITOMASTER. Available online: https://www.mitomap.org/foswiki/bin/view/MITOMASTER/WebHome (accessed on 20 December 2021).
40. Bachmakov, N. Expert in Antique Restoration in New York, New York, NY, USA. Personal communication, 2020.
41. Rogaev, I.E.; Ovchinnikov, I.V.; Dzhorzh-Khislop, P.; Rogaeva, A.E. Comparison of mitochondrial DNA sequences of T.N. Kulikovski? -Romanov, the nephew of Tsar Nikola? II Romanov, with DNA from the putative remains of the Tsar. *Генетика* **1996**, *32*, 1690–1692.
42. Comas, D.; Pääbo, S.; Bertranpetit, J. Heteroplasmy in the control region of human mitochondrial DNA. *Genome Res.* **1995**, *5*, 89–90. [CrossRef]
43. Bendall, K.E.; Macaulay, V.A.; Sykes, B.C. Variable Levels of a Heteroplasmic Point Mutation in Individual Hair Roots. *Am. J. Hum. Genet.* **1997**, *61*, 1303–1308. [CrossRef]
44. Alonso, A.; Salas, A.; Albarrán, C.; Arroyo-Pardo, E.; Castro, A.; Crespillo, M.; di Lonardo, A.M.; Lareu, M.V.; Cubría, C.L.; Soto, M.L.; et al. Results of the 1999–2000 collaborative exercise and proficiency testing program on mitochondrial DNA of the GEP-ISFG: An inter-laboratory study of the observed variability in the heteroplasmy level of hair from the same donor. *Forensic Sci. Int.* **2002**, *125*, 1–7. [CrossRef]
45. Sekiguchi, K.; Sato, H.; Kasai, K. Mitochondrial DNA heteroplasmy among hairs from single individuals. *J. Forensic Sci.* **2004**, *49*, 986–991. [CrossRef]
46. Tully, G.; Barritt, S.; Bender, K.; Brignon, E.; Capelli, C.; Dimo-Simonin, N.; Eichmann, C.; Ernst, C.; Lambert, C.; Lareu, M.; et al. Results of a collaborative study of the EDNAP group regarding mitochondrial DNA heteroplasmy and segregation in hair shafts. *Forensic Sci. Int.* **2004**, *140*, 1–11. [CrossRef]
47. Van Der Gaag, K.J.; Desmyter, S.; Smit, S.; Prieto, L.; Sijen, T. Reducing the Number of Mismatches between Hairs and Buccal References When Analysing mtDNA Heteroplasmic Variation by Massively Parallel Sequencing. *Genes* **2020**, *11*, 1355. [CrossRef]
48. Desmyter, S.; Bodner, M.; Huber, G.; Dognaux, S.; Berger, C.; Noël, F.; Parson, W. Hairy matters: MtDNA quantity and sequence variation along and among human head hairs. *Forensic Sci. Int. Genet.* **2016**, *25*, 1–9. [CrossRef]

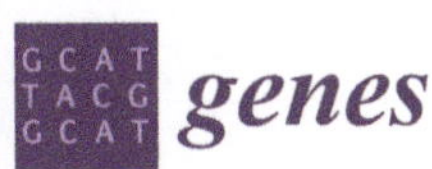

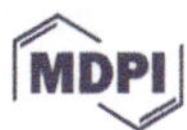

Article

Prediction of Eye Colour in Scandinavians Using the EyeColour 11 (EC11) SNP Set

Olivia Strunge Meyer [1,*,†], Nina Mjølsnes Salvo [2,†], Anne Kjærbye [1], Marianne Kjersem [2], Mikkel Meyer Andersen [3], Erik Sørensen [4], Henrik Ullum [5], Kirstin Janssen [2], Niels Morling [1], Claus Børsting [1], Gunn-Hege Olsen [2] and Jeppe Dyrberg Andersen [1]

[1] Section of Forensic Genetics, Department of Forensic Medicine, Faculty of Health and Medical Sciences, University of Copenhagen, 2100 Copenhagen, Denmark; anne.kjaerbye@sund.ku.dk (A.K.); niels.morling@sund.ku.dk (N.M.); claus.boersting@sund.ku.dk (C.B.); jeppe.dyrberg.andersen@sund.ku.dk (J.D.A.)

[2] Centre for Forensic Genetics, Department of Medical Biology, UiT–The Arctic University of Norway, 9037 Tromsø, Norway; nina.mjolsnes@uit.no (N.M.S.); marianne.kjersem@uit.no (M.K.); kirstin.janssen@uit.no (K.J.); gunn-hege.olsen@uit.no (G.-H.O.)

[3] Department of Mathematical Sciences, Aalborg University, 9220 Aalborg, Denmark; mikl@math.aau.dk

[4] Department of Clinical Immunology, Copenhagen University Hospital, Rigshospitalet, 2100 Copenhagen, Denmark; erik.soerensen@regionh.dk

[5] Statens Serum Institut, 2300 Copenhagen, Denmark; heul@ssi.dk

* Correspondence: olivia.meyer@sund.ku.dk

† These authors contributed equally.

Citation: Meyer, O.S.; Salvo, N.M.; Kjærbye, A.; Kjersem, M.; Andersen, M.M.; Sørensen, E.; Ullum, H.; Janssen, K.; Morling, N.; Børsting, C.; et al. Prediction of Eye Colour in Scandinavians Using the EyeColour 11 (EC11) SNP Set. *Genes* 2021, 12, 821. https://doi.org/10.3390/genes12060821

Academic Editor: Fulvio Cruciani

Received: 12 May 2021
Accepted: 25 May 2021
Published: 27 May 2021

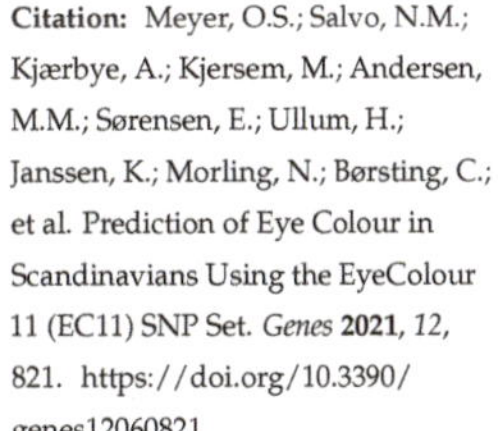
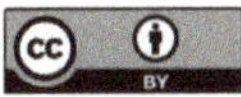

Abstract: Description of a perpetrator's eye colour can be an important investigative lead in a forensic case with no apparent suspects. Herein, we present 11 SNPs (Eye Colour 11-EC11) that are important for eye colour prediction and eye colour prediction models for a two-category reporting system (blue and brown) and a three-category system (blue, intermediate, and brown). The EC11 SNPs were carefully selected from 44 pigmentary variants in seven genes previously found to be associated with eye colours in 757 Europeans (Danes, Swedes, and Italians). Mathematical models using three different reporting systems: a quantitative system (PIE-score), a two-category system (blue and brown), and a three-category system (blue, intermediate, brown) were used to rank the variants. SNPs with a sufficient mean variable importance (above 0.3%) were selected for EC11. Eye colour prediction models using the EC11 SNPs were developed using leave-one-out cross-validation (LOOCV) in an independent data set of 523 Norwegian individuals. Performance of the EC11 models for the two- and three-category system was compared with models based on the IrisPlex SNPs and the most important eye colour locus, rs12913832. We also compared model performances with the IrisPlex online tool (IrisPlex Web). The EC11 eye colour prediction models performed slightly better than the IrisPlex and rs12913832 models in all reporting systems and better than the IrisPlex Web in the three-category system. Three important points to consider prior to the implementation of eye colour prediction in a forensic genetic setting are discussed: (1) the reference population, (2) the SNP set, and (3) the reporting strategy.

Keywords: forensic genetics; eye colour; rs12913832; pigmentation; DNA phenotyping

1. Introduction

Prediction of physical traits (externally visible characteristics) from DNA can be important in criminal cases with no apparent suspects. Multiple assays for forensic prediction of eye colour, hair colour, skin colour, and biogeographic ancestry have been developed with varying accuracies [1–5]. Prediction of biogeographic ancestry can give an indirect indication of a person's appearance. However, for individuals of European ancestry, there are large variations in eye colour. A direct description of the eye colour of a perpetrator could aid police investigators in focusing on a smaller group of individuals. The most widely known system for eye colour prediction is the IrisPlex assay [3], which is based on six SNPs in six genes (*HERC2, OCA2, SLC24A4, SLC45A2, TYR*, and *IRF4*) that are associated with eye colour variation. The IrisPlex predicts eye colour in three categories: blue, intermediate, and brown [3,6]. It is well known that a single SNP in *HERC2*, rs12913832, is almost perfectly associated with blue and brown eye colour [7,8]. The SNP is located in the promoter region of *OCA2* and strongly associated with *OCA2* expression [9]. In 2012, Visser and co-workers demonstrated that the *OCA2* expression was increased in melanocytes carrying the rs12913832: A allele and decreased in melanocytes carrying the rs12913832: G allele. Hence, individuals carrying a rs12913832: A allele (genotypes rs12913832: AA and rs12913832:AG) are expected to have brown eye colour, and individuals carrying the genotype rs12913832:GG are expected to have blue eye colour. Eye colour prediction using the IrisPlex relies heavily on rs12913832 [10]. Thus, the IrisPlex prediction shows high accuracies for blue and brown eye colour but low accuracy for intermediate eye colour [3]. Some individuals do not follow the expected genotype–phenotype patterns of rs12913832, and for these individuals, the IrisPlex eye colour predictions are incorrect [10,11]. We previously performed in-depth sequencing analyses of individuals with incorrect IrisPlex eye colour predictions and identified variants in *OCA2, TYRP1, TYR*, and *SLC24A4* that may explain the incorrectly predicted eye colours [11,12]. In this study, we typed those variants and the IrisPlex SNPs in 757 European individuals and selected 11 SNPs for a new eye colour prediction model, named Eye Colour 11 (EC11). We modelled and tested the EC11 in an independent data set of 523 Norwegian individuals and compared the predictions with a model solely based on the rs12913832 SNP and a model based on the six IrisPlex SNPs (called IrisPlex Norway) using different reporting systems. Lastly, we compared the results with those obtained with the IrisPlex online prediction tool (IrisPlex Web) [3].

2. Materials and Methods

2.1. Samples and DNA Extraction

A total of 757 healthy individuals residing in Denmark, Sweden, or Italy comprised the variant discovery data set. The model data set included 523 healthy individuals living in Tromsø and Bodø (Norway). Blood samples were collected from employees and students at universities, residents and employees at health care centres, employees at hospitals, and through the Danish Blood Donor Study as described elsewhere [10,13,14]. DNA was extracted using the QIAamp DNA Blood Mini Kit (Qiagen, Hilden, Germany), the QIAsymphony DNA Midi Kit (Qiagen, Hilden, Germany), or the PrepFiler™ Express DNA Extraction kit (Thermo Fisher Scientific, Waltham, MA, USA) following instructions from the manufacturers. The use of material was approved by the Danish Ethical Committee (M-20090237, H-4-2009-125, and H-3-2012-023), the Ethical Committee of Azienda Ospedaliera Ospedal Sant'Anna di Como (U.0026484.23-11-2012), the Ethical Committee of the University of Milan-Bicocca (P.U. 0033373/12), and the Faculty of Health Sciences, UiT–The Arctic University of Norway (2021/2034). All participants gave signed and informed consent and all samples were anonymised.

2.2. Quantitative Eye Colour Measurements and Eye Colour Categorisation

A digital photograph of one of the eyes of each participant was taken as described previously [13]. The pixel index of the eye score (PIE-score) was calculated from jpeg images 639 × 426 pixels as: (number of blue pixels–number of brown pixels)/(number of blue pixels + number of brown pixels) using the Digital Iris Analysis Tool (DIAT) [13]. The PIE-scores ranged from −1 to 1; eye colour photos with a PIE-score of 1 had only blue pixels, and eye colour photos with a PIE-score of −1 had only brown pixels. Eye colour was also categorised in a two-category (blue and brown) and a three-category (blue, intermediate, and brown) system. The categorisation was based on the PIE-score and our recent study on the perception of blue and brown eye colours [15]. In the two-category system, eye colours with PIE-score > 0.2 were categorised as blue, and eye colours with

PIE-score ≤ 0.2 were categorised as brown. In the three-category system, eye colours with PIE-score > 0.8 were categorised as blue, eye colours with PIE-score ≤ 0.8 and ≥ -0.5 were categorised as intermediate, and eye colours with PIE-score < -0.5 were categorised as brown. The number of individuals in each eye colour category and the mean PIE-score in the discovery data set and the model data set are shown in Table 1.

Table 1. Eye colour variation in the variant discovery and model data sets.

	Quantitative System [1]	Two-Category System [2]		Three-Category System [3]		
	Mean PIE-Score	Blue	Brown	Blue	Intermediate	Brown
Discovery data set (n = 757)	0.24	447 (59%)	310 (41%)	368 (49%)	148 (20%)	241 (31%)
Model data set (n = 523)	0.44	376 (72%)	147 (28%)	293 (56%)	123 (24%)	107 (20%)

[1] Statistically significant difference in mean PIE-scores between the two data sets ($p < 0.05$). [2] PIE-score > 0.2: blue, and PIE-score ≤ 0.2: brown. [3] PIE-score > 0.8: blue, PIE-score ≤ 0.8 to ≥ -0.5: intermediate, and PIE-score < -0.5: brown.

2.3. Variant Typing (Discovery Data Set)

A total of 44 pigmentary variants were investigated. The variants included all six IrisPlex SNPs [3], five variants in *OCA2* found to be associated with blue eye colour in individuals with the rs12913832:GA genotype [11], as well as 33 variants in *IRF4*, *TYRP1*, *SLC24A4*, and *TYR*, associated with brown eye colour in individuals with the rs12913832: GG genotype [12]. We included three variants in *TYRP1* (rs201447946, rs74606098, and rs79586719, $r^2 \geq 0.91$) to tag one large haploblock associated with eye colour [12]. Two variants in *TYR* were also in strong LD (rs1126809 and rs1393350, $r^2 = 0.92$). rs1393350 was part of the IrisPlex [3], and rs1126809 was found to be of importance in individuals with brown eye colour [12]. The 757 individuals in the variant discovery data set were previously typed for the IrisPlex SNPs and the five *OCA2* variants [10,11]. The 33 variants in *IRF4*, *TYRP1*, *SLC24A4*, and *TYR* were typed using two multiplexes, a 24 plex and an 11 plex, respectively (Table S1). The 24 plex included rs12913832 and 23 variants in *SLC24A4* and *TYRP1* (rs10131374, rs12590749, rs12880508, rs12894551, rs17128288, rs17128324, rs34755843, rs35617057, rs4904887, rs4904891, rs4904897, rs4904927, rs59977926, rs7144273, rs7152962, rs7401792, rs10491745, rs1408799, rs201447946, rs62538950, rs62538956, rs74606098, and rs79586719). The 11 plex comprised rs1393350 from the IrisPlex and 10 variants in *IRF4* and *TYR* (rs1393350, rs1050976, rs10530949, rs12211228, rs9378807, rs11018509, rs1126809, rs2047512, rs34749698, rs7120151, and rs9919559). Samples were typed with the iPLEX™ Assay (Agena Bioscience, Hamburg, Germany) and analysed with matrix-assisted laser desorption-ionization time of flight mass spectrometry (MALDI-TOF MS) using the MassARRAY Analyzer 4 System (Agena Bioscience, Hamburg, Germany). The PCRs contained 0.5 µL 10X PCR buffer, 0.4 µL MgCl2 (25 mM), 0.1 µL dNTP mix (25 mM), 0.2 µL PCR Enzyme, 1 µL primer mix (1 µM of each primer), and 1 µL DNA (≥ 1 ng). Thermal cycling comprised initial denaturation for 2 min at 94 °C followed by 45 cycles of denaturation at 94 °C for 20 s, annealing at 56–58 °C for 30 s (56 °C for the 11 plex and 58 °C for the 24 plex), and extension at 72 °C for 1 min. A final extension step at 72 °C for 3 min was included. Shrimp alkaline phosphate (SAP) treatment, single-base extension (SBE) reactions, and preparation for mass analysis was carried out following the manufacturer's recommendations. In the MassARRAY Nanodispenser RS1000, 5–15 nl sample was robotically spotted onto a SpectroCHIP® II (Agena Bioscience, Hamburg, Germany). Mass analysis was carried out using the MassARRAY Analyzer 4, and the mass spectra were analysed with the Typer 4.0 software (Agena Bioscience, Hamburg, Germany). The Hardy–Weinberg equilibrium (HWE) and pairwise r^2 values for linkage disequilibrium (LD) were calculated with HaploView version 4.2 [16].

2.4. Selection of Variants for Eye Colour Prediction Model (Discovery Data Set)

Eye colour was considered in three different reporting systems, the quantitative system (PIE-score), the two-category system, and the three-category system. For numerical reasons (statistical modelling and stability), the PIE-score (values from −1 to 1) in the quantitative system was transformed to resemble unbounded values. The transformation had an inverse, such that any real number could be transformed into a PIE-score. The PIE-score, r, was transformed by:

$$y = f(r) = logit\ (0.5 + r*0.499)$$

Genotypes were coded as 0, 1, or 2 according to the number of minor alleles, where the minor alleles were determined based on the allele frequencies in all samples. Due to low allele frequency, the two variants rs121918166 and rs74653330 were combined [11]. rs12913832 was considered dominant with AA and AG as 0 and GG as 1. For stability, the discovery data set (757 individuals) was randomly divided into a training set (2/3) and a test set (1/3). This was repeated 100 times. If a training set resulted in fixed variants (i.e., only one genotype observed at a base position), a new set was randomly selected. In the quantitative system (transformed PIE-score) and in the two-category system, data were analysed with three different mathematical models: (i) LASSO model with main effects [17,18]; (ii) LASSO model (with the distribution family depending on the system; Gaussian for the quantitative system and binomial for the two-category system) with main effects and all pairwise interactions between rs12913832 and all other variants (still obeying the hierarchical principle such that the main effects must also be included); and (iii) a regression tree [19]. In the three-category system, data were analysed with a classification tree [19]. All seven mathematical models were fitted on the training set, which was also used to compute variable importance of the top 20 variables (variants). The test data were used for testing and estimating the test error. For LASSO regressions, the variables were standardised (such that all had a standard deviation of (1)), and the tuning parameter was chosen by cross-validation with 10 folds to get the most regularised model with an error within one standard error of the minimum error amongst the folds. For LASSO regressions, the absolute value of the estimated effect was used as variable importance. For regression and classification trees, the variable importances provided by the R package *rpart* version 4.1–15 were used [19]. Variable importances were standardised by dividing the importance of each variant with the sum of importances within each model. The mean variable importance (across all models) was used to rank variables (i.e., the variants). The top 12 performing variants were selected for an eye colour prediction model.

2.5. Variant Typing (Model Data Set)

The 12 selected variants and two non-selected SNPs from the IrisPlex [3] were typed with SNaPshot (rs12913832, rs12896399, rs16891982, rs1800407, rs10131374, rs1126809, rs121918166, rs1408799, rs1800401, rs4904927, rs7120151, rs74653330, rs12203592, and rs1393350) in the model data set comprising 523 Norwegian individuals (Table S2). DNA was amplified in one multiplex reaction (14-plex) using the Qiagen Multiplex PCR kit (Qiagen, Hilden, Germany) in a final reaction volume of 10 µL. The PCR comprised denaturation for 15 min at 95 °C followed by 35 cycles of 94 °C for 30 s, 58 °C for 30 s, 72 °C for 30 s, and a final extension step of 72 °C for 10 min. A total of 5 µL amplified DNA/PCR product was treated with 2 µL ExoSAP-IT™ (Thermo Fisher Scientific, Waltham, MA, USA) for 60 min at 37 °C and 15 min at 75 °C. Single-base extension was performed with 1 µL cleaned PCR product, 2 µL SNaPshot™ Multiplex Ready Reaction Mix, 1 µL nuclease-free water (G-Biosciences), and 1 µL SBE primer mix (Table S2). Thermal cycling comprised 30 cycles of 96 °C for 10 s, 55 °C for 5 s, and 60 °C for 30 s. SBE products were treated with 1 µL SAP (Thermo Fisher Scientific, Waltham, MA, USA) for 60 min at

37 °C and 15 min at 75 °C. Separation and detection of SBE products were carried out on an ABI 3500 Genetic Analyser (Thermo Fisher Scientific, Waltham, MA, USA) using the FragmentAnalysis36_POPxl run module (POP-4™ polymer, 36 cm capillary, Dye Set E5). Capillary electrophoresis was performed with 1 μL SAP-treated SBE products and 20 μL Hi-Di formamide mixed with GeneScan™-120 LIZ® Size Standard (200:1). The results were analysed with GeneMapper® ID-X v.1.5 (Thermo Fisher Scientific, Waltham, MA, USA). One of the selected variants, rs7120151, could not be typed and was excluded. Hence, we used 11 selected variants for the eye colour prediction model (EC11).

2.6. Eye Colour Prediction Modelling (Model Data Set)

Eye colour prediction models were modelled with leave-one-out cross-validation (LOOCV) using the model data set (523 Norwegian individuals) and the selected variants. For observation number i, all observations except number i were used to train the model. The model was used to predict the eye colour of observation i, and the predicted and observed values were compared. Three different reporting systems were used (quantitative system, two-category system, and three-category system), and thereby three different ways of measuring the prediction error were employed. For the quantitative system, a linear regression model was used where the prediction error was the mean squared error. For the two-category system, a logistic regression model was used where blue was chosen as 1 and brown as 0 (without loss of generality). The prediction error for a predicted probability (p) was log(p) if the true eye colour was blue, and log(1-p) if the true eye colour was brown. For the three-category system, a multinomial logistic regression model was used [20]. The prediction error was the Kullback–Leibler divergence between the observed distribution (the observed eye colour has probability 1, and the other two categories probability 0) and the estimated probabilities. All prediction errors were out-of-sample prediction errors. For each reporting system, the modelling was performed with three different variant (SNP) sets: the six IrisPlex SNPs, the 11 SNPs selected in this study (EC11), and rs12913832 alone. This resulted in a total of nine models. Lastly, we used the IrisPlex online tool (model called IrisPlex Web) (https://hirisplex.erasmusmc.nl/, accessed 1 July 2020) to predict eye colour in three categories.

3. Results

3.1. Allele Frequencies of 44 Variants in the Discovery Data Set

We investigated 44 pigmentary variants in our discovery data set of 757 individuals. In this work, we typed 33 variants [12] in two multiplexes using single-base extension. Eleven variants were typed in previous studies [11,13]. The allele frequencies of the 44 variants are shown in Table 2. The allele frequencies were similar in the Danish, Swedish, and Italian populations with small discrepancies between the Scandinavian (Danish and Swedish) and Italian populations, especially in rs12913832 and rs1800407 (Table S3). Moreover, two variants, rs12913832 and rs16891982, deviated significantly from the Hardy–Weinberg equilibrium (HWE) (p-value < 0.001) in the discovery data set. This could be explained by positive selection in the European population or a lack of random mating between the Scandinavian (Danish and Swedish) and the Italian populations.

Table 2. Allele frequencies of 44 variants typed in the discovery data set and 13 variants typed in the model data set.

Gene	Variant [1]	Reference Allele	Variant Allele	Variant Allele Frequency	
				Discovery Data Set (n = 757)	**Model Data Set (n = 523)**
HERC2	**rs12913832 ***	**A**	**G**	0.74	0.83
IRF4	rs1050976	C	T	0.44	
IRF4	rs10530949	TCT	-	0.43	
IRF4	rs12211228	G	C	0.14	
IRF4	rs9378807	C	T	0.49	
TYR	rs11018509	T	A	0.29	
TYR	**rs1126809**	**G**	**A**	**0.24**	**0.24**
TYR	rs1393350 *	G	A	0.23	0.23
TYR	rs2047512	T	C	0.35	
TYR	rs34749698	T	C	0.23	
TYR	**rs7120151 [2]**	**A**	**G**	**0.74**	**NA**
TYR	rs9919559	T	C	0.33	
SLC24A4	**rs10131374**	**G**	**A**	**0.14**	**0.15**
TYRP1	rs10491745	T	C	0.82	
SLC24A4	rs12590749	C	A	0.37	
SLC24A4	rs12880508	C	T	0.74	
SLC24A4	rs12894551	T	C	0.65	
TYRP1	**rs1408799**	**T**	**C**	**0.68**	**0.69**
SLC24A4	rs17128288	A	G	0.30	
SLC24A4	rs17128324	C	T	0.17	
TYRP1	rs201447946	T	TA	0.06	
SLC24A4	rs34755843	CGACTCT	-	0.16	
SLC24A4	rs35617057	G	T	0.41	
SLC24A4	rs4904887	C	G	0.36	
SLC24A4	rs4904891	G	C	0.35	
SLC24A4	rs4904897	C	T	0.22	
SLC24A4	**rs4904927**	**A**	**G**	**0.87**	**0.89**
SLC24A4	rs59977926	T	C	0.18	
TYRP1	rs62538950	A	T	0.10	
TYRP1	rs62538956	T	C	0.11	
SLC24A4	rs7144273	C	T	0.49	
SLC24A4	rs7152962	G	A	0.23	
SLC24A4	rs7401792	G	A	0.62	
TYRP1	rs74606098	C	T	0.06	
TYRP1	rs79586719	G	A	0.06	
OCA2	**rs1800407 ***	**C**	**T**	**0.07**	**0.03**
IRF4	rs12203592 *	C	T	0.08	0.09
SLC24A4	**rs12896399 ***	**G**	**T**	**0.49**	**0.52**
SLC45A2	**rs16891982 ***	**C**	**G**	**0.93**	**0.95**
OCA2	**rs1800401**	**G**	**A**	**0.04**	**0.05**
OCA2	rs1800414	T	C	<0.01	
OCA2	rs62008729	C	T	0.09	
OCA2	**rs121918166 [2]**	**C**	**T**	**<0.01**	**0.01**
OCA2	**rs74653330 [2]**	**C**	**T**	**<0.01**	**0.02**

[1] Variants in bold were part of the EC11 SNPs and typed in the model data set. rs7120151 was not included in the final prediction modelling. [2] The combined frequency of rs121918166 and rs74653330 was 0.01 in the discovery data set. * Part of the IrisPlex prediction model [3]. NA: not analysed.

3.2. Selection of Variants for Eye Colour Prediction (Discovery Data Set)

The discovery data set with information on eye colour and the 44 pigmentary variants was analysed with seven different mathematical models. Variants were ranked according to the mean variable importance across the mathematical models (Table 3 and Table S4). rs12913832 was the top-performing SNP in all seven mathematical models and ranked number one (Table 3). The mean variable importance for rs12913832 was 74.6% (Table 3). rs121918166 and rs74653330 were combined as one variable and ranked second (Table 3). We saw a drop in mean variable importance after rank 11 (Table S4). Hence, we selected the top 11 performing variables (comprising 12 variants) for a new eye colour SNP set (Table 3). These variants had mean variable importances of at least 0.3% (Table 3 and Table S4). Four of six variants in the IrisPlex assay [3] were among the selected variants (rs12913832, rs16891982, rs1800407, and rs12896399), whereas the *TYR* variant rs1393350 (ranked 18) and the *IRF4* variant rs12203592 (not in top 20) from the IrisPlex were not selected.

Table 3. Twelve variants selected for the EC11 SNP set.

Rank	Gene	Variant	Mean Variable Importance
1	*HERC2*	rs12913832 *	74.63%
2	*OCA2*	rs121918166 + rs74653330	8.54%
3	*SLC45A2*	rs16891982 *	6.23%
4	*OCA2*	rs1800407 *	5.26%
5	*TYRP1*	rs1408799	1.54%
6	*SLC24A4*	rs4904927	1.19%
7	*SLC24A4*	rs12896399 *	0.68%
8	*TYR*	rs1126809	0.47%
9	*TYR*	rs7120151 [1]	0.46%
10	*SLC24A4*	rs10131374	0.32%
11	*OCA2*	rs1800401	0.32%

[1] Variant not included in the final prediction modelling. * Part of the IrisPlex prediction model [3].

3.3. Typing of Selected Variants and IrisPlex SNPs (Model Data Set)

The 12 selected variants (SNPs) were typed with single-base extension in an independent data set, the model data set of 523 Norwegians (bold in Tables 2 and 3). To enable comparison with the IrisPlex, we included two SNPs from the IrisPlex assay, rs12203592 and rs1393350, in a multiplex comprising 14 SNPs. One SNP, rs7120151, that was ranked as number 9 (Table 3), was excluded due to poor amplification of the A allele. We obtained 523 complete profiles, including the 11 selected SNPs (EC11) (Table 2) and the two additional IrisPlex SNPs.

3.4. Eye Colour Prediction Models with EC11, IrisPlex SNPs, and rs12913832

We constructed nine different eye colour prediction models based on the model data set with 523 Norwegians by using three different reporting systems and three different SNP sets (Tables 2 and 3). We also used the IrisPlex Web for eye colour prediction using the three-category system. Prediction errors for each eye colour prediction model are presented in Table 4. Since we used three different reporting systems, the models within each system have their own measure of prediction error. Therefore, the performance of SNP sets (including prediction errors) can only be directly compared within the same but not across different reporting systems. The EC11 models had the smallest error under all reporting systems, followed by IrisPlex Norway and rs12913832. Under the three-category system, the IrisPlex Web resulted in the highest prediction error (Table 4).

Table 4. Prediction errors for the nine eye colour prediction models (three reporting systems modelled with three SNP sets) and the IrisPlex online tool (IrisPlex Web).

Eye Colour Prediction Model	Quantitative System [1]	Two-Category System [2]	Three-Category System [3]
EC11	5.07	0.26	0.59
IrisPlex Norway	5.90	0.30	0.66
rs12913832	6.96	0.32	0.69
IrisPlex Web *	NA	NA	0.80

[1] Prediction error is the mean squared error. [2] Prediction error for a predicted probability, p, is log(p) if the true eye colour was blue, and log(1-p) if the true eye colour was brown. [3] Prediction error is the Kullback–Leibler divergence. * The IrisPlex Web predicts eye colour according to a three-category system. NA: not analysed.

The sensitivity and specificity of eye colour prediction models in the two-category and the three-category reporting systems were determined without applying a probability threshold (pmax) (Tables 5 and 6). Hence, the predicted eye colour was the eye colour with the highest probability value. The rs12913832 and IrisPlex Norway models showed the same sensitivity and specificity (0.92 and 0.84, respectively) in the two-category system. The EC11 was slightly more sensitive (0.96), and in turn, slightly less specific (0.82) (Table 5 and Table S5).

Table 5. Sensitivity and specificity of eye colour prediction models in the two-category reporting system modelled with three SNP sets. No probability threshold was applied (pmax).

Two-Category System	Sensitivity [1]	Specificity [1]
rs12913832	0.92	0.84
IrisPlex Norway	0.92	0.84
EC11	0.96	0.82

[1] Reference is blue eye colour.

Table 6. Sensitivity and specificity of eye colour prediction models in the three-category reporting system modelled with three SNP sets and the IrisPlex Web model. No probability threshold was applied (pmax).

Three-Category System		Sensitivity [1]	Specificity [1]
rs12913832	Blue	0.95	0.61
	Intermediate	0.00	1.00
	Brown	0.95	0.87
IrisPlex Norway	Blue	0.94	0.61
	Intermediate	0.10	0.97
	Brown	0.86	0.90
EC11	Blue	0.95	0.59
	Intermediate	0.15	0.95
	Brown	0.88	0.96
IrisPlex Web	Blue	0.95	0.60
	Intermediate	0.00	1.00
	Brown	0.95	0.88

[1] Reference is blue eye colour.

In the three-category system, the sensitivity was highest for blue and brown eye colours and lowest for intermediate eye colour with all three SNP sets and the IrisPlex Web (Table 6). The rs12913832 and IrisPlex Web predictions resulted in the highest sensitivity for brown eye colour: 0.95, whereas the IrisPlex Norway and EC11 models had slightly lower sensitivities (Table 6). For blue eye colour, the sensitivities were similar for all models. No individuals were predicted to have intermediate eye colour with either rs12913832 or the IrisPlex Web. Hence, the sensitivity was 0, and the specificity was 1 (Table 6). Of the individuals with intermediate eye colours, 69% and 72% were incorrectly predicted to have blue eye colours with the two models, respectively (Table S6). In contrast, intermediate eye colour predictions were obtained with IrisPlex Norway and EC11. However, only 48% and 46% of the predictions were correct (Table S6). Thus, the sensitivity was low (0.10 and 0.15, respectively), and the specificity was high (0.97 and 0.95, respectively) (Table 6).

Figure 1 shows the percentages of correct, incorrect, and inconclusive predictions for prediction models in the two-category reporting system. Using pmax, 89% of the predictions with both rs12913832 and IrisPlex Norway were correct (Figure 1, Table S5). The EC11 model resulted in 92% correct predictions (Figure 1). Here, 93% of the blue eye colour predictions and 90% of the brown eye colour predictions were correct (Table S5). We also evaluated the prediction with a probability threshold of 0.7 in the two-category reporting system (Figure 1). If the highest prediction value was below 0.7, the prediction was defined as inconclusive. No eye colours were inconclusive with rs12913832 (Figure 1). The IrisPlex Norway and EC11 resulted in 9% and 5% inconclusive predictions, respectively (Figure 1). With the IrisPlex Norway, 62% of the inconclusive eye colours were brown according to the PIE score. With EC11, it was only 46% (Table S5).

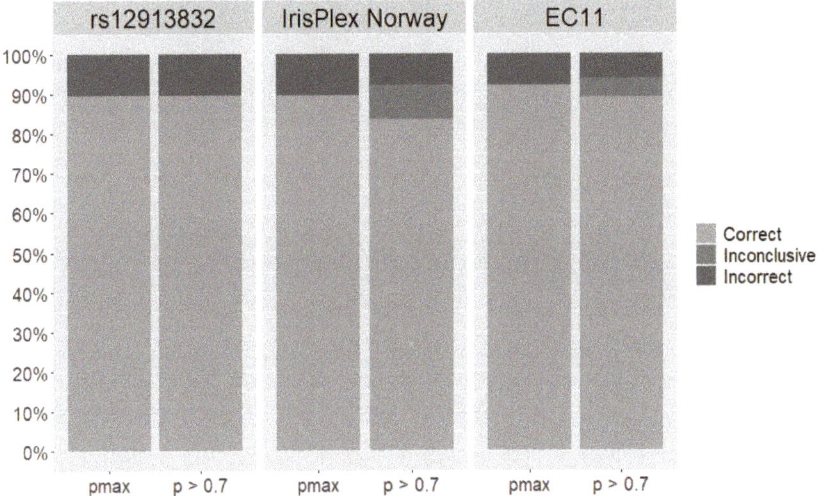

Figure 1. Performance of eye colour prediction models in the two-category reporting system modelled with three SNP sets: rs12913832, IrisPlex Norway, and EC11. Bars represent the percentage of correct, incorrect, and inconclusive predictions with no probability threshold (pmax) and a probability threshold of 0.7 (p > 0.7).

In the three-category reporting system, we tested the prediction with pmax, a probability threshold of 0.5, and a probability threshold of 0.7 (Figure 2). With no probability threshold, the rs12913832, IrisPlex Norway, and IrisPlex Web models all resulted in 72% correct predictions (Figure 2, Table S6). The EC11 model resulted in a slightly higher number of correct predictions (75%) (Figure 2, Table S6). When applying a probability threshold of 0.5, predictions with rs12913832 were unchanged compared with predictions without probability threshold (Figure 2). Predictions with the IrisPlex Web tool were also similar though 3% of the total predictions were inconclusive. There was a slight decrease in the number of correct and incorrect predictions with EC11 and IrisPlex Norway as both models resulted in 2% inconclusive predictions (Figure 2). When applying a probability threshold of 0.7, blue eye colour was correctly predicted in 95% of the blue-eyed individuals with rs12913832, but no individuals were predicted to have brown eye colours (Table S6). Thus, the total number of correct predictions with rs12913832 was only 53%. The number of correct predictions using the 0.7 probability threshold was highest with IrisPlex Web (Figure 2). However, the IrisPlex Web also resulted in the highest percentage of incorrect predictions (20%) and resulted in 15% inconclusive predictions (Figure 2). The IrisPlex Norway model resulted in only 8% incorrect predictions but a high number of inconclusive predictions (51%) (Figure 2). Prediction with EC11 resulted in 12% incorrect predictions, 32% inconclusive predictions, and only 54% correct predictions (Figure 2). Of the 32% inconclusive eye colour predictions, 49% had blue eye colour, 39% had intermediate eye colour, and only 12% had brown eye colour based on the PIE-score (Table S6). Especially the percentage of brown-eyed individuals with inconclusive predictions was much lower than compared with rs12913832, IrisPlex Norway, and IrisPlex Web. For these models, the percentages were 32–65% (Table S6).

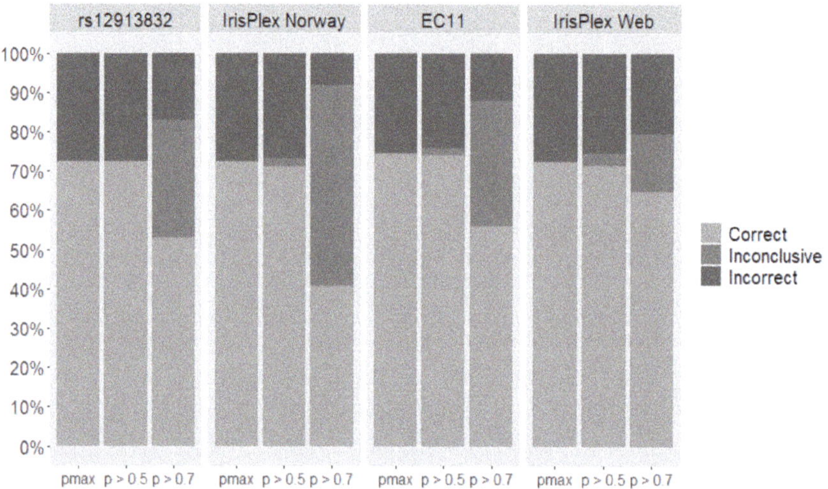

Figure 2. Performance of eye colour prediction models in the three-category reporting system modelled with three SNP sets: rs12913832, IrisPlex Norway and EC11, as well as performance of the IrisPlex Web prediction model. Bars represent the percentage of correct, incorrect, and inconclusive predictions with no probability threshold (pmax), probability threshold of 0.5 (p > 0.5), and probability threshold of 0.7 (p > 0.7).

4. Discussion

In this study, we selected 11 SNPs (EC11) for eye colour prediction and developed new eye colour prediction models for a two-category and a three-category system that performed better than the corresponding IrisPlex and rs12913832 prediction models. The 11 SNPs in EC11 were selected from a group of 44 pigmentary variants that were originally identified in eye colour association studies [3,6] and from detailed sequence analyses of individuals with eye colours that deviated from the expected eye colour based on the genotype of rs12913832 [11,12]. The 44 variants were typed in 757 Europeans whose eye colours were quantitatively determined. Seven different mathematical models were used to rank the variants according to informativeness, and all variants with more than 0.3% mean variable importance were selected. Four of the six SNPs in the IrisPlex assay [3] were included in EC11. However, the *TYR* SNP, rs1393350 (ranked 18), was replaced by another *TYR* SNP, rs1126809 (ranked 8), and the *IRF4* gene represented by the SNP rs12203592 (not in top 20) from the IrisPlex, was not included in EC11. For the selection of SNPs, we combined individuals of Scandinavian (Danish and Swedish) and Italian descent and treated these as one population. We are aware that we may had selected different SNPs if the selection was performed solely on either the Scandinavian or the South European population. We typed the EC11 SNPs and the two additional IrisPlex SNPs in an independent data set of 523 Norwegians whose eye colours were determined with the same quantitative method as the 757 individuals in the discovery data set. We modelled nine different eye colour prediction models on the Norwegian population using the LOOCV method. Each eye colour prediction model consisted of a combination of one of three reporting systems: the quantitative system (prediction of PIE score), the two-category system (blue and brown), and the three-category system (blue, intermediate, brown), and one of three SNP sets: EC11, IrisPlex SNPs, and rs12913832. We also evaluated the IrisPlex Web model for prediction of eye colour in three categories. Based on the analysis of error rates, sensitivity, and specificity of the different eye colour prediction models, there are three main points to consider prior to implementation of eye colour prediction in a forensic genetic setting: (1) the reference population, (2) the SNP set, and (3) the reporting strategy.

4.1. The Reference Population

The rs12913832, IrisPlex Norway, and IrisPlex Web models showed almost identical results in the three-category system (Figure 2, Table 6). Nevertheless, a detailed comparison between the three-category IrisPlex Norway and the IrisPlex Web models highlights the importance of the reference population. The two models were based on the exact same SNPs. However, the IrisPlex Norway model was developed on the Norwegian population, which was the intended target population, whereas the IrisPlex Web model was developed on 9466 individuals of primarily European descent [6,21,22]. The two models resulted in the same number of correct predictions (72%) when no probability threshold was applied. With probability thresholds, inconclusive results were possible, and the IrisPlex Web model resulted in a higher number of correct predictions than the IrisPlex Norway model (Figure 2). However, when applying the recommended threshold for the IrisPlex Web model (p > 0.7) [21], the number of incorrect predictions was also higher (Figure 2). The two models showed similar sensitivities and specificities for blue and brown eye colour but differed for the intermediate eye colour category (Table 6). A total of 123 Norwegian individuals had intermediate eye colours according to the PIE-score (Table 1). Intermediate eye colour predictions were obtained with the IrisPlex Norway model using both pmax and p > 0.5 (Table S6), whereas no individuals were predicted to have intermediate eye colours with the IrisPlex Web model (Table S6). Hence, the IrisPlex Norway model showed an overall lower prediction error than the IrisPlex Web model (Table 4), and this emphasises the importance of modelling a prediction model on the appropriate reference population. This is in agreement with previous evaluations of the IrisPlex model which showed that prediction models based on the intended target population (the reference population) performed better than the IrisPlex Web tool [23,24]. However, it is important to note that the differences between the IrisPlex Web and the IrisPlex Norway models may not only be due to the different reference populations. Different strategies on phenotyping and categorisation of eye colour may also have contributed here. In our study, we determined the eye colour quantitatively, and the eye colour prediction models were modelled accordingly. For the IrisPlex Web model, the eye colour was evaluated by a medical researcher who categorised eye colours in blue, brown, and non-blue/non-brown (called intermediate) categories [3,6,21,22].

4.2. The SNP Set

The eye colour prediction models based on EC11 had the lowest prediction error rates in all three reporting systems and consistently performed better than the rs12913832, IrisPlex Norway, and IrisPlex Web models in the Norwegian population (Table 4). In the three-category reporting system, only EC11 and IrisPlex Norway were able to predict intermediate eye colours (Table 6, Table S6). For the EC11 model, intermediate eye colour predictions were even obtained with a probability threshold of 0.7 (Table S6). We did expect the prediction errors to decrease when the number of loci increased. However, the prediction errors obtained with EC11 (11 SNPs) were only slightly smaller than with IrisPlex Norway (six SNPs), closely followed by rs12913832 (one SNP) and IrisPlex Web (six SNPs) (Table 4). This shows that a single SNP, rs12913238, may be sufficient for prediction of eye colour. This SNP was ranked as number one across all mathematical models with a mean variable importance of 74.6% (Table 3). We modelled rs12913832 in a dominant matter and acknowledge that it is unreasonable to predict eye colour in three categories with a predictor variable containing only two levels (AA/AG and GG). However, even in the three-category reporting system, prediction with rs12913832 showed a lower prediction error than prediction with the IrisPlex Web (Table 4). In both the three-category reporting system and the two-category reporting system, prediction with rs12913832 and IrisPlex Norway performed almost identically (Figure 1, Figure 2). This stresses the importance of rs12913832 for prediction of eye colour and shows that the remaining five SNPs in the IrisPlex SNP set have very small effects on the outcome of the eye colour prediction in the studied population.

4.3. The Reporting Strategy

In this work, we tested three different eye colour categorisation systems: the quantitative system (prediction of PIE score), the two-category system (blue and brown), and the three-category system (blue, intermediate, and brown). Although it is possible to report the predicted eye colour in the form of a PIE-score, this likely requires that the end-user or the reporting laboratory translate the PIE-score into an eye colour category. Therefore, the use of a quantitative system for reporting is not relevant in a forensic genetic setting. The difference between the two- and three-category system is the definition of the intermediate eye colour, which is very difficult to perceive. When multiple individuals were asked to evaluate eye colours categorised as intermediate, they often disagreed, whereas they agreed much more frequently when eye colours were blue or brown [15]. Intermediate eye colour is predicted as the most likely eye colour (without any probability threshold) for only 8% (60 out of 729) and 14% (7.508 out of 52,488) of the possible genotype combinations in the IrisPlex Web and EC11 models, respectively [10] (Table S7). For the IrisPlex Web, the maximum probability value for prediction of intermediate eye colour is 0.62 [10]. With EC11, it is 0.94 (Table S7). In this study, we did observe intermediate eye colour predictions with EC11 with high probability values (maximum: 0.82). However, the intermediate eye colour predictions were incorrect more than half of the time (Table S6). Overall, eye colour prediction in two categories resulted in more correct predictions than eye colour prediction in three categories (92% vs. 75% for EC11; 89% vs. 72% for IrisPlex Norway and 89% vs. 72% for rs12913832) (Figures 1 and 2). Hence, the definition of an intermediate eye colour category is counterintuitive, as it is both difficult to identify and predict. A recent study discusses the need for standardised methods for reporting forensic DNA phenotyping predictions to the police [25]. Reducing the complexity of eye colour predictions to only two categories results in only two hypotheses (H_1: The person has brown eyes and H_2: The person has blue eyes). Hence, it is possible to report the weight of the evidence with a single likelihood ratio, which resembles standard STR-profiling reports. The likelihood ratio could be supplemented with picture examples of eye colours represented by each category. This may overcome any misunderstandings or subjective opinions of eye colour interpretation, especially for eye colours that may appear non-blue and non-brown.

4.4. DNA Phenotyping in Forensic Genetics

The Section of Forensic Genetics in Denmark recently began offering eye colour prediction to the police using the two-category system based on the genotype of rs12913832. Prediction of EVCs can cause ethical concerns as discussed in [26]. This is especially apparent if the genetic markers used for prediction a certain trait are also linked to diseases [26]. That is not the case for rs12913832. The SNP is included in the Precision ID Ancestry Panel (Thermo Fisher Scientific, Waltham, MA, USA), which has already been validated for case work [5,27,28]. The weight of the evidence for both ancestry and eye colour predictions are reported as likelihood ratios. For eye colour predictions in the Danish population, LR = (rs12913832:GG | H_1 / rs12913832:GG | H_2) = 0.1, LR = (rs12913832:AG | H_1 / rs12913832:AG | H_2) = 19, and LR = (rs12913832:AA | H_1 / rs12913832:AA | H_2) = 54 [15], where H_1: The person has brown eyes and H_2: The person has blue eyes. The EC11 model may be implemented at the Section of Forensic Genetics in Denmark in the future once the EC11 markers are included in a validated massively parallel sequencing (MPS) assay. The most important shortcoming of the rs12913832 two-category prediction model is the lack of information gained when including the two *OCA2* variants, rs121918166 and rs74653330. These variants were previously shown to be of importance for blue eye colour in Scandinavians with the rs12913832:AG genotype [11]. The variants had low frequencies in Danes and Swedes and were completely absent in Italians [11] (Table S3). These variants combined were ranked as second most important, with a mean variable importance of 8.5% (Table 3). In the Norwegian data set, 30 individuals with the rs12913832:AG genotype had blue eye colours according to the PIE-score. Seventeen of the 30 individuals had at least one of the *OCA2* variants and were correctly predicted to have blue eyes using the EC11 two-category model. By contrast, only one of the 30 individuals was correctly predicted with the IrisPlex Norway model, and none were correctly predicted with rs12913832. Moreover, two Norwegians with the rs12913832:AA genotype had blue eye colours according to the PIE-score. One of the two individuals was correctly predicted to have blue eye colour with the EC11 two-category model. This individual was homozygous for the rs74653330 variant. We hypothesise that the second individual has other variants in or around the *OCA2* gene that could explain the formation of blue eye colour in the rs12913832:AA genotype background. Both individuals were incorrectly predicted to have brown eye colours with the IrisPlex Norway and rs12913832 models. Lastly, 10 Norwegians with the rs12913832:GG genotype had brown eyes according to the PIE-score. Only one of them was correctly predicted to have brown eyes with the two-category EC11 and IrisPlex Norway models. This shows that we do not fully understand the formation of brown eye colour in rs12913832:GG individuals and that the EC11 model may have to be expanded further.

Supplementary Materials: The following are available online at https://www.mdpi.com/2073-4425/12/6/821/s1; Table S1: Primer sequences and primer concentrations for 24 plex and 11 plex typed in the variant discovery data set; Table S2: Primer sequences and primer concentrations for 14 plex typed with SNaPshot in the model data set; Table S3: Allele frequencies of 44 variants typed in the discovery data set comprising Danish, Swedish, and Italian individuals (DK/SWE/ITA) and 13 variants typed in the model data set comprising Norwegian individuals (NO); Table S4: Mean variable importance of top 20 variants; Table S5: Confusion matrices for two-category system prediction models; one for each SNP set and each threshold (pmax and p > 0.7); Table S6: Confusion matrices for three-category system prediction models; one for each SNP set and each threshold (pmax, p > 0.5, and p > 0.7); Table S7: Eye colour prediction outcomes for 52,488 possible genotype combinations using the EC11 three-category model.

Author Contributions: Conceptualization, O.S.M., N.M., C.B. and J.D.A.; formal analysis, O.S.M. N.M.S, A.K., M.K. and M.M.A.; data curation, E.S. and H.U .; writing—original draft prep-aration, O.S.M. and N.M.S.; writing—review and editing, A.K., M.K., M.M.A., E.S., H.U., K.J., N.M., C.B., G.-H.O. and J.D.A. All authors have read and agreed to the published version of the manuscript.

Funding: This research received no external funding.

Institutional Review Board Statement: The study was conducted according to the guidelines of the Declaration of Helsinki, and approved by the Danish Ethical Committee (M-20090237, H-4-2009-125, and H-3-2012-023), the Ethical Committee of Azienda Ospedaliera Ospedal Sant'Anna di Como (U.0026484.23-11-2012), the Ethical Committee of the University of Milan-Bicocca (P.U. 0033373/12), and the Faculty of Health Sciences, UiT–The Arctic University of Norway (2021/2034).

Informed Consent Statement: Informed consent was obtained from all subjects involved in the study.

Data Availability Statement: The data generated in the present study are included within the manuscript and its supplementary files.

Acknowledgments: The authors thank A. L. J. and N. J. for their technical assistance.

Conflicts of Interest: The authors declare no conflict of interest.

References

1. Walsh, S.; Liu, F.; Wollstein, A.; Kovatsi, L.; Ralf, A.; Kosiniak-Kamysz, A.; Branicki, W.; Kayser, M. The HIrisPlex system for simultaneous prediction of hair and eye colour from DNA. *Forensic Sci. Int. Genet.* **2013**, *7*, 98–115. [CrossRef] [PubMed]
2. Chaitanya, L.; Breslin, K.; Zuñiga, S.; Wirken, L.; Pośpiech, E.; Kukla-Bartoszek, M.; Sijen, T.; de Knijff, P.; Liu, F.; Branicki, W.; et al. The HIrisPlex-S system for eye, hair and skin colour prediction from DNA: Introduction and forensic developmental validation. *Forensic Sci. Int. Genet.* **2018**, *35*, 123–135. [CrossRef] [PubMed]
3. Walsh, S.; Liu, F.; Ballantyne, K.N.; van Oven, M.; Lao, O.; Kayser, M. IrisPlex: A sensitive DNA tool for accurate prediction of blue and brown eye colour in the absence of ancestry information. *Forensic Sci. Int. Genet.* **2011**, *5*, 170–180. [CrossRef] [PubMed]
4. Ruiz, Y.; Phillips, C.; Gomez-Tato, A.; Alvarez-Dios, J.; Casares de Cal, M.; Cruz, R.; Maroñas, O.; Söchtig, J.; Fondevila, M.; Rodriguez-Cid, M.; et al. Further development of forensic eye color predictive tests. *Forensic Sci. Int. Genet.* **2013**, *7*, 28–40. [CrossRef] [PubMed]
5. Mogensen, H.S.; Tvedebrink, T.; Børsting, C.; Pereira, V.; Morling, N. Ancestry prediction efficiency of the software GenoGeographer using a z-score method and the ancestry informative markers in the Precision ID Ancestry Panel. *Forensic Sci. Int. Genet.* **2020**, *44*, 102154. [CrossRef]
6. Liu, F.; van Duijn, K.; Vingerling, J.R.; Hofman, A.; Uitterlinden, A.G.; Janssens, A.C.J.; Kayser, M. Eye color and the prediction of complex phenotypes from genotypes. *Curr. Biol.* **2009**, *19*, R192–R193. [CrossRef] [PubMed]
7. Sturm, R.A.; Duffy, D.L.; Zhao, Z.Z.; Leite, F.P.; Stark, M.; Hayward, N.K.; Martin, N.; Montgomery, G.W. A single SNP in an evolutionary conserved region within Intron 86 of the HERC2 gene determines human blue-brown eye color. *Am. J. Hum. Genet.* **2008**, *82*, 424–431. [CrossRef]
8. Eiberg, H.; Troelsen, J.T.; Nielsen, M.; Mikkelsen, A.; Mengel-From, J.; Kjaer, K.W.; Hansen, L. Blue eye color in humans may be caused by a perfectly associated founder mutation in a regulatory element located within the HERC2 gene inhibiting OCA2 expression. *Hum. Genet.* **2008**, *123*, 177–187. [CrossRef]
9. Visser, M.; Kayser, M.; Palstra, R.-J. HERC2 rs12913832 modulates human pigmentation by attenuating chromatin-loop formation between a long-range enhancer and the OCA2 promoter. *Genome Res.* **2012**, *22*, 446–455. [CrossRef]
10. Pietroni, C.; Andersen, J.D.; Johansen, P.; Andersen, M.M.; Harder, S.; Paulsen, R.R.; Børsting, C.; Morling, N. The effect of gender on eye colour variation in European populations and an evaluation of the IrisPlex prediction model. *Forensic Sci. Int. Genet.* **2014**, *11*, 1–6. [CrossRef]
11. Andersen, J.D.; Pietroni, C.; Johansen, P.; Andersen, M.M.; Pereira, V.; Børsting, C.; Morling, N. Importance of nonsynonymous OCA 2 variants in human eye color prediction. *Mol. Genet. Genom. Med.* **2016**, *4*, 420–430. [CrossRef]
12. Meyer, O.S.; Lunn, M.M.B.; Garcia, S.L.; Kjærbye, A.B.; Morling, N.; Børsting, C.; Andersen, J.D. Association between brown eye colour in rs12913832:GG individuals and SNPs in TYR, TYRP1, and SLC24A4. *PLoS ONE* **2020**, *15*, e0239131. [CrossRef] [PubMed]
13. Andersen, J.D.; Johansen, P.; Harder, S.; Christoffersen, S.R.; Delgado, M.C.; Henriksen, S.T.; Nielsen, M.M.; Sørensen, E.; Ullum, H.; Hansen, T.; et al. Genetic analyses of the human eye colours using a novel objective method for eye colour classification. *Forensic Sci. Int. Genet.* **2013**, *7*, 508–515. [CrossRef]
14. Salvo, N.M.; Janssen, K.; Kirsebom, M.K.; Meyer, O.S.; Berg, T.; Olsen, G.-H. Forensic DNA phenotyping—Predicting eye and hair colour in a Norwegian population using Verogen's ForenSeqTM DNA Signature Prep Kit. *Forensic Sci. Int. Genet.* **2021**, submitted.
15. Meyer, O.S.; Børsting, C.; Andersen, J.D. Perception of blue and brown eye colours for forensic DNA phenotyping. *Forensic Sci. Int. Genet. Suppl. Ser.* **2019**, *7*, 476–477. [CrossRef]
16. Barrett, J.C.; Fry, B.; Maller, J.; Daly, M.J. Haploview: Analysis and visualization of LD and haplotype maps. *Bioinformatics* **2005**, *21*, 263–265. [CrossRef] [PubMed]
17. Santosa, F.; Symes, W.W. Linear inversion of band-limited reflection seismograms. *SIAM J. Sci. Stat. Comput.* **1986**, *7*, 1307–1330. [CrossRef]
18. Tibshirani, R. Regression shrinkage and selection via the Lasso. *J. R. Stat. Soc. Ser. B* **1996**, *58*, 267–288. [CrossRef]
19. Breiman, L.; Friedman, J.H.; Olshen, R.A.; Stone, C.J. *Classification and Regression Trees*; Taylor & Francis: Abingdon, UK, 1984; ISBN 9781351460491.
20. Venables, W.N.; Ripley, B.D. *Modern Applied Statistics with S*, 4th ed.; Springer: New York, NY, USA, 2002; pp. 435–446.
21. Walsh, S.; Wollstein, A.; Liu, F.; Chakravarthy, U.; Rahu, M.; Seland, J.H.; Soubrane, G.; Tomazzoli, L.; Topouzis, F.; Vingerling, J.R.; et al. DNA-based eye colour prediction across Europe with the IrisPlex system. *Forensic Sci. Int. Genet.* **2012**, *6*, 330–340. [CrossRef] [PubMed]
22. Walsh, S.; Chaitanya, L.; Breslin, K.; Muralidharan, C.; Bronikowska, A.; Pospiech, E.; Koller, J.; Kovatsi, L.; Wollstein, A.; Branicki, W.; et al. Global skin colour prediction from DNA. *Qual. Life Res.* **2017**, *136*, 847–863. [CrossRef]

23. Dembinski, G.M.; Picard, C.J. Evaluation of the IrisPlex DNA-based eye color prediction assay in a United States population. *Forensic Sci. Int. Genet.* **2014**, *9*, 111–117. [CrossRef]
24. Salvoro, C.; Faccinetto, C.; Zucchelli, L.; Porto, M.; Marino, A.; Occhi, G.; de los Campos, G.; Vazza, G. Performance of four models for eye color prediction in an Italian population sample. *Forensic Sci. Int. Genet.* **2019**, *40*, 192–200. [CrossRef]
25. Atwood, L.; Raymond, J.; Sears, A.; Bell, M.; Daniel, R. From identification to intelligence: An assessment of the suitability of forensic DNA phenotyping service providers for use in Australian law enforcement casework. *Front. Genet.* **2021**, *11*, 11. [CrossRef]
26. Kayser, M. Forensic DNA phenotyping: Predicting human appearance from crime scene material for investigative purposes. *Forensic Sci. Int. Genet.* **2015**, *18*, 33–48. [CrossRef] [PubMed]
27. Pereira, V.; Mogensen, H.S.; Børsting, C.; Morling, N. Evaluation of the precision ID Ancestry Panel for crime case work: A SNP typing assay developed for typing of 165 ancestral informative markers. *Forensic Sci. Int. Genet.* **2017**, *28*, 138–145. [CrossRef] [PubMed]
28. Tvedebrink, T.; Eriksen, P.S.; Mogensen, H.S.; Morling, N. Weight of the evidence of genetic investigations of ancestry informative markers. *Theor. Popul. Biol.* **2018**, *120*, 1–10. [CrossRef] [PubMed]

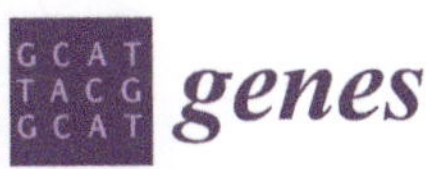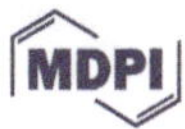

Evaluation of Different Cleaning Strategies for Removal of Contaminating DNA Molecules

Martina Nilsson [1], Hanne De Maeyer [2] and Marie Allen [2,*]

[1] Forensic Section, Division of Investigation, Stockholm Police Region, Swedish Police Authority, 106 75 Stockholm, Sweden; martina.nilsson@polisen.se

[2] Department of Immunology, Genetics and Pathology, Uppsala University, 751 08 Uppsala, Sweden; hanne.demaeyer@igp.uu.se

[*] Correspondence: marie.allen@igp.uu.se

Abstract: Decontamination strategies and their efficiencies are crucial when performing routine forensic analysis, and many factors influence the choice of agent to use. In this study, the effects of ten different cleaning strategies were evaluated to compare their ability to remove contaminating DNA molecules. Cell-free DNA or blood was deposited on three surfaces (plastic, metal, and wood) and decontaminated with various treatments. The quantities of recovered DNA, obtained by swabbing the surfaces after cleaning using the different strategies, was analyzed by real-time PCR. Large differences in the DNA removal efficiencies were observed between different cleaning strategies, as well as between different surfaces. The most efficient cleaning strategies for cell-free DNA were the different sodium hypochlorite solutions and Trigene®, for which a maximum of 0.3% DNA was recovered on all three surfaces. For blood, a maximum of 0.8% of the deposited DNA was recovered after using Virkon® for decontamination. The recoveries after using these cleaning strategies correspond to DNA from only a few cells, out of 60 ng of cell-free DNA or thousands of deposited blood cells.

Keywords: DNA molecules; decontamination; cleaning strategies

Citation: Nilsson, M.; De Maeyer, H.; Allen, M. Evaluation of Different Cleaning Strategies for Removal of Contaminating DNA Molecules. *Genes* **2022**, *13*, 162. https://doi.org/10.3390/genes13010162

Academic Editor: Niels Morling

Received: 15 December 2021
Accepted: 11 January 2022
Published: 17 January 2022

Publisher's Note: MDPI stays neutral with regard to jurisdictional claims in published maps and institutional affiliations.

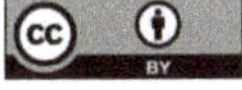

1. Introduction

DNA analysis of trace evidence can present many challenges in a forensic investigation, such as samples that contain low quantities of biological material and degraded DNA. However, improved typing kits for forensic analysis may allow STR profiling on DNA extracted from only a few cells [1,2]. In addition, using mitochondrial DNA (mtDNA) instead of nuclear DNA (nDNA) markers allows testing of even lower DNA input amounts, due to the high copy number of mtDNA in each cell [3,4]. Another challenge, especially when analyzing mtDNA, is that exogenous DNA can be present in the samples and cause ambiguous or erroneous results. Contaminating DNA may be introduced to a sample by the first responding officers, rescue workers, or crime scene investigators present at the crime scene, archaeologists during excavations or later by laboratory personnel during DNA analysis [5–7]. Contamination may also originate from other samples processed at the same laboratory (cross-contamination) [6,8] or even from disposables and consumables contaminated during manufacturing [9,10].

Several preventive measures should be taken to reduce the risk of contamination in order to assure a high quality of DNA profiling results. Contamination is monitored by establishing elimination databases with DNA profiles from staff [11], periodic wipe tests, and the use of no template control (NTC) reactions [8]. Moreover, personal protective clothing, disposable consumables, aerosol resistant tips, and dedicated instruments are used to prevent the introduction of contaminating DNA into the laboratory environment and casework samples. A laboratory construction with designated pre- and post-PCR rooms equipped with dead-air cabinets and a unidirectional workflow is also important. In addition, several decontamination strategies (e.g., chemical cleaning agents and ultraviolet radiation [UV]) can be used for the decontamination of laboratory surfaces and equipment. While decontamination agents have various DNA damaging mechanisms, UV radiation is destructive because it oxidizes bases to introduce single- and double-strand breaks in the DNA molecules [12–18].

This study evaluates the decontamination efficiency of ten different cleaning strategies: ethanol, UV radiation, ethanol in combination with UV radiation, fresh and stored household bleach, DAX Ytdesinfektion Plus, Rely+On™ Virkon®, Trigene®, DNA Remover®, and sodium hypochlorite. Most forensic materials have a majority of the DNA present within cells, but it also exists in free form, so-called cell-free DNA. As cells deteriorate with time and in challenging environments, the cell walls become disrupted, resulting in a release of cell content, including the DNA [19,20]. Therefore, both cell-free (extracted DNA) and cell-contained DNA (blood) were placed on three different surfaces (plastic, metal, and wood) in the experiments. The artificially contaminated surfaces were cleaned with the different treatments and then swabbed for residual DNA. Real-time PCR quantification of mtDNA extracted from the collected samples was thereafter used to compare the efficiency of the different cleaning strategies.

2. Materials and Methods

Human male DNA in a 10 µL volume (6 ng/µL, PE Biosystems, Foster City, CA, USA) was deposited on different surfaces. The applied DNA solution consisted of 60 ng DNA, with approximately 18 million mtDNA copies, assuming 2000 mtDNA copies per cell. The mtDNA and nuclear DNA (nDNA) ratio for the DNA sample used in this study was estimated previously (by comparison to a plasmid clone of mtDNA) [21]. As cell-contained DNA, 10 µL of whole blood (unknown DNA concentration) from one anonymous donor was deposited on several surfaces. The sample solutions were deposited in marked 25 mm-wide circles on plastic, metal, or wood surfaces. The wood consisted of a skirting board with one layer of water-based transparent white base paint, the metal of aluminum foil and the plastic of plastic document folders. These surfaces were chosen to mimic common types of material in surfaces of workbenches and equipment in the laboratory environment. The liquid was spread with a pipette tip within the circle and left to dry for two hours.

The different decontaminating strategies to be evaluated were chosen following an informal survey of the most commonly used treatments among European forensic laboratories. The ten strategies selected are described in detail in Supplementary Materials, Table S1. Briefly, the strategies consisted of 70% aqueous ethanol, UV radiation (20 min at a distance of 60 to 70 cm, 254 nm), 70% aqueous ethanol in combination with UV radiation, 15% freshly diluted Klorin Original household bleach (Colgate-Palmolive AB, New York, NY, USA), (3.6% sodium hypochlorite diluted to 0.54%), 15% stored Klorin household bleach (2.7% sodium hypochlorite diluted to 0.4%), DAX Ytdesinfektion Plus, 1% Rely+On™ Virkon®, 10% Trigene® Disinfectant Cleaner, DNA Remover®, and 0.4% freshly diluted sodium hypochlorite. The commercial cleaning agents were prepared according to the manufacturers' instructions. The stability of diluted sodium hypochlorite for longer periods has been discussed as the concentration of available chlorine decreases with time [22]. Therefore, both diluted household bleach stored in a dark refrigerator at 8 °C for 80 days and freshly made dilutions were evaluated.

The liquid cleaning agents were administered to the artificially contaminated surfaces by one spray from a calibrated spray bottle. The calibration was performed by weighing five replicates of sprayed volumes followed by adjustments when needed. The cleaned areas were wiped in three circular movements in a similar manner and were performed by the same person using dust-free paper. The cleaned areas were thereafter left to dry for 120 min, with the exception of areas cleaned with Trigene®, which was sprayed with a single spray of water before wiping, and then left for 10 min. The entire marked area for each sample was swabbed with a cotton swab (Selefa, OneMed, Danderyd, Sweden) moistened in 0.9% sodium chloride. Five replicates were collected for each test parameter (surface and treatment). No-treatment controls, consisting of the addition of DNA or blood without any decontamination treatment, were collected in three replicates for each surface. The no-treatment controls revealing a maximum DNA yield were used to estimate the ability of the cleaning strategies to remove DNA contamination by comparing the percentage of recovered DNA for the different cleaning strategies. Negative control swabs (background controls) were obtained by sampling three replicates from surfaces without addition of DNA or blood. Thus, at least three replicates were available and analyzed for all different tests.

DNA extraction was performed using the DNeasy Blood and Tissue kit (Qiagen, Hilden, Germany), with the final extracts being eluted in a total volume of 100 μL. Mitochondrial DNA was quantified using a real-time PCR based assay described by Andréasson et al. [21]. This assay was chosen in order to achieve a highly sensitive DNA quantification allowing determination of trace residues of DNA left after cleaning. The PCR reaction consisted of 2X SsoAdvanced™ Universal SYBR Green Supermix (Bio-Rad Laboratories Inc., Hercules, CA, USA), 400 nM each primer (mt-8294F/mt-8436R), and 5 μL DNA extract in a total reaction volume of 25 μL [21]. Real-time PCR was performed using the Bio-Rad CFX96™ Real-Time System (C1000 Touch Thermal Cycler, Bio-Rad Laboratories, Hercules, CA, USA) and Bio-Rad CFX Manager 2.1 software. The PCR conditions consisted of 98 °C for 2 min followed by 40 cycles at 95 °C for 5 s, 60 °C for 20 s, and 95 °C for 5 s. Negative controls were included in all extraction (no swabs added) and quantification (water instead of DNA added) steps.

Data analysis was performed using Microsoft® Excel (version 2019). The $1.5 \times$ interquartile rule was applied to the five biological replicates for each condition to identify potential outliers. Data with and without removal of outliers are presented in Tables S2 and S3. The efficiencies of the cleaning strategies were calculated as a percentage of the positive controls. RStudio® (version 1.3.1093) was used to produce Figures 1 and 2 using the following packages: stats [23], tidyverse, dplyr, ggpubr, ggplot2, and bibtex.

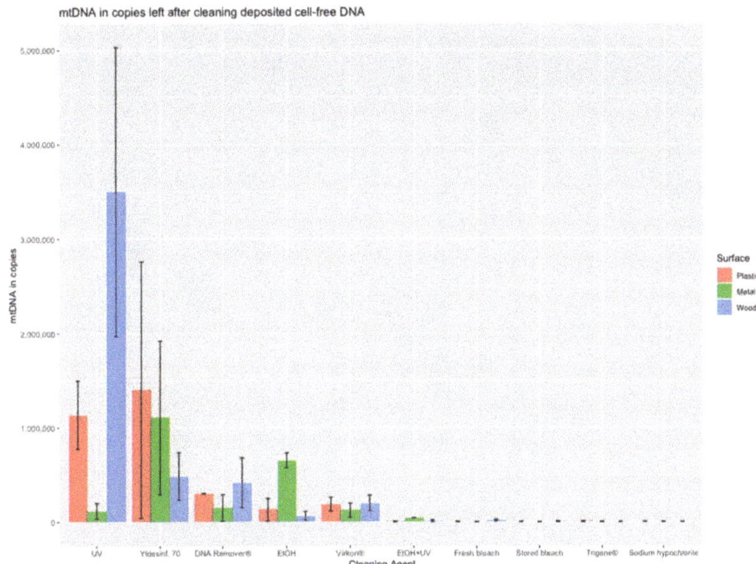

Figure 1. The amount of mtDNA recovered from cell-free DNA deposited on the different surfaces following cleaning with the different strategies. The results are presented as the mean of mtDNA copies (and standard deviations) for a minimum of three replicates recovered from each surface after using the cleaning treatments. The agents are displayed according to the mean recovery for the three surfaces from the highest to the lowest recoveries.

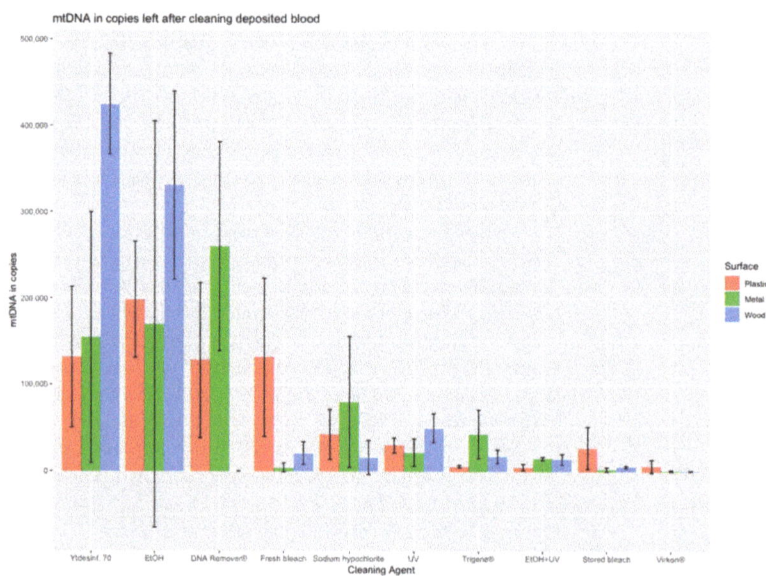

Figure 2. The amount of mtDNA recovered from blood deposited on the different surfaces following cleaning with the different strategies. The results are presented as the mean of mtDNA copies (and standard deviation) for a minimum of three replicates recovered from each surface after using the cleaning treatments. The agents are displayed according to the mean recovery for the three surfaces from the highest to the lowest recoveries.

3. Results

An evaluation of the decontamination efficiency of ten cleaning strategies was performed by quantifying the amount of mitochondrial DNA (from both cell-free DNA and cell-contained DNA) recovered after the cleaning of contaminated plastic, metal, and wood surfaces. The mtDNA quantification results for each combination of cleaning treatment and surface are illustrated in Figures 1 and 2 and Supplementary Materials, Tables S2 and S3. In general, there were large differences in the efficiency of DNA removal between the tested cleaning strategies.

For the cell-free DNA, recoveries of approximately 52, 32, and 27% of the total 60 ng DNA deposited were observed for the no-treatment controls on the plastic, metal, and wood surfaces, respectively. These quantities were used to compare the recovery after the different cleaning strategies. The background controls generated less than 400 mtDNA copies (out of 18 million copies deposited) and were, therefore, ignored in the further evaluation. The recoveries expressed in mtDNA copies and the percent of recovery relative to the no-treatment controls are shown in Table 1.

The cleaning procedures of ethanol and UV were quite inefficient when used alone, with DNA recoveries of up to 11% and 73%, respectively, from all surfaces. However, the combination of both treatments was much more efficient, with recoveries between 0.1 to 0.7% from the three surfaces. Moreover, fresh bleach, stored bleach, Trigene®, and sodium hypochlorite were very efficient in removing DNA, with recoveries from 0.0 to 0.3% from all surfaces. These five decontamination strategies (EtOH+UV, fresh bleach, stored bleach, Trigene®, and sodium hypochlorite) resulted in less than 1% of the DNA recovered from the surface. In addition, if accepting up to 5% recovered DNA, Virkon® is also efficient. The least efficient decontamination strategies were UV and DAX Ytdesinfektion Plus, with up to 73% and 19% DNA recovered, respectively.

Table 1. The efficiency of cell-free DNA removal after cleaning with different treatments on plastic, metal, and wood surfaces. The table is summarizing the mean in mtDNA copies (and standard deviation) per category (3 to 5 biological replicates). The efficiency (Yield) is expressed as the percentage of recovered mtDNA copies of the no-treatment controls.

Cell-Free DNA/Surface	PLASTIC			METAL			WOOD		
Cleaning Agent	Mean	SD	Yield	Mean	SD	Yield	Mean	SD	Yield
No-treatment controls	9,396,667	4,074,633		5,701,333	4,395,753		4,792,667	3,528,892	
EtOH	131,640	120,771	1.4%	655,333	78,520	11.4%	63,460	45,714	1.3%
UV	1,136,000	361,494	12.1%	115,507	84,110	2.0%	3,500,000	1,530,768	73.0%
EtOH+UV	4724	3020	0.1%	42,567	1570	0.7%	11,480	8569	0.2%
Fresh bleach	1991	2900	0.0%	23	30	0.0%	15,313	8443	0.3%
Stored bleach	918	1238	0.0%	85	77	0.0%	4337	5040	0.1%
DAX Ytdesinfektion Plus	1,399,800	1,357,424	14.9%	1,108,198	812,671	19.2%	486,000	252,391	10.1%
Virkon®	188,720	75,615	2.0%	123,350	77,649	2.1%	201,400	84,417	4.2%
DNA Remover®	304,333	3055	3.2%	149,910	142,169	2.6%	416,000	265,640	8.7%
Trigene®	4223	4026	0.0%	970	1657	0.0%	0	0	0.0%
Sodium hypochlorite	199	151	0.0%	0	0	0.0%	8	16	0.0%
Background controls	15	26		37	65		354	352	

For cell-contained DNA in the form of blood, the recoveries expressed in mtDNA copies and the percent of recovery relative to the no-treatment controls are shown in Table 2. Also, for blood, the cleaning procedures of UV and ethanol were relatively inefficient when used alone, with recoveries of up to 11% and 70%, respectively, from all surfaces. Again, the combination of both treatments (EtOH+UV) was much more efficient, with recoveries between 0.6 to 2.9% from the three surfaces, representing the second most efficient strategy for blood. The most efficient strategy was Virkon®, with recoveries between 0.0 and 0.8% for the three different surfaces. If accepting up to 5% recovered DNA, also stored bleach fulfils the criterion. The least efficient decontamination strategy was DAX Ytdesinfektion Plus, with up to 91% DNA recovered after cleaning.

Large differences were observed between the DNA removal of both DNA sources (cell-free DNA and blood) from the plastic, metal, and wood surfaces, indicating differences in surface absorbance and sampling efficiency. On the wood surface, more than 70% of the added DNA was recovered, and, thus, not efficiently removed by the cleaning with ethanol (for blood), UV (for cell-free DNA,) and DAX Ytdesinfektion Plus (for blood). For these three decontamination strategies, the recoveries differed at least 40% between wood and the other surfaces, indicating that the porous wood presents a challenge for decontamination with large amounts of DNA remaining on the surface (Tables 1 and 2). For cell-free DNA, UV radiation left the highest amount of mtDNA copies (73% on wood), followed by the second highest, which was DNA in blood left by DAX Ytdesinfektion Plus (27% on metal). DAX Ytdesinfektion Plus left the highest DNA amount from blood (91% on wood) of all agents, followed by aqueous ethanol (70% of blood DNA on wood) and DNA Remover® (43% of blood DNA on metal). It was observed that decontamination of DNA is less efficient in general for DNA from blood compared to cell-free DNA, which may be a result of the protection by the nucleus and the cell wall (Tables 1 and 2). This is illustrated by the fact that more of the decontamination agents exceed 5% of recovered DNA for blood than for cell-free DNA. Moreover, recovery of more than 5% of DNA from blood was observed on all three surfaces for DAX Ytdesinfektion Plus (ranging from 18 to 91%) and EtOH (ranging from 28 to 70%).

Table 2. The efficiency of cell-contained DNA (blood) removal after cleaning with different treatments on plastic, metal, and wood surfaces. The table is summarizing the mean in mtDNA copies (and standard deviation) per category (3 to 5 biological replicates). The efficiency (Yield) is expressed as the percentage of recovered mtDNA copies of the no-treatment controls.

Blood/Surface	PLASTIC			METAL			WOOD		
Cleaning Agent	Mean	SD	Yield	Mean	SD	Yield	Mean	SD	Yield
No-treatment controls	720,000	66,144		607,667	345,048		469,333	150,111	
EtOH	198,200	67,277	27.5%	170,078	235,148	28.0%	330,600	108,933	70.4%
UV	29,640	8644	4.1%	21,308	15,775	3.5%	49,660	16,808	10.6%
EtOH+UV	4530	3678	0.6%	14,475	1987	2.4%	13,624	6104	2.9%
Fresh bleach	131,380	91,357	18.3%	4028	5124	0.7%	20,465	13,006	4.4%
Stored bleach	26,898	24,457	3.7%	2118	2527	0.4%	5003	1221	1.1%
DAX Ytdesinfektion Plus	131,880	81,201	18.3%	154,488	145,119	25.4%	425,000	58,151	90.6%
Virkon®	5824	7503	0.8%	395	790	0.1%	160	321	0.0%
DNA Remover®	128,060	89,646	17.8%	260,000	121,290	42.8%	0	0	0.0%
Trigene®	5598	1517	0.8%	42,775	28,180	7.0%	16,960	7688	3.6%
Sodium hypochlorite	42,310	28,842	5.9%	79,700	75,524	13.1%	15,618	19,392	3.3%
Background controls	15	26		37	65		354	352	

The most successful decontamination strategies identified in this study for cell-free DNA were fresh and stored bleach, Trigene® and sodium hypochlorite. These cleaning strategies resulted in 0.3% or less of cell-free DNA being recovered from all surfaces, which is equivalent to 0.05 ng DNA or approximately 15,000 mtDNA copies (approximately eight cells) out of the 18 million mtDNA copies initially deposited on the surface. In addition, the combination of EtOH and UV was highly efficient on all three surfaces (0.1 to 0.7%). For blood, the best decontamination efficiency was obtained by Virkon® (0.0 to 0.8%). Thus, some of the decontamination treatments were demonstrated as highly efficient in this study, while others were less efficient in removing contamination.

4. Discussion

Our results demonstrate that using different cleaning strategies on three different surfaces can remove between 27 and 100% of cell-free DNA and between 9 and 100% of the DNA in the blood. While most treatments showed moderate differences between the recoveries from the three surfaces, the DNA recoveries following UV treatment ranged from 2 to 73% for cell-free DNA and from 4 to 11% for DNA in the blood (Tables 1 and 2). The differences in the DNA recoveries from the three surfaces may be attributed to the different structures, absorbances, and porousness of the materials as well as the efficiencies of the different treatments. In addition, the agents may result in a chemical reaction with components of the surface, causing for example, corrosion.

In addition to the type of cleaning agents, several other factors can influence the efficiency of removing contaminating DNA during the cleaning process. For example, the mechanical energy from the wiping action, combined with the chemicals used, may enhance the cleaning effect [24]. Moreover, substantial DNA loss is expected in the sampling by swabbing and the extraction process [25]. In this study, the sampling and extraction efficiency was demonstrated by the no-treatment positive controls, resulting in a loss of 48, 68, and 73% of cell-free DNA from the plastic, metal and wood surfaces, respectively. It is important to note, however, that most extraction kits are developed for the purification of cell-contained DNA and not cell-free DNA, which may result in larger losses in this case than for other sample types. The amount of DNA to simulate contamination to be removed or destroyed was very high in this study, with a total of 60 ng of DNA or 10 µL of blood added to the surface. The high amounts of DNA were used to compensate for expected loss in the initial sample preparation process and to challenge the different cleaning strategies efficiently. The added DNA amount is excessively more than expected from most contamination events by aerosols or touched surfaces (without gloves) and may only be possible to transfer to laboratory surfaces by contamination from a concentrated DNA extract or items with relatively fresh blood stains. Despite all factors that may cause variation, this study could demonstrate decontamination efficiency, by measurements of DNA quantities made before and after cleaning.

Apart from efficiency, several parameters are important when choosing a decontamination strategy, such as simplicity of use, safety, and cost. Ethylene oxide is a highly efficient but poisonous agent and, therefore, unsuitable for decontamination in a laboratory environment [26]. Moreover, certain combinations of agents and strategies may be hazardous, such as 1% sodium hypochlorite and 70% ethanol, which form gaseous chlorine and chloroform when combined [17]. It is also essential to allow practical and straightforward daily routines. A commonly used decontaminating agent in laboratories is 1–10% sodium hypochlorite solutions, and a low-cost solution can easily be prepared by diluting household bleach. [17]. A low-cost hypochlorite solution can easily be prepared by diluting household bleach. In this study, the in-house sodium hypochlorite dilutions were made at 15% for easy preparations. Due to discontinuation of the stock solution used for the stored bleach, the bleach solutions were prepared from two different variants of the same brand, Klorin Original and Klorin, with sodium hypochlorite concentrations of 3.6 and 2.7%, respectively. Thus, the 15% dilutions resulted in final Cl_2 ion concentrations of 0.54 and 0.4% for fresh and stored bleach, respectively. It is, therefore, important to note that the ratio between the fresh and the stored bleach is 1:0.74 rather than 1:1 when comparing the decontamination efficiencies. To further simplify the routines, the lasting properties of diluted household bleach are important. The available chlorine concentration may be affected in hypochlorite solutions when exposed to light, air, and heat, among other factors. This may reduce the stability, but it has been shown that solutions stored up to 200 days at 4 °C are stable [22]. Our study demonstrated that a hypochlorite solution stored at 8 °C for 80 days is not less efficient than the freshly made solution. Therefore, preparing a new solution is not needed more often than every second month if stored properly.

Many cleaning agent solutions contain hazardous chemical compounds listed in their safety data sheets. The treatments used in this study have a variety of health risks. Some are safe (e.g., DNA Remover®) with no risks listed, while others present several risks (Supplementary Materials, Table S1). Health risks are very important, but also, the cost is a relevant parameter. For example, DNA Remover® costs 100 times more than household bleach. In contrast, Trigene® has a low cost but is associated with multiple health and environmental hazards. Another important aspect is that the cleaning agent might inhibit the PCR reaction and affect the downstream profiling process. An inhibitory effect has been observed for minute amounts of Trigene® introduced into the PCR reaction, whereas Virkon® or ethanol did not affect STR profiling [14]. All this may influence laboratories final choice of decontamination agent.

Although sodium hypochlorite is highly efficient for the removal of DNA contamination, there are several drawbacks, such as corrosion of metal instruments (e.g., scissors and tweezers). For this reason, alternatives to bleach may be preferred for repeated decontamination of metal items. We performed a limited experiment with metal scissors (stainless steel) submerged in 15% household bleach, DNA Remover®, Virkon®, and water. Preliminary observations showed that corrosion was apparent after only one day in the bleach solution and after five days for water, while no corrosion was observed after 14 days in DNA Remover® or Virkon® (Table S4).Thus, as Virkon® appears to have a high DNA removal ability, this agent may be a good option when decontaminating metal instruments, despite a somewhat lower ability to remove cell-free contaminating DNA compared to household bleach. However, disposable instruments for evidence sampling and recovery (e.g., single-use scalpels or plastic tweezers) may eliminate the need for a non-corrosive decontamination treatment either completely or at least to some extent. Alternatively, if using sodium hypochlorite for decontamination, rinsing or wiping the surface with distilled water should be performed to avoid corrosion [17].

To conclude, this study showed large differences in the decontamination efficiency between commonly used cleaning strategies on different surfaces and types of traces, cell-free or cell-contained. Of all cleaning agents, six left around 1% or less of either cell-free DNA or DNA in blood on all surfaces. For cell-free DNA, EtOH+UV, fresh bleach, stored bleach, Trigene®, and sodium hypochlorite demonstrated the highest efficiency. Out of these, the highest remaining DNA amounts of 0.7% (on metal and with removal of outliers) correspond to 0.14 ng or around 43,000 copies of mtDNA. For cell-contained DNA as blood, Virkon® left less than 1% DNA and the highest remaining amount corresponds to 0.025 ng or around 7500 mtDNA copies. In addition to efficiency, parameters such as health hazards, simplicity, and cost should also be considered. Therefore, different agents or a combination of treatments may be optimal for the decontamination in laboratories performing forensic DNA analysis. Considering our own requirements and priorities, the updated routines for our laboratory will be to perform decontamination with a 15% dilution of stored household bleach for laboratory work surfaces and with Virkon® for metal instrumentation to avoid corrosion.

Supplementary Materials: The following are available online at https://www.mdpi.com/article/10.3390/genes13010162/s1: Table S1, Overview of the cleaning strategies; Table S2, Overview of the mtDNA data in copies from cell-free DNA samples; and Table S3, Overview of the mtDNA data in copies from blood samples; Table S4: Cleaning of scissors_HDM.

Author Contributions: Conceptualization, M.A. and M.N.; methodology, M.A. and M.N.; software, H.D.M.; validation, M.A., M.N. and H.D.M.; resources, M.N.; data curation, H.D.M.; writing—original draft preparation, M.A., M.N. and H.D.M.; writing—review and editing, M.A., M.N. and H.D.M. All authors have read and agreed to the published version of the manuscript.

Funding: M.A. and MN received financial support from VINNOVA (The Swedish Governmental Agency for Innovation Systems) and UU Innovation, Verifiering för samverkan (VFS) collaboration grant, 2021, UFV2020/32.

Institutional Review Board Statement: The study was conducted in accordance with the Declaration of Helsinki. Use of human samples was approved by the Ethical Review Agency (Etikprövningsmyndigheten, Linköping, dnr 2019-03878 on dnr 2020-06776 on 2020-12-09).

Informed Consent Statement: Informed consent was obtained from all subjects involved in the study.

Data Availability Statement: Not applicable.

Acknowledgments: We want to thank Kristina Gawelin for excellent technical assistance in this project.

Conflicts of Interest: The authors declare no conflict of interest.

References

1. Ludeman, M.J.; Zhong, C.; Mulero, J.J.; Lagacé, R.E.; Hennessy, L.K.; Short, M.L.; Wang, D.Y. Developmental Validation of GlobalFiler™ PCR Amplification Kit: A 6-Dye Multiplex Assay Designed for Amplification of Casework Samples. *Int. J. Leg. Med.* **2018**, *132*, 1555–1573. [CrossRef] [PubMed]
2. McLaren, R.S.; Bourdeau-Heller, J.; Patel, J.; Thompson, J.M.; Pagram, J.; Loake, T.; Beesley, D.; Pirttimaa, M.; Hill, C.R.; Duewer, D.L.; et al. Developmental Validation of the PowerPlex® ESI 16/17 Fast and PowerPlex® ESX 16/17 Fast Systems. *Forensic Sci. Int. Genet.* **2014**, *13*, 195–205. [CrossRef]
3. Bogenhagen, D.; Clayton, D.A. The Number of Mitochondrial Deoxyribonucleic Acid Genomes in Mouse L and Human HeLa Cells. Quantitative Isolation of Mitochondrial Deoxyribonucleic Acid. *J. Biol. Chem.* **1974**, *249*, 7991–7995. [CrossRef]
4. Allen, M.; Engström, A.-S.; Meyers, S.; Handt, O.; Saldeen, T.; von Haeseler, A.; Pääbo, S.; Gyllensten, U. Mitochondrial DNA Sequencing of Shed Hairs and Saliva on Robbery Caps: Sensitivity and Matching Probabilities. *J. Forensic Sci.* **1998**, *43*, 453–464. [CrossRef]
5. Kloosterman, A.; Sjerps, M.; Quak, A. Error Rates in Forensic DNA Analysis: Definition, Numbers, Impact and Communication. *Forensic Sci. Int. Genet.* **2014**, *12*, 77–85. [CrossRef]

6. Codes of Practice and Conduct. Protocol: DNA contamination detection—The management and use of staff elimination DNA databases. In *Forensic Science Regulator, FSR-P-302, Issue 1*; 2014; p. 49. Available online: https://assets.publishing.service.gov.uk/government/uploads/system/uploads/attachment_data/file/915377/302-Elimination_database_protocol_v2.pdf (accessed on 15 November 2021).

7. Fonneløp, A.E.; Johannessen, H.; Egeland, T.; Gill, P. Contamination during Criminal Investigation: Detecting Police Contamination and Secondary DNA Transfer from Evidence Bags. *Forensic Sci. Int. Genet.* **2016**, *23*, 121–129. [CrossRef] [PubMed]

8. Gill, P. Role of Short Tandem Repeat DNA in Forensic Casework in the UK-Past, Present, and Future Perspectives. *BioTechniques* **2002**, *32*, 366–385. [CrossRef] [PubMed]

9. Neuhuber, F.; Dunkelmann, B.; Höckner, G.; Kiesslich, J.; Klausriegler, E.; Radacher, M. Female Criminals—It's Not Always the Offender! *Forensic Sci. Int. Genet. Suppl. Ser.* **2009**, *2*, 145–146. [CrossRef]

10. Daniel, R.; van Oorschot, R.A.H. An Investigation of the Presence of DNA on Unused Laboratory Gloves. *Forensic Sci. Int. Genet. Suppl. Ser.* **2011**, *3*, e45–e46. [CrossRef]

11. Lapointe, M.; Rogic, A.; Bourgoin, S.; Jolicoeur, C.; Séguin, D. Leading-Edge Forensic DNA Analyses and the Necessity of Including Crime Scene Investigators, Police Officers and Technicians in a DNA Elimination Database. *Forensic Sci. Int. Genet.* **2015**, *19*, 50–55. [CrossRef]

12. Gefrides, L.A.; Powell, M.C.; Donley, M.A.; Kahn, R. UV Irradiation and Autoclave Treatment for Elimination of Contaminating DNA from Laboratory Consumables. *Forensic Sci. Int. Genet.* **2010**, *4*, 89–94. [CrossRef]

13. Preuße-Prange, A.; Renneberg, R.; Schwark, T.; Poetsch, M.; Simeoni, E.; von Wurmb-Schwark, N. The Problem of DNA Contamination in Forensic Case Work-How to Get Rid of Unwanted DNA? *Forensic Sci. Int. Genet. Suppl. Ser.* **2009**, *2*, 185–186. [CrossRef]

14. Bright, J.A.; Cockerton, S.; Harbison, S.A.; Russell, A.; Samson, O.; Stevenson, K. The Effect of Cleaning Agents on the Ability to Obtain DNA Profiles Using the Identifiler™ and PowerPlex® Y Multiplex Kits. *J. Forensic Sci.* **2011**, *56*, 181–185. [CrossRef] [PubMed]

15. Hoofstat, V.; Groote, D.; Van Thuyne, S.; Haerinck, N. Sources of DNA Contamination and Decontamination Procedures in the Forensic Laboratory. *J. Forensic Res.* **2011**, *2*, 1. [CrossRef]

16. Champlot, S.; Berthelot, C.; Pruvost, M.; Andrew Bennett, E.; Grange, T.; Geigl, E.M. An Efficient Multistrategy DNA Decontamination Procedure of PCR Reagents for Hypersensitive PCR Applications. *PLoS ONE* **2010**, *5*, e13042. [CrossRef] [PubMed]

17. Ballantyne, K.N.; Salemi, R.; Guarino, F.; Pearson, J.R.; Garlepp, D.; Fowler, S.; Van Oorschot, R.A.H. DNA Contamination Minimisation-Finding an Effective Cleaning Method. *Aust. J. Forensic Sci.* **2015**, *47*, 428–439. [CrossRef]

18. Shaw, K.; Sesardić, I.; Bristol, N.; Ames, C.; Dagnall, K.; Ellis, C.; Whittaker, F.; Daniel, B. Comparison of the Effects of Sterilisation Techniques on Subsequent DNA Profiling. *Int. J. Leg. Med.* **2008**, *122*, 29–33. [CrossRef] [PubMed]

19. Vandewoestyne, M.; Van Hoofstat, D.; Franssen, A.; Van Nieuwerburgh, F.; Deforce, D. Presence and Potential of Cell Free DNA in Different Types of Forensic Samples. *Forensic Sci. Int. Genet.* **2013**, *7*, 316–320. [CrossRef] [PubMed]

20. Quinones, I.; Daniel, B. Cell Free DNA as a Component of Forensic Evidence Recovered from Touched Surfaces. *Forensic Sci. Int. Genet.* **2012**, *6*, 26–30. [CrossRef]

21. Andréasson, H.; Gyllensten, U.; Allen, M. Real-Time DNA Quantification of Nuclear and Mitochondrial DNA in Forensic Analysis. *BioTechniques* **2002**, *33*, 402–411. [CrossRef] [PubMed]

22. Piskin, B.; Türkün, M. Stability of Various Sodium Hypochlorite Solutions. *J. Endod.* **1995**, *21*, 253–255. [CrossRef]

23. R Core Team. *R: A Language and Environment for Statistical Computing*; R Foundation for Statistical Computing: Vienna, Austria, 2021. Available online: https://www.R-project.org (accessed on 13 December 2021).

24. Forensic Science Community. *Comparison Study of Disinfectants for Decontamination Project Information Stakeholder Information Photos*; National Forensic Science Technology Center: Largo, FL, USA, 2011; No. 727.

25. Verdon, T.J.; Mitchell, R.J.; van Oorschot, R.A.H. Swabs as DNA Collection Devices for Sampling Different Biological Materials from Different Substrates. *J. Forensic Sci.* **2014**, *59*, 1080–1089. [CrossRef] [PubMed]

26. Wilson-Wilde, L.; Yakovchyts, D.; Neville, S.; Maynard, P.; Gunn, P. Investigation into Ethylene Oxide Treatment and Residuals on DNA and Downstream DNA Analysis. *Sci. Justice* **2017**, *57*, 13–20. [CrossRef] [PubMed]

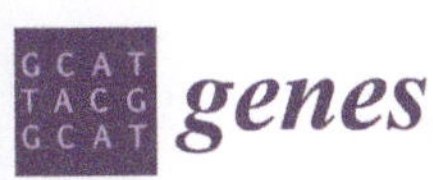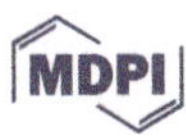

Article

Analysis of Skin Pigmentation and Genetic Ancestry in Three Subpopulations from Pakistan: Punjabi, Pashtun, and Baloch

Muhammad Adnan Shan [1,2,*,†], **Olivia Strunge Meyer** [1,†], **Mie Refn** [1], **Niels Morling** [1], **Jeppe Dyrberg Andersen** [1] and **Claus Børsting** [1]

[1] Section of Forensic Genetics, Department of Forensic Medicine, Faculty of Health and Medical Sciences, University of Copenhagen, 2100 Copenhagen, Denmark; olivia.meyer@sund.ku.dk (O.S.M.); mrefn@sund.ku.dk (M.R.); niels.morling@sund.ku.dk (N.M.); jeppe.dyrberg.andersen@sund.ku.dk (J.D.A.); claus.boersting@sund.ku.dk (C.B.)

[2] Centre for Applied Molecular Biology (CAMB), University of the Punjab, Lahore 54590, Pakistan

* Correspondence: forensic.genetics@sund.ku.dk

† Authors contributed equally.

Citation: Shan, M.A.; Meyer, O.S.; Refn, M.; Morling, N.; Andersen, J.D.; Børsting, C. Analysis of Skin Pigmentation and Genetic Ancestry in Three Subpopulations from Pakistan: Punjabi, Pashtun, and Baloch. *Genes* **2021**, *12*, 733. https://doi.org/10.3390/genes12050733

Academic Editor: Adriano Tagliabracci

Received: 10 April 2021
Accepted: 11 May 2021
Published: 13 May 2021

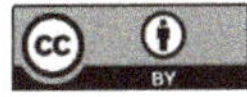

Abstract: Skin pigmentation is one of the most prominent and variable phenotypes in humans. We compared the alleles of 163 SNPs and indels from the Human Pigmentation (HuPi) AmpliSeq™ Custom panel, and biogeographic ancestry with the quantitative skin pigmentation levels on the upper arm, lower arm, and forehead of 299 Pakistani individuals from three subpopulations: Baloch, Pashtun, and Punjabi. The biogeographic ancestry of each individual was estimated using the Precision ID Ancestry Panel. All individuals were mainly of mixed South-Central Asian and European ancestry. However, the Baloch individuals also had an average proportion of Sub-Saharan African ancestry of approximately 10%, whereas it was <1% in the Punjabi and Pashtun individuals. The pairwise genetic distances between the Pashtun, Punjabi, and Baloch subpopulations based on the ancestry markers were statistically significantly different. Individuals from the Pashtun subpopulation had statistically significantly lower skin pigmentation than individuals from the Punjabi and Baloch subpopulations ($p < 0.05$). The proportions of European and Sub-Saharan African ancestry and five SNPs (rs1042602, rs10831496, rs1426654, rs16891982, and rs12913832) were statistically significantly associated with skin pigmentation at either the upper arm, lower arm or forehead in the Pakistani population after correction for multiple testing ($p < 10^{-3}$). A model based on four of these SNPs (rs1426654, rs1042602, rs16891982, and rs12913832) explained 33% of the upper arm skin pigmentation. The four SNPs and the proportions of European and Sub-Saharan African ancestry explained 37% of the upper arm skin pigmentation. Our results indicate that the four likely causative SNPs, rs1426654, rs1042602, rs16891982, and rs12913832 located in *SLC24A5, TYR, SLC45A2*, and *HERC2*, respectively, are essential for skin color variation in the admixed Pakistani subpopulations.

Keywords: biogeographic ancestry; pigmentation; skin color; forensic DNA phenotyping; externally visible characteristics

1. Introduction

Human pigmentation is one of the most variable externally visible characteristics (EVCs). Prediction of EVCs may result in helpful leads early in a police investigation by providing a 'genetic eye witness' of a possible perpetrator and may allow the police investigators to focus their attention on specific groups of individuals and decrease the number of potential suspects [1–3]. The genetics of human pigmentation is a field of great interest in forensic genetics because it offers a prediction of three prominent EVCs: hair, eye, and skin color [4,5]. Skin pigmentation is strongly associated with biogeographic ancestry [6] and influenced by environmental factors (e.g., UV radiation) [7], which complicates the identification of causative variants and the reliability of the predictions. Prediction of the biogeographic ancestry may indicate skin pigmentation of the individual. However, skin color prediction based on the assumption that biogeographic ancestry and skin color are well correlated only offers an indirect prediction, and the assumption is not necessarily true in admixed populations [8,9]. Studies of admixed individuals from North and South American populations showed that the correlation between ancestry and skin pigmentation varied considerably and explained 20–65% of the skin pigmentation [3,6,10,11]. Nevertheless, admixed populations are ideal for studying the effect of genetic variants associated with skin pigmentation because they have a wide range of skin colors, and the ancestry proportions of each individual may be estimated using standard population genetic methods.

The Pakistani population is an admixed population with several subpopulations and ethnic groups. Pakistan is situated at the junction of the Middle East, Central Asia, and Southeast Asia. This area was the home of various ancient cultures, including the Bronze Age Indus Valley Civilization [12]. The region was ruled by dynasties and empires of different religions and cultures, including Muslims, Turco-Mongols, Hindus, Indo-Greeks, Sikhs, and Afghans [13]. Hence, the Pakistani population is well suited for studying biogeographic ancestry and skin pigmentation genetics.

We studied the associations among pigmentary variants, biogeographic ancestry, and quantitative skin pigmentation in three admixed subpopulations from Pakistan ($n = 299$). We evaluated the individuals' ancestry with the Precision ID Ancestry Panel (Thermo Fisher Scientific, Waltham, MA, USA) [14–16] and investigated the association between skin pigmentation and genetic pigmentary variants in the HuPi AmpliSeq™ Custom panel [17]. We also analyzed the correlation between skin pigmentation and the 36 HIrisPlex-S SNPs [18,19] as well as nine SNPs found to be associated with skin pigmentation variation in an admixed Brazilian population [3]. Lastly, we analyzed the efficiency of the skin color prediction using the HIrisPlex-S prediction model [18,19].

2. Materials and Methods

2.1. Samples, DNA Extraction, and DNA Quantification

Buccal swabs were collected from 299 unrelated healthy Pakistani individuals and stored on FTA cards. The individuals belonged to three major Pakistani subpopulations: 107 Baloch from Baluchistan, 103 Pashtuns from Khyber Pakhtunkhwa, and 89 Punjabis from northern Punjab. Signed informed consent was obtained from all participants, and the samples were anonymized. The study was approved by the Review Board/Ethical Committee of the University of the Punjab, Pakistan (D/No. 019/DFEMS). Genomic DNA was extracted using the Qiagen BioRobot® EZ1 Workstation and the EZ1 DNA investigator kit (Qiagen, Hilden, Germany). Purified DNA was quantified using the Qubit™ dsDNA HS Assay Kit and a Qubit® 4.0 Fluorometer (Thermo Fisher Scientific, Waltham, MA, USA) according to the manufacturer's recommendations.

2.2. Measurement of Quantitative Skin Pigmentation

The UV-Optimize Scientific 555 (Chromo Light APS, Vedbæk, Denmark) calibrated with a white standard (ISO 2469) was used to measure quantitative skin pigmentation. Quantitative skin pigmentation was determined as the pigment protection factor, PPF, which is a measure for skin pigmentation levels [20,21]. The skin pigmentation of each individual was measured in triplicates from skin areas on the lower inner forearm (lower arm), upper inner arm (upper arm), and forehead. The median PPF-value for each measuring site was used for further analysis. All skin measurements were taken from areas without hair, freckles, nevi, or tattoos.

2.3. Typing with the Precision ID Ancestry Panel and the Human Pigmentation (HuPi) AmpliSeq™ Custom Panel

DNA was amplified with the Precision ID Ancestry Panel (Thermo Fisher Scientific, Waltham, MA, USA) and the Human Pigmentation (HuPi) AmpliSeq™ Custom panel [17] in two separate reactions. The Precision ID Ancestry Panel targets 165 ancestry-informative markers (AIMs). The HuPi AmpliSeq™ Custom panel targets 183 SNPs and indels, which were previously found to be associated with human pigmentary variation [17]. Sequencing libraries were prepared with the Ion AmpliSeq™ Library Kit 2.0 (Thermo Fisher Scientific, Waltham, MA, USA) using half volume of all reagents but otherwise following the manufacturer's instructions. Amplification of targets was carried out using approximately 1 ng DNA (1–3 µL) and 24 and 26 cycles for the Precision ID Ancestry Panel and the HuPi AmpliSeq™ Custom panel, respectively. Sequencing libraries were purified using the Biomek 3000 pipetting robot [22]. Purified libraries were quantified using the Qubit™ 4.0 Fluorometer with the Qubit™ dsDNA HS Assay kit (Thermo Fisher Scientific, Waltham, MA, USA) and pooled in equimolar concentrations to a final volume of 28 pM for the Precision ID Ancestry panel and 35–60 pM for the HuPi AmpliSeq™ Custom Panel. Template preparation was performed with the Ion Chef™ instrument (Thermo Fisher Scientific, Waltham, MA, USA) using the Ion S5™ Precision ID Chef Kit (Thermo Fisher Scientific, Waltham, MA, USA) following the manufacturer's recommendations (Thermo Fisher Scientific, Waltham, MA, USA). Sequencing was carried out with Ion 530™ Chips and Ion S5™ Precision ID Sequencing Reagents on the Ion S5™ (Thermo Fisher Scientific, Waltham, MA, USA) with up to 80 samples per chip.

2.4. Analysis of Sequencing Data

The data were initially analyzed with the Torrent Suite Software v.5.10.1 (Thermo Fisher Scientific, Waltham, MA, USA). For the Precision ID Ancestry panel, data were analyzed with the HID_SNP_Genotyper_v5_2_2 plugin using GRCh37 (hg19) as the reference genome and default parameters (Thermo Fisher Scientific, Waltham, MA, USA). The data obtained with the HuPi AmpliSeq™ Custom Panel were analyzed with the VariantCaller v5.10.1.20 plugin and the GRCh38.p2 (hg38) reference genome. The "Down-sample to coverage" was changed from 400 to 10,000 reads. Otherwise, the analyses were performed with the default parameters (Thermo Fisher Scientific, Waltham, MA, USA). The resulting Excel-files were processed using R v.4.0.2 (R core team, https://www.R-project.org/, accessed on 1 November 2020) and an in-house developed script. The data quality control comprised evaluation of the locus balance, heterozygote balance (Hb), and noise levels for each target. Hb was calculated as the number of reads for one nucleotide divided by the number of reads for the other nucleotide in the order A, C, G, and T. Genotypes were accepted when a locus had $\geq$45 reads and the Hb was between 0.3 and 3. SNPs with 30–44 reads were inspected and accepted if the Hb was between 0.7 and 1.5 or if the noise did not exceed one read for homozygous genotype calls. Genotypes that did not meet the criteria were annotated as NN. For both panels, loci with NNs in more than 15% of the samples were excluded. Moreover, samples with more than 15% missing data (NN) were excluded from further analysis. Hardy–Weinberg Equilibrium (HWE) and pairwise linkage disequilibrium (LD) were calculated with Haploview v. 4.2 [23], and pairwise F_{ST}-values were calculated using Arlequin v3.5.2.2 software [24].

2.5. Classification of Biogeographic Ancestry

The alleles of the AIM-SNPs in each sample were investigated using STRUCTURE v.2.3.4.21 [25,26]. The analyses were carried out using 100,000 steps of burn-in followed by 100,000 repetitions for the MCMC. The 'admixture' and the 'correlated allele frequencies' models were used [25,26]. After testing the number of clusters (K) from K = 3 to K = 6, K was set to 4, corresponding to the Sub-Saharan African, South-Central Asian, European, and East Asian populations. The results were visualized using CLUMPP v.1.1.222 [27] and Distruct v.1.1.23 [28]. Principal component analysis (PCA) was carried out using an in-house written Python script. Reference population data (Supplementary Table S1) were collected as previously described [14,29]. Four SNPs, rs1800414, rs12913832, rs1426654, and rs16891982, were included in both the Precision ID Ancestry Panel and the HuPi AmpliSeq™ Custom panel. One SNP, rs10954737, lacked genotype data in all reference populations. Hence, these five SNPs were not considered in the PCA and STRUCTURE analyses and were not used to classify ancestry.

2.6. Correlations between Biogeographic Ancestry, Pigmentary Variants, and Skin Pigmentation

We excluded monomorphic genetic variants (i.e., variants with only one observed genotype) and variants in LD ($r^2 > 0.8$) with other variants in the HuPi AmpliSeq™ Custom Panel. Hence, the dataset was limited to 102 genetic variants and four metapopulations (Sub-Saharan Africa, South-Central Asia, Europe, and East Asia). Differences in skin pigmentation levels of the lower arm, upper arm, and forehead, as well as differences in skin pigmentation of the three subpopulations, were investigated using Student's *t*-test for paired data or the Welch two-sample *t*-test for unpaired data. The correlations among skin pigmentation levels, genetic variants in the HuPi AmpliSeq™ Custom Panel, and the estimation of the ancestry proportions were carried out using multiple linear regression (MLR). The correlation was evaluated using the adjusted R^2. To select a subset of variants, backwards model selection was performed using MLR with Akaike Information Criterion (AIC) using the *stepAIC* function in the MASS R-package [30].

We also evaluated the correlation between skin pigmentation and the genotypes of the 36 HIrisPlex-S SNPs [18,19], and between skin pigmentation and nine SNPs (rs1426654, rs1448484, rs16891982, rs4424881, rs10831496, rs6119471, rs12913832, rs10424065, and rs1408799) previously found to explain up to 65% of the skin pigmentation variation in a Brazilian population of primarily European ancestry [3].

2.7. Prediction of Skin Colour Using the HIrisPlex-S

Prediction of skin color using the HIrisPlex-S model was carried out with the online web-tool (https://hirisplex.erasmusmc.nl/, accessed on 1 Novmber 2020). The HIrisPlex-S model predicts skin color in five categories: Very pale, Pale, Intermediate, Dark, and Dark to Black [18,19]. The skin color category with the highest predictive value was used as the skin pigmentation prediction. The HIrisPlex-S skin color prediction and the quantitative skin pigmentation measurements were compared.

2.8. Statistical Methods

The statistical methods used are described in each section. When multiple comparisons were performed, the statistical significance was corrected with the Bonferroni method.

3. Results

3.1. Skin Pigmentation Measurements

Quantitative skin pigmentation measurements were performed for the 299 Pakistani individuals, Baloch ($n = 107$), Pashtun ($n = 103$), and Punjabi ($n = 89$). The lowest pigmentation levels were observed on the upper arm (mean PPF of 11.08), followed by the lower arm (mean PPF of 12.30) and the forehead (mean PPF of 12.43). We observed statistically significant differences between the pigmentation levels on the upper arm and lower arm ($p < 0.05$) and the upper arm and forehead ($p < 0.05$) among all subpopulations. Statistically significant difference between pigmentation levels of the lower arm and forehead was only observed in the Baloch subpopulation ($p < 0.05$).

Individuals from the Pashtun subpopulation showed statistically significant ($p < 0.05$) lower pigmentation levels than individuals in the Baloch and Punjabi subpopulations on all measured areas (Figure 1).

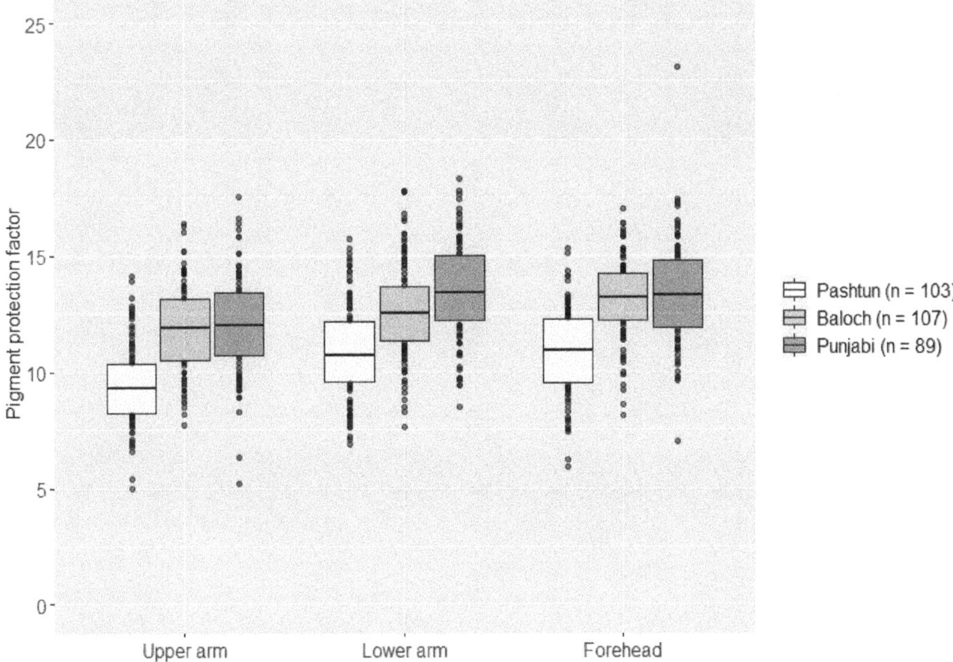

Figure 1. Boxplots of skin pigmentation measurements (pigment protection factor) of the upper arm, lower arm, and forehead in three Pakistani subpopulations. The pigment protection factor was measured in triplicate at each measured skin area.

3.2. The Precision ID Ancestry Panel

The allele frequencies for the 165 loci in the Punjabi, Pashtun, and Baloch populations are presented in Supplementary Table S2. The median number of reads per target was 493 (range: 45–12,105), the median Hb was 1.0 (range: 0.3–3.0) for heterozygous SNPs, and the median level of noise was 0.0% (range: 0–14.3%). One locus, rs2070586, deviated from HWE ($p < 10^{-3}$) in the Baloch population. The loci rs3811801 and rs671 were monomorphic in all three populations, rs1871534 and rs2814778 were monomorphic in Pashtuns and Punjabis, and rs1800414 was monomorphic in the Baloch. No pairwise LD (pairwise $r^2 > 0.8$) was detected in any of the three populations. The observed values of pairwise F_{ST} genetic distances were statistically significantly different among all subpopulations ($p < 10^{-5}$) (Supplementary Table S3).

3.3. Proportion of Ancestry Components

The biogeographic ancestry of each individual was investigated with STRUCTURE and PCA using reference data from 34 populations grouped into six metapopulations: Sub-Saharan African, North African, European, Middle Eastern, South-Central Asian, and East Asian (Supplementary Table S1). The results of the STRUCTURE analysis with K = 4 are shown in Figure 2. The Baloch, Punjabi, and Pashtun subpopulations were admixed populations with major contributions from South-Central Asian and European populations. The Baloch differed from the other two subpopulations due to approximately 10% Sub-Saharan African genetic contribution, whereas the Sub-Saharan African contribution was <1% in the Punjabis and Pashtuns. The Baloch had the lowest proportion of South-Central Asian ancestry (44.7%), followed by the Pashtuns (56.6%) and the Punjabis (69.3%).

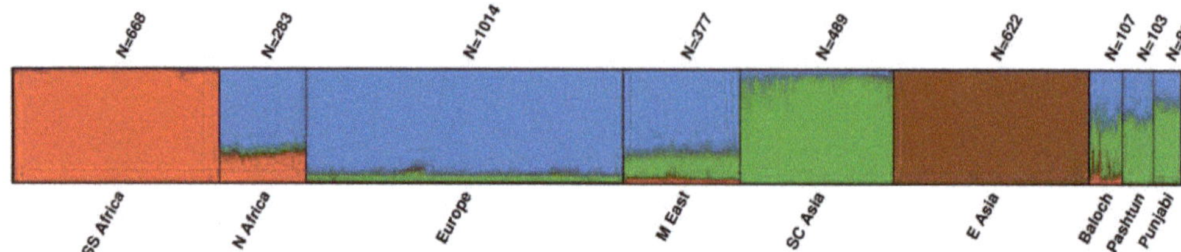

Figure 2. STRUCTURE analysis with K = 4 using 160 ancestry informative markers (AIMs) and six meta-populations. Each cluster (K) is represented by a color. Population abbreviations used: SS Africa: Sub-Saharan Africa; N Africa: North Africa; M East: Middle East; SC Asia: South-Central Asia; E Asia: East Asia.

The first two principal components (PC1 and PC2) in the PCA analysis separated the Sub-Saharan African, European, and East Asian populations from each other (Supplementary Figure S1). The North Africans clustered closest to the European and Middle Eastern populations, while the South-Central Asian populations clustered between the East Asian and European populations. The positions of the three Pakistani subpopulations, Punjabis, Pashtuns, and the Baloch, overlapped with each other and the South-Central Asian and Middle Eastern populations. The Baloch individuals clustered closer to the African populations than the Pashtuns and Punjabis. In contrast, the Punjabis clustered closer to the South-Central Asian populations than the Pashtuns and Baloch, supporting the STRUCTURE analysis conclusions.

3.4. The HuPi AmpliSeq™ Custom Panel

A total of 163 variants were successfully typed with the HuPi AmpliSeq™ Custom Panel (Supplementary Table S4). The median number of reads was 597 (range: 60–1532) per target. The median Hb for heterozygous SNP calls was 1.0 (range: 0.35–2.86). The median level of noise was 0.0% (range: 0–12.7%). The allele frequencies of rs4778241 in *OCA2* deviated statistically significantly from HWE ($p < 10^{-3}$). Twelve variants were monomorphic (Supplementary Table S4), and these data were removed from the subsequent analysis. For the correlation measurements between skin pigmentation and genetic variants, only independent genetic variants were considered (pairwise $r^2 < 0.8$), reducing the number of genetic variants to 102 (Supplementary Table S4).

3.5. Correlation between Skin Pigmentation and Biogeographic Ancestry

The proportions of Sub-Saharan African, European, South-Central Asian, and East Asian ancestry were compared with the skin pigmentation at each measured site using MLR. We found statistically significant ($p < 10^{-3}$) adjusted R^2-values for the upper arm: 0.10, lower arm: 0.13, and forehead: 0.12 when comparing the full ancestry profiles with the skin pigmentation (Supplementary Table S5). We found statistically significant ($p < 0.05$) negative correlations between the proportion of European ancestry and skin pigmentation at all three measured sites (adjusted R^2: 0.04–0.09) and statistically significant positive correlation ($p < 0.05$) between Sub-Saharan African ancestry and skin pigmentation at the upper arm and forehead (adjusted R^2 = 0.06 and 0.07, respectively). In contrast, the proportions of East Asian and South-Central Asian ancestry showed no statistically significant correlation with skin pigmentation (Supplementary Table S5). We analyzed the correlation between the proportions of only European and Sub-Saharan African ancestry with skin pigmentation at all three measuring sites using MLR. The resulting adjusted R^2-values were 0.10 ($p < 10^{-3}$), 0.13 ($p < 10^{-6}$), and 0.12 ($p < 10^{-6}$) for the upper arm, lower arm, and forehead pigmentation, respectively (Supplementary Table S5).

3.6. Correlations among Skin Pigmentation, Pigmentary Variants, and Biogeographic Ancestry

Each of the independent variants typed with the HuPi AmpliSeq™ Custom Panel was compared with the skin pigmentation at the upper arm, lower arm, and forehead using linear regression. We observed statistically significant ($p < 0.05$) correlations between skin pigmentation on either the upper arm, lower arm, or forehead and the SNPs rs1042602 in *TYR* and rs10831496 in *GRM5*, rs1426654 in *SLC24A5*, rs16891982 in *SLC45A2*, and rs12913832 in *HERC2* (Table 1). Only rs1426654 and rs1042602 were statistically significantly correlated with skin pigmentation at all three sites ($p < 10^{-3}$) (Table 1).

Table 1. Five SNPs with statistically significant association with skin pigmentation on the upper arm, lower arm, or forehead in 299 Pakistani individuals from three subpopulations (Baloch, Pashtun, and Punjabi).

		Upper Arm		Lower Arm		Forehead	
Gene	SNP	Adjusted R^2	Sign.[1]	Adjusted R^2	Sign.[1]	Adjusted R^2	Sign.[1]
TYR	rs1042602	0.13	***	0.11	**	0.071	**
GRM5	rs10831496	0.029	–	0.047	*	0.014	–
HERC2	rs12913832	0.025	–	0.016	–	0.064	*
SLC24A5	rs1426654	0.16	***	0.10	**	0.082	**
SLC45A2	rs16891982	0.075	**	0.028	–	0.058	**

[1] Statistical significance (Sign.) after Bonferroni correction: * $p < 0.05$, ** $p < 10^{-3}$, *** $p < 10^{-6}$.

The five SNPs were compared with skin pigmentation using MLR, and the adjusted R^2 ranged from 0.24 to 0.33 ($p < 10^{-6}$) (Table 2). Subsequently, model selection was performed using stepwise AIC, giving the best model with rs1426654, rs1042602, rs16891982, and rs12913832 for all three sites (upper arm, lower arm, and forehead). When the proportions of European and Sub-Saharan African ancestry were included, the adjusted R^2-values increased slightly (Table 2, Figure 3). The cumulative correlations between (1) the four SNPs and ancestry and (2) the skin pigmentation are shown in Figure 3. The four SNPs, ancestry, and the upper arm pigmentation showed the highest adjusted R^2-values (Table 2 and Figure 3).

Table 2. Multiple loci correlations with skin pigmentation on the upper arm, lower arm, or forehead in 299 Pakistani individuals from three subpopulations (Baloch, Pashtun, and Punjabi).

	Upper Arm		Lower Arm		Forehead	
	Adjusted R^2	Sign.[1]	Adjusted R^2	Sign.[1]	Adjusted R^2	Sign.[1]
Five SNPs [2]	0.33	***	0.24	***	0.24	***
Best model [3]	0.33	***	0.23	***	0.24	***
Best model + ancestry [4]	0.37	***	0.28	***	0.30	***

[1] Statistical significance (Sign.): *** $p < 10^{-6}$. [2] rs1042602, rs10831496, rs12913832, rs1426654, and rs16891982. [3] rs1042602, rs12913832, rs1426654, and rs16891982. [4] Ancestry is the estimated proportion of European and Sub-Saharan African ancestry.

3.7. Correlation of Skin Pigmentation with SNPs from Existing Skin Colour Models

The skin pigmentation in the Pakistani individuals was compared with nine SNPs previously found to be associated with skin pigmentation in a Brazilian population of primarily European ancestry [3]. The nine SNPs included rs10831496, rs12913832, rs1426654, and rs16891982, which were associated with skin pigmentation in the Pakistani population (Table 1), as well as rs1448484 in *OCA2*, rs4424881 in *APBA2*, rs6119471 in *ASIP*, rs1408799 in *TYRP1*, and rs10424065 in *MFSD12*, which were not associated with skin pigmentation in our study. In the Pakistani population, these nine SNPs explained up to 26% of the skin pigmentation (upper arm). The adjusted R^2-values were 0.26 ($p < 0.05$), 0.15 ($p < 0.05$), and 0.19 ($p < 0.05$) for the upper arm, lower arm, and forehead pigmentation, respectively.

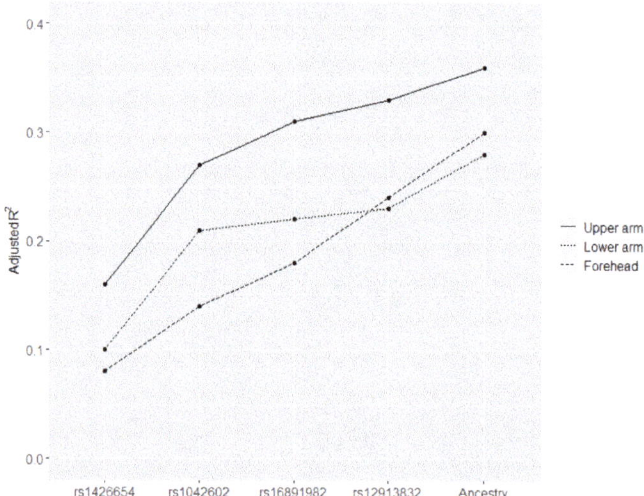

Figure 3. Cumulative correlations between (1) four SNPs and ancestry and (2) upper arm, lower arm, and forehead pigmentation. The SNPs were ranked based on their correlations with skin color (adjusted R^2). Ancestry is the proportion of Sub-Saharan African and European ancestry.

We also correlated the HIrisPlex-S SNPs with the skin pigmentation on the upper arm, lower arm, and forehead using MLR. Four SNPs in the *MC1R*-gene, rs3212355, rs1805006, rs11547464, and rs1110400 were monomorphic and excluded from the analysis. Thus, the correlation was based on 32 of the 36 skin color predictive SNPs in the HIrisPlex-S. The adjusted R^2-values were 0.36 ($p < 10^{-6}$), 0.29 ($p < 10^{-6}$), and 0.27 ($p < 10^{-6}$), for pigmentation on the upper arm, lower arm, and forehead, respectively.

Lastly, we evaluated the performance of the HIrisPlex-S model that is a forensically validated skin color prediction model [18,19]. The predicted skin colors of the 299 Pakistani individuals were: Intermediate: 102, Dark: 167, and Black: 30. No individual was predicted to have very pale or pale skin colors. Comparisons between the predicted skin color categories and the quantitative skin pigmentation measurements are shown in Figure 4.

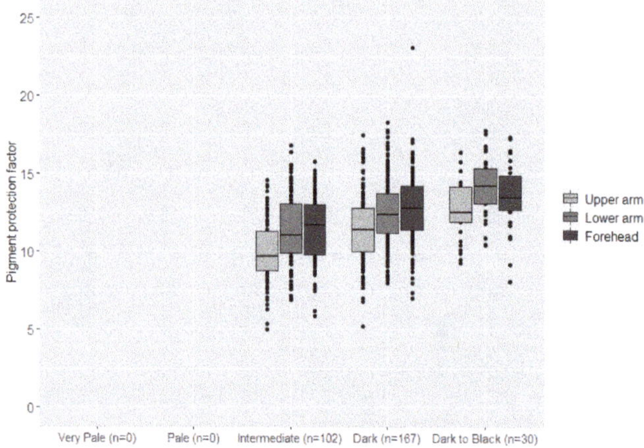

Figure 4. Boxplots showing the skin color category predicted with the HIrisPlex-S prediction model and the pigmentation protection factor on the upper arm, lower arm, and forehead.

4. Discussion

The pairwise genetic distances calculated among the three subpopulations were statistically significantly different (Supplementary Table S3). The Baloch were more distant from Punjabis and Pashtuns than Punjabis were from Pashtuns. The results agreed with our previous results obtained with short tandem repeats that depicted genetic differences between the Baloch and other subpopulations from Pakistan [31]. The STRUCTURE analysis (Figure 2) showed that all three subpopulations from Pakistan were admixed, mainly with South-Central Asian and European genetic contributions. However, the Baloch population also had a genetic contribution from Sub-Saharan African populations, which may be remnants of African individuals settling in the Indian subcontinent [32,33].

The proportion of European and Sub-Saharan African ancestry affected the skin pigmentation, whereas the proportion of South-Central Asian ancestry did not (Supplementary Table S5). However, the proportions of European and Sub-Saharan African ancestry only explained approximately 10% of the variation (Supplementary Table S5) and only influenced the adjusted R^2-values of the MLR model marginally (Table 2). This showed that ancestry was a relatively poor predictor of skin pigmentation in the highly admixed Pakistani populations. It also indicated that any association between a locus and skin pigmentation levels would most likely come from causative SNPs or indels, and not be a consequence of population genetic differences.

Of the 163 variants that were previously shown to be associated with pigmentary traits, five SNPs were statistically significantly correlated with the skin pigmentation levels of the investigated individuals from the Pakistani subpopulations (Table 1). These five SNPs are located in five genes, *TYR, GRM5, SLC24A5, SLC45A2,* and *HERC2.* Four of the five SNPs, rs1042602 in *TYR,* rs1426654 in *SLC24A5,* rs16891982 in *SLC45A2,* and rs12913832 in *HERC2,* explained 33% of the skin pigmentation variation on the upper arm area and 23–24% of the skin pigmentation variation on the lower arm and forehead that are less protected from UV irradiation (Table 2). Three of the SNPs, rs1426654 (ranked 1), rs1042602 (ranked 2), and rs16891982 (ranked 3), were previously found to be associated with skin pigmentation in individuals of South Asian descent [7,34,35]. In agreement with our results, the *SLC24A5* SNP rs1426654 had the most pronounced effect on skin pigmentation levels [7,34,36]. The *HERC2* SNP rs12913832 (ranked 4) has not previously reported to be associated with skin pigmentation in South Asian populations. However, it was reported to be associated with skin color in other populations [11,19]. The fifth SNP, *GRM5* rs10831496 (ranked 5), did not increase the cumulative adjusted R^2-value of the MLR model at any of the measured pigmentation areas. This SNP is highly polymorphic and located in intron 3 of the *GRM5* gene, 340 kbp upstream of the *TYR* gene on chromosome 11. *GRM5* rs10831496 was previously reported to be associated with tanning response after exposure to sunlight [37]. In our study, it was associated with skin pigmentation on the lower arm.

The three highest ranking SNPs, rs1426654, rs1042602, and rs16891982, are non-synonymous variants: Thr111Ala in *SLC24A5,* Ser192Tyr in *TYR,* and Phe374Leu in *SLC45A2,* respectively, and they all influence melanin production. In human primary melanocytes that were homozygous for the *SLC24A5* 111Ala variant, the TYR activity, melanin content, and the number of mature melanosomes were decreased [38]. The 192Tyr *TYR* variant reduced the TYR activity by 40% [39] and the number of primary melanocytes, and human skin tissue samples that were homozygous for the 192Tyr variant had reduced TYR activity and expression [40]. The *SLC45A2* 374Leu variant was found in increased frequency in non-European populations, and 374Leu homozygous melanocytes had higher TYR activity and melanin content than melanocytes that were homozygous for the 374Phe variant [38]. The fourth-ranking SNP, *HERC2* rs12913832, is the most important variant for eye color determination [41–43]. It is positioned in a key enhancer element of the *OCA2* pigmentary gene [44]. Human primary melanocytes that were homozygous for the derived rs12913832 G allele had reduced TYR activity, melanin content, and numbers of mature melanosomes [38]. When we analyzed five additional SNPs that were previously found to be associated with pigmentation in an admixed Brazilian population with primarily European and Sub-Saharan African genetic contributions [3], the correlation with skin pigmentation of the upper arm was reduced from 33% to 26%. This indicates that the biogeographic background of an individual is important for the selection of markers that eventually will give the best prediction of skin color, which is well in line with the knowledge that some genetic markers are associated with skin pigmentation in certain populations and not in others [45]. It also indicates that the estimation of the biogeographic background should be the first step in the estimation of skin pigmentation levels from DNA samples of unknown individuals. The second step should be to investigate causative variants found to be associated with skin pigmentation in the most likely biogeographic background of the collected trace sample and these variants should form the basis for the estimation of skin pigmentation.

In forensics genetic casework, ancestry inference can provide helpful information about an unidentified perpetrator who left a biological trace sample at a crime scene. Several well-established AIM panels that successfully differentiate the major human populations, including Europeans, East Asians, South Central Asians, Native Americans, Sub-Saharan Africans, and Oceanians, have been developed [14,46–49]. Ancestry information may also provide indications on EVCs that are typical for a given population. However, caution must be taken when using ancestry to infer the phenotypes of an individual. An individual of mixed ancestry may have AIM alleles inherited from one parental population, but phenotypic characteristics, e.g., skin color, of the other parental population [3,9]. Thus, skin color and other EVCs should be estimated using causative genetic variants. We identified four likely causative variants that influence skin pigmentation in Pakistanis and are included in the leading skin color prediction model, HIrisPlex-S [18,19]. However, the variants only explained approximately one-third of the skin pigmentation variation and the remaining SNPs of the HIrisPlex-S only slightly increased the adjusted R^2-values underlining the need for additional genetic studies of human skin pigmentation.

Supplementary Materials: The following are available online at https://www.mdpi.com/2073-442 5/12/5/733/s1, Figure S1: PCA plot of the studied populations and selected reference populations, Table S1: Reference data used in the population comparison analysis, Table S2: Allele frequencies of 165 variants typed with the Precision ID Ancestry panel in 299 Pakistani individuals from three subpopulations (Baloch, Pashtun, and Punjabi), Table S3: Pairwise FST-values among the three Pakistani subpopulations Baloch, Pashtun, and Punjabi based on the allele frequencies of 165 AIMs typed with the Precision ID Ancestry panel, Table S4: Allele frequencies of 163 variants typed with the Human Pigmentation (HuPi) AmpliSeq™ Custom panel in 299 Pakistani individuals from three subpopulations (Baloch, Pashtun, and Punjabi), Table S5: Estimated ancestry proportions associated with skin pigmentation on the upper arm, lower arm, or forehead in 299 Pakistani individuals from three subpopulations (Baloch, Pashtun, and Punjabi).

Author Contributions: Conceptualization, C.B., J.D.A., M.A.S., N.M., and O.S.M.; analysis and interpretation, M.A.S., M.R., and O.S.M.; drafting the work, M.A.S. and O.S.M.; critically revising the work for important intellectual content, C.B., J.D.A., M.R., and N.M. All authors have read and agreed to the published version of the manuscript.

Funding: The study was supported by an overseas research grant to Muhammad Adnan Shan from the University of the Punjab, Pakistan (No. D-1829-Est-I/2017).

Institutional Review Board Statement: The study was conducted according to the guidelines of the Declaration of Helsinki and approved by the Review Board/Ethical Committee of the University of the Punjab, Pakistan (D/No. 019/DFEMS). The project was notified to the Ethics Committee for the Capital Region of Denmark (Journal no. H-20024636). According to the Danish Act on Research Ethics Review of Health Research Projects, the work did not require approval by the Ethics Committee.

Informed Consent Statement: Informed consent was obtained from all subjects involved in the study.

Data Availability Statement: The data generated in the present study are included within the manuscript and its supplementary file.

Acknowledgments: The authors would like to thank Nadia Jochumsen for laboratory assistance and Vania Pereira for help with the population genetic analyses. We thank Kenneth Kidd and his staff for providing the genotype SNP data of the reference populations assembled from publicly available data.

Conflicts of Interest: The authors declare no conflict of interest.

References

1. Kayser, M.; Schneider, P.M. DNA-based prediction of human externally visible characteristics in forensics: Motivations, scientific challenges, and ethical considerations. *Forensic Sci. Int. Genet.* **2009**, *3*, 154–161. [CrossRef] [PubMed]

2. Samuel, G.; Prainsack, B. Forensic DNA phenotyping in Europe: Views "on the ground" from those who have a professional stake in the technology. *New Genet. Soc.* **2019**, *38*, 119–141. [CrossRef]

3. Andersen, J.D.; Meyer, O.S.; Simão, F.; Jannuzzi, J.; Carvalho, E.; Andersen, M.M.; Pereira, V.; Børsting, C.; Morling, N.; Gusmão, L. Skin pigmentation and genetic variants in an admixed Brazilian population of primarily European ancestry. *Int. J. Legal Med.* **2020**, *134*, 1569–1579. [CrossRef]

4. Kayser, M.; De Knijff, P. Improving human forensics through advances in genetics, genomics and molecular biology. *Nat. Rev. Genet.* **2011**, *12*, 179–192. [CrossRef] [PubMed]

5. Maroñas, O.; Phillips, C.; Söchtig, J.; Gomez-Tato, A.; Cruz, R.; Alvarez-Dios, J.; de Cal, M.C.; Ruiz, Y.; Fondevila, M.; Carracedo, Á.; et al. Development of a forensic skin colour predictive test. *Forensic Sci. Int. Genet.* **2014**, *13*, 34–44. [CrossRef]

6. Parra, E.J.; Kittles, R.A.; Shriver, M.D. Implications of correlations between skin color and genetic ancestry for biomedical research. *Nat. Genet.* **2004**, *36*, S54–S60. [CrossRef] [PubMed]

7. Stokowski, R.P.; Pant, P.V.K.; Dadd, T.; Fereday, A.; Hinds, D.A.; Jarman, C.; Filsell, W.; Ginger, R.S.; Green, M.R.; Van Der Ouderaa, F.J.; et al. A genomewide association study of skin pigmentation in a South Asian population. *Am. J. Hum. Genet.* **2007**, *81*, 1119–1132. [CrossRef]

8. Shriver, M.D.; Parra, E.J.; Dios, S.; Bonilla, C.; Norton, H.; Jovel, C.; Pfaff, C.; Jones, C.; Massac, A.; Cameron, N.; et al. Skin pigmentation, biogeographical ancestry and admixture mapping. *Hum. Genet.* **2003**, *112*, 387–399. [CrossRef] [PubMed]

9. Valenzuela, R.K.; Henderson, M.S.; Walsh, M.H.; Garrison, N.; Kelch, J.T.; Cohen-Barak, O.; Erickson, D.T.; John Meaney, F.; Bruce Walsh, J.; Cheng, K.C. Predicting phenotype from genotype: Normal pigmentation. *J. Forensic Sci.* **2010**, *55*, 315–322. [CrossRef]

10. Beleza, S.; Johnson, N.A.; Candille, S.I.; Absher, D.M.; Coram, M.A.; Lopes, J.; Campos, J.; Araújo, I.I.; Anderson, T.M.; Vilhjálmsson, B.J.; et al. Genetic Architecture of Skin and Eye Color in an African-European Admixed Population. *PLOS Genet.* **2013**, *9*, e1003372. [CrossRef]

11. Lona-Durazo, F.; Hernandez-Pacheco, N.; Fan, S.; Zhang, T.; Choi, J.; Kovacs, M.A.; Loftus, S.K.; Le, P.; Edwards, M.; Fortes-Lima, C.A.; et al. Meta-analysis of GWA studies provides new insights on the genetic architecture of skin pigmentation in recently admixed populations. *BMC Genet.* **2019**, *20*, 59. [CrossRef]

12. Wright, R.P. *The Ancient Indus: Urbanism, Economy, and Society*; Case Studies in Early Societies; Cambridge University Press: Cambridge, UK, 2010; ISBN 9780521576529.

13. Wynbrandt, J. *A Brief History of Pakistan*; Brief history; Infobase Publishing: New York, NY, USA, 2009; ISBN 9780816061846.

14. Pereira, V.; Mogensen, H.S.; Børsting, C.; Morling, N. Evaluation of the Precision ID Ancestry Panel for crime case work: A SNP typing assay developed for typing of 165 ancestral informative markers. *Forensic Sci. Int. Genet.* **2017**, *28*, 138–145. [CrossRef] [PubMed]

15. Mogensen, H.S.; Tvedebrink, T.; Børsting, C.; Pereira, V.; Morling, N. Ancestry prediction efficiency of the software GenoGeographer using a z-score method and the ancestry informative markers in the Precision ID Ancestry Panel. *Forensic Sci. Int. Genet.* **2020**, *44*, 102154. [CrossRef] [PubMed]

16. Al-Asfi, M.; McNevin, D.; Mehta, B.; Power, D.; Gahan, M.E.; Daniel, R. Assessment of the Precision ID Ancestry panel. *Int. J. Legal Med.* **2018**, *132*, 1581–1594. [CrossRef] [PubMed]

17. Meyer, O.S.; Andersen, J.D.; Børsting, C. Presentation of the Human Pigmentation (HuPi) AmpliSeq™ custom panel. *Forensic Sci. Int. Genet. Suppl. Ser.* **2019**, *7*, 478–479. [CrossRef]

18. Walsh, S.; Chaitanya, L.; Breslin, K.; Muralidharan, C.; Bronikowska, A.; Pospiech, E.; Koller, J.; Kovatsi, L.; Wollstein, A.; Branicki, W.; et al. Global skin colour prediction from DNA. *Hum. Genet.* **2017**, *136*, 847–863. [CrossRef]

19. Chaitanya, L.; Breslin, K.; Zuñiga, S.; Wirken, L.; Pośpiech, E.; Kukla-Bartoszek, M.; Sijen, T.; de Knijff, P.; Liu, F.; Branicki, W.; et al. The HIrisPlex-S system for eye, hair and skin colour prediction from DNA: Introduction and forensic developmental validation. *Forensic Sci. Int. Genet.* **2018**, *35*, 123–135. [CrossRef] [PubMed]

20. Kongshoj, B.; Thorleifsson, A.; Wulf, H.C. Pheomelanin and eumelanin in human skin determined by high-performance liquid chromatography and its relation to in vivo reflectance measurements. *Photodermatol. Photoimmunol. Photomed.* **2006**, *22*, 141–147. [CrossRef] [PubMed]

21. Ravnbak, M.H. Objective determination of Fitzpatrick skin type. *Dan. Med. Bull.* **2010**, *57*, B4153.

22. Farzad, M.S.; Pedersen, B.M.; Mogensen, H.S.; Børsting, C. Development of an automated AmpliSeq™ library building workflow for biological stain samples on the Biomek(®) 3000. *Biotechniques* **2020**, *68*, 342–344. [CrossRef]

23. Barrett, J.C.; Fry, B.; Maller, J.; Daly, M.J. Haploview: Analysis and visualization of LD and haplotype maps. *Bioinformatics* **2005**, *21*, 263–265. [CrossRef]

24. Excoffier, L.; Lischer, H.E.L. Arlequin suite ver 3.5: A new series of programs to perform population genetics analyses under Linux and Windows. *Mol. Ecol. Resour.* **2010**, *10*, 564–567. [CrossRef] [PubMed]

25. Falush, D.; Stephens, M.; Pritchard, J.K. Inference of population structure using multilocus genotype data: Linked loci and correlated allele frequencies. *Genetics* **2003**, *164*, 1567–1587. [CrossRef]

26. Pritchard, J.K.; Stephens, M.; Donnelly, P. Inference of Population Structure Using Multilocus Genotype Data. *Genetics* **2000**, *155*, 945–959. [CrossRef]

27. Jakobsson, M.; Rosenberg, N.A. CLUMPP: A cluster matching and permutation program for dealing with label switching and multimodality in analysis of population structure. *Bioinformatics* **2007**, *23*, 1801–1806. [CrossRef] [PubMed]

28. Rosenberg, N.A. DISTRUCT: A program for the graphical display of population structure. *Mol. Ecol. Notes* **2004**, *4*, 137–138. [CrossRef]

29. Simayijiang, H.; Børsting, C.; Tvedebrink, T.; Morling, N. Analysis of Uyghur and Kazakh populations using the Precision ID Ancestry Panel. *Forensic Sci. Int. Genet.* **2019**, *43*, 102144. [CrossRef] [PubMed]

30. Venables, W.N.; Ripley, B.D. *Modern Applied Statistics with S*; Springer: New York, NY, USA, 2002.

31. Shan, M.A.; Børsting, C.; Morling, N. Forensic application and genetic diversity of 21 autosomal STR loci in five major population groups of Pakistan. *Int. J. Legal Med.* **2021**, *135*, 775–777. [CrossRef]

32. Korn, A.; Nourzaei, M. "Those were the hungry years": A glimpse of Coastal Afro-Balochi. *J. R. Asiat. Soc.* **2018**, *28*, 661–695. [CrossRef]

33. Siddiqi, M.H.; Akhtar, T.; Rakha, A.; Abbas, G.; Ali, A.; Haider, N.; Ali, A.; Hayat, S.; Masooma, S.; Ahmad, J.; et al. Genetic characterization of the Makrani people of Pakistan from mitochondrial DNA control-region data. *Leg. Med.* **2015**, *17*, 134–139. [CrossRef] [PubMed]

34. Mallick, C.B.; Iliescu, F.M.; Möls, M.; Hill, S.; Tamang, R.; Chaubey, G.; Goto, R.; Ho, S.Y.W.; Gallego Romero, I.; Crivellaro, F.; et al. The light skin allele of SLC24A5 in South Asians and Europeans shares identity by descent. *PLoS Genet.* **2013**, *9*, e1003912. [CrossRef]

35. Jonnalagadda, M.; Faizan, M.A.; Ozarkar, S.; Ashma, R.; Kulkarni, S.; Norton, H.L.; Parra, E. A Genome-Wide Association Study of Skin and Iris Pigmentation among Individuals of South Asian Ancestry. *Genome Biol. Evol.* **2019**, *11*, 1066–1076. [CrossRef]

36. Lamason, R.L.; Mohideen, M.-A.P.K.; Mest, J.R.; Wong, A.C.; Norton, H.L.; Aros, M.C.; Jurynec, M.J.; Mao, X.; Humphreville, V.R.; Humbert, J.E.; et al. SLC24A5, a Putative Cation Exchanger, Affects Pigmentation in Zebrafish and Humans. *Science* **2005**, *310*, 1782–1786. [CrossRef]

37. Nan, H.; Kraft, P.; Qureshi, A.A.; Guo, Q.; Chen, C.; Hankinson, S.E.; Hu, F.B.; Thomas, G.; Hoover, R.N.; Chanock, S.; et al. Genome-wide association study of tanning phenotype in a population of European ancestry. *J. Investig. Dermatol.* **2009**, *129*, 2250–2257. [CrossRef] [PubMed]

38. Cook, A.L.; Chen, W.; Thurber, A.E.; Smit, D.J.; Smith, A.G.; Bladen, T.G.; Brown, D.L.; Duffy, D.L.; Pastorino, L.; Bianchi-Scarra, G. Analysis of cultured human melanocytes based on polymorphisms within the SLC45A2/MATP, SLC24A5/NCKX5, and OCA2/P loci. *J. Investig. Dermatol.* **2009**, *129*, 392–405. [CrossRef]

39. Chaki, M.; Sengupta, M.; Mondal, M.; Bhattacharya, A.; Mallick, S. Molecular and functional studies of tyrosinase variants among Indian oculocutaneous albinism type 1 patients. *J. Investig. Dermatol.* **2011**, *131*, 260–262. [CrossRef]

40. Jagirdar, K.; Smit, D.J.; Ainger, S.A.; Lee, K.J.; Brown, D.L.; Chapman, B.; Zhen Zhao, Z.; Montgomery, G.W.; Martin, N.G.; Stow, J.L. Molecular analysis of common polymorphisms within the human Tyrosinase locus and genetic association with pigmentation traits. *Pigment Cell Melanoma Res.* **2014**, *27*, 552–564. [CrossRef] [PubMed]

41. Eiberg, H.; Troelsen, J.; Nielsen, M.; Mikkelsen, A.; Mengel-From, J.; Kjaer, K.W.; Hansen, L. Blue eye color in humans may be caused by a perfectly associated founder mutation in a regulatory element located within the HERC2 gene inhibiting OCA2 expression. *Hum. Genet.* **2008**, *123*, 177–187. [CrossRef] [PubMed]

42. Sturm, R.A.; Duffy, D.L.; Zhao, Z.Z.; Leite, F.P.N.; Stark, M.S.; Hayward, N.K.; Martin, N.G.; Montgomery, G.W. A single SNP in an evolutionary conserved region within intron 86 of the HERC2 gene determines human blue-brown eye color. *Am. J. Hum. Genet.* **2008**, *82*, 424–431. [CrossRef]

43. Liu, F.; van Duijn, K.; Vingerling, J.R.; Hofman, A.; Uitterlinden, A.G.; Janssens, A.C.J.W.; Kayser, M. Eye color and the prediction of complex phenotypes from genotypes. *Curr. Biol.* **2009**, *19*, R192–R193. [CrossRef] [PubMed]

44. Visser, M.; Kayser, M.; Palstra, R.-J. HERC2 rs12913832 modulates human pigmentation by attenuating chromatin-loop formation between a long-range enhancer and the OCA2 promoter. *Genome Res.* **2012**, *22*, 446–455. [CrossRef] [PubMed]

45. Pavan, W.J.; Sturm, R.A. The genetics of human skin and hair pigmentation. *Annu. Rev. Genomics Hum. Genet.* **2019**, *20*, 41–72. [CrossRef]

46. Kosoy, R.; Nassir, R.; Tian, C.; White, P.A.; Butler, L.M.; Silva, G.; Kittles, R.; Alarcon-Riquelme, M.E.; Gregersen, P.K.; Belmont, J.W.; et al. Ancestry informative marker sets for determining continental origin and admixture proportions in common populations in America. *Hum. Mutat.* **2009**, *30*, 69–78. [CrossRef] [PubMed]

47. Kidd, K.K.; Speed, W.C.; Pakstis, A.J.; Furtado, M.R.; Fang, R.; Madbouly, A.; Maiers, M.; Middha, M.; Friedlaender, F.R.; Kidd, J.R. Progress toward an efficient panel of SNPs for ancestry inference. *Forensic Sci. Int. Genet.* **2014**, *10*, 23–32. [CrossRef]

48. Phillips, C.; Parson, W.; Lundsberg, B.; Santos, C.; Freire-Aradas, A.; Torres, M.; Eduardoff, M.; Børsting, C.; Johansen, P.; Fondevila, M.; et al. Building a forensic ancestry panel from the ground up: The EUROFORGEN Global AIM-SNP set. *Forensic Sci. Int. Genet.* **2014**, *11*, 13–25. [CrossRef]
49. Phillips, C.; McNevin, D.; Kidd, K.K.; Lagacé, R.; Wootton, S.; de la Puente, M.; Freire-Aradas, A.; Mosquera-Miguel, A.; Eduardoff, M.; Gross, T.; et al. MAPlex—A massively parallel sequencing ancestry analysis multiplex for Asia-Pacific populations. *Forensic Sci. Int. Genet.* **2019**, *42*, 213–226. [CrossRef] [PubMed]

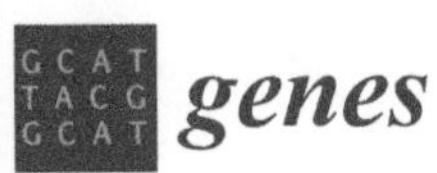

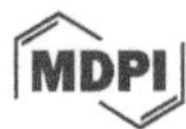

Article

Evaluation of OpenArray™ as a Genotyping Method for Forensic DNA Phenotyping and Human Identification

Michele Ragazzo [1], Giulio Puleri [1], Valeria Errichiello [1], Laura Manzo [1], Laura Luzzi [1], Saverio Potenza [2], Claudia Strafella [1,3], Cristina Peconi [3], Fabio Nicastro [4], Valerio Caputo [1] and Emiliano Giardina [1,3,*]

1 Department of Biomedicine and Prevention, Tor Vergata University of Rome, 00133 Rome, Italy; michele.ragazzo@uniroma2.it (M.R.); giuliopuleri@gmail.com (G.P.); valeria.errichiello@uniroma2.it (V.E.); laura.manzo@uniroma2.it (L.M.); lauraluzzi92@gmail.com (L.L.); claudia.strafella@gmail.com (C.S.); v.caputo91@gmail.com (V.C.)
2 Department of Biomedicine and Prevention, Section of Legal Medicine, Social Security and Forensic Toxicology, University of Rome Tor Vergata, 00133 Rome, Italy; potenza@med.uniroma2.it
3 Genomic Medicine Laboratory UILDM, IRCCS Santa Lucia Foundation, 00179 Rome, Italy; cristinapeconi@gmail.com
4 Austech, 00153 Rome, Italy; f.nicastro@austech-italy.com
* Correspondence: emiliano.giardina@uniroma2.it

Abstract: A custom plate of OpenArray™ technology was evaluated to test 60 single-nucleotide polymorphisms (SNPs) validated for the prediction of eye color, hair color, and skin pigmentation, and for personal identification. The SNPs were selected from already validated subsets (Hirisplex-s, Precision ID Identity SNP Panel, and ForenSeq DNA Signature Prep Kit). The concordance rate and call rate for every SNP were calculated by analyzing 314 sequenced DNA samples. The sensitivity of the assay was assessed by preparing a dilution series of 10.0, 5.0, 1.0, and 0.5 ng. The OpenArray™ platform obtained an average call rate of 96.9% and a concordance rate near 99.8%. Sensitivity testing performed on serial dilutions demonstrated that a sample with 0.5 ng of total input DNA can be correctly typed. The profiles of the 19 SNPs selected for human identification reached a random match probability (RMP) of, on average, 10^{-8}. An analysis of 21 examples of biological evidence from 8 individuals, that generated single short tandem repeat profiles during the routine workflow, demonstrated the applicability of this technology in real cases. Seventeen samples were correctly typed, revealing a call rate higher than 90%. Accordingly, the phenotype prediction revealed the same accuracy described in the corresponding validation data. Despite the reduced discrimination power of this system compared to STR based kits, the OpenArray™ System can be used to exclude suspects and prioritize samples for downstream analyses, providing well-established information about the prediction of eye color, hair color, and skin pigmentation. More studies will be needed for further validation of this technology and to consider the opportunity to implement this custom array with more SNPs to obtain a lower RMP and to include markers for studies of ancestry and lineage.

Keywords: TaqMan SNP genotyping; OpenArray™ system; forensic DNA phenotyping; forensic DNA typing

Citation: Ragazzo, M.; Puleri, G.; Errichiello, V.; Manzo, L.; Luzzi, L.; Potenza, S.; Strafella, C.; Peconi, C.; Nicastro, F.; Caputo, V.; et al. Evaluation of OpenArray™ as a Genotyping Method for Forensic DNA Phenotyping and Human Identification. *Genes* **2021**, *12*, 221. https://doi.org/10.3390/genes12020221

Academic Editor: Niels Morling
Received: 11 December 2020
Accepted: 1 February 2021
Published: 3 February 2021

Publisher's Note: MDPI stays neutral with regard to jurisdictional claims in published maps and institutional affiliations.

1. Introduction

Short tandem repeats (STRs) are genetic variants widely used in forensic investigations for the identification of offenders and in cases concerning relationship testing [1,2]. However, the multiplexing capacity of STRs is relatively low because of the need for capillary electrophoresis and inability to accommodate large numbers of markers. In the genomic era, it is well known that STRs are not the only source of genetic variation in humans [3]. Single-nucleotide polymorphisms (SNPs) are the most common type of genetic variation among people and can provide additional information such as the inferred ancestry of a DNA sample and phenotypes (eye and hair color) [4]. From a technical point of view,

SNPs can be used to support forensic DNA analyses because of an abundance of potential markers, amenability to automation, and potential reduction in required fragment length to only 60–80 bp [5–7].

Forensic analysis usually involves comparisons between genetic profiles extracted from biological samples collected from a crime scene, and objects and suspects which are thought to be associated to that crime. In the absence of suspects, the power of forensic DNA analysis has been enhanced through the development of DNA databases, allowing the identification of unknown offenders and serial offenders by linking different crimes [1,8,9]. However, in criminal cases without an STR profile match, police investigation can be aided by different kinds of genetic tests.

In this context, the analysis of SNPs for the study of phenotypic variability (forensic DNA phenotyping, FDP) and for the determination of biogeographical origin is particularly promising [1,10]. The main advantage of such analysis is to narrow down the number of potential crime scene trace donors to a smaller group of people who most likely have the externally visible characteristics and biogeographic ancestry that were inferred from the crime scene DNA [11].

Forensic DNA phenotyping is explicitly regulated and permitted by law in two EU member states (the Netherlands and Slovakia) and practiced in compliance with existing laws in six more (Poland, Czech Republic, Sweden, Hungary, Austria, and Spain) and the United Kingdom [11].

In the "omic era", different approaches have been developed to test thousands of genetic variations for forensic purposes (phenotype, ancestry, and identification). Real-time PCR using TaqMan chemistry is a well-known technology routinely used in the workflow of forensic laboratories to quantify the DNA extracted from biological samples [12,13]. The OpenArray™ system (Thermo Fisher Scientific, Waltham, MA, USA) applies TaqMan chemistry for the simultaneous and massive study of samples and SNPs [14,15].

Here we report a pilot study aimed at evaluating the applicability of OpenArray™ technology (Thermo Fisher Scientific, Waltham, MA, USA) for the testing of SNPs for human identification and for inferring phenotypes. To this end, we selected the entire panel of 41 SNPs for eye, hair, and skin color prediction from the validated tool HIrisPlex-S and 19 SNPs for individual identification from the Precision ID Identity SNP Panel (Thermo Fisher Scientific, Waltham, MA, USA) and ForenSeq DNA Signature Prep Kit (Verogen Inc, San Diego, CA, USA). A total of 314 samples were typed to test the genotyping accuracy of OpenArray™ through comparison with resequencing data.

The sensitivity of the platform was assessed using four serial dilutions of DNA consisting of 10, 5, 1, and 0.5 ng [16–18].

2. Materials and Methods

2.1. Selection of SNPs

In this work we selected 41 SNPs for eye, hair, and skin color prediction from the HIrisPlex-S system and 19 SNPs from a universal individual identification SNPs panel validated for forensic purposes [16–19]. The SNPs for human identification were selected based on their chromosomal location (each SNP is mapped to a different chromosome to avoid linkage and linkage disequilibrium effects). These genetic variants were included in a customized panel of 60 SNPs able to provide both human identification and phenotyping information in the same analytical session. The TaqMan probe related to rs1805008 could not be developed. Therefore, rs11538871 was chosen because of its complete linkage disequilibrium (LD) with rs1805008 [20].

The selected SNPs are summarized in Table 1.

Table 1. Single-nucleotide polymorphism (SNP) details. FDP: forensic DNA phenotyping; ID: SNPs for forensic identification [16–19].

Reference SNP Number	Assay Name	Call Rate (%)	Concordance Rate (%)	FDP/ID
rs3114908	C__27458355	100%	100%	skin
rs1800414	C___8866240_10	100%	100%	skin
rs10756819	C_____69643_10	97.8%	97.5%	skin
rs2238289	C__26683035_10	97.8%	97.5%	skin
rs17128291	C__34508041_10	100%	100%	skin
rs6497292	C__31479145_10	97.8%	100%	skin
rs1129038	C____489033_10	97.8%	100%	skin
rs1667394	C__26683195_10	97.8%	100%	skin
rs1126809	C_175675702_10	100%	100%	skin
rs1470608	C___8866144_10	97.8%	100%	skin
rs1426654	C___2908190_10	100%	100%	skin
rs6119471	C__30035872_10	100%	100%	skin
rs1545397	C__11751858_10	100%	100%	skin
rs6059655	C_189135912_10	100%	100%	skin
rs12441727	C___1289851_10	97.8%	100%	skin
rs8051733	C__43670381_20	100%	100%	skin
rs3212355	C__32390816_10	100%	100%	hair
rs312262906/rs796296176	C_339644346_10	100%	100%	hair
rs11547464	C__27541634_10	100%	100%	hair
rs885479	C___7519060_20	100%	100%	hair
rs1805008 (rs11538871)	C_175977481_10	100%	100%	hair
rs1805005	C___7519054_10	100%	100%	hair
rs1805006	C___7519055_20	100%	100%	hair
rs1805007	C___2033404_30	97.8%	100%	hair
rs1805009	C___1010501_30	100%	100%	hair
rs201326893	C_190249836_20	100%	100%	hair
rs2228479	C___2033405_20	97.8%	100%	hair
rs1110400	ANKCDY2	97.8%	100%	hair
rs28777	C___2390574_10	100%	100%	hair
rs12821256	C__26988870_10	100%	100%	hair
rs4959270	C__29334795_10	97.8%	100%	hair
rs1042602	C___8362862_10	95.7%	100%	hair
rs2402130	C__27204528_20	100%	100%	hair
rs2378249	C__16003674_10	100%	100%	hair
rs683	C___3119206_10	97.8%	100%	hair
rs16891982	C___2842665_10	100%	100%	eye
rs12203592	C__31918199_10	100%	100%	eye
rs1800407	C___8866200_10	97.8%	97.5%	eye
rs12913832	C__30724404_10	97.8%	100%	eye
rs12896399	C___3244615_10	100%	100%	eye
rs1393350	C___9491300_10	100%	100%	eye
rs10488710	C___2450075_30	97.8%	100%	ID
rs2920816	C__16156638_10	97.8%	100%	ID
rs6955448	C__29220288_10	100%	100%	ID
rs1058083	C___1619935_1_	95.7%	97.4%	ID
rs221956	C____824925_10	100%	100%	ID
rs13182883	C___2556113_10	100%	100%	ID
rs1821380	C__11673733_10	100%	100%	ID
rs6811238	C__11245682_10	100%	100%	ID
rs430046	C___9603287_10	100%	100%	ID
rs576261	C____788229_10	97.8%	100%	ID
rs10092491	C___2049946_10	95.7%	100%	ID
rs560681	C___1006721_1_	100%	100%	ID
rs1736442	C___3285337_1_	91.3%	97.3%	ID
rs4364205	C__26449463_10	95.7%	100%	ID
rs445251	C___2997607_10	100%	100%	ID
rs7041158	C__29060279_10	97.8%	100%	ID
rs13218440	C___9371416_10	100%	100%	ID
rs9786184	C__29554891_10	100%	100%	ID
rs2032652	C___2259382_10	100%	100%	ID

2.2. Ethical Committee Approval

These investigations were carried out following the rules of the Declaration of Helsinki of 1975, revised in 2013. According to Point 23 of this declaration, approval from the ethical committee of Policlinico Tor Vergata (protocol number: Prot. CE/PROG.177/20) was obtained.

2.3. Reference DNA Samples

A total of 314 reference DNA samples were used. In particular, 114 genomic DNA samples were obtained from the 1000 Genomes Project (Coriell Institute for Medical Research, Camden, NJ, USA) and 200 blood samples were obtained from the Laboratory of Genomic Medicine UILDM (Italian Muscular Dystrophy Association) Santa Lucia Foundation [21]. The 114 samples from 1000 Genomes were selected from a small town near Florence in the Tuscany region of Italy. The genotype data of genomic DNA samples from 1000 Genomes were extracted from the Ensembl genome browser [22]. An additional four volunteer donors were used for the sensitivity testing.

2.4. Biological Samples from Real Cases

We analyzed a total of 21 samples of biological evidence that had single STR profiles generated during the routine workflow and that were assigned to their reference perpetrator. This evidence was from different tissues (10 from saliva, 2 from semen, 7 from blood, 2 from urine) and was attributed to 8 different subjects from different tissues [23,24]. All samples were marked with a specific internal code, as shown in Table 2 [2]. The forensic samples were loaded in the same plate twice with the purpose of verifying the reproducibility of genotyping assignation.

Table 2. Details of forensic biological samples. Subject A (SubjA), Subject B (SubjB), Subject C (SubjC), Subject D (SubjD), Subject E (SubjE), Subject F (SubjF), Subject G (SubjG), and Subject H (SubjH).

Sample	Source	Subject	[ng/μL]	Call Rate (%)	Predicted Phenotype	Real Phenotype
20–352	Saliva	SubjA	9.483	97.5	blue eyes; brown hair/dark hair; pale skin	confirmed
20–367	Blood	SubjA	1.263	91.7		
20–368	Blood	SubjB	2.322	93.3	blue eyes; blond hair/light hair; intermediate skin	confirmed
20–369	Blood	SubjC	6.609	97.5	brown eyes; brown hair/dark hair; dark skin	confirmed
20–361	Saliva	SubjD	18.493	95.8	brown eyes; brown hair/dark hair; intermediate skin	confirmed
20–370	Blood	SubjD	2.178	94.2		
20–364	Saliva	SubjE	36.327	96.7	brown eyes; red hair; intermediate skin	confirmed
20–371	Blood	SubjE	1.657	95.0		
20–144	Blood	SubjF	0.078	16.7	blue eyes; blond hair/light hair; intermediate skin	confirmed
20–145	Semen	SubjF	7.022	92.5		
20–146	Urine	SubjF	0.009	4.2		
20–147	Saliva	SubjF	5.534	95.0		
20–148	Blood	SubjG	4.994	96.7	brown eyes; brown hair/light hair; intermediate skin	confirmed
20–149	Semen	SubjG	0.642	52.5		
20–150	Urine	SubjG	0.012	0.8		
20–151	Saliva	SubjG	20.448	99.2		
20–065	Saliva	SubjH	18.562	97.5	brown eyes; brown hair/dark hair; intermediate skin	confirmed
20–069	Saliva	SubjH	19.640	97.5		
20–071	Saliva	SubjH	13.438	98.3		
20–072	Saliva	SubjH	12.512	97.5		
20–074	Saliva	SubjH	10.603	97.5		

2.5. DNA Purification and Quantification

In accordance with the quality standards of forensic laboratories that require the use of automatized instruments, the genomic DNA of 225 samples were extracted using the Maxwell®16 MDx Instrument (Promega, Madison, WI, USA) and the DNA IQ Casework Pro Kit for Maxwell®16 (Promega, Madison, WI, USA).

Each DNA sample was quantified using the Quantifiler®Trio DNA Quantification Kit (Thermo Fisher Scientific, Waltham, MA, USA).

2.6. OpenArray™ Technology

OpenArray™ Technology (Thermo Fisher Scientific, Waltham, MA, USA) is a high-throughput real-time PCR genotyping method that allows for rapid screening of several TaqMan assays in many samples [13]. This real-time method involves the use of an array composed of 3072 through-holes running on the QuantStudio 12K Flex Real Time

PCR System (Thermo Fisher Scientific, Waltham, MA, USA) with an OpenArray™ block. The OpenArray™ system is composed of a specific plate (OpenArray™ plate) enabling 192 samples to be typed in a single run [14].

For each sample, 5 ng (volume of 3 µL) of extracted DNA from the reference samples and 3 µL of 2× TaqMan OpenArray™ Genotyping Master Mix were manually loaded into 384 well-plates according to the manufacturer's instructions (Thermo Fisher Scientific, Waltham, MA, USA). A negative control was obtained by adding 3 µL of pure distilled water to the Master Mix. The QuantStudio 12K Flex OpenArray™ AccuFill System transferred the previously generated mix to the TaqMan OpenArray™ plate. The amplification was performed using the QuantStudio 12K Flex Real Time PCR System (Thermo Fisher Scientific, Waltham, MA, USA) instrument, and the results were analyzed using TaqMan Genotyper Software (Thermo Fisher Scientific, Waltham, MA, USA) [14]. For each SNP, the call rate and concordance rate were calculated as described in Section 2.7 [25].

2.7. Sensitivity

For sensitivity studies, genotyping results from four volunteer donors were assessed from serial dilutions of DNA consisting of 10 ng, 5 ng, 1 ng, and 0.5 ng. These four volunteer donors provided a total of one sample (buccal swab) each.

2.8. Resequencing Analysis

The genotyping accuracy was assessed through comparison with resequencing data. Resequencing data were available from the Ensembl genome browser for the 1000 Genomes Project samples and from an internal database for the Laboratory of Genomic Medicine UILDM Santa Lucia Foundation samples. The PCR sequence reactions were performed with BigDye Terminator v3.1 (Thermo Fisher Scientific, Waltham, MA, USA) and the purification with BigDyeXTerminator (Thermo Fisher Scientific, Waltham, MA, USA) according to the manufacturer's instructions. The samples were run on ABI3130xl (Thermo Fisher Scientific, Waltham, MA, USA) and the obtained sequences were read by Sequencing Analysis software v5.2 (Thermo Fisher Scientific, Waltham, MA, USA) [13].

2.9. Statistical Analysis

At the end of the analytical assay, TaqMan Genotyper Software indicated the percentage of successful genotyping, reported as the call rate. The call rate is defined as the percentage of SNPs that were assigned a genotype call by the software out of the total number of SNPs typed. According to the software's instructions, a successful call rate is more than 90%. The concordance rate is defined as the proportion of SNPs typed by OpenArray™ confirming the resequencing data. This value was determined by comparing the allele calls generated by OpenArray™ technology with the genotypes resulting from resequencing data [25]. Concordance is the percentage of SNPs with identical results using both OpenArray™ and resequencing.

For phenotypic characterization of biological forensic samples ($n = 17$), we constructed a statistical prediction model using HIrisPlex-S webtool systems, available at https://hirisplex.erasmusmc.nl/ (accessed on 20 January 2021). Each phenotype was predicted by applying established algorithms for the color of the eyes, hair, and skin, which returns a p-value (prediction probability) [19]. In terms of eye color, the highest p-value is assigned to the most probable phenotype [19,26]. For the interpretation of hair color, we considered the hair color prediction guide developed by Walsh S. et al. [23,27]. This guide examines categorical hair color probabilities in combination with light/dark hair color shade probabilities as obtained from genotype data [23,27]. For the interpretation of skin color, we used the guide developed by L. Chaitanya et al. [16]. This guide considers the highest p-value in combination with the second highest p-value [16,28]. For example, if in the pale category we obtained a p-value greater than 0.7, this phenotypic characteristic depends on the effect of the second highest category if this p-value is greater than 0.15. In particular, it will appear darker if the second most likely category is intermediate, whereas it will appear lighter if the second most likely category is pale [16].

Prior visual phenotyping was performed by two blind assessments (two independent individuals from our laboratory not involved in this study) to verify the validity of the software prediction.

In order to verify the discrimination power of 17 human identification SNPs (not including rs9786184 and rs2032652 on the Y chromosome), we determined the random match probability (RMP) [29]. The random match probability is the estimated frequency of a genetic profile in the reference population and is calculated using allele frequencies from that population group. Therefore, the RMP is a useful value for evaluating the discriminating power of a DNA profiling system, and it indicates the probability of obtaining a match between two distinct and unrelated individuals [29].

3. Results

3.1. Genotyping of the Control Sample and Concordance

The OpenArray™ System (Thermo Fisher Scientific, Waltham, MA, USA) successfully analyzed 100% of the reference DNA samples. The average call rate and the average concordance rate were 96.9 ± 1.72 and 99.8 ± 0.56, respectively [25]. The call rate was also calculated for each SNP. The average SNP call rate was 98.9% ± 1.67, with values from 91.3–100% (Table 1).

3.2. Sensitivity Study

The results of the sensitivity study are shown in Table 3. A call rate higher than or equal to 90% was obtained for all samples. The results obtained demonstrated that the system is able to correctly type DNA evidence in quantities starting from 0.5 ng.

Table 3. The call rate and concordance rate obtained from the sensitivity study.

Sample	Call Rate (%)	Concordance Rate (%)
SAMPLE_1_10 ng	100	100
SAMPLE_1_5 ng	100	100
SAMPLE_1_1 ng	100	100
SAMPLE_1_0.5 ng	100	100
SAMPLE_2_10 ng	95	100
SAMPLE_2_5 ng	98.3	100
SAMPLE_2_1 ng	96.7	100
SAMPLE_2_0.5 ng	96.7	100
SAMPLE_3_10 ng	96.7	100
SAMPLE_3_5 ng	95	100
SAMPLE_3_1 ng	90	98.21
SAMPLE_3_0.5 ng	91.7	100
SAMPLE_4_10 ng	96.7	100
SAMPLE_4_5 ng	95	100
SAMPLE_4_1 ng	91.7	98.28
SAMPLE_4_0.5 ng	95	100

3.3. Genotyping of Biological Evidence from Real Cases

A total of 21 single biological evidence samples from different tissues (10 from saliva, 2 from semen, 7 from blood, 2 from urine), previously assigned to their reference perpetrator, were analyzed using the OpenArray™ System. This evidence was attributed to eight different subjects [23,24] (Table 2). A total of 17 samples presented call rates higher than 90%, with only 4 samples showing call rates below 90% (Table 2). As expected, these 4 samples were characterized by an extremely low starting concentration (Table 2).

We typed two replicates of each sample to verify the genotype call reliability. We obtained concordant results between the two replicates for all samples.

3.3.1. Predicting Human Appearance from Forensic Samples

Once the correct allelic call was ascertained for all subjects, it was possible to carry out predictive analysis on the HIrisPlex-S System software [19].

The data reported in Supplementary Table S1 describe the outputs (*p*-values) obtained by the HIrisPlex-S System Software for each subject [19].

Table 2 reports the phenotype predictions given by the HIrisPlex-S System software [19].

3.3.2. RMP Calculation

Calculation of the random match probability (RMP) was performed. The calculation considered 17 SNPs located on the autosomal chromosomes. The frequencies relating to the European (EUR), African (AFR), and East Asian (EAS) populations of the 1000 Genomes Project, available on the Ensembl genome browser, were used [22].

Table 4 shows the RMP values obtained for each subject.

Table 4. The random match probability (RMP) values relating to the eight subjects. European (EUR), African (AFR), and East Asian (EAS).

Subject	RMP_{EUR}	RMP_{AFR}	RMP_{EAS}
SubjA	2.67×10^{-8}	1.48×10^{-8}	1.56×10^{-8}
SubjB	5.60×10^{-9}	1.57×10^{-9}	3.51×10^{-9}
SubjC	1.15×10^{-7}	2.49×10^{-8}	4.51×10^{-8}
SubjD	4.24×10^{-7}	1.91×10^{-7}	1.37×10^{-7}
SubjE	2.89×10^{-8}	1.51×10^{-8}	2.81×10^{-8}
SubjF	1.80×10^{-9}	6.07×10^{-10}	3.27×10^{-10}
SubjG	2.23×10^{-7}	8.95×10^{-8}	1.19×10^{-7}
SubjH	4.26×10^{-8}	2.30×10^{-8}	6.44×10^{-8}

These values show that the discriminatory power of the analyzed SNPs is not sufficient to uniquely identify a subject in the world population but can be used to verify genetic compatibility with suspects to be confirmed by traditional STR analysis [30,31].

4. Discussion

To the best of our knowledge this is the first application of the OpenArray™ System in the forensic field. We designed a panel of 60 SNPs for phenotype estimation and personal identification [2]. SNPs for eye, hair, and skin color prediction were directly selected from the HIrisPlex-S system, while SNPs for human identification were selected from already validated subsets (the Precision ID Identity SNP Panel (Thermo Fisher Scientific, Waltham, MA, USA) and ForenSeq DNA Signature Prep Kit (Verogen Inc, San Diego, CA, USA) [16–19]. These SNPs were first tested on 314 reference samples, revealing an average call rate of 96.9% and a concordance rate near 99.8%.

Sensitivity testing performed on serial dilutions demonstrated that samples with 0.5 ng of total input DNA can be correctly typed.

Of 21 biological evidence samples from different tissues (10 from saliva, 2 from semen, 7 from blood, 2 from urine), a total of 17 were correctly typed using OpenArray™, revealing a call rate higher than 90%.

Regarding identification purposes, since most SNPs are biallelic, they are less informative for identity testing than STR analyses [32]. Thus, many more SNPs will be needed to achieve the same level of discrimination afforded by the commonly used STR loci [33]. However, our system is not intended to replace the present STR analysis for human identification. Despite the reduced discrimination power of this system compared to STR based kits, the OpenArray™ System can be used to exclude suspects, to prioritize samples for downstream analyses providing well-established information about the prediction of eye color, hair color, and skin pigmentation.

It should be used primarily as a tool for phenotype prediction, while identification should also be supported by traditional methods. A total of 17 SNPs for human identification were used in this study, yielding a mean RMP of approximately 10^{-8}.

It is important to outline that our work was intended to provide a new tool, based on previously validated SNPs, for phenotype prediction and prioritizing samples for downstream analyses for human identification [16–19,34,35]. The HIrisPlex-S panel and the related software were previously validated elsewhere [16,19]. Thus, our work was aimed at verifying the ability of OpenArray™ to correctly type the selected SNPs.

The main strengths of the OpenArray™ System are the speed of the analysis (less than four hours against the current 24–48 h), the standardized interpretation of the results, the low cost for the analysis of a single sample (about 10 euros, in the region of 20% of the current average) and the opportunity to provide both a first evaluation of biological compatibility and phenotypic information. Moreover, TaqMan chemistry is a well-known technology routinely used in the workflow of forensic laboratories to quantify the DNA extracted from biological samples.

Current weaknesses are that it is necessary to analyze the samples with a second system based on traditional STRs to determine biological compatibility. Furthermore, the OpenArray™ System is not used in the workflow of forensic genetics laboratories, limiting its availability for routine use.

5. Conclusions

To the best of our knowledge, this study represents the first application of the OpenArray™ System as a genotyping tool in forensic genetics. In particular, the results obtained suggest that the OpenArray™ System is robust and reliable and is suitable for use in forensic genotyping. Herein, we developed a panel for phenotypic prediction and human identification. Although the 19 SNPs used provide useful information for personal identification, a greater number of SNPs is required for the reliable identification of a subject.

The quality of the results obtained from biological evidence also promotes the application of this system in forensic laboratories to assist investigators in resolving cases.

Finally: these data suggest the applicability of this system as a genotyping method in the forensic field. In particular, it could be suitable as a first line method to verify the presence of genetic compatibility between evidence and suspects and to achieve rapid investigative information also providing well-founded predictions of eye color, hair color, and skin pigmentation. More studies will be needed for further validation of this technology and to consider opportunities to implement this custom array with more SNPs to lower the RMP and to include markers for studies of ancestry and lineage.

Supplementary Materials: The following are available online at https://www.mdpi.com/2073-4425/12/2/221/s1. Table S1. The output obtained by the HIrisPlex-S System Software for Subject A (SubjA), Subject B (SubjB), Subject C (SubjC), Subject D (SubjD), Subject E (SubjE), Subject F (SubjF), Subject G (SubjG), and Subject H (SubjH).

Author Contributions: Conceptualization, M.R. and E.G.; writing—original draft preparation, M.R., and E.G.; software and formal analysis, G.P., V.E., L.M., L.L., S.P., C.S., C.P., F.N. and V.C.; methodology and validation, G.P., V.E., L.M. and V.C.; data curation, M.R., G.P., V.E., L.M., and V.C.; supervision and project administration, E.G. All authors contributed to the revision of the manuscript and approved the final version. All authors have read and agreed to the published version of the manuscript.

Funding: This research received no external funding.

Institutional Review Board Statement: The study was conducted according to the guidelines of the Declaration of Helsinki and approved by the Ethics Committee of Policlinico Tor Vergata (protocol number: Prot. CE/PROG.177/20).

Informed Consent Statement: Informed consent was obtained from all subjects involved in the study.

Data Availability Statement: The data generated in the present study are included within the manuscript and its supplementary file.

Conflicts of Interest: The authors declare no conflict of interest.

References

1. Kayser, M. Forensic DNA Phenotyping: Predicting human appearance from crime scene material for investigative purposes. *Forensic Sci. Int. Genet.* **2015**, *18*, 33–48. [CrossRef] [PubMed]
2. Ragazzo, M.; Carboni, S.; Caputo, V.; Buttini, C.; Manzo, L.; Errichiello, V.; Puleri, G.; Giardina, E. Interpreting Mixture Profiles: Comparison between Precision ID GlobalFiler™ NGS STR Panel v2 and Traditional Methods. *Genes* **2020**, *11*, 591. [CrossRef] [PubMed]
3. Cascella, R.; Strafella, C.; Caputo, V.; Errichiello, V.; Zampatti, S.; Milano, F.; Potenza, S.; Mauriello, S.; Novelli, G.; Ricci, F.; et al. Towards the application of precision medicine in Age-Related Macular Degeneration. *Prog. Retin. Eye Res.* **2018**, *63*, 132–146. [CrossRef] [PubMed]
4. Giardina, E.; Spinella, A.; Novelli, G. Past, present and future of forensic DNA typing. *Nanomedicine* **2011**, *6*, 257–270. [CrossRef] [PubMed]
5. Giardina, E.; Pietrangeli, I.; Martone, C.; Zampatti, S.; Marsala, P.; Gabriele, L.; Ricci, O.; Solla, G.; Asili, P.; Arcudi, G.; et al. Whole genome amplification and real-time PCR in forensic casework. *BMC Genom.* **2009**, *10*, 159. [CrossRef]
6. Oldoni, F.; Podini, D. Forensic molecular biomarkers for mixture analysis. *Forensic Sci. Int. Genet.* **2019**, *41*, 107–119. [CrossRef]
7. Schwark, T.; Meyer, P.; Harder, M.; Modrow, J.-H.; von Wurmb-Schwark, N. The SNPforID Assay as a Supplementary Method in Kinship and Trace Analysis. *Transfus. Med. Hemother.* **2012**, *39*, 187–193. [CrossRef]
8. Machado, H.; Granja, R. DNA Databases and Big Data. In *Forensic Genetics in the Governance of Crime*; Palgrave Pivot: Singapore, 2020; pp. 57–70. [CrossRef]
9. Amankwaa, A.O. Trends in forensic DNA database: Transnational exchange of DNA data. *Forensic Sci. Res.* **2019**, *5*, 8–14. [CrossRef]
10. Butler, J.M.; Willis, S. Interpol review of forensic biology and forensic DNA typing 2016–2019. *Forensic Sci. Int. Synerg.* **2020**, *2*, 352–367. [CrossRef]
11. Schneider, P.M.; Prainsack, B.; Kayser, M. The Use of Forensic DNA Phenotyping in Predicting Appearance and Biogeographic Ancestry. *Dtsch. Arztebl. Int.* **2019**, *51–52*, 873–880. [CrossRef]
12. Butler, J.M. DNA Quantitation. In *Advanced Topics in Forensic DNA Typing: Methodology*; Butler, J.M., Ed.; Academic Press: Cambridge, MA, USA, 2012; pp. 49–67. [CrossRef]
13. Cascella, R.; Strafella, C.; Ragazzo, M.; Manzo, L.; Costanza, G.; Bowes, J.; Hüffmeier, U.; Potenza, S.; Sangiuolo, F.; Reis, A.; et al. *KIF3A* and *IL-4* are disease-specific biomarkers for psoriatic arthritis susceptibility. *Oncotarget* **2017**, *8*, 95401–95411. [CrossRef] [PubMed]
14. Broccanello, C.; Gerace, L.; Stevanato, P. QuantStudio™ 12K Flex OpenArray®System as a Tool for High-Throughput Genotyping and Gene Expression Analysis. In *Quantitative Real-Time PCR Methods in Molecular Biology*; Biassoni, R., Raso, A., Eds.; Humana: New York, NY, USA, 2020; Volume 2065, pp. 199–208. [CrossRef]
15. Pomeroy, R.; Duncan, G.; Sunar-Reeder, B.; Ortenberg, E.; Ketchum, M.; Wasiluk, H.; Reeder, D. A low-cost, high-throughput, automated single nucleotide polymorphism assay for forensic human DNA applications. *Anal. Biochem.* **2009**, *395*, 61–67. [CrossRef] [PubMed]
16. Chaitanya, L.; Breslin, K.; Zuñiga, S.; Wirken, L.; Pośpiech, E.; Kukla-Bartoszek, M.; Sijen, T.; Knijff, P.; Liu, F.; Branicki, W.; et al. The HIrisPlex-S system for eye, hair and skin colour prediction from DNA: Introduction and forensic developmental validation. *Forensic Sci. Int. Genet.* **2018**, *35*, 123–135. [CrossRef] [PubMed]
17. Pakstis, A.J.; Speed, W.C.; Fang, R.; Hyland, F.C.; Furtado, M.R.; Kidd, J.R.; Kidd, K.K. SNPs for a universal individual identification panel. *Hum. Genet.* **2010**, *127*, 315–324. [CrossRef]
18. Ochiai, E.; Minaguchi, K.; Nambiar, P.; Kakimoto, Y.; Satoh, F.; Nakatome, M.; Miyashita, K.; Osawa, M. Evaluation of Y chromosomal SNP haplogrouping in the HID-Ion AmpliSeq™ Identity Panel. *Leg. Med.* **2016**, *22*, 58–61. [CrossRef]
19. HIrisPlex-S Eye. Hair and Skin Colour DNA Phenotyping Webtool. Available online: https://hirisplex.erasmusmc.nl/ (accessed on 28 September 2020).
20. rs1805008 SNP. Available online: http://www.ensembl.org/Homo_sapiens/Variation/HighLD?db=core;r=16:89919236-89920236;v=rs1805008;vdb=variation;vf=22711199#373537_tablePanel (accessed on 30 November 2020).
21. 1000 Genomes Project Consortium; Abecasis, G.R.; Altshuler, D.; Auton, A.; Brooks, L.D.; Durbin, R.M.; Gibbs, R.A.; Hurles, M.E.; McVean, G.A. A map of human genome variation from population-scale sequencing. *Nature* **2010**, *467*, 1061–1073. [CrossRef]
22. Yates, A.D.; Achuthan, P.; Akanni, W.; Allen, J.; Allen, J.; Alvarez-Jarreta, J.; Amode, M.R.; Armean, I.M.; Azov, A.G.; Bennett, R.; et al. Ensembl 2020. *Nucleic Acids Res.* **2020**, *48*, D682–D688. [CrossRef]
23. Walsh, S.; Chaitanya, L.; Clarisse, L.; Wirken, L.; Draus-Barini, J.; Kovatsi, L.; Maeda, H.; Ishikawa, T.; Sijen, T.; de Knijff, P.; et al. Developmental validation of the HIrisPlex system: DNA-based eye and hair colour prediction for forensic and anthropological usage. *Forensic Sci. Int. Genet.* **2014**, *9*, 150–161. [CrossRef]

24. Cascella, R.; Stocchiy, L.; Strafella, C.; Mezzaroma, I.; Mannazzu, M.; Vullo, V.; Montella, F.; Parruti, G.; Borgiani, P.; Sangiuolo, F.C.; et al. Comparative analysis between saliva and buccal swabs as source of DNA: Lesson from *HLA-B*57:01* testing. *Pharmacogenomics* **2015**, *16*, 1039–1046. [CrossRef]

25. Ragazzo, M.; Melchiorri, S.; Manzo, L.; Errichiello, V.; Puleri, G.; Nicastro, F.; Giardina, E. Comparative Analysis of ANDE 6C Rapid DNA Analysis System and Traditional Methods. *Genes* **2020**, *11*, 582. [CrossRef]

26. Walsh, S.; Liu, F.; Ballantyne, K.N.; van Oven, M.; Lao, O.; Kayser, M. IrisPlex: A sensitive DNA tool for accurate prediction of blue and brown eye colour in the absence of ancestry information. *Forensic Sci. Int. Genet.* **2011**, *5*, 170–180. [CrossRef] [PubMed]

27. Walsh, S.; Liu, F.; Wollstein, A.; Kovatsi, L.; Ralf, A.; Kosiniak-Kamysz, A.; Branicki, W.; Kayser, M. The HIrisPlex system for simultaneous prediction of hair and eye colour from DNA. *Forensic Sci. Int. Genet.* **2013**, *7*, 98–115. [CrossRef] [PubMed]

28. Walsh, S.; Chaitanya, L.; Breslin, K.; Muralidharan, C.; Bronikowska, A.; Pospiech, E.; Koller, J.; Kovatsi, L.; Wollstein, A.; Branicki, W.; et al. Global skin colour prediction from DNA. *Hum. Genet.* **2017**, *136*, 847–863. [CrossRef] [PubMed]

29. Butler, J.M. Statistical Interpretation Overview. In *Advanced Topics in Forensic DNA Typing: Interpretation*; Butler, J.M., Ed.; Academic Press: Cambridge, MA, USA, 2014; pp. 213–237. [CrossRef]

30. Sanchez, J.J.; Phillips, C.; Børsting, C.; Balogh, K.; Bogus, M.; Fondevila, M.; Harrison, C.D.; Musgrave-Brown, E.; Salas, A.; Syndercombe-Court, D.; et al. A multiplex assay with 52 single nucleotide polymorphisms for human identification. *Electrophoresis* **2006**, *27*, 1713–1724. [CrossRef]

31. Kidd, K.K.; Soundararajan, U.; Rajeevan, H.; Pakstis, A.J.; Moore, K.N.; Ropero-Miller, J.D. The redesigned Forensic Research/Reference on Genetics-knowledge base, FROG-kb. *Forensic Sci. Int. Genet.* **2018**, *33*, 33–37. [CrossRef] [PubMed]

32. Yang, J.; Lin, D.; Deng, C.; Li, Z.; Pu, Y.; Yu, Y.; Li, K.; Li, D.; Chen, P.; Chen, F. The advances in DNA mixture interpretation. *Forensic Sci. Int.* **2019**, *301*, 101–106. [CrossRef]

33. King, J.L.; Churchill, J.D.; Novroski, N.M.M.; Zeng, X.; Warshauer, D.H.; Seah, L.H.; Budowle, B. Increasing the discrimination power of ancestry- and identity-informative SNP loci within the ForenSeq™ DNA Signature Prep Kit. *Forensic Sci. Int. Genet.* **2018**, *36*, 60–76. [CrossRef]

34. Palencia-Madrid, L.; Xavier, C.; de la Puente, M.; Hohoff, C.; Phillips, C.; Kayser, M.; Parson, W. Evaluation of the VISAGE Basic Tool for Appearance and Ancestry Prediction Using PowerSeq Chemistry on the MiSeq FGx System. *Genes* **2020**, *11*, 708. [CrossRef]

35. Breslin, K.; Wills, B.; Ralf, A.; Ventayol Garcia, M.; Kukla-Bartoszek, M.; Pospiech, E.; Freire-Aradas, A.; Xavier, C.; Ingold, S.; de La Puente, M.; et al. HIrisPlex-S system for eye, hair, and skin color prediction from DNA: Massively parallel sequencing solutions for two common forensically used platforms. *Forensic Sci. Int. Genet.* **2019**, *43*, 102152. [CrossRef]

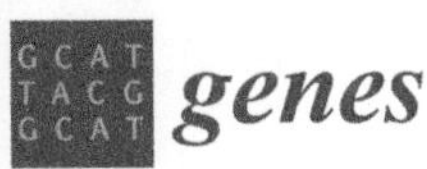

Article

Efficient DNA Sampling in Burglary Investigations

Colin Charles Tièche [1], Markus Dubach [2] and Martin Zieger [1,*]

1   Forensic Molecular Biology Department, Institute of Forensic Medicine, University of Bern, Murtenstrasse 26, 3008 Bern, Switzerland; colin.tieche@irm.unibe.ch

2   Bern Cantonal Police, Nordring 30, 3001 Bern, Switzerland; pmad@police.be.ch

*   Correspondence: martin.zieger@irm.unibe.ch; Tel.: +41-31-684-01-89

Abstract: In terms of crime scene investigations by means of forensic DNA-analyses, burglaries are the number one mass crime in Switzerland. Around one third of the DNA trace profiles registered in the Swiss DNA database are related to burglaries. However, during the collection of potential DNA traces within someone's residence after a burglary, it is not known whether the sampled DNA originated from the perpetrator or from an inhabitant of said home. Because of the high incidence of burglaries, crime scene investigators usually do not collect reference samples from all the residents for economical and administrative reasons. Therefore, the presumably high probability that a DNA profile belonging to a person authorized to be at the crime scene ends up being sent to a DNA database for comparison, has to be taken into account. To our knowledge, no investigation has been made to evaluate the percentage of these non-perpetrator profiles straying into DNA databases. To shed light on this question, we collected reference samples from residents who had been victims of recent burglaries in their private homes. By comparing the profiles established from these reference samples with the profiles generated from trace DNA, we can show that the majority of the DNA samples collected in burglary investigations belong to the residents. Despite the limited number of cases included in the study, presumably due to a crime decline caused by the pandemic, we further show that trace DNA collection in the vicinity of the break and entry area, in particular window and door glasses, is most promising for sampling perpetrator instead of inhabitant DNA.

Keywords: burglary; CODIS; touch DNA; forensic genetics; crime scene; authorized; sampling

Citation: Tièche, C.C.; Dubach, M.; Zieger, M. Efficient DNA Sampling in Burglary Investigations. *Genes* **2022**, *13*, 26. https://doi.org/10.3390/genes13010026

Academic Editor: Niels Morling

Received: 14 December 2021
Accepted: 21 December 2021
Published: 23 December 2021

1. Introduction

Burglaries, usually coming along as a mixture of property damage, trespassing, and theft, are a severe type of property crime, the impact being increased by the feeling of insecurity left among the victims. In Switzerland and probably many other countries, burglaries constitute the number one volume crime investigated by means of forensic genetics. On one hand, it is a frequent type of property crime with 24,010 registered cases in Switzerland in 2020 (about 9% of all registered offences against property) [1] and on the other hand, burglaries are particularly suited for the sampling of DNA traces, compared to other volume crimes such as fraud. In the department for Forensic Molecular Biology of the Institute of Forensic Medicine, in which the present study was conducted, "touch" DNA traces from burglaries and burglary attempts make up for more than 50% of the overall number of traces analyzed.

Given the time spent within a household, one can expect that the majority of the DNA traces left on site actually originated from the respective inhabitants. However, despite the large number of cases, we rarely obtain reference samples from inhabitants to avoid having their profiles established from DNA traces sampled at the crime scene sent to the Swiss DNA database for comparison via CODIS. Assuming an average of 2–3 persons per household or even more for workspaces, when taking burglaries in business environments into account, routine sampling of reference swabs from all residents would cause enormous financial and administrative costs.

However, ignoring the fact that a large number of resident profiles end up registered in CODIS as traces profiles creates a couple of problems: (a) The police run the risk of spoiling investigations through the presentation of inadmissible evidence. The following real case might serve as an example to illustrate this particular problem: Two persons, a man and a woman living together, were assaulted by three men. From the jacket of the woman, a DNA mixture containing a female and a male component was recovered and sent to CODIS. The female component belonged to the female victim, as inferred by crosschecking all samples in the same case. The male component, however, resulted in profile matches with DNA traces from two burglaries. The police therefore started investigations against the male victim of the assault. The Bern Cantonal High Court, however, prohibited all the evidence gathered in this case from being used, since the investigation was launched based on inadmissible evidence given by two random and case unrelated DNA matches that could have been avoided by taking reference samples [2]. The verdict prevented the assailants from being brought to justice and the affaire became a cold case. (b) A lack of prior exclusion might prevent crime victims from contacting the police. The risk of being associated with a past crime or a juvenile sin, e.g., illegal graffiti spraying, might discourage people from contacting the police, once they have become victims themselves. In Switzerland, trace DNA sampling is legitimate in cases of property damage having caused more than 10,000 CHF of pecuniary damage, a sum that is easily reached through graffiti spraying. We can imagine a 16-year-old graffiti sprayer, who becomes a victim in a more serious crime and who refrains from contacting the police, because he fears that through incidental DNA matches, his past or present spraying activities might be revealed to the police. (c) The database becomes inflated. DNA trace profiles caused by residents will normally not generate hits in forensic databases, at least not with profiles of convicted individuals. Therefore, the traces will remain in the database for years and create candidate matches with newly added suspect profiles or trace profiles from other cases. DNA mixture profiles frequently lead to candidate matches that have to be verified by the submitting lab. The lab than decides whether the "candidate match" is considered as a true match ("HIT"), or not. For mixture profiles, most of the verifications result in "NO HIT" verdicts. The control of those candidate matches is time consuming and constitutes a possible source of error, justifying a cleanup of the database from profiles from crime-authorized people.

From controlled studies on DNA transfer and persistence [3–6], we expect a high number of the DNA trace profiles generated in burglary investigations to be from the inhabitants. However, no figures are available on how many of the profiles in real case scenarios stem from residents. To get an impression of those figures, we focused on burglaries in private households, because access is more restricted than in stores or other business environments. We collected the reference samples from the inhabitants and compared them to the DNA profiles generated from the crime scene traces before sending them for comparison into the Swiss DNA database.

2. Materials and Methods

2.1. Sampling

Sampling for crime scene traces in burglaries was performed by the Bern Cantonal Police in accordance with their usual practice. The police officers individually decided ad hoc at the scene where DNA from the offender could be expected and took samples accordingly. Reference samples from residents of private households were collected between November 2020 and April 2021. Residents present during the crime scene investigation were asked for reference samples. Consenting residents were handed out a written agreement form with explanations concerning the procedure, the modalities for the usage of their DNA profiles and information on why prior exclusion of their profiles would be in their favor. The police officer further registered the number of persons living in the household and whether there had been any visitors at the house within the last 7 days prior to the burglary. For all inhabitants not present at the apartment or house during the crime scene sampling, the police officer left a set of documents, buccal swabs, and a prepaid reply envelope on-site, so the absent inhabitants could send their reference swabs directly to the DNA laboratory by mail. All samples were given a pseudonymized family role (such as "father" or "man") under which they were subsequently processed in the DNA laboratory. Buccal swabs were collected with Sarstedt Forensic Swab L. (Sarstedt AG, Nümbrecht, Germany), crime scene traces were collected using the forensiX Cardboard Evidence Collection Kit (Art. Nr. 9021040; Prionics, Schlieren, Switzerland). One or two partially moistened swabs were used for the sampling of one trace.

2.2. Analysis

DNA from buccal swabs was extracted by Chelex 100 (Bio-Rad Laboratories, Hercules, CA, USA). Samples were placed in 1500 µL of 20% Chelex 100, put for two times 30 s at 5900 rpm on a Precellys®24 homogenizer (Bertin instruments, Montigny-le-Bretonneux, France), incubated at 100 °C for 10 min and subsequently centrifuged at 13,000 rpm on an Eppendorf Minispin centrifuge (Eppendorf, Hamburg, Germany). DNA extracted from buccal swabs was quantified using a Qubit fluorometer (Thermo Fisher, Waltham, MA, USA). DNA profiles were established in 12.5 µL reaction volume by multiplex-PCR using the AmpFlSTR® NGM Select Express™ (Thermo Fisher, Waltham, MA, USA) and PowerPlex® ESI17 Fast kits (Promega, Madison, WI, USA). DNA from trace samples was extracted with the AutoMateExpress™ device and the PrepFiler Express™ Kit (both Thermo Fisher, Waltham, MA, USA), with an elution volume of 50 µL, representing our standard lab procedure for swabs from touched surfaces [7]. DNA was quantified by Real-Time-PCR (qPCR) using the Quantifiler® HP Kit from Thermo Fisher on a 7500 RT PCR System (Thermo Fisher, Waltham, MA, USA). DNA profiles were established by multiplex-PCR using the AmpFlSTR® NGM Select™ and NGMDetect™ Kits (Thermo Fisher, Waltham, MA, USA) in a total reaction volume of 25 µL (at least two independent amplifications). A maximum of 0.5 ng DNA was amplified per reaction, using the maximum sample volume of 10 µL for samples with DNA-concentrations below 50 pg/µL. In line with our standard operating procedures for casework, all samples with a DNA concentration below 20 pg/µL were amplified with 32 instead of 30 PCR cycles. Capillary electrophoresis was run either on a 3130 xl or on a 3500 xl genetic analyzer (Thermo Fisher, Waltham, MA, USA). Signal interpretation was performed with Genemapper ID-X, v1.4 (Thermo Fisher, Waltham, MA, USA). All peaks above 50 rfu (3130 xl) and 100 rfu (3500 xl) were considered as true alleles.

2.3. Criteria for a Submission to Swiss CODIS Database

The Swiss DNA database uses the CODIS (combined DNA index system) software v7.0. Switzerland has defined by law the 16 loci included in the AmpFlSTR® NGMSelect/NGMDetect and PowerPlex® ESI17/ESX17 kits as database core loci [8]. More or less all offences leading to ordinary criminal proceedings are recordable, except misdemeanors penalized with a fine. Familial searches are permitted for all offences penalized with a prison sentence of more than three years and can be ordered by the public prosecutor. If reference samples are collected, the generated profiles are used only for the exclusion of people with lawful right of access to the scene. Reference profiles are not registered in CODIS. Profile exclusion is performed locally in the laboratory, before sending the trace profile to CODIS. The entry criteria for a regular database search in Switzerland are a minimum of 6 loci for single or major component profiles and 8 loci for two person mixtures. The sex locus Amelogenin can be entered, but is not searched for in CODIS. Apparent major components are selected, if no two-person mixture can be clearly distinguished. A submission was considered when the lab internal quality conditions were met, i.e., a minimum ratio of 3:1 for major to minor component and heterozygote peak balance of at least 60%. Profiles that did not fulfill our lab or the search criteria for CODIS, although they could possibly still be interpreted, e.g., by probabilistic genotyping [9,10], were not investigated any further. It is important to note that our study targets the investigative phase of burglary investigations and not the evaluative phase [11].

3. Results

3.1. Samples Obtained

We had a bad timing for our study, since we registered in the relevant timeframe between November 2020 and April 2021 an unusual low number of burglaries in private households. This was presumably due to the COVID-19 pandemic. As part of the measures taken in the fight against the pandemic, e.g., restrictions in cross-border traffic or the obligation of working in the home office, people spent more time at home. In 2020, we temporarily observed a workload drop of about 80%. From November to April, our lab registered 226 burglaries in private housings; attempts and sneak-in thefts not included. In 55 of those cases, so approximately one-quarter, we obtained the reference samples from the inhabitants. We analyzed 144 trace samples in total, what corresponds to 2.6 traces per burglary. We obtained a total of 118 references samples (50 women, 47 men, and 21 children), so in average about 2.14 reference samples per case, corresponding well with the average household size in Switzerland of 2.2 persons [12].

3.2. Sample Categories

Samples were classified into three categories: (a) furniture, e.g., handles from cupboards, pieces of furniture that had been moved by the offenders; (b) portable items, e.g., keys or jewelry; and (c) samples taken around the entry of the offender, e.g., door or window. The majority, about 65%, of the samples were taken in the vicinity of the entry (Figure 1a). The samples around the entry were further divided into subcategories (Figure 1b). Half of them (n = 46) were collected from window glass or glass fragments.

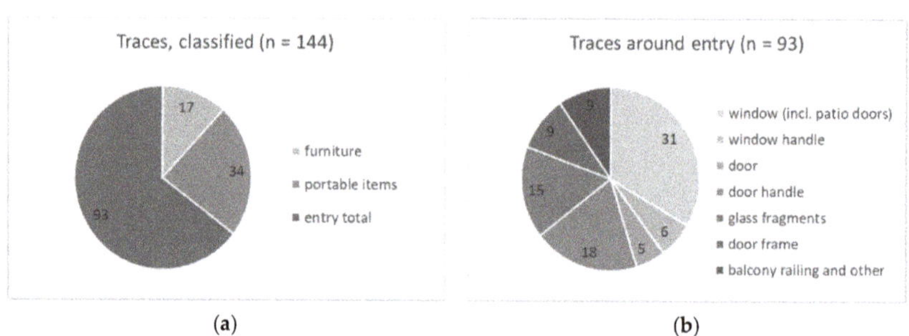

(a) (b)

Figure 1. (**a**) All samples classified in three categories; (**b**) samples from entry divided in several sub-classes.

3.3. Typing Success

We were able to establish DNA profiles suitable for submission to CODIS from 48 traces, what corresponds to an overall success rate of 33% (Figure 2).

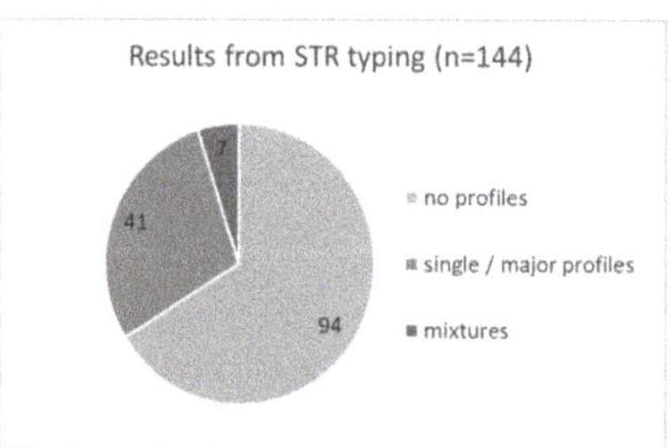

Figure 2. The STR typing results for all 144 crime scene samples summarized. The category "no profiles" includes all profiles not fulfilling the CODIS entry criteria.

Figure 3 shows the distribution of the total amount of DNA extracted from each sample of all 144 samples (Figure 3a) and of the 48 samples that resulted in CODIS-suitable profiles (Figure 3b). We were able to establish DNA profiles for database entry for all traces with a total DNA amount of more than 1 ng. Around 85% of the traces with less than 0.5 ng total DNA did not result in CODIS-suitable profiles.

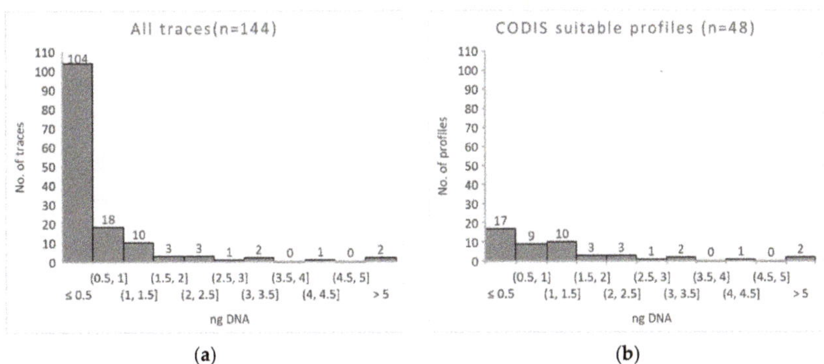

Figure 3. Histograms of the distributions of DNA amounts in ng obtained from: (**a**) all samples and (**b**) samples for which we were able to establish CODIS-suitable DNA profiles.

The DNA typing success rate of samples taken from furniture and portable items reaches 70% and 50%, respectively, whereas only about 30% of traces taken around the entry resulted in CODIS-suitable profiles (Figure 4).

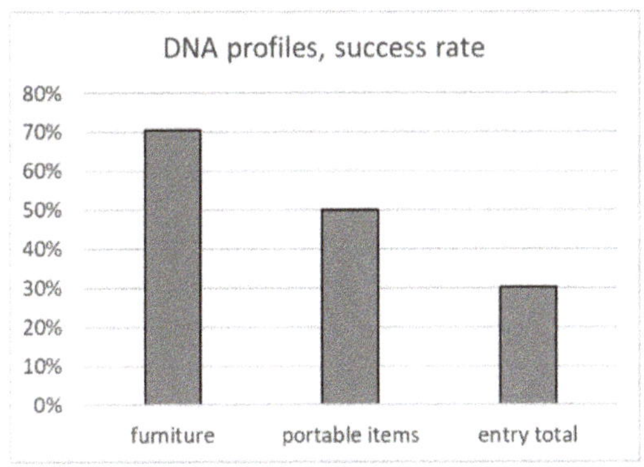

Figure 4. Fraction of samples of the respective class that resulted in CODIS-suitable DNA profiles.

3.4. Comparison with Reference Samples

The 48 CODIS-suitable profiles include interpretable components from 57 DNA contributors. We obtained 41 single or major component profiles and 7 two-person mixtures. Two of the major component profiles showed a reproducible (at least three PCR amplifications conducted) minor component with more than five but less than eight alleles. Therefore, those three minor components are not suitable for CODIS as a mixture, but would be sufficient according to the Swiss CODIS criteria for interpretation, the reason why we included them in our interpretation. Of those 57 trace donors, 17 were detected on portable items, 12 on furniture and 28 on samples around the entry, half of which were from windows glass (Figure 5a). Of those 57 trace contributors, 43 (75%) were identified as crime scene authorized persons, i.e., inhabitants.

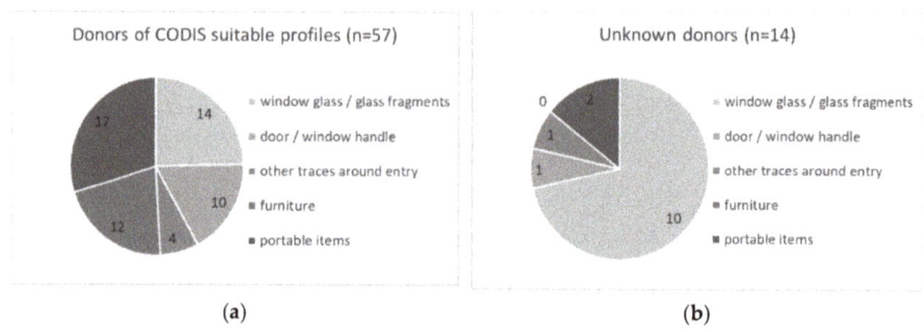

(a) (b)

Figure 5. (**a**) Donors of the 48 CODIS-suitable profiles, according to trace class. (**b**) Unknown donors according to trace class. There were 0 unknown donors on furniture.

If we have a closer look on the different sample categories, we can see that traces from window glass clearly outperform the rest of the samples (Figure 5b). Whereas 71% of the interpretable traces detected on window glass and glass fragments are from unknown contributors, and therefore from possible suspects, less than 10% of the contributors from all other traces were from unknown individuals. The ratio of unknown vs. known contributors is depicted in Figure 6.

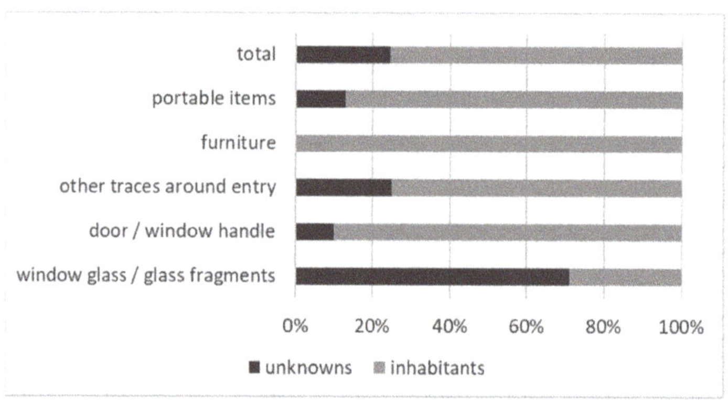

Figure 6. Ratios between unknown contributors and inhabitants detected on the different types of traces.

4. Discussion

The 33% success rate for DNA typing of contact ("touch") traces in burglaries are in line with the approximate 25% overall typing efficiency we have observed in our lab in recent years. It also corresponds with the success rate from casework published by another Swiss laboratory, therefore operating within the same national and regulatory framework [13]. Their average success rate for "touch" DNA traces of 26% is slightly lower than the one for the samples from our study, but we have to take into account the higher sensitivity of the multiplex kits nowadays, since the study from 2008 used AmpFlSTR® SGM Plus™ and we used the more sensitive NGMSElect™ and NGMDetect™ kits.

Around 70% of the profiles established from window glass and glass fragments were from unknown individuals. A low level of background DNA on windows has been reported in a previous study, which suggests windows as premium choice for DNA sampling in burglary cases. However, no numbers were presented by the authors of this study from 2008 [14]. The results from our study confirm that windows have a comparatively low background of resident DNA and are therefore most suited for DNA trace analysis. We can see that the police officers of the Bern Cantonal Police are already focusing on the most promising sampling spots, since 32% of the traces we received were taken from windows or glass fragments.

Even though the data shown in Figure 6 seem to be very strong in favor of the sampling of window glass, we have to keep one limitation in mind, concerning the pre-selection effectuated by the police officer handling the case. This pre-selection is twofold: First, the officer will select the traces appearing most promising to him or her at the crime scene. Second, he or she will make a subsequent selection as to which samples to send for analysis to the DNA laboratory. If the analysis of the first samples sent to the lab do not result in interpretable DNA profiles, the case-managing officer might decide to send additional samples for analysis. Therefore, we encounter some risk of bias if samples from window glass are prioritized and no other samples are analyzed in the case. If we assume that the unknown profiles we can recover are maybe from "less prudent" burglars, than we might also possibly expect more of their profiles on other items in the apartment. However, we would not see those suspect profiles, because we do not analyze additional samples after having successfully established a profile from window glass.

In the years from 2009 to 2017, between 30 to 40% of all the DNA trace profiles submitted every year to the Swiss DNA database originated from burglary cases [15]. From our study, we would expect that at least 75% of those profiles originate from residents. The number of non-suspect profiles could even be higher, because we cannot be sure that we obtained reference samples from all people authorized to the crime scene, e.g., visitors or first responding local police officers, and DNA might also be transferred and subsequently picked up [3–6].

In routine casework, we usually do not obtain reference samples from inhabitants. From the 144 samples in the present study, we normally would have sent 44 unique profiles into CODIS (redundant profiles from the same case would not be submitted and were subtracted). After the comparison with the reference samples, we ended up submitting 11 profiles (10 single/major component profiles and 1 mixture). To date (10 December 2021), six of those profiles generated hits with profiles from persons registered in the Swiss DNA database, five of which originated from samples taken from window glass, underlining the high potential of this trace type to advance burglary investigations.

To date, the Swiss DNA database contains around 100,000 trace DNA profiles. Therefore, extrapolating the results from of our study, we expect that around 25,000 trace DNA profiles registered in the database actually originate from inhabitants. Not being excluded from a trace DNA profile as a resident bears the risk of being associated with other offences by a trace-to-trace match in CODIS, as mentioned in the introduction. However, a lack of prior exclusion interferes also with the privacy of the residents in a more general way. Today, the standard STR profiles contain only little personal information. However, potentially more privacy intrusive techniques, such as forensic DNA phenotyping (FDP) are on the rise [16]. Even though we consider such a development as not very probable, privacy issues for crime scene authorized individuals might increase in situations where FDP could also be employed for volume crimes in the future.

5. Conclusions

More than 70% of all profiles generated from window glass in the vicinity of the break-in site were caused by unknown individuals, whereas less than 10% of all other traces led to unknown, and therefore possible suspect profiles. Therefore, traces from (broken) windows should be prioritized in crime scene sampling for the generation of investigative leads. To minimize the inclusion of DNA profiles originating from crime scene authorized individuals in CODIS, the collection of reference samples should at least be considered for traces that were not sampled from window glass.

Author Contributions: Conceptualization, M.Z.; formal analysis, C.C.T. and M.Z.; data curation, C.C.T. and M.Z.; writing—original draft preparation, M.Z.; writing—review and editing, C.C.T. and M.Z.; project administration, M.D. and M.Z. All authors have read and agreed to the published version of the manuscript.

Funding: This research received no external funding.

Institutional Review Board Statement: The study involves casework samples and does not fall under the scope of the Swiss Federal Act on Research involving Human Beings. No identifiable personal data has been used for this publication.

Informed Consent Statement: Informed consent was obtained from all reference persons.

Data Availability Statement: DNA quantification data are stored at the University of Bern and may be made available upon request. No access to DNA profiles will be provided to anyone.

Acknowledgments: We would like to thank all the residents who provided a reference sample, all the police officers implicated in collecting samples, C. Düllmann and D. Leuenberger (Institute of Forensic Medicine) for administrative support and Z. Lechissa and P. Selitaj (Institute of Forensic Medicine) for analyzing the reference samples. We also thank S. Utz (Institute of Forensic Medicine), D. Comment and C. Zingg (Bern Cantonal Police) for their general support.

Conflicts of Interest: The authors declare no conflict of interest.

References

1. Polizeiliche Kriminalstatistik (PKS). *Jahresbericht 2020 der Polizeilich Registrierten Straftaten*; Swiss Federal Statistical Office: Neuchâtel, Switzerland, 2021.
2. Bern Cantonal High Court. *BK 2015 62—DNA-Analyse (Leitentscheid)*; Judgment of the Bern Cantonal High Court; Bern Cantonal High Court: Bern, Switzerland, 2015.
3. Meakin, G.; Jamieson, A. DNA transfer: Review and implications for casework. *Forensic Sci. Int. Genet.* **2013**, *7*, 434–443. [CrossRef]
4. van Oorschot, R.A.H.; Szkuta, B.; Meakin, G.E.; Kokshoorn, B.; Goray, M. DNA transfer in forensic science: A review. *Forensic Sci. Int. Genet.* **2019**, *38*, 140–166. [CrossRef] [PubMed]
5. Burrill, J.; Daniel, B.; Frascione, N. A review of trace "Touch DNA" deposits: Variability factors and an exploration of cellular composition. *Forensic Sci. Int. Genet.* **2019**, *39*, 8–18. [CrossRef] [PubMed]
6. Gosch, A.; Courts, C. On DNA transfer: The lack and difficulty of systematic research and how to do it better. *Forensic Sci. Int. Genet.* **2019**, *40*, 24–36. [CrossRef] [PubMed]
7. Zieger, M.; Schneider, C.; Utz, S. DNA recovery from gelatin fingerprint lifters by direct proteolytic digestion. *Forensic Sci. Int.* **2019**, *295*, 145–149. [CrossRef]
8. DNA-Analyselaborverordnung EJPD. Available online: https://www.fedlex.admin.ch/eli/cc/2014/605/de (accessed on 20 December 2021).
9. Bright, J.-A.; Richards, R.; Kruijver, M.; Kelly, H.; McGovern, C.; Magee, A.; McWhorter, A.; Ciecko, A.; Peck, B.; Baumgartner, C.; et al. Internal validation of STRmix™—A multi laboratory response to PCAST. *Forensic Sci. Int. Genet.* **2018**, *34*, 11–24. [CrossRef] [PubMed]
10. Bleka, Ø.; Storvik, G.; Gill, P. EuroForMix: An open source software based on a continuous model to evaluate STR DNA profiles from a mixture of contributors with artefacts. *Forensic Sci. Int. Genet.* **2016**, *21*, 35–44. [CrossRef] [PubMed]
11. ENFSI Guideline for Evaluative Reporting in Forensic Science. 2015. Available online: https://enfsi.eu/wp-content/uploads/2016/09/m1_guideline.pdf (accessed on 22 December 2021).
12. Swiss Federal Statistical Office. Households. 2020. Available online: https://www.bfs.admin.ch/bfs/de/home/statistiken/bevoelkerung/stand-entwicklung/haushalte.html (accessed on 22 December 2021).
13. Castella, V.; Mangin, P. DNA profiling success and relevance of 1739 contact stains from caseworks. *Forensic Sci. Int.-Genet. Suppl. Ser.* **2008**, *1*, 405–407. [CrossRef]
14. Raymond, J.J.; Walsh, S.J.; van Oorschot, R.A.H.; Gunn, P.R.; Evans, L.; Roux, C. Assessing trace DNA evidence from a residential burglary: Abundance, transfer and persistence. *Forensic Sci. Int. Genet. Suppl. Ser.* **2008**, *1*, 442–443. [CrossRef]
15. Killias, M.; Gut, M.; Biberstein, L.; Walser, S. *DNA-Analysen im Strafverfahren: Entwicklung, Umfang und Wirkungen*; Killias Research & Consulting: Zürich, Switzerland, 2018.
16. Scudder, N.; McNevin, D.; Kelty, S.F.; Walsh, S.J.; Robertson, J. Massively parallel sequencing and the emergence of forensic genomics: Defining the policy and legal issues for law enforcement. *Sci. Justice J. Forensic Sci. Soc.* **2018**, *58*, 153–158. [CrossRef]

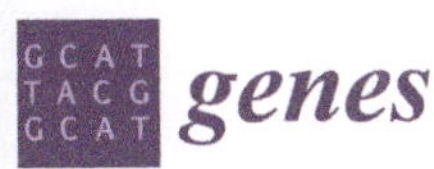

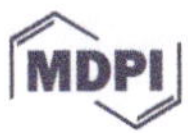

Article

The FORCE Panel: An All-in-One SNP Marker Set for Confirming Investigative Genetic Genealogy Leads and for General Forensic Applications

Andreas Tillmar [1,2,*], Kimberly Sturk-Andreaggi [3,4,5], Jennifer Daniels-Higginbotham [3,4], Jacqueline Tyler Thomas [3,4] and Charla Marshall [3,4,6,*]

[1] Department of Forensic Genetics and Forensic Toxicology, National Board of Forensic Medicine, SE-587 58 Linköping, Sweden
[2] Department of Biomedical and Clinical Sciences, Faculty of Medicine and Health Sciences, Linköping University, SE-582 25 Linköping, Sweden
[3] Armed Forces Medical Examiner System's Armed Forces DNA Identification Laboratory (AFMES-AFDIL), Dover Air Force Base, Dover, DE 19902, USA; kimberly.s.andreaggi.ctr@mail.mil (K.S.-A.); jennifer.l.higginbotham3.ctr@mail.mil (J.D.-H.); jacqueline.t.thomas2.ctr@mail.mil (J.T.T.)
[4] SNA International, LLC, Contractor Supporting the AFMES-AFDIL, Alexandria, VA 22314, USA
[5] Department of Immunology, Genetics and Pathology, Uppsala University, SE-751 08 Uppsala, Sweden
[6] Forensic Science Program, The Pennsylvania State University, State College, PA 16802, USA
[*] Correspondence: andreas.tillmar@rmv.se (A.T.); charla.k.marshall.ctr@mail.mil (C.M.); Tel.: +46-104834143 (A.T.); +1-302-3468-519 (C.M.)

Citation: Tillmar, A.; Sturk-Andreaggi, K.; Daniels-Higginbotham, J.; Thomas, J.T.; Marshall, C. The FORCE Panel: An All-in-One SNP Marker Set for Confirming Investigative Genetic Genealogy Leads and for General Forensic Applications. *Genes* **2021**, *12*, 1968. https://doi.org/10.3390/genes12121968

Academic Editor: Niels Morling

Received: 29 November 2021
Accepted: 8 December 2021
Published: 10 December 2021

Publisher's Note: MDPI stays neutral with regard to jurisdictional claims in published maps and institutional affiliations.

Abstract: The FORensic Capture Enrichment (FORCE) panel is an all-in-one SNP panel for forensic applications. This panel of 5422 markers encompasses common, forensically relevant SNPs (identity, ancestry, phenotype, X- and Y-chromosomal SNPs), a novel set of 3931 autosomal SNPs for extended kinship analysis, and no clinically relevant/disease markers. The FORCE panel was developed as a custom hybridization capture assay utilizing ~20,000 baits to target the selected SNPs. Five non-probative, previously identified World War II (WWII) cases were used to assess the kinship panel. Each case included one bone sample and associated family reference DNA samples. Additionally, seven reference quality samples, two 200-year-old bone samples, and four control DNAs were processed for kit performance and concordance assessments. SNP recovery after capture resulted in a mean of ~99% SNPs exceeding 10X coverage for reference and control samples, and 44.4% SNPs for bone samples. The WWII case results showed that the FORCE panel could predict first to fifth degree relationships with strong statistical support (likelihood ratios over 10,000 and posterior probabilities over 99.99%). To conclude, SNPs will be important for further advances in forensic DNA analysis. The FORCE panel shows promising results and demonstrates the utility of a 5000 SNP panel for forensic applications.

Keywords: SNP; kinship; massively parallel sequencing; next generation sequencing; hybridization capture; bone

1. Introduction

Forensic DNA databases were built around the use of non-coding DNA markers for human identification, primarily short tandem repeat (STR) loci from autosomal and Y-chromosomal targets [1]. By using a core set of DNA markers with almost no significance outside the medico-legal system, forensic DNA profiling was set to evolve independently from, and in parallel to, other fields of genetics sans overlap. This technological independence was rapidly breached, however, with the adoption of investigative genetic genealogy (IGG) and high-density single nucleotide polymorphism (SNP) genotyping for solving high-profile criminal cases (e.g., the Golden State Killer) and for identifications of unknown human remains [2]. Extant direct to consumer (DTC) SNP databases provided an exponentially growing, vast resource that could produce a genetic trail to anyone whose relatives participated in the consumer DNA testing market and opted into genealogical DNA databases such as GEDmatch [3,4]. The IGG method involves determining an extended DNA profile from a crime scene (or other forensic) sample using high-density SNP genotyping microarrays [5] or whole-genome sequencing (WGS) [6]. Then the SNP genotype dataset is searched in a public DNA database to identify matches with significant DNA sharing, indicating a familial relationship. Genealogists reconstruct family trees from the matches, identifying branches that could represent possible suspects that are provided to law enforcement. Once the "investigative lead" is identified, the next phase in the DNA profiling reverts back to using the forensic DNA core markers (i.e., STRs) to confirm the identification. DNA from the person of interest is obtained for testing, and the suspect's STR profile is compared to the STR profile produced from the crime scene sample. The final DNA-based identification rests on the court-admissible STR results, which constitute the definitive forensic evidence from the case.

Confirmatory STR testing is feasible when the DNA from a forensic sample is of standard forensic quality. Yet certain sample types contain degraded DNA, making them unsuitable for STR profiling, most notably rootless hair shafts and aged skeletal remains. Furthermore, confirmatory STR testing is limited when direct/reference samples are lacking and distant relationships must be inferred, as in historical remains identifications. In such cases, mitochondrial DNA (mtDNA) analysis is often used to recover a DNA profile, as mtDNA is higher in copy number than nuclear DNA (nDNA); thus, the chances of recovering a mtDNA target are higher. Since mtDNA is a non-recombining lineage marker whose DNA sequence is shared amongst maternal relatives, the utility of mtDNA is limited forensically because its discrimination power is fairly weak. Therefore, mtDNA best serves degraded DNA cases that can be bolstered by other types of evidence, DNA, or otherwise. Recent methods for mitogenome massively parallel sequencing (MPS) have been applied to degraded DNA samples and validated for forensic use, including mini-amplicon PCR [7,8], primer extension capture (PEC) [9], and hybridization capture [10]. Such methods are very sensitive and capable of providing authentic mtDNA data from the most challenging of forensic specimens. These MPS workflows have also been adapted for SNP profiling of degraded DNA specimens [11–15]. Large SNP multiplexes suitable for extended kinship analysis can be readily enriched using custom hybridization capture [14]. However, such large panels may not be suitable for routine forensic casework due to the markers that may be linked and/or associated with pathogenic variants.

To provide an enrichment approach for the generation of a large number of SNPs from all sample types, the FORensic Capture Enrichment (FORCE) panel was designed as an all-in-one SNP panel for forensic applications. This panel encompasses all forensically relevant SNP markers (identity, ancestry, phenotype, X- and Y-chromosomal SNPs) and presents a novel kinship SNP set for distant relationship inference. The relatively small size of the FORCE panel minimizes the number of primers/probes per reaction to reduce the enrichment cost. The FORCE panel can be adapted to various enrichment methods, including hybridization capture, PEC, and possibly multiplexed PCR, making it a viable option for both high quality and degraded DNA samples. The enriched SNP targets can be sequenced on a variety of downstream MPS platforms. By limiting the number of SNPs, fewer MPS reads are required to obtain per-SNP coverage requirements, and thus sequencing efficiency is maximized. The FORCE panel SNPs were sub-selected from SNPs on the genotyping microarrays used by DTC DNA testing companies, enabling cross-compatibility with externally developed SNP data. This is important for forensic validation purposes to demonstrate concordance and genotyping accuracy. Medically relevant SNPs were excluded from the FORCE panel design in order to mitigate genetic privacy issues around FORCE panel DNA databanks. Y-SNPs were included for high-resolution Y-chromosome haplogroup inference, which may be informative for both identification and ancestry prediction purposes [16]. X-SNPs were included due to their potential kinship informative value for cases scenarios in which one may make use of the X-chromosomal specific mode of inheritance [17]. Aside from general forensic sample use, the FORCE panel is ideally suited to confirm investigative leads gained with genetic genealogy that cannot be confirmed with STR typing, such as those from degraded DNA.

2. Materials and Methods

2.1. FORCE Panel Design

A kinship SNP panel was designed to provide maximum kinship resolution with minimal SNPs for enhanced sequencing efficiency. Kinship SNPs were selected based on the following criteria (Table 1): (1) Inclusion in three commonly used Illumina SNP genotyping chips (Table 2; San Diego, CA, USA), (2) minor allele frequency (MAF) between 0.2 and 0.8 in the major 1000 Genomes continental populations (African (AFR), Admixed American (AMR), East Asian (EAS), European (EUR), and South Asian (SAS)) [18], (3) at least 0.5-cm genetic distance between selected SNPs, (4) linkage disequilibrium (LD) metric r^2 smaller than 0.1, and (5) frequency difference of less than 0.35 between the 1000 Genomes five continental populations. Using the same parameters as the autosomal kinship SNPs, X-SNPs were selected for cases requiring X-chromosomal information. Pre-existing SNP marker sets were added to the FORCE panel to offer cross-compatibility with commercial SNP assays (Table 2). Identity-informative SNPs (iiSNPs) were compiled from the ForenSeq DNA Signature Prep Kit (Primer Mix A; San Diego, CA, USA), the Precision ID Identity Panel (Thermo Fisher Scientific, Waltham, MA, USA), and a published QIAseq panel (QIAGEN) [19]. The ancestry- and phenotype-informative SNPs (aiSNPs and piSNPs, respectively) were compiled from the ForenSeq kit (Primer Mix B), the Precision ID Ancestry Panel (Thermo Fisher Scientific), and markers identified by the VISAGE consortium [20]. To increase the Y haplogroup resolution beyond the 34 Y-SNPs in the Precision ID Identify Panel, 884 Y-SNPs targeted by the amplicons of the Ralf et al. [16]. AmpliSeq panel (Thermo Fisher Scientific) were included in the assay. All of the selected FORCE panel SNPs were compared with American College of Medical Genetics (ACMG) secondary findings (SF) 2.0 genes to test for clinical relevance [21]. SNPs listed the ACMG SF 2.0 were omitted from the panel. Tri-allelic SNPs were omitted from the panel and autosomal microhaplotypes were not included to simplify the data analysis.

Table 1. Kinship SNP selection criteria and resulting viable SNPs.

Kinship Panel Criterion	Number of Remaining SNPs
1. Included on all major SNP array chips (Table 2)	116,544
2. MAF 0.2–0.8 in 1000 Genomes populations	34,851
3. Minimum 0.5 cm distance	5426
4. LD metric $r^2 < 0.1$	5376
5. Maximum 35% frequency difference between 1000 Genomes populations	3937

A custom myBaits-20,000 kit (Arbor Biosciences, Ann Arbor, MI, USA) was designed for hybridization capture of the selected SNPs. The design included four baits per autosomal SNP (right flank, left flank, and each allele) and two baits per X/Y SNP (each allele). A BLAST [22] analysis was then performed to filter out non-specific baits. A total of 228 baits failed to meet the BLAST analysis requirements. Most of these failed baits (139/228) came from the AmpliSeq Y-SNP marker set [16], including 61 Y-SNPs for which both baits failed. The remaining failed baits targeted autosomal markers (74 SNPs with one failed bait, six SNPs with two failed baits, and one SNP with three failed baits). The failed baits were removed from the kit, thus eliminating 61 of the 884 Y-SNPs. Overall, there were 97 SNP markers with at least one failed bait and thus may show reduced coverage in the SNP capture results. The α version of the myBaits FORCE capture assay tested in this study included 5446 SNPs (Table S1), targeted by 19,526 unique baits. There were 24 SNPs included in the α panel but ultimately excluded from analysis due to the outlined criteria. The excluded SNPs were six kinship SNPs with clinical relevance, 15 triallelic aiSNPs (one of which also had clinical relevance), one Y-SNP from the Precision ID Identity Panel with no Y haplogroup association, and two uninformative autosomal SNPs. A summary of the marker types comprising the 5422 FORCE panel SNP targets analyzed in this study is presented in Figure 1 and detailed marker information is provided in Table S1.

Table 2. Commercial and/or published SNP panels utilized for the FORCE panel selection. iiSNP = identity-informative SNP; aiSNP = ancestry-informative SNP; piSNP = phenotype-informative SNP; X-SNP = X-chromosomal SNP; Y-SNP = Y-chromosomal SNP.

Marker Type	SNP Panels (# SNPs)
Kinship SNP/ X-SNP	Infinium Global Screening Array (654,027), Infinium Omni Express (710,000), Infinium CytoSNP-850K (850,000)
iiSNP	ForenSeq DNA Signature Prep Kit: Primer Mix A (94)
	Precision ID Identity Panel (90)
	QIAseq Investigator 140 SNP panel (140)
aiSNP	ForenSeq DNA Signature Prep Kit: Primer Mix B (56)
	Precision ID Ancestry Panel (165)
	VISAGE panel (115)
piSNP	ForenSeq DNA Signature Prep Kit: Primer Mix B (24)
	VISAGE panel (41)
Y-SNP	Precision ID Identity Panel (34)
	AmpliSeq (884)

2.2. Simulated Panel Performance

A simulation approach was used to study expected likelihood ratio (LR) distributions for various kinship case scenarios based on the kinship SNPs included in the FORCE panel. Five different kinship case scenarios were selected, representing second to sixth degrees of pairwise relatedness (i.e., half siblings, first cousins, first cousins once removed, second cousins, and second cousins once removed). The simulations were performed with the complete kinship SNP set (the initial 3937 SNPs including the six that were ultimately excluded). Simulations were also performed with 75% and 25% of the kinship SNPs in order to mimic situations for which only partial SNP profiles are available.

The simulations were performed using the software Merlin [23]. Merlin was used both to create the pedigree-based DNA data and to calculate likelihoods for the tested hypotheses. European allele frequencies from [18] were used and genetic linkage was accounted for using genetic position information from Rutgers map [24]. For each simulated kinship case scenario, the likelihood ratio was calculated as LR = Pr (DNA | H1)/Pr (DNA | H2), where H1 was the hypothesis representing the related case scenario, and H2 was the hypothesis representing the alternative, in which the tested individuals are unrelated. For each case scenario and true hypothesis, 10,000 simulation events were performed. A front-end script written in R [25] was used to format and manage input files, and R was also used to handle the outputs from Merlin and for plotting the distribution curves (R package *ggplot2*).

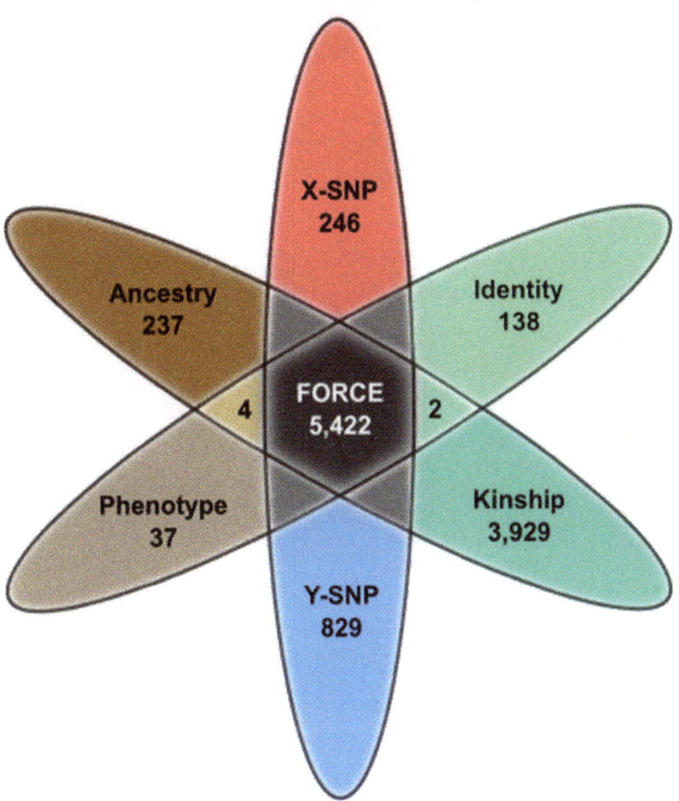

Figure 1. FORCE panel SNP marker summary ($n = 5422$).

2.3. SNP Capture Assay Laboratory Testing

2.3.1. Sample Selection

The samples utilized in this study originated from non-probative Defense Personnel Accounting Agency (DPAA) cases that were previously processed by the Armed Forces Medical Examiner System's Armed Forces DNA Identification Laboratory (AFMES-AFDIL). These cases involve skeletal samples from five previously identified World War II (WWII) male service members and their associated family reference specimens. One or more DNA extracts from a single skeletal element per service member was included in this study, along with two or three family reference samples for each service member (Table 3). The five cases were chosen to range in sample quality and degree of relationship. In addition to the case samples included for testing the effectiveness of the kinship SNPs, further non-probative samples were evaluated for concordance and/or SNP performance (Table 4). These included seven reference samples, a 19th century bone sample from a previously identified individual (sample 25, JB55 [12]), an additional 19th century bone sample associated with JB55 (sample 26), and four control DNAs.

Table 3. Non-probative case descriptions. Each of the five cases includes one or more DNA extracts from a degraded bone sample (~70 years) of a previously identified World War II (WWII) service member, along with two or three family reference specimens (buccal swabs). DOR = degree of relatedness.

Case	WWII Context	Sample	Sample Type	Relationship to Service Member (DOR)
A	USS *Oklahoma*	1	Buccal swab	Grandniece (3)
		2	Buccal swab	Nephew (2)
		3	Left femur	Self
B	USS *Oklahoma*	4	Buccal swab	Nephew (2)
		5	Buccal swab	Great grandnephew (4)
		6	Buccal swab	Great grandniece (4)
		7.1	Left femur	Self
		7.2		
C	Austria	8	Buccal swab	First cousin twice removed, male (5)
		9	Buccal swab	Nephew (2)
		10	Buccal swab	Daughter (1)
		11.1	Long bone	Self
		11.2		
D	Italy	12	Buccal swab	Sister (1)
		13	Buccal swab	Grandniece (3)
		14.1	Right parietal	Self
		14.2		
		14.3		
E	Tarawa	15	Buccal swab	Son (1)
		16	Buccal swab	Daughter (1)
		17.1	Right tibia	Self
		17.2		

All living sample donors provided informed consent for their samples to be used in research and quality improvement activities. The use of these reference and bone samples was approved by the Defense Health Agency Office of Research Protections (Protocol # DHQ-20-2073).

2.3.2. DNA Extraction and Quantitation

Existing DNA extracts and associated reagent blanks (RBs) from the five skeletal samples as well as JB55 [12] were obtained. During previous processing of these samples, DNA was extracted from 0.2–1.0 g bone powder. Samples were first digested overnight at 56 °C in a buffer containing 0.5 M EDTA, 1% lauroylsarcosine and 200 µL of 20 mg/mL proteinase K. DNA extraction was achieved using either an organic protocol or a double QIAquick PCR Purification Kit method (QIAGEN, Hilden, Germany), as described in [26]. Purification was performed on all organic extracts using the QIAGEN MinElute PCR Purification Kit, followed by elution in 50 to 100 µL of Tris-EDTA (10 mM Tris, (pH 7.5) 0.1 mM EDTA). An unknown skeletal sample from the same historical context as JB55, along with associated RB, underwent a modified Dabney DNA extraction. This Dabney protocol followed the method using large volume silica columns [27]; however, overnight digestion was performed at 56 °C.

Table 4. Additional non-probative samples tested: seven reference samples with self-reported phenotypic and ancestry information (18–24), two historical bone samples ~200 years postmortem (25 and 26), and four control DNA samples (2800M, K562, NA12877, and NA12878).

Sample	Sample Type	Sex
18	Buccal swab	Female
19	Buccal swab	Female
20	Buccal swab	Male
21	Buccal swab	Female
22	Buccal swab	Female
23	Buccal swab	Male
24	Buccal swab	Male
25 (JB55)	Femoral bone (~200 years)	Male
26	Unknown bone (~200 years)	Unknown
2800M	Whole blood	Male
K562	Cell line	Female
NA12877	Cell line	Male
NA12878	Cell line	Female

DNA was isolated from the buccal swabs using the QIAGEN EZ1 DNA Investigator Kit automated on an EZ1 Advanced XL instrument following the manufacturer's Trace or Tip Dance Protocol. The final elution volume for all samples ranged from 50 to 100 µL of Tris-EDTA. DNA was quantified with the dsDNA High Sensitivity (HS) Assay Kit on the Qubit 2.0 or Qubit 3.0 Fluorometer (Thermo Fisher Scientific, Waltham, MA, USA) to determine input into library preparation.

2.3.3. Library Preparation

Samples were divided into three sets for laboratory processing and sequencing, and each set included library negative and positive controls to evaluate library and capture success. The first sample set (bone) included ten DNA extracts from the WWII bone samples and one of the historical bone samples (26) plus two associated RBs. The bone set positive control was 1 ng of fragmented K562 control DNA as previously described in [10]. JB55 was processed separately from the other bone samples in its own set, which included an associated RB, library negative control, and K562 positive control as used in the bone sample set. Lastly, the reference sample set included the 12 family references, seven additional reference-type samples, and three control DNAs (2800M, NA12877, and NA12878). Associated RBs and a library negative control were included in the reference sample set.

The bone libraries were prepared in a dedicated low copy DNA laboratory using the KAPA Hyper Prep Kit (Roche Sequencing, Wilmington, MA, USA). Library preparation followed the manufacturer's recommendations using 15-µM 8-bp dual-indexed adapters. A target DNA extract volume of 50 µL was used for library preparation, with a maximum DNA input of 1 µg. Some of the previously existing DNA extracts had limited volume available; therefore, Tris-EDTA was added to create a total volume of 50 µL. Reference sample libraries were prepared with the KAPA HyperPlus Kit (Roche Sequencing), as fragmented DNA is required for successful library preparation. Library preparation was performed in accordance with the manufacturer's protocol with a 20-min fragmentation and ligation of dual-indexed 8-bp adapters (Integrated DNA Technologies, Coralville, IA, USA). The library PCR reactions for the bone samples utilized KAPA HiFi HotStart Uracil + ReadyMix (Roche Sequencing) to accommodate for uracils present in the native DNA molecule from cytosine deamination. The reference/control sample libraries were amplified with the KAPA HiFi HotStart ReadyMix (Roche Sequencing). Library amplification was completed following the manufacturer's recommendations, using a total of 12 cycles of PCR for each of the sample sets (bone and reference/control). Samples were purified using a 1.0× AMPure XP (Beckman Coulter, Indianapolis, ID, USA) bead-based cleanup and were then eluted in 20 µL of Tris-EDTA. The quality of the libraries was checked on the 2100 Bioanalyzer instrument (Agilent Technologies, Santa Clara, CA, USA) using the Agilent DNA 7500 Kit. For the bone sample and control DNA libraries, an aliquot of the purified library product was reserved for WGS (described below).

2.3.4. Hybridization Capture

Hybridization capture with the α version of the FORCE capture panel was completed using the myBaits 1-20K Custom DNA Hybridization Capture kit (Arbor Biosciences, Ann Arbor, MI, USA). The procedure followed the manufacturer's recommended v5 protocol using a single capture and 5 µL of custom SNP baits. Samples were allowed to incubate overnight for approximately 24 h at 62 °C with a heated lid (72 °C) using a Veriti thermal cycler (Thermo Fisher Scientific, Waltham, MA, USA). PCR amplification was achieved using duplicate PCR reactions to make use of the entire capture product. The post-capture PCR reactions were completed with 19 PCR cycles using the KAPA HiFi HotStart ReadyMix following the manufacturer's recommendations. The two amplified capture products were combined for each sample and then purified with the MinElute PCR Purification Kit, eluting in 25 µL of Tris-EDTA.

2.3.5. Normalization, Pooling, and High Throughput Sequencing

Purified capture product was quantified using the 2100 Bioanalyzer instrument with the Agilent DNA 7500 Kit to determine DNA molarity. As in library preparation and hybridization capture, the three sample sets (bone, JB55, and reference) were pooled separately to minimize the impact of crosstalk between samples of disparate quality during sequencing [10]. The bone set positive control (K562) was omitted from the bone sample sequencing pool and instead added to the reference sample pool for sequencing. The JB55 sample pool included JB55 and its associated RB, as well as an additional library from a different JB55 DNA extract. (Since both JB55 libraries produced similar results; only the data from the DNA extract that also underwent WGS are presented below.) The JB55 library controls were not sequenced; but they were assessed with the Bioanalyzer for contamination and quality control purposes.

Pooling was achieved by individually normalizing captured libraries to the same concentration as the least concentrated sample (nM) in the set, then adding equal volume of all samples to the pool along with maximum RB and negative control volumes. The captured library pools were quantified using the Agilent DNA 7500 Kit on the 2100 Bioanalyzer. The bone and reference captured library pools were diluted to 1 pM with a 5% spike-in of PhiX Control V3 (Illumina) for sequencing on a NextSeq 550 (Illumina) using NextSeq 500/550 High Output Kits, v2.5 (150 cycles). Paired-end sequencing (75 × 75 cycles) was performed for the bone sample pool (14 captured libraries), while single-end data (150 cycles) were generated for the reference and control DNA samples (26 captured libraries). The JB55 pool was diluted to 12 pM including 5% PhiX control V3, and paired-end sequencing (75 × 75 cycles) was completed on a Verogen MiSeq FGx in RUO mode using a MiSeq Reagent Kit, v3 (150 cycles).

To gauge capture efficiency for the non-probative bone sample and control DNA libraries, baseline WGS data were produced on an Illumina NextSeq 550. WGS was not performed for any of the reference samples. Sequencing was completed with NextSeq 500/550 High Output Kits, v2.5 (150 cycles) using the same approach as the captured libraries (75 × 75 cycles for the bone sample pool and 1 × 150 cycles for the control DNA pool). For direct comparison with the JB55 capture data, WGS of one JB55 library was performed on a MiSeq FGx using RUO mode and paired-end (75 × 75 cycles) sequencing on a v3 cartridge (150 cycles).

2.3.6. Sequence Data Analysis

FASTQ files were imported into the CLC Genomics Workbench v12.0.1 (QIAGEN) and all sample data were analyzed with a custom workflow. The workflow, which was applied to all samples, included five steps. (1) Reads were trimmed based on quality (including ambiguous bases) as well as adapter read-through (for paired reads only). (2) Trimmed reads were then mapped to the GRCh38 human reference genome using stringent mapping parameters designed to prevent off-target mapping of exogenous DNA (e.g., bacterial DNA). Modifications to the default mapping parameters were a length fraction of 0.85 and stringency fraction of 0.95, and non-specific reads (i.e., reads that produce an equal alignment score for multiple mapping regions) were ignored. (3) Duplicate mapped reads were removed with 20% maximum representation of minority sequence. (4) Local realignment of unaligned ends was performed to improve indel alignment in the mapping. (5) The alleles observed at each of the 5422 FORCE SNPs was determined using the Identify Known Mutations from Mappings tool, ignoring broken pairs in the bone set sequence data. Various analysis metrics such as the total number of reads, percent mapped, and percent duplicate reads were reported throughout the workflow using different CLC Genomics Workbench quality control (e.g., QC for Targeted Sequencing) tools.

A custom Microsoft Excel (Redmond, WA, USA) template was developed for genotype generation based on the CLC Identify Known Mutations from Mappings output. The targeted SNP had to be covered by a minimum of 10 reads for analysis. Furthermore, in order for a FORCE SNP to be called (i.e., used for downstream analyses), genotypes required allele frequency of 90% or greater to be called as a homozygote and heterozygous genotypes needed at least 30% MAF. SNPs meeting the minimum coverage requirement (10X) but with imbalanced alleles (10–30% MAF) that could not be confidently called homozygote or heterozygote were noted as "imbalanced" and excluded from further analyses. The called SNPs were separated by type (e.g., kinship SNPs, aiSNPs, piSNPs) for analysis and interpretation as described below.

2.3.7. SNP Concordance Assessment

The genotypes derived from the FORCE capture data of the four control DNAs (2800M, K562, NA12877, and NA12878) and one of the historical bone samples (JB55) were compared to previously published data. For 2800M, data from the ForenSeq DNA Library Preparation Kit were used for comparison [28], taking into account reverse strand orientation at 52 markers. For the remaining control DNA samples, published variant call format (VCF) files from WGS data were used for the concordance assessment ([29] for K562, [30,31] for NA12877 and NA12878). The VCF files for K562 and NA12877 included only those positions in which a variant was detected; thus, the genotype was assumed to be homozygous for the reference allele at SNPs missing from the VCF for the purpose of this comparison. A preliminary assessment identified a few issues in the published control DNA datasets that impacted concordance. There was an error in the K562 VCF for rs10892689, and the genotype for this SNP was determined by visual inspection of the associated BAM [29]. The NA12878 VCF included all SNP positions regardless of the detection of a non-reference allele. Five FORCE SNPs were missing from the NA12878 VCF, and the associated BAM [30,31] was used to confirm the genotype at those positions. Additionally, strand orientation was corrected in the published genotypes at two SNP markers (rs6670984 and rs4922532).

For JB55, published genotypes produced with the Precision ID Ancestry Panel (n = 165) and targeted Y-SNP typing (n = 4) as described in [12] were used for comparison to the FORCE profile. The genotype with the highest coverage was utilized when discordant data were observed between the two Precision ID replicates analyzed in the previously published study. Additionally, there were 16 SNPs without sufficient coverage (<10X) in either Precision ID replicate; these markers were excluded from the concordance assessment.

Supplementary to called SNPs, "imbalanced" FORCE genotypes were also compared to the published data. Imbalanced genotypes were observed at SNPs with sufficient coverage ($\geq$10X), but where the allele frequency thresholds for homozygote/heterozygote calling were not met. When the minor allele(s) was observed with base quality <20 and <10% forward reverse balance, indicating sequencing error, the artifact (minor) allele was removed, and the observed genotype noted for the imbalanced SNP was modified. This was only performed for the concordance assessment. No imbalanced SNPs were utilized in downstream analyses (e.g., ancestry predictions, kinship comparisons).

When discordance was observed between the FORCE and published genotype, the FORCE BAM and the BAM associated with the published data were reviewed to confirm the genotypes at the SNP marker. If the genotypes were still inconsistent after further review, the cause of the discrepancy was investigated.

2.3.8. Biogeographical Ancestry Predictions

Biogeographical ancestry predictions, based on the aiSNPs, were performed with two different methods: principal component analysis (PCA) and naïve Bayes analysis. An R script [25] was developed, in which the R package *prcomp* [32] was used for the PCA analysis with SNP profiles from the 1000 Genomes project [18] to train the PCA model. In the same script we included the naïve Bayes [33] analysis method by calculating the likelihood Pr (DNA | Population X), for each major continental population group (EUR, EAS, AMR, SAS, and AFR). Allele frequencies from the 1000 Genomes project [18] were used for these likelihood calculations. Since the allele frequencies were missing for one aiSNP (rs10954737) in the 1000 Genomes dataset, this marker was excluded from analysis and ancestry predictions were based on 240 aiSNPs. Posterior probabilities were calculated assuming a flat prior. These previously characterized aiSNPs allow for clear separation of the major population groups EUR, AFR, EAS, and SAS [34].

2.3.9. Phenotype Predictions

The 41 piSNPs included in the FORCE panel are consistent with the markers of the HirisPlex-S System [35]. Using the Excel template described in Section 2.3.6, the genotypes from sequence data were converted into the correct allele orientation and assigned "0", "1", "2", or "N/A" based upon a customized R script [36]. The converted genotypes were then submitted to the HirisPlex-S System webtool for phenotype prediction [37]. The Excel template organizes the converted genotypes of the piSNPs either for easy manual entry or for batch analysis using the file upload functionality. The FORCE data were uploaded as a single file and the HirisPlex-S output was downloaded. The results were compared to self-reported eye color and hair color for the seven additional non-probative reference samples (18–24; Table 4).

2.3.10. Y Haplogroup Predictions

Y haplogroups were predicted based upon the 829 Y-SNPs included in the FORCE panel. Called Y-SNPs were compared to the Yleaf WGS HG38 Position file [38,39] within the Excel template and variants (non-reference alleles) were denoted with the corresponding Y haplogroup. Identified haplogroups were reviewed manually and the most refined Y haplogroup was reported. The results were further inspected to ensure that the variants observed were expected based upon the predicted Y haplogroup (e.g., variants associated with ancestral haplogroups of the reported haplogroup). Though not utilized in this study, Yleaf offers automated Y haplogroup predictions [38]. Yleaf can analyze both FASTQ and BAM files; however, current functionality does not allow for duplicate removal, and therefore it is recommended to utilize FORCE BAM files after mapped duplicate removal for haplogroup predictions performed with the Yleaf software.

2.3.11. Kinship Statistics (Kinship SNP and X-SNP)

Pairwise kinship calculations (kinship SNPs). Likelihoods were calculated based on observed kinship SNP data given seven different relationship hypotheses (parent/offspring, full siblings, half siblings, first cousins, first cousins once removed, second cousins, and second cousins once removed) and one hypothesis representing no genetic relationship between the two compared individuals (i.e., unrelated). From these likelihoods, likelihood ratios (LRs) were calculated for each related hypothesis using the unrelated hypothesis as the alternative hypothesis (i.e., LR = Pr (DNA I H1)/Pr (DNA I H2), where H1 was the hypothesis representing one of the related relationships given above and H2 was the unrelated hypothesis). These kinship calculations were performed in a pairwise fashion between all reference samples as well as between each "Unknown" (i.e., WWII bone sample) and each reference sample. Posterior probabilities were calculated assuming a flat prior. The likelihoods were calculated using Merlin with the preferences described above (Section 2.2). R was again used to format and manage input files (e.g., filter SNPs when having partial SNP profiles) as well as to handle the outputs from Merlin and for the plotting of distribution curves.

Pedigree kinship calculations (kinship SNPs). In addition to the pairwise kinship calculation, kinship statistics were also calculated in a pedigree fashion. Here, SNP profiles for all reference individuals, in each reference family, were included in the likelihood calculations. In this approach each unknown sample was tested as the missing person in each reference pedigree (Figure S1). For each such pedigree, the LR was calculated as LR = Pr (DNA I "H1: The tested unknown sample comes from the missing person")/Pr (DNA I "H2: The tested unknown sample comes from an individual unrelated to the reference pedigree"). The likelihoods were calculated using Merlin with the preferences described above (Section 2.2). As previously noted, a front-end script was written in R to format input files and to handle the outputs from Merlin. Kinship predictions with strong statistical support were defined as those that met the following two criteria: LR $\geq$ 10,000 (log 10 LR $\geq$ 4) and posterior probability $\geq$ 99.99% given equal priors for the tested hypotheses.

Kinship calculations using X-SNPs. In order to demonstrate the possibility to calculate kinship statistics solely based on X-SNPs, two samples were selected from family D: sample 12 ("reference") and sample 14.1 ("unknown"). These two individuals are full siblings (Figure 2) and their X-SNP genotypes were used to calculate the LR = Pr (DNA I "Sample 12 and sample 14.1 come from two full siblings)/Pr (DNA I "Sample 12 and sample 14.1 come from two unrelated individuals"). The X-specific version of Merlin ("MINX") calculated the likelihoods of the two hypotheses, using European allele frequencies and genetic positions obtained from Rutgers map [18,24]. As previously noted, R was used to format input files and to handle the outputs from Merlin.

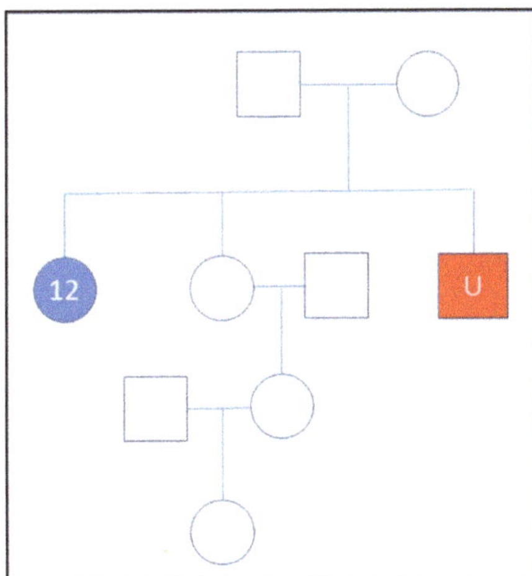

Figure 2. Pedigree of unknown (sample 14.1) and the reference sample (12) from family D utilized in X-SNP kinship assessment.

3. Results and Discussion

3.1. Simulated Panel Performance

The results from the kinship simulations clearly demonstrate that the kinship SNPs could be used to solve the majority of kinship case scenarios down to first cousins, including cases with partial SNP profiles (Figure 3). Furthermore, this set of kinship SNPs can be informative in cases involving a more distant relationship issue (such as second cousins) (Figure S2); however, the LR distribution curves for such cases for true related and true unrelated cases are overlapping.

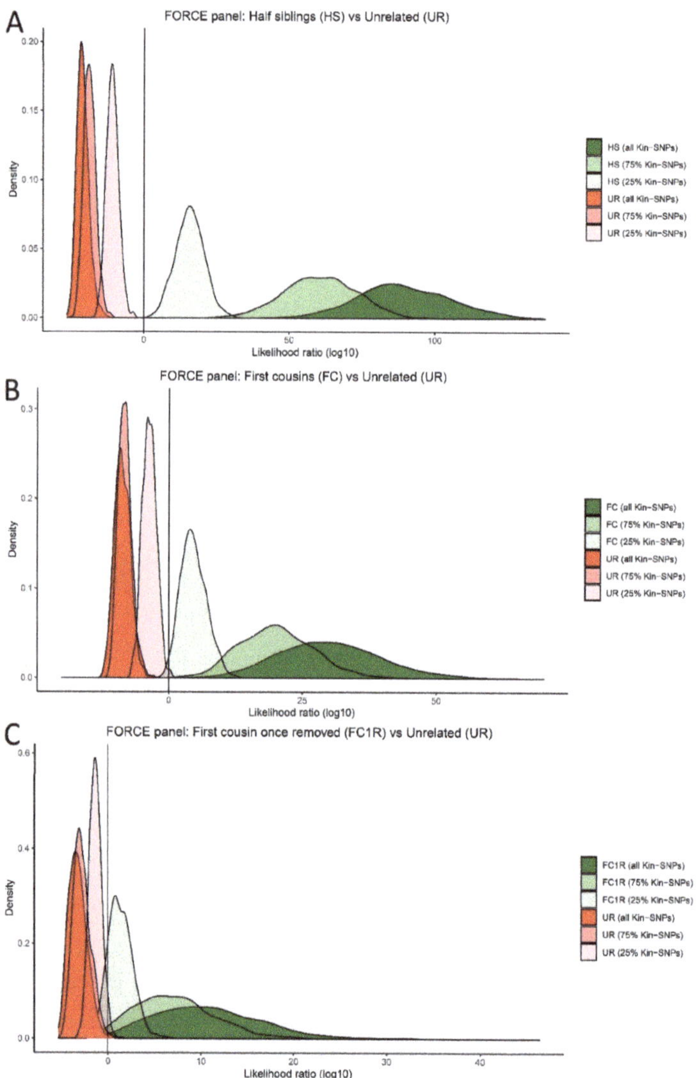

Figure 3. Simulation results for pairwise kinship predictions. Simulations were performed between an unknown sample at varying levels of kinship SNP recovery (100%, 75%, and 25%) compared to a complete reference sample profile. (**A**) Second degree (half siblings) vs. unrelated (UR); (**B**) third degree (first cousins) vs. UR; (**C**) fourth degree (first cousins once removed) vs. UR. Simulation results for additional relationships (first degree and fifth degree) are presented in Figure S2.

3.2. SNP Capture Assay Laboratory Testing

Detailed sequencing and SNP coverage metrics for all samples can be found in Table S2. The number of called SNPs, which met the 10X coverage and allele frequency requirements for homozygotes and heterozygotes, varied by sex due to the number of Y-SNPs in the assay. The maximum number of called SNPs was 5422 for males and 4593 for females. All reference and control DNA SNP profiles were 94.7–99.8% complete when accounting for sex, with an average of 5355 SNPs for males and 4552 SNPs for females (Table 5). The average coverage of the called SNPs in reference/control samples was 225X (Table S2). The standard deviation of called SNPs in the reference/control samples was approximately 42% of the average coverage. As noted in the methods, some SNPs had fewer probes than others. Hence, average coverage by bait count was investigated (Figure S3). For autosomal SNPs having all four baits (n = 4267), the average coverage across the reference/control samples was 241X. The average coverage dropped to 180X for autosomal SNPs with three baits (n = 73) and 122X for autosomal SNPs with two baits (n = 6). The single autosomal (kinship) SNP (rs4847178) with one bait (right flank) produced an average coverage of 157X, with called data for 100% of the reference/control samples. All 246 X-SNPs were targeted by two baits, averaging 166X in coverage for females and 89X for males. The 812 Y-SNPs with two baits produced an average coverage of 105X in male reference/control samples, with the reduced coverage observed at the 17 Y-SNPs with only one bait (50X). There were 13 SNPs (including two kinship SNPs, one iiSNP and ten Y-SNPs) that failed to produce sufficient coverage (10X) for any sample (Table S3). An additional 17 SNPs (six kinship SNPs, one iiSNP, five X-SNPs, and five Y-SNPs) had no call for a majority (>50%) of reference/control samples. Of these 30 poor performing SNPs, four had one bait that failed during the kit design. Three of these four SNPs with one failed bait were Y-SNPs (which consequently failed in all samples due to Y-SNPs only targeted by two baits per SNP). In all three cases, the failed bait was associated with the reference allele. The fourth poorly performing SNP that also had a failed bait (rs662185) had coverage and allele imbalance issues in the reference/control samples (see Section 3.3 below). Other factors such as the specific baits included (e.g., reference allele, alternate allele, right flank, or left flank) and the surrounding sequence motif (e.g., insertions and deletions impacting alignment) may have affected SNP performance. As a result of these findings, the capture kit will be modified in the future to remove poor performing SNPs. The modified/"β" FORCE kit will also eliminate baits targeting SNPs that were later discovered to lack one or more of the FORCE panel criteria (e.g., clinical relevance or triallelic SNPs).

Table 5. Summary of the number and proportion of called SNPs after capture of the FORCE panel targets. The results are broken down by sample type. High quality includes family references, additional non-probative reference samples, and control DNAs.

Sample Type	Count	Maximum Possible SNPs	Called SNPs *					
			Count			Percentage		
			Minimum	Maximum	Average	Minimum	Maximum	Average
Male, high quality	11	5422	5133	5395	5355	94.7%	99.5%	98.8%
Female, high quality	12	4593	4396	4582	4552	95.7%	99.8%	99.1%
Bone (all male)	12	5422	11	5361	2407	0.2%	98.9%	44.4%
Control blank	7	5422	0	26	4	0.0%	0.5%	0.1%

* ≥10X coverage, homozygous genotype ≥ 90% allele frequency; heterozygous genotype ≥ 30% minor allele frequency.

The bone sample results varied considerably, ranging from 11–5361 called SNPs and an average of 44.4% of the possible 5422 SNPs across the 12 DNA extracts (Table S2). To compare the number of called SNPs per bone, the results from each DNA extract were averaged for bone samples with multiple DNA extracts (Figure 4). Four of the seven bone samples produced 3719 or more SNPs (two USS *Oklahoma* (3 and 7) and the two historical bones (JB55 and sample 26)). These four samples were extracted with either PCIA followed by MinElute purification or the Dabney DNA extraction method. In contrast, the bone samples that were extracted with QIAquick produced fewer called SNPs. The three QIAquick replicates from the Italy bone sample (14) yielded 282–5121 called SNPs, for an average of 2308. The Austria (11) and Tarawa (17) bone samples, which were also extracted with QIAquick, produced only 50 and 14 called SNPs on average, respectively. The Tarawa bone sample was likely chemically treated with formalin, which was the standard postmortem procedure during WWII. Such chemically treated samples have been shown to produce poor DNA sequencing results [10]. The bone from Austria may have also received the same standard WWII postmortem chemical treatment. It is important to note that the variable results obtained from the bone samples may be due to a combination of differing factors, including separate case contexts, the DNA extraction method utilized, as well as the remaining DNA extract volume available for library preparation. The sample selection strategy for this study had prioritized known, non-probative samples with available DNA extracts from both the bone sample and associated family reference samples. Therefore, it was not possible to control for DNA extract preparation and other variables that may have a considerable impact on SNP capture results. An investigation into DNA extraction methods for downstream SNP capture success is an area of future research.

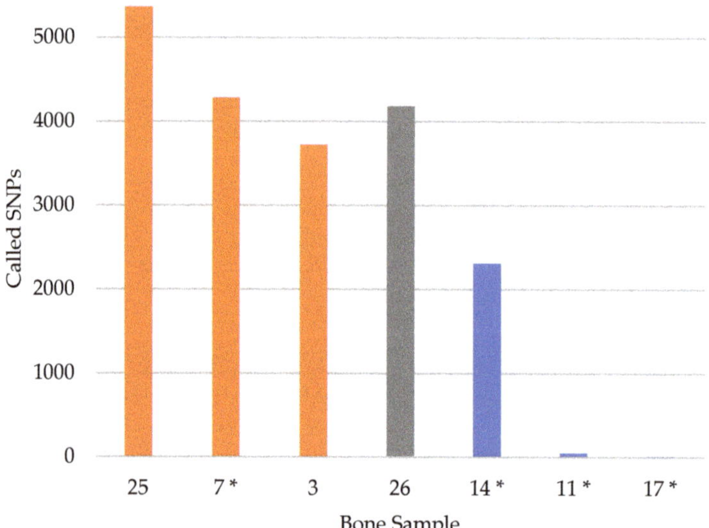

Figure 4. The number of called SNPs per bone sample (maximum 5422). An asterisk (*) represents the average number of called SNPs for a bone sample with multiple DNA extracts. The color indicates the DNA extraction method: orange = phenol chloroform isoamyl alcohol (PCIA) extracts purified with MinElute; gray = Dabney; blue = QIAquick.

In the absence of capture, the bone DNA extracts produced 2–1539 SNPs at 1X coverage and zero SNPs met the 10X calling threshold. These details and the remaining shotgun sequencing results are shown in Table S4. The proportion of reads aligning to the FORCE panel regions (i.e., mapped read specificity) was significantly increased by capture, from an average of 0.03% in the shotgun data to 11.4% in the capture data. The capture procedure thus resulted in a 380-fold increase in mapped read specificity over shotgun sequencing. Of note, shotgun sequencing of the four control DNAs produced only partial 10X FORCE SNP profiles. Thus, the capture enrichment was necessary for all samples, including references and control DNAs, in order to meet the 10X coverage requirement for SNP calling. The improved SNP profiling of the captured libraries demonstrates the efficacy of the enrichment step in obtaining on-target FORCE panel SNPs.

3.3. Concordance with Published SNP Data

Overall, 14,519 (99.97%) SNPs were concordant between the 14,524 called FORCE genotypes and published data of the four control DNA samples (Figure 5; Table S5). Complete concordance (100%) was observed for 2800M across the 170 SNPs overlapping called FORCE and expected ForenSeq genotypes. High concordance (99.98%) was also observed for both NA12877 and NA12878 when considering the called FORCE genotypes for each sample (5383 and 4576 SNPs, respectively). Though slightly lower, FORCE data of K562 produced concordant genotypes with published data at 99.93% of the 4395 compared SNPs.

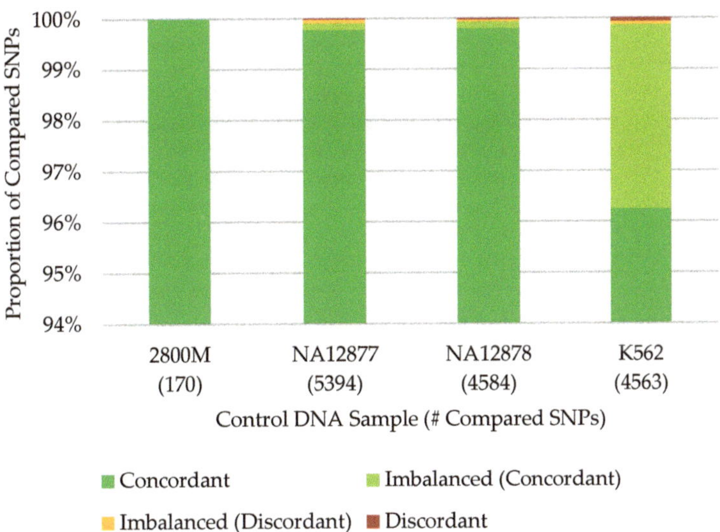

Figure 5. SNP concordance of FORCE capture data compared to published genotypes from the four control DNA samples.

The five discordant called FORCE genotypes were all kinship SNPs, and each discordance was observed in only one control DNA sample (Table S6). The greatest proportion of discordant calls (60%) was observed in the K562 data. Two of three discordant called SNPs produced high-coverage homozygote genotypes in the FORCE data, while heterozygote genotypes were observed in the published K562 BAM but with allele imbalance (MAF ~20%). The third K562 discordance may be the result of incorrect genotyping based on the published data, as all reads at the SNP location in the published BAM were forward-oriented and unpaired. The greater discordance observed in the K562 data compared to the other control samples is likely due to well-known immortalization effects [29] as well as lot-to-lot variability of this cell line [40]. For NA12877, there was one difference between the called FORCE SNP and the published data at rs229352. Insufficient coverage (<10X) at this same SNP was observed for many reference/control samples (n = 7). Interestingly, NA12878 and K562 were expected to be homozygous for the alternate allele (GG) at rs229352 based on the published data (this marker is not included in ForenSeq and therefore the expected genotype for 2800M is unknown). Analysis of the rs229352 bait design identified that the alternate allele (G) or left flank did not map under the stringent mapping parameters utilized in the developed workflow. Furthermore, review of the published BAM showed a 5-bp insertion located 30 bp upstream (5′) of the SNP on the reads with the G allele at rs229352. For NA12878, the discordant called SNP (rs662185) was identified as a poor performing SNP in Section 3.2, with nearly half (47.8%) of the reference/control samples failing to produce sufficient coverage (<10X) and an additional 17.4% with imbalanced genotypes (Table S3). In NA12878, significantly lower coverage (10X) was observed at rs662185 compared to the average coverage of the other FORCE SNPs (>250X for called SNPs; Table S2). Similar to rs229352, the published NA12878 BAM showed a 4-bp deletion associated with the G allele at rs662185 located 5 bp downstream (3′) of the SNP. Additionally, evaluation of the three baits for this marker (the right flank bait failed during design) revealed that the alternate allele bait included in the kit was incorrect (T instead of G). Inspection of the baits for all targets identified an additional 522 markers with the incorrect alternate allele. However, these errors in the bait design appeared to have little to no impact on the SNP performance, as only seven (1.3%) of the 523 SNPs with the wrong alternate allele bait performed poorly (<75% called) in reference/control samples (Table S3). Therefore, the discordances observed at rs229352 and rs662185 are likely due to the indel clusters associated with the alternate allele, which may impact the probe hybridization efficacy and/or prevent mapping under the stringent parameters applied.

Though not utilized for other analyses in this study, the concordance of the 187 observed genotypes at imbalanced FORCE SNPs was assessed for the four control DNA samples. It is noted that 95.19% (178) of the observed imbalanced genotypes were consistent with the published data (Table S5). Unsurprisingly, a majority (168 of 187; ~90%) of the imbalanced genotypes were detected in K562 (Table S5). As stated above, stochastic variation is expected in the K562 cell line, resulting in allele imbalance and loss of heterozygosity [29]. Furthermore, these cell line artifacts may be exacerbated by the relatively low input (1 ng) into library preparation [10]. Of the nine discordances found in the imbalanced genotypes, rs169250 accounted for three instances. The imbalanced FORCE genotypes at rs169250 were discordant for three of the control DNA samples (NA12877, NA12878, and K562; this marker is not targeted by ForenSeq and therefore no published genotype was available for 2800M). Further investigation of the BAMs revealed that rs169250 is located in the middle of a 12-bp polycytosine stretch, and thus the complexity of the region for sequencing and/or alignment likely caused discordant genotypes. As a result, future designs of the FORCE panel may exclude rs169250 to ensure successful and accurate genotyping. The remaining imbalanced FORCE genotypes for NA12877 ($n = 3$) and NA12878 ($n = 1$) that were discordant with the published data appear to be the result of non-specific mapping in the FORCE data. The last two discordances involving imbalanced FORCE genotypes were found in K562. One appeared to be the result of non-specific mapping in the published BAM (rs241408), while the other (rs7117433) could not be resolved and may be due to cell line artifacts previously discussed.

In the end, considering both called and imbalanced FORCE genotypes, a total of 99.90% (14,697 out of 14,711) SNPs were in agreement between the FORCE and published control DNA datasets (Table S5). There were, however, a total of 69 genotypes could not be compared out of a maximum of 14,780 possible SNPs (Table S5) because no call was possible for the FORCE or published data (<10X). Most (68) of the failed SNPs were observed in the FORCE data, while one SNP for K562 had low coverage (5X) in the published BAM that prevented the associated published genotype from being confirmed. The number of failed SNPs varied by sample: two of 172 SNPs for 2800M, nine of 4593 SNPs for NA12878, 28 of 5422 SNPs for NA12877, and 30 of 4593 SNPs for K562. Of note, FORCE data from all four control DNA samples failed to produce called genotypes for 16 SNPs. Thirteen of these SNPs failed to produce sufficient coverage for any samples (Table S3), as previously noted in Section 3.2. The three additional poor performing SNPs included two X-SNPs and one Y-SNP. Most (~70%) reference samples failed to produce called genotypes at the two X-SNPs, with no called data in the bone samples. The Y-SNP produced greater reference/control samples success (>65% of male references/controls with a called genotype), but 0% SNP recovery for the bone samples.

Published and FORCE data for JB55, the only bone sample evaluated for concordance, enabled the comparison of 153 SNPs. Sixteen of the 169 overlapping SNPs were excluded from comparison due to insufficient coverage (<10X) in the published Precision ID data. JB55 had 151 of 153 (98.69%) concordant genotypes, and two discordant aiSNPs were observed (Table S6). The FORCE genotype (CC) for the first discordant marker (rs1879488) was inconsistent with the highest coverage Precision ID replicate from the published study (AC with 395X in replicate 2); however, the FORCE results were concordant with the replicate with slightly lower coverage (CC with 236X in replicate 1). The second difference was observed at a SNP with low coverage in both Precision ID replicates (8X and 16X), potentially the result of non-specific amplification and/or mapping. In the case of these two discordant SNPs, stricter parameters such as a higher coverage threshold or heterozygote threshold than what was used for the previous JB55 study ($\geq$6X and $\geq$10% MAF) [12] may have improved the concordance for JB55.

3.4. Ancestry, Phenotype, and Y Haplogroup Predictions

The completeness of the reference and control sample profiles allowed for ancestry, phenotype, and Y-chromosomal haplogroup predictions, which were consistent with available metadata (Table S7). The predictive results from the bone sample DNA extracts were much more variable due to the wide range of SNPs obtained. As an example of the bone sample data, the ancestry of sample 7.2 was predicted to be 100% European from 210 called aiSNPs (Figure 6). Phenotype predictions were also possible for this bone sample (7.2) using 33 called piSNPs, which estimated blue eyes (93.2% probability), blond-brown hair (66.0% and 27.4% probabilities, respectively), light hair shade (92.8% probability), and pale-intermediate skin (54.1% and 41.6% probabilities, respectively). The Y haplogroup was predicted to be R1a1a1b1a2b~ from 370 Y-SNPs, which was the same Y haplogroup that was predicted for the paternal nephew (sample 4). These predictions were possible even with the partial SNP profile (4165, or 76.8%, of possible 5422 called SNPs) generated from this degraded USS *Oklahoma* sample. Thus, hybridization capture was effective in producing sufficient SNPs from the multiple marker types included within the FORCE panel to allow for predictive information to be gained.

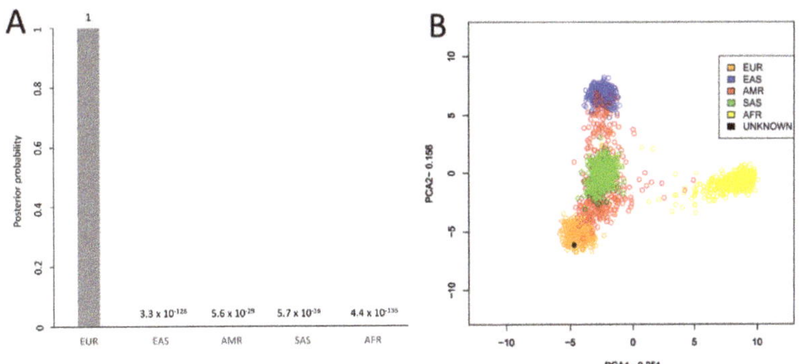

Figure 6. An illustration of ancestry predictions, here exemplified with predictions for sample 7.2. Individuals from the 1000 Genomes project (grouped into the five different continental groups: EUR (European), EAS (East Asian), AMR (American), SAS (South Asian), and AFR (African)) were used as reference data. (**A**) Posterior probabilities using a naïve Bayes approach; (**B**) Prediction using a PCA.

3.5. Kinship Predictions

The related reference to reference sample kinship prediction results are shown in Figure 7. The first degree (parent/offspring and full sibling) predictions produced log 10 LRs from 287.7–439.3 with well over 99.99% posterior probabilities, demonstrating extremely strong statistical support of these predictions. The log 10 LRs for the third degree reference to reference predictions were 34.4 and 37.8 with over 99.99% posterior probability, indicating very strong statistical support. The two fifth degree relationship predictions produced log 10 LRs of 3.8 and 6.5, with 99.98% and 99.99% posterior probabilities, respectively. Thus, the kinship analysis was capable of correctly predicting fifth degree relatives from reference quality FORCE panel profiles. The two sixth degree relationship predictions were supported with over 99% posterior probability, but with log 10 LRs of 2.2 and 2.6, indicating moderate statistical support. Considering the four examples of fifth–sixth degree relationships, log 10 LRs corresponding to moderate statistical support [41] were obtained in a majority (75%) of the fifth–sixth degree comparisons. Interestingly, sample 4 (fifth degree comparison) had the lowest SNP recovery of the references (95%) and sample 8 (sixth degree comparison) also had reduced SNP recovery (98%). All but one of the remaining references had >99% complete FORCE profiles (sample 13 at 98%). Therefore, the ability to obtain stronger statistical support for these more distant degrees of relatedness (as in the case of samples 4 and 8) could be possible when complete FORCE panel profiles are obtained. Regardless, the simulation studies indicated considerable overlap in expected versus unrelated relationships when testing 5th degree relatives and beyond. When pairwise kinship predictions were performed in a blind search fashion allowing up to either third degree or sixth degree relatedness, zero incorrect (false positive) relationships with strong statistical support were observed (Table S8).

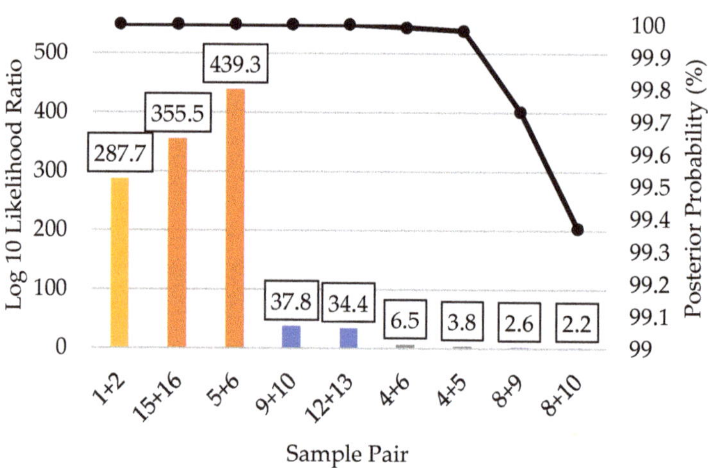

Figure 7. Pairwise kinship prediction log 10 likelihood ratio (LR) (left y-axis; bars) and posterior probabilities (right y-axis; black line) of reference-to-reference comparisons. All predictions compared the expected (known) relationships vs. unrelated. Parent/offspring = yellow (sample pair 1 + 2); full siblings = orange (sample pairs 15 + 16 and 5 + 6); third degree = blue (sample pairs 9 + 10 and 12 + 13); fifth degree = gray (sample pairs 4 + 6 and 4 + 5); and sixth degree = purple (sample pairs 8 + 9 and 8 + 10).

Unknown to reference pairwise kinship predictions from bone sample DNA extracts that produced 1000 (~25%) or more kinship SNPs are presented in Figure 8. Similar to what was observed in the reference to reference pairwise comparisons, the unknown to reference full sibling predictions had extremely strong statistical support. The log 10 LRs of these first degree relationship predictions were 120.7 and 492.8, with posterior probabilities over 99.99%. The three second degree relationship predictions produced log 10 LRs between 65.4 and 82.3 and posterior probabilities over 99.99%, also indicating extremely strong statistical support. Two of the three third degree relationship predictions (for sample pairs 3 + 1 and 14.1 + 13) were consistent with the reference to reference predictions. These two had log 10 LRs of 32.8 and 41.1 with posterior probabilities over 99.99%, indicating extremely strong statistical support. The other third degree prediction (14.2 + 13) also had a posterior probability over 99.99% but with a log 10 LR of 5.5, which was much lower than that of the other two third degree predictions. This LR indicating strong statistical support was made from a bone sample profile with only 1324 (33.7%) kinship SNPs. It is likely that a higher LR would have been obtained if sample 14.2 had greater SNP recovery. The four fourth degree relationship predictions had log 10 LRs from 4.5 to 11.8, and all had posterior probabilities over 99.99%. These fourth degree unknown to reference predictions would be classified as having strong to very strong support.

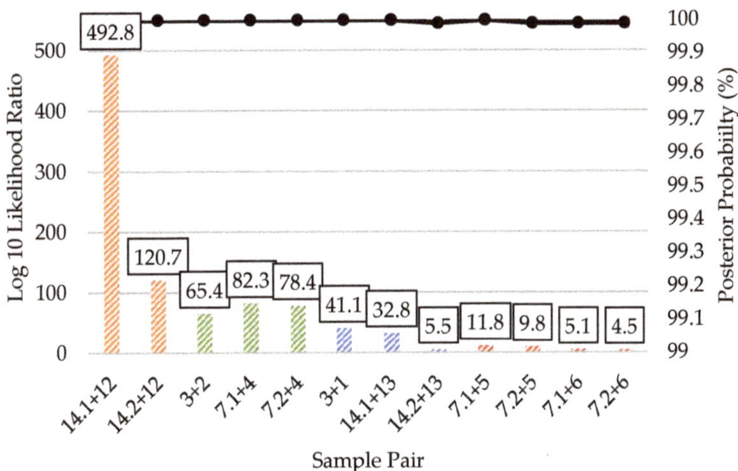

Figure 8. Pairwise kinship prediction log 10 likelihood ratio (LR) (left y-axis; bars) and posterior probabilities (right y-axis; black line) of unknown to reference comparisons. Results are presented for each bone sample DNA extract that produced 1000 (~25%) or more kinship SNPs. All predictions compared the expected (known) relationships vs. unrelated. Full siblings = orange (sample pairs 14.1 + 12 and 14.2 + 12); second degree = green (sample pairs 3 + 2, 7.1 + 4, and 7.2 + 4); third degree = blue (sample pairs 3 + 1, 14.1 + 13, and 14.2 + 13); fourth degree = red (sample pairs 7.1 + 5, 7.2 + 5, 7.1 + 6, and 7.2 + 6).

The five bone sample DNA profiles with >25% kinship SNPs were utilized for kinship predictions in a pedigree scenario, as presented in Figure 9. All of the predicted relationships indicated relatedness between the unknown and the expected family members. These pedigree scenario relationship predictions were supported by log 10 LRs greater than 91.3 (and up to 503.7) with posterior probabilities exceeding 99.99%. Thus, the pedigree scenarios yielded extremely strong statistical support when bone sample profiles yielded ~25% or more kinship SNPs.

When bone sample profiles produced minimal SNP data (10–247 kinship SNPs), the kinship predictions were expectedly weaker overall (Figure 10). Only two bone sample profiles yielded predictions that would indicate strong statistical support, and both involved first degree relationships. Unknown (bone) sample 11.2 had 73 kinship SNPs, and its parent/offspring relationship with sample 10 was strongly supported by a log 10 LR of 5.2 and a posterior probability > 99.99%. Sample 14.3 had 247 kinship SNPs, and its full sibling relationship with sample 12 was very strongly supported by a log 10 LR of 15.8 and posterior probability > 99.99%. The remaining six relationship pairs shown in Figure 10 had low log 10 LRs (1.2 or less) and posterior probabilities (<95%). The pedigree scenario kinship predictions did not significantly improve the log 10 LRs or posterior probabilities of the bone sample profiles with 10–247 called SNPs (Figure 11). Additionally, samples 17.1 and 17.2 yielded <15 kinship SNPs each, with some SNPs that were inconsistent with the profiles of the associated child reference (one son and one daughter of the unknown) in these parent/offspring relationships. As a result of the poor SNP recovery, bone samples 17.1 and 17.2 were excluded altogether from the pairwise and pedigree scenario kinship predictions. Regardless of the number of kinship SNPs in the bone sample profiles, there were no incorrect (false positive) relationship predictions between unknowns and unrelated reference samples with strong statistical support in blind search scenarios (Table S9).

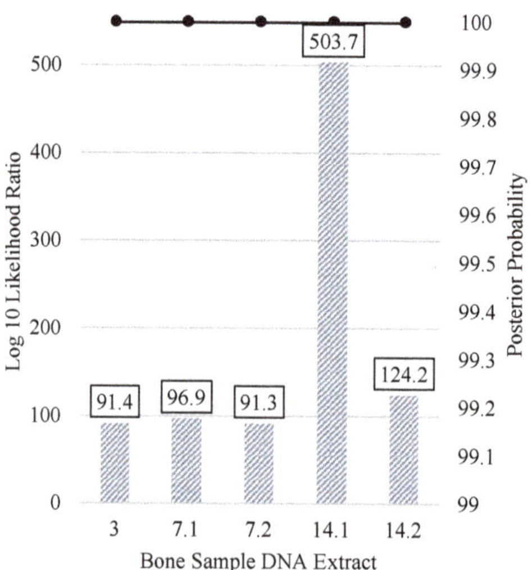

Figure 9. Pedigree scenario kinship prediction results of all bone samples with more than 1000 (~25%) kinship SNPs. All predictions compared the unknown when situated in the expected (known) pedigree vs. unrelated. The log 10 likelihood ratio (LR) (left y-axis; bars) and posterior probabilities (right y-axis; black line) are shown.

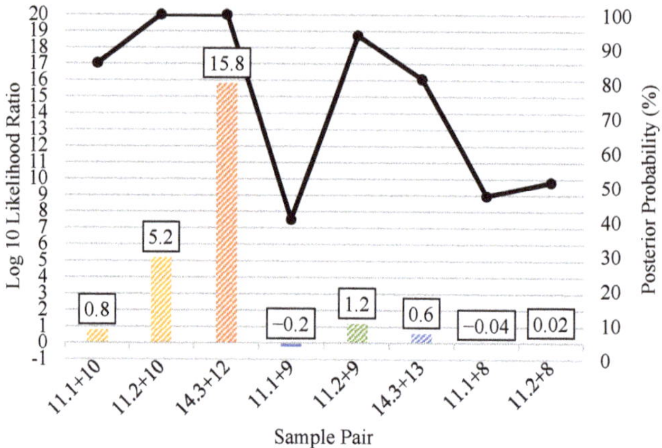

Figure 10. Pairwise kinship prediction log 10 likelihood ratio (LR) (left y-axis; bars) and posterior probabilities (right y-axis; black line) of unknown to reference comparisons. Results are presented for each bone sample DNA extract that produced 10–247 kinship SNPs (all results <25% called SNPs). Samples 17.1 and 17.2 yielded <15 kinship SNP calls that were inconsistent with the expected parent/offspring relationships; therefore 17.1 and 17.2 and were excluded altogether. All predictions compared the expected (known) relationships vs. unrelated. Parent/offspring = yellow (sample pairs 11.1 + 10 and 11.2 + 10), full siblings = orange (sample pair 14.3 + 12); second degree = green (sample pairs 11.1 + 9 and 11.2 + 9); third degree = blue (sample pair 14.3 + 13); and fifth degree = gray (sample pairs 11.1 + 8 and 11.2 + 8).

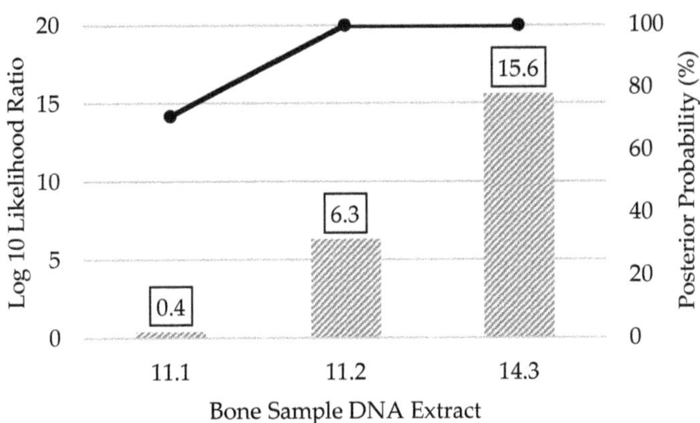

Figure 11. Pedigree scenario kinship prediction results of bone sample DNA extracts that produced 10–247 kinship SNPs. All predictions compared the expected (known) pedigree vs. unrelated. The log 10 likelihood ratio (LR) (left y-axis; bars) and posterior probabilities (right y-axis; black line) are shown. Samples 17.1 and 17.2 yielded <15 kinship SNP calls that were inconsistent with the expected parent/offspring relationships; therefore, 17.1 and 17.2 were excluded altogether.

Supplementary to the autosomal SNPs, 246 X-SNPs were targeted in the panel for kinship testing in specific case contexts. The X-SNPs included in the panel were used to connect individual 12 with the remains from individual 14.1 in family D. The log 10 LR (for them being full siblings versus being unrelated) was calculated to be 6.7 and a posterior probability > 99.99%; thus, the X-SNP data showed to be clearly informative in the case example. The use of X-chromosomal data may be especially informative in kinship testing due to its particular mode of inheritance. For example, when comparing two alleged paternal half-sisters or an alleged paternal grandmother and a granddaughter, the exclusion power for X-chromosomal markers are not zero, in contrast to autosomal markers [17].

4. Conclusions

This study demonstrates the utility of the 5422-SNP FORCE panel for forensic applications. This panel was designed to exclude clinically relevant markers to alleviate privacy concerns with DNA databanking. The SNPs included in the FORCE panel are found on microarray genotyping chips used for genetic genealogy, enabling cross-compatibility with externally produced data that will be useful in validation studies. Moreover, large reference databases are available for all of the markers included in the kit, unlike other marker types such as microhaplotypes. The FORCE panel includes kinship SNPs with forensic iiSNPs, aiSNPs, piSNPs, Y-SNPs, and X-SNPs. The hybridization capture method was capable of recovering SNP profiles from high quality reference and historical bone samples alike. A high degree of concordance (>99.9%) was observed when comparing FORCE profiles with previously published data. The few underperforming SNPs that were identified in the present study can be removed from future designs of the FORCE panel to improve efficiency. Ancestry and phenotype predictions were possible and consistent with self-reported data from reference sample donors. Additionally, high-resolution Y-haplogroup prediction was possible from 829 Y-SNPs. The novel kinship marker set of 3931 SNPs was shown to be effective for 4th degree relationship predictions with strong statistical support. Furthermore, known case examples involving previously identified WWII service members and associated family reference samples resulted in kinship predictions consistent with expected relationships. Future efforts involving the FORCE panel will entail an inter-laboratory study incorporating alternate enrichment methods for SNP profiling. This will be pertinent before the FORCE panel can be used in routine casework.

Supplementary Materials: The following are available online at https://www.mdpi.com/article/10.3390/genes12121968/s1, Table S1: The 5446 SNPs targeted by the α version of the custom FORCE capture panel; Table S2: Detailed sequencing and SNP coverage metrics after FORCE capture; Table S3: SNPs with called FORCE genotypes for less than 75% of the reference/control samples; Table S4: Shotgun sequencing and SNP coverage metrics; Table S5: Concordance of FORCE genotypes and published genotypes for the four control DNA samples as well as historical bone sample JB55; Table S6: Discordances observed between the FORCE and published genotypes of the four control DNA samples and historical bone sample JB55; Table S7: Ancestry, phenotype, and Y-chromosomal haplogroup predictions of reference and control DNA samples; Table S8: Blind search reference to reference pairwise comparison results; Table S9: Blind search unknown to reference pairwise comparison results; Figure S1: Pedigree scenarios evaluated for the five WWII cases; Figure S2: Additional kinship simulations; Figure S3: SNP coverage based on the number of baits.

Author Contributions: Conceptualization, A.T., K.S.-A. and C.M.; kinship SNP selection and simulations, A.T.; hybridization capture panel design, K.S.-A. in collaboration with Arbor Biosciences; hybridization capture data generation, J.D.-H. and J.T.T.; formal analysis, A.T., K.S.-A. and C.M.; writing—original draft preparation, A.T., K.S.-A., J.D.-H. and C.M.; writing—review and editing, all authors. All authors have read and agreed to the published version of the manuscript.

Funding: This research received no external funding.

Institutional Review Board Statement: The study was conducted in accordance with the guidelines of the Declaration of Helsinki, and approved by the Defense Health Agency Office of Research Protections on 20 November 2020 (Protocol # DHQ-20-2073).

Informed Consent Statement: All living sample donors provided informed consent for their samples to be used in research and quality improvement activities.

Data Availability Statement: Data are stored at the AFMES-AFDIL and may be made available to approved laboratories upon written request.

Acknowledgments: The authors would like to thank Timothy McMahon (AFMES-AFDIL) for administrative support and resources; Ursula Zipperer for anonymizing samples; Cassandra R. Taylor for assistance with laboratory experiments.

Conflicts of Interest: The authors declare no conflict of interest.

Disclaimer: The assertions herein are those of the authors and do not necessarily represent the official position of the United States Department of Defense, the Defense Health Agency, or its entities including the Armed Forces Medical Examiner System. Any mention of commercial products was done for scientific transparency and should not be viewed as an endorsement of the product or manufacturer.

References

1. Butler, J.M.; Hill, C.R. Biology and Genetics of New Autosomal STR Loci Useful for Forensic DNA Analysis. *Forensic Sci. Rev.* **2012**, *24*, 15–26.
2. Kling, D.; Phillips, C.; Kennett, D.; Tillmar, A. Investigative genetic genealogy: Current methods, knowledge and practice. *Forensic Sci. Int. Genet.* **2021**, *52*, 102474. [CrossRef] [PubMed]
3. Erlich, Y.; Shor, T.; Pe'er, I.; Carmi, S. Identity inference of genomic data using long-range familial searches. *Science* **2018**, *362*, 690–694. [CrossRef]
4. GEDmatch. Available online: https://pro.gedmatch.com/user/login (accessed on 11 November 2021).
5. Greytak, E.M.; Moore, C.; Armentrout, S.L. Genetic genealogy for cold case and active investigations. *Forensic Sci. Int.* **2019**, *299*, 103–113. [CrossRef]
6. Tillmar, A.; Fagerholm, S.A.; Staaf, J.; Sjolund, P.; Ansell, R. Getting the conclusive lead with investigative genetic genealogy—A successful case study of a 16 year old double murder in Sweden. *Forensic Sci. Int. Genet.* **2021**, *53*, 102525. [CrossRef] [PubMed]
7. Cuenca, D.; Battaglia, J.; Halsing, M.; Sheehan, S. Mitochondrial Sequencing of Missing Persons DNA Casework by Implementing Thermo Fisher's Precision ID mtDNA Whole Genome Assay. *Genes* **2020**, *11*, 1303. [CrossRef]
8. Holt, C.L.; Stephens, K.M.; Walichiewicz, P.; Fleming, K.D.; Forouzmand, E.; Wu, S.F. Human Mitochondrial Control Region and mtGenome: Design and Forensic Validation of NGS Multiplexes, Sequencing and Analytical Software. *Genes* **2021**, *12*, 599. [CrossRef] [PubMed]

9. Eduardoff, M.; Xavier, C.; Strobl, C.; Casas-Vargas, A.; Parson, W. Optimized mtDNA Control Region Primer Extension Capture Analysis for Forensically Relevant Samples and Highly Compromised mtDNA of Different Age and Origin. *Genes* **2017**, *8*, 237. [CrossRef]

10. Marshall, C.; Sturk-Andreaggi, K.; Daniels-Higginbotham, J.; Oliver, R.S.; Barritt-Ross, S.; McMahon, T.P. Performance evaluation of a mitogenome capture and Illumina sequencing protocol using non-probative, case-type skeletal samples: Implications for the use of a positive control in a next-generation sequencing procedure. *Forensic Sci. Int. Genet.* **2017**, *31*, 198–206. [CrossRef]

11. Bose, N.; Carlberg, K.; Sensabaugh, G.; Erlich, H.; Calloway, C. Target capture enrichment of nuclear SNP markers for massively parallel sequencing of degraded and mixed samples. *Forensic Sci. Int. Genet.* **2018**, *34*, 186–196. [CrossRef]

12. Daniels-Higginbotham, J.; Gorden, E.M.; Farmer, S.K.; Spatola, B.; Damann, F.; Bellantoni, N.; Gagnon, K.S.; de la Puente, M.; Xavier, C.; Walsh, S.; et al. DNA Testing Reveals the Putative Identity of JB55, a 19th Century Vampire Buried in Griswold, Connecticut. *Genes* **2019**, *10*, 636. [CrossRef]

13. Marshall, C.; Sturk-Andreaggi, K.; Gorden, E.M.; Daniels-Higginbotham, J.; Sanchez, S.G.; Basic, Z.; Kruzic, I.; Andelinovic, S.; Bosnar, A.; Coklo, M.; et al. A Forensic Genomics Approach for the Identification of Sister Marija Crucifiksa Kozulic. *Genes* **2020**, *11*, 938. [CrossRef]

14. Gorden, E.M.; Greytak, E.M.; Sturk-Andreaggi, K.; Cady, J.; McMahon, T.P.; Armentrout, S.; Marshall, C. Ex-tended kinship analysis of historical remains using SNP capture. *Forensic Sci. Int. Genet.* **2021**, *57*, 102636. [CrossRef]

15. Turchi, C.; Previdere, C.; Bini, C.; Carnevali, E.; Grignani, P.; Manfredi, A.; Melchionda, F.; Onofri, V.; Pelotti, S.; Robino, C.; et al. Assessment of the Precision ID Identity Panel kit on challenging forensic samples. *Forensic Sci. Int. Genet.* **2020**, *49*, 102400. [CrossRef] [PubMed]

16. Ralf, A.; van Oven, M.; Montiel Gonzalez, D.; de Knijff, P.; van der Beek, K.; Wootton, S.; Lagace, R.; Kayser, M. Forensic Y-SNP analysis beyond SNaPshot: High-resolution Y-chromosomal haplogrouping from low quality and quantity DNA using Ion AmpliSeq and targeted massively parallel sequencing. *Forensic Sci. Int. Genet.* **2019**, *41*, 93–106. [CrossRef]

17. Tillmar, A.O.; Kling, D.; Butler, J.M.; Parson, W.; Prinz, M.; Schneider, P.M.; Egeland, T.; Gusmao, L. DNA Commission of the International Society for Forensic Genetics (ISFG): Guidelines on the use of X-STRs in kinship analysis. *Forensic Sci. Int. Genet.* **2017**, *29*, 269–275. [CrossRef] [PubMed]

18. Genomes Project, C.; Auton, A.; Brooks, L.D.; Durbin, R.M.; Garrison, E.P.; Kang, H.M.; Korbel, J.O.; Marchini, J.L.; McCarthy, S.; McVean, G.A.; et al. A global reference for human genetic variation. *Nature* **2015**, *526*, 68–74. [CrossRef]

19. Grandell, I.; Samara, R.; Tillmar, A.O. A SNP panel for identity and kinship testing using massive parallel sequencing. *Int. J. Legal Med.* **2016**, *130*, 905–914. [CrossRef]

20. Xavier, C.; de la Puente, M.; Mosquera-Miguel, A.; Freire-Aradas, A.; Kalamara, V.; Vidaki, A.; Gross, T.E.; Revoir, A.; Pospiech, E.; Kartasinska, E.; et al. Development and validation of the VISAGE AmpliSeq basic tool to predict appearance and ancestry from DNA. *Forensic Sci. Int. Genet.* **2020**, *48*, 102336. [CrossRef] [PubMed]

21. Kalia, S.S.; Adelman, K.; Bale, S.J.; Chung, W.K.; Eng, C.; Evans, J.P.; Herman, G.E.; Hufnagel, S.B.; Klein, T.E.; Korf, B.R.; et al. Recommendations for reporting of secondary findings in clinical exome and genome sequencing, 2016 update (ACMG SF v2.0): A policy statement of the American College of Medical Genetics and Genomics. *Genet. Med. Off. J. Am. Coll. Med. Genet.* **2017**, *19*, 249–255. [CrossRef]

22. Altschul, S.F.; Gish, W.; Miller, W.; Myers, E.W.; Lipman, D.J. Basic local alignment search tool. *J. Mol. Biol.* **1990**, *215*, 403–410. [CrossRef]

23. Abecasis, G.R.; Cherny, S.S.; Cookson, W.O.; Cardon, L.R. Merlin–rapid analysis of dense genetic maps using sparse gene flow trees. *Nat. Genet.* **2002**, *30*, 97–101. [CrossRef]

24. Matise, T.C.; Chen, F.; Chen, W.; De La Vega, F.M.; Hansen, M.; He, C.; Hyland, F.C.; Kennedy, G.C.; Kong, X.; Murray, S.S.; et al. A second-generation combined linkage physical map of the human genome. *Genome Res.* **2007**, *17*, 1783–1786. [CrossRef]

25. R Core Team. *R: A Language and Environment for Statistical Computing*; R Foundation for Statistical Computing: Vienna, Austria, 2013.

26. Edson, S.M. Extraction of DNA from Skeletonized Postcranial Remains: A Discussion of Protocols and Testing Modalities. *J. Forensic Sci.* **2019**, *64*, 1312–1323. [CrossRef] [PubMed]

27. Rohland, N.; Glocke, I.; Aximu-Petri, A.; Meyer, M. Extraction of highly degraded DNA from ancient bones, teeth and sediments for high-throughput sequencing. *Nat. Protoc.* **2018**, *13*, 2447–2461. [CrossRef] [PubMed]

28. *ForenSeq DNA Signature Prep Reference Guide, Rev C*; Verogen: San Diego, CA, USA, 2020.

29. Zhou, B.; Ho, S.S.; Greer, S.U.; Zhu, X.; Bell, J.M.; Arthur, J.G.; Spies, N.; Zhang, X.; Byeon, S.; Pattni, R.; et al. Comprehensive, integrated, and phased whole-genome analysis of the primary ENCODE cell line K562. *Genome Res.* **2019**, *29*, 472–484. [CrossRef] [PubMed]

30. Illumina Platinum Genomes. Available online: https://www.illumina.com/platinumgenomes.html (accessed on 13 November 2021).

31. Eberle, M.A.; Fritzilas, E.; Krusche, P.; Kallberg, M.; Moore, B.L.; Bekritsky, M.A.; Iqbal, Z.; Chuang, H.Y.; Humphray, S.J.; Halpern, A.L.; et al. A reference data set of 5.4 million phased human variants validated by genetic inheritance from sequencing a three-generation 17-member pedigree. *Genome Res.* **2017**, *27*, 157–164. [CrossRef] [PubMed]

32. Prcomp. Available online: https://stat.ethz.ch/R-manual/R-devel/library/stats/html/prcomp.html (accessed on 13 November 2021).

33. Santos, C.; Phillips, C.; Gomez-Tato, A.; Alvarez-Dios, J.; Carracedo, A.; Lareu, M.V. Inference of Ancestry in Forensic Analysis II: Analysis of Genetic Data. *Methods Mol. Biol.* **2016**, *1420*, 255–285. [CrossRef]
34. de la Puente, M.; Ruiz-Ramirez, J.; Ambroa-Conde, A.; Xavier, C.; Pardo-Seco, J.; Alvarez-Dios, J.; Freire-Aradas, A.; Mosquera-Miguel, A.; Gross, T.E.; Cheung, E.Y.Y.; et al. Development and Evaluation of the Ancestry Informative Marker Panel of the VISAGE Basic Tool. *Genes* **2021**, *12*, 1284. [CrossRef] [PubMed]
35. Chaitanya, L.; Breslin, K.; Zuniga, S.; Wirken, L.; Pospiech, E.; Kukla-Bartoszek, M.; Sijen, T.; Knijff, P.; Liu, F.; Branicki, W.; et al. The HIrisPlex-S system for eye, hair and skin colour prediction from DNA: Introduction and forensic developmental validation. *Forensic Sci. Int. Genet.* **2018**, *35*, 123–135. [CrossRef]
36. Hpsconvertsonline. Available online: https://walshlab.sitehost.iu.edu/hpsconvertsonline.R (accessed on 13 November 2021).
37. HirisPlex-S System Webtool. Available online: https://hirisplex.erasmusmc.nl/ (accessed on 13 November 2021).
38. Ralf, A.; Gonzalez, D.M.; Zhong, K.; Kayser, M. Yleaf: Software for Human Y-Chromosomal Haplogroup Inference from Next-Generation Sequencing Data. *Mol. Biol. Evol.* **2018**, *35*, 1820. [CrossRef] [PubMed]
39. Yleaf Position File. Available online: https://github.com/genid/Yleaf/blob/master/Position_files/WGS_hg38.txt (accessed on 13 November 2021).
40. Dimery, I.W.; Ross, D.D.; Testa, J.R.; Gupta, S.K.; Felsted, R.L.; Pollak, A.; Bachur, N.R. Variation amongst K562 cell cultures. *Exp. Hematol.* **1983**, *11*, 601–610. [PubMed]
41. SWGDAM. *Recommendations of the SWGDAM ad hoc Working Group on Genotyping Results Reported as Likelihood Ratios*; Federal Bureau of Investigation's Scientific Working Group on DNA Analysis Methods (SWGDAM): Quantico, VA, USA, 2018.

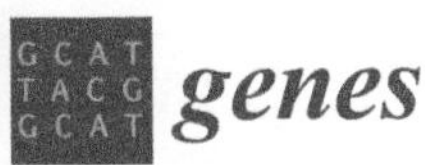

Article

Ancient DNA Methods Improve Forensic DNA Profiling of Korean War and World War II Unknowns

Elena I. Zavala [1,*,†], Jacqueline Tyler Thomas [2,3,†], Kimberly Sturk-Andreaggi [2,3,4], Jennifer Daniels-Higginbotham [2,3], Kerriann K. Meyers [2,3], Suzanne Barrit-Ross [2], Ayinuer Aximu-Petri [1], Julia Richter [1], Birgit Nickel [1], Gregory E. Berg [5], Timothy P. McMahon [2,3], Matthias Meyer [1] and Charla Marshall [2,3,6,*]

1   Department of Evolutionary Genetics, Max Planck Institute for Evolutionary Anthropology, 04103 Leipzig, Germany; aximu_ayinuer@eva.mpg.de (A.A.-P.); julia_richter@eva.mpg.de (J.R.); nickel@eva.mpg.de (B.N.); mmeyer@eva.mpg.de (M.M.)
2   Armed Forces Medical Examiner System's Armed Forces DNA Identification Laboratory (AFMES-AFDIL), Dover Air Force Base, Dover, DE 19902, USA; jacqueline.t.thomas2.ctr@mail.mil (J.T.T.); kimberly.s.andreaggi.ctr@mail.mil (K.S.-A.); jennifer.l.higginbotham3.ctr@mail.mil (J.D.-H.); kerriann.k.meyers.ctr@mail.mil (K.K.M.); suzanne.m.barritt-ross.civ@mail.mil (S.B.-R.); Timothy.p.mcmahon10.civ@mail.mil (T.P.M.)
3   SNA International, Contractor Supporting the Armed Forces Medical Examiner System, Alexandria, VA 22314, USA
4   Department of Immunology, Genetics and Pathology, Uppsala University, SE-751 08 Uppsala, Sweden
5   Defense Personnel Accounting Agency, Central Identification Laboratory, Hickam Air Force Base, Oahu, HI 96853, USA; gregory.e.berg2.civ@mail.mil
6   Forensic Science Program, Pennsylvania State University, State College, PA 16802, USA
*   Correspondence: elena_zavala@eva.mpg.de (E.I.Z.); charla.k.marshall.ctr@mail.mil (C.M.)
†   These authors contributed equally to this work.

Citation: Zavala, E.I.; Thomas, J.T.; Sturk-Andreaggi, K.; Daniels-Higginbotham, J.; Meyers, K.K.; Barrit-Ross, S.; Aximu-Petri, A.; Richter, J.; Nickel, B.; Berg, G.E.; et al. Ancient DNA Methods Improve Forensic DNA Profiling of Korean War and World War II Unknowns. *Genes* **2022**, *13*, 129. https://doi.org/10.3390/genes13010129

Academic Editor: Niels Morling

Received: 15 December 2021
Accepted: 7 January 2022
Published: 11 January 2022

Publisher's Note: MDPI stays neutral with regard to jurisdictional claims in published maps and institutional affiliations.

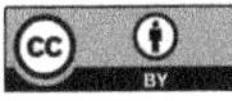

Abstract: The integration of massively parallel sequencing (MPS) technology into forensic casework has been of particular benefit to the identification of unknown military service members. However, highly degraded or chemically treated skeletal remains often fail to provide usable DNA profiles, even with sensitive mitochondrial (mt) DNA capture and MPS methods. In parallel, the ancient DNA field has developed workflows specifically for degraded DNA, resulting in the successful recovery of nuclear DNA and mtDNA from skeletal remains as well as sediment over 100,000 years old. In this study we use a set of disinterred skeletal remains from the Korean War and World War II to test if ancient DNA extraction and library preparation methods improve forensic DNA profiling. We identified an ancient DNA extraction protocol that resulted in the recovery of significantly more human mtDNA fragments than protocols previously used in casework. In addition, utilizing single-stranded rather than double-stranded library preparation resulted in increased attainment of reportable mtDNA profiles. This study emphasizes that the combination of ancient DNA extraction and library preparation methods evaluated here increases the success rate of DNA profiling, and likelihood of identifying historical remains.

Keywords: degraded DNA; massively parallel sequencing (MPS); mitochondrial DNA; forensic DNA profiling; ancient DNA; human identification

1. Introduction

Massively parallel sequencing (MPS), also known as next-generation sequencing (NGS), has only recently begun integration into the forensic field. MPS was first accepted in a court case in the Netherlands in 2019 [1]. The technology has also been approved for use within the U.S. criminal justice system for both STR profiling and mitochondrial (mt) DNA sequencing [2]. Furthermore, whole genome (shotgun) sequencing and genome-wide SNP arrays are often used for investigative genetic genealogy to provide leads in active and cold cases [3]. While more challenging cases involving historical skeletal remains, including historical figures, unmarked graves, and unidentified war victims, have seen some advances in DNA profiling with MPS, success rates are still low [4–6]. This may be due to the fact that successful forensic DNA profiling typically requires relatively large DNA fragments (greater than ~100 base pairs) with current methods, which are not always available in sufficient number in degraded samples.

One set of historical remains that exemplifies the challenges faced by historical identification cases is Unknowns from the Korean War buried in the National Memorial Cemetery of the Pacific (NMCP) in Honolulu, Hawaii [7]. These remains contain poorly preserved DNA due to extensive chemical treatment that was standard postmortem military practice in the 1940s and 1950s. The war dead were initially collected in temporary graves (Figure 1a) by the Army Graves Registration Service. They were then transferred to the United Nations Cemetery in Tanggok, Republic of Korea [8,9] where they were treated with insecticide and deodorant. The remains were subsequently shipped to the Army's Central Identification Unit in Kokura, Japan [7,10]. At this location, the remains were soaked in 40–50% formaldehyde solution for three to five days (Figure 1b). Formaldehyde is known to lead to the formation of cross-linked complexes between DNA molecules or between DNA and proteins, complicating DNA extraction [11]. In addition, Hawaii has a warm and wet environment, while Korea is climatically diverse with temperatures fluctuating from freezing to extremely hot. Such environmental conditions involving high heat have been found to increase DNA degradation, specifically deamination and fragmentation rates [12]. After further treatment with fungicide and a powdered hardening compound (Figure 1c), bodies were wrapped and casketed. In total, the remains of 859 unidentified Korean War service members were shipped to Hawaii in 1956 and buried as Unknowns at the NMCP, also known as the Punchbowl [7]. In 1999, the then Central Identification Laboratory, Hawaii (CILHI, now called the Defense POW/MIA Accounting Agency (DPAA)) [13], undertook a fledgling exhumation program focused on identifying Korean War Unknowns at NMCP. Working in concert with the CILHI, the Armed Forces DNA Identification Laboratory (a division of the Armed Forces Medical Examiner System (AFMES-AFDIL)) attempted DNA testing of the first five exhumed cases using standard forensic DNA profiling techniques [14]. However, the results were not reproducible and therefore determined to be unreliable.

In 2016 the AFMES-AFDIL validated a novel MPS protocol for mitochondrial genome (mitogenome) sequencing using a probe capture and Illumina sequencing approach. This method was shown to be more amenable to the crosslinked and severely fragmented DNA from NMCP Unknowns, which was detailed in a 2017 performance evaluation [4]. As a result of this MPS mitogenome sequencing validation, the AFMES-AFDIL became the first accredited laboratory to adopt MPS for forensic casework worldwide. The study showed severe degradation of the DNA from Korean War NMCP Unknowns, which averaged <70 base pairs (bp) in length. The validated MPS methods are now routinely applied to all chemically treated or severely degraded DNA samples at the AFMES-AFDIL, regardless of the military conflict. These include remains from U.S. military WWII cemetery exhumations with similar preservation problems to those encountered with the Korean War unknowns from the NMCP. To date, over 3000 samples have been tested using the validated mitogenome MPS protocol with a success rate of ~60%. While this is a marked improvement from before the integration of MPS into the casework workflow (6% success rate with PCR and Sanger sequencing), the sample failure rate is still substantial, even when targeting mtDNA, which is high in copy number relative to nuclear DNA. Additional advancements to improve MPS sensitivity could elevate success rates in reportable mitogenome profile generation and may furthermore enable SNP profiling for extended kinship analysis [15].

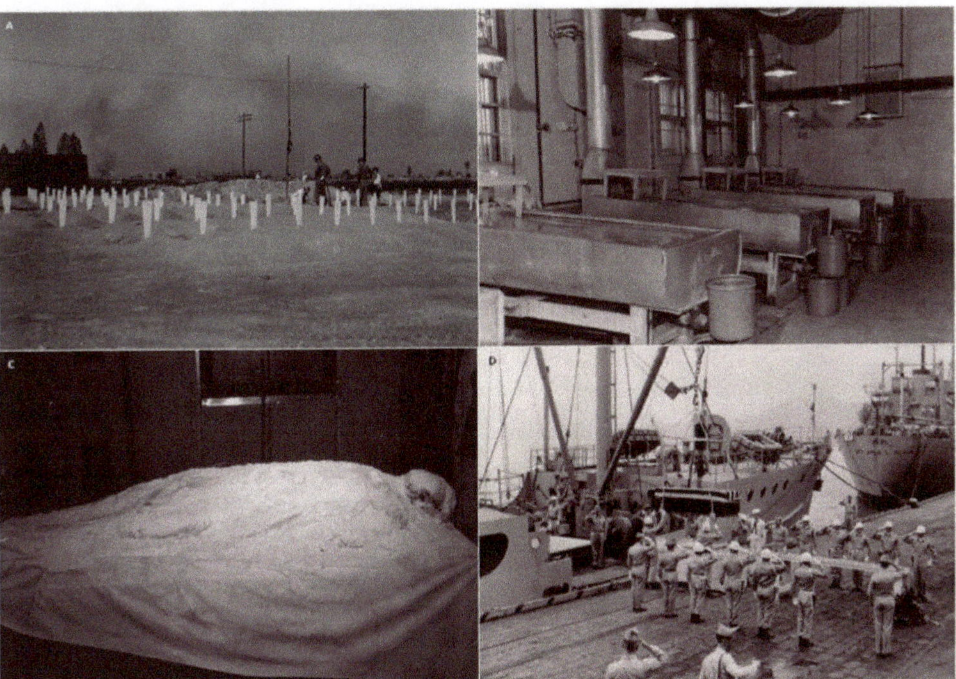

Figure 1. These historical photographs show some of the important events that occurred after service members were killed in action during the Korean War. (**A**) In this photograph, taken on 19 August 1950, a battlefield cemetery in Daegu (formerly Taegu), Korea, contains dozens of temporary graves where the bodies of soldiers killed in action were laid to rest. This image was reprinted with permission of the U.S. Army Quartermaster Museum in Fort Lee, Virginia. (**B**) This photograph of the Kokura embalming laboratory was originally printed in the American Graves Registration Service Group 8204th Army Unit APO 3 Brochure, April 1955. Examination tables were equipped with exhaust systems for formaldehyde treatment. (**C**) These remains from a Korean War service member were covered with a powdered hardening compound prior to shipment to the United States. This photograph was reprinted courtesy of the DPAA. (**D**) In Operation GLORY, the first of the United Nations war dead from North Korea were received at Moji Port near Kokura, Japan (ca. fall of 1954). This photograph was originally printed in the American Graves Registration Service Group 8204th Army Unit APO 3 Brochure, April 1955.

While the forensic field has faced obstacles in generating DNA profiles from historical remains, the ancient DNA field has been successful in recovering authentic DNA from very old and degraded samples from a variety of substrates and environments. Advancements in the extraction [16,17], library preparation [18], and enrichment of target DNA [19,20] have enabled the generation of hominin nuclear and mtDNA sequence profiles from skeletal elements as well as sediment over 300,000 years old [21–23]. Of particular importance in these developments was an extraction protocol that can recover DNA fragments <50 bp in length [16] and transitioning from double- to single-stranded DNA library preparation [24], a method that has also been shown to improve the recovery of DNA molecules from formalin-fixed samples [25–27]. However, the focus for method development for forensic casework and ancient DNA studies is different. This is due to the consistent, degraded nature of ancient DNA samples that motivates the foundation for methodological advancements in the field. Forensic samples, by contrast, are much more heterogeneous in terms of DNA quality. Novel forensic methods are largely aimed to improve DNA profiling of traditional forensic targets that exceed 100 bp in size. Furthermore, new forensic DNA methods must meet rigorous validation standards, making it difficult to test and adopt new protocols. These differing forces that drive the two fields have positioned ancient DNA considerably ahead of forensics in terms of method development. Yet both fields share the common problem of analyzing DNA that is (or can be) highly degraded. This commonality prompted the question if methods from the ancient DNA field could improve success rates for generating mtDNA profiles for historical identifications, which has been suggested in recent studies and reviews [28–30]. Therefore, we tested the feasibility of integrating ancient DNA methods into a forensic casework workflow by comparing different DNA extraction and library preparation protocols using fifteen skeletal remains with DNA of varying quality as determined by previous testing. We then evaluated the success of each protocol based on the number of informative sequences, completeness of mtDNA profiles, and concordance with expected profiles when available. This study lays the groundwork for further developments that will advance DNA profiling and identification of the poorest quality historical remains samples.

2. Materials and Methods

2.1. Skeletal Samples

Fifteen non-probative skeletal samples were utilized for DNA testing in this study (Table 1). The samples originated from disinterred burials of World War II and Korean War service members that were likely to have been chemically treated, either with formalin or with chemical powder (deodorant or insecticide) application. All fifteen samples were previously processed in routine casework at the AFMES-AFDIL using the validated mitogenome sequencing methods outlined in [4]. Samples were selected based on DNA quality in order to cover a range in quality types and not based on skeletal element. The samples ranged in DNA quality based on casework sequencing success: seven failed with <10-fold average coverage, four provided mtDNA sequences with 10-35-fold (low) average coverage, and four yielded high coverage mtDNA data (100-360-fold).

Table 1. Sample descriptions and case contexts. World War II (WWII) conflict locations are shown, as well as the cemetery of disinterment. Formalin treatment was not documented, but was noted as being likely in certain cases. Powder application was evidenced by visible powder on the remains. Casework results were based on the coverage of the revised Cambridge Reference Sequence (rCRS) [31] produced from the same skeletal sample using the methods outlined in [4].

Sample ID	Skeletal Element	Context	Cemetery of Disinterment	Formalin Treatment	Powder Application	Casework Results
2224	Tibia	WWII-Tarawa	NMCP [1]	Unknown	Not visible	High Coverage
0858	Temporal	WWII-USS Oklahoma	NMCP [1]	No, Oil Soaked	Likely	High Coverage
0994	Femur	WWII-Buna	MAC [2]	Unknown	Not visible	High Coverage
2255	Humerus	WWII-Cabanatuan	MAC [2]	Unknown	Not visible	High Coverage
0899	Humerus	WWII-Tarawa	NMCP [1]	Unknown	Yes	Low Coverage
0100	Femur	Korea	NMCP [1]	Likely	Yes	Low Coverage
1001	Os coxa	WWII-Yugoslavia	SRAC [3]	Unknown	Not visible	Low Coverage
3140	Radius	WWII-Burma	NMCP [1]	Unknown	Yes	Low Coverage
0378	Femur	WWII-Tarawa	NMCP [1]	Unknown	Yes	Failed
1837	Tibia	WWII-Tarawa	NMCP [1]	Unknown	Yes	Failed
1198	Tibia	Korea	NMCP [1]	Likely	Yes	Failed
1964	Humerus	Korea	NMCP [1]	Likely	Yes	Failed
0917	Tibia	Korea	NMCP [1]	Likely	Yes	Failed
3825	Radius	Korea	NMCP [1]	Likely	Yes	Failed
1487	Femur	WWII-Italy	SRAC [3]	Unknown	Yes	Failed

[1] National Memorial Cemetery of the Pacific, Honolulu, Hawaii, USA; [2] Manila American Cemetery, Philippines; [3] Sicily-Rome American Cemetery, Italy.

2.2. DNA Extraction

All DNA extractions were performed at the AFMES-AFDIL in a clean, pre-PCR room with positive pressure, per standard ancient and forensic DNA practices. Under sterile conditions, each bone was sanded to remove the external surface, washed in ethanol, and then powdered using a blender cup. Bone powder samples were digested and a reagent blank (RB) was initiated for each extraction set. DNA was extracted using one of the conditions outlined in Table 2. As described in Edson et al. [32], the AFDIL method utilized 1.0 g of bone powder incubated overnight at 56 °C in 7.5 mL digestion buffer (0.5 M EDTA, 1% lauroylsarcosine) with 200 µL proteinase K (20 mg/mL). DNA was then isolated using an organic DNA extraction protocol with phenol chloroform isoamyl alcohol (PCIA), followed by concentration and buffer exchange using an Amicon Ultra-4 (molecular weight cut-off 30 kDa) (MilliporeSigma, Burlington, MA, USA). The resulting DNA extracts were divided into three aliquots to assess the effect of DNA repair on the sequence data. The following repair conditions were evaluated: (1) no repair, (2) USER (New England Biolabs (NEB), Ipswich, MA, USA) treatment to remove uracil residues resulting from cytosine deamination, and (3) NEBNext FFPE DNA Repair Mix (NEB) to remove uracils and also repair nicks, gaps, oxidized bases, and blocked 3' ends [33]. Repair treatments followed their respective manufacturer protocols. All three DNA extracts (no repair, USER, and FFPE DNA Repair) underwent MinElute (QIAGEN, Hilden, Germany) purification after repair. This resulted in a total of three different PCIA-based protocols that were tested (PM: no repair, PUM: USER, and PFM: FFPE DNA Repair).

Table 2. DNA extraction methods tested.

Method	Bone Powder (g)	Digestion Buffer	Digestion Buffer Volume (mL)	Proteinase K (20 mg/mL) (µL)	Incubation Temperature (°C)	DNA Purification	Repair Protocol
AFDIL (PM)	1.0	Demin buffer [1]	7.5	200	56	PCIA with buffer exchange	NA (MinElute purification)
AFDIL-USER (PUM)	1.0	Demin buffer [1]	7.5	200	56	PCIA with buffer exchange	USER (NEB, Ipswich, MA, USA)
AFDIL-FFPE (PFM)	1.0	Demin buffer [1]	7.5	200	56	PCIA with buffer exchange	NEBNext FFPE DNA Repair Mix (NEB)
Dabney—37 (aDNA37)	0.2	Dabney buffer [2]	1.0	25	37	Silica column and PB Buffer	NA
Dabney—56 (aDNA56)	Dabney 37 remaining pellet	Dabney buffer [2]	1.0	25	56	Silica column and PB Buffer	NA
AFDIL-Dabney (A_D)	0.2	Demin buffer [1]	4.0	200	56	Silica column and PB Buffer	NA

[1] Demin buffer: 0.5 M EDTA, 1% lauroyl sarcosine; [2] Dabney buffer: 0.45 M, 0.5% Tween 20.

The ancient DNA extraction protocol followed was the Dabney method [16] as described in Rohland et al. [17], substituting the binding buffer 'D' with QIAGEN PB buffer. This method utilized 0.2 g bone powder digested at 37 °C in 1 mL 0.45 M EDTA with 0.05% Tween 20 and 25 µL proteinase K (20 mg/mL). Unlike the AFDIL digestion, there was not a complete digestion of bone powder. Therefore, the bone powder pellets remaining after the initial 37 °C Dabney extraction were re-digested overnight with 1.0 mL buffer at 56 °C, which resulted in the powder going into solution. Purification was then performed with the Roche High Pure Spin Column (a large volume silica column) (Pleasanton, CA, USA). This resulted in two ancient DNA extractions, although each were from the same bone powder aliquot (first digestion: aDNA37 and second digestion: aDNA56).

Finally, a hybrid "AFDIL-Dabney" DNA extraction method was performed following the AFMES-AFDIL digestion procedures (i.e., 1.0 g of bone powder incubated overnight at 56 °C in 7.5 mL digestion buffer and 200 µL proteinase K) and Dabney purification (i.e., High Pure Spin Column).

2.3. Library Preparation

2.3.1. In House MPI Method

This single-stranded DNA library preparation was performed as described in [19] on a Bravo NGS Workstation (Agilent Technologies) at the Max Planck Institute for Evolutionary Anthropology (MPI-EVA) in Leipzig, Germany from 5µL of each sample extract and RB. In short, the DNA was denatured by heat, and then the 5′ and 3′ phosphate groups were removed. T4 DNA ligase was used to ligate an adapter oligonucleotide with a 3′ biotin to the 3′ end of each DNA fragment, aided by a splinter oligonucleotide. This product was then immobilized on streptavidin magnetic beads and a wash was performed at 45 °C to remove the splinter. Primer and the *E.coli* DNA polymerase I Klenow fragment was added to make a copy of the template strand from the attached adapter. A bead wash was then performed to remove excess primers and prevent adapter dimer formation. Next, T4 DNA ligase was used for a blunt-end ligation of a second, double-stranded adapter. Heat denaturation at 95 °C was then used to release the library products from the beads. Library amplification and indexing was performed with AccuPrime Pfx DNA polymerase with the following cycling parameters: 95 °C for 2 min, then 35 cycles of 95 °C for 20 s, 60 °C for 30 s and 68 °C for 1 min, with a final additional 5 min at 68 °C. Post-amplification purification was performed using the MinElute PCR purification kit. Libraries were generated from all 15 samples, one RB, one library positive control and one library negative control.

2.3.2. SRSLY Kit

The SRSLY single-stranded DNA library preparations were performed manually at the AFMES-AFDIL using Claret's SRSLY PicoPlus Library Prep Kit for Illumina (Santa Cruz, CA, USA). Unless otherwise noted, library preparation was carried out according to the manufacturer protocol for ancient and highly degraded DNA samples, including purification steps with AMPure XP (Beckman Coulter, Brea, CA, USA) for maximum short fragment retention [34]. In summary, 5 µL of extract was used for library preparation, and a positive control and negative control were included with each sample set. The positive control was enzymatically fragmented K562 cell line with 1 ng library input, as described in [4]. An initial denaturation step rendered all DNA single-stranded and then stabilized by a single-stranded binding protein, followed by adapter ligation at 37 °C (lid 45 °C) for 1 h with splinted adapters that retain the original strand orientation. AMPure XP purification after adapter ligation included the addition of isopropanol and 10 mM Tris-HCl pH 8.5 with a final ratio of 0.54× (0.99× ratio to library prior to isopropanol and Tris-HCl addition). The full library volume was amplified in a single reaction using Claret unique dual indexes (undiluted) and KAPA HiFi HotStart Uracil+ ReadyMix (Roche) according to the manufacturer recommendations. Uracil+ was selected in order to tolerate uracil bases present in the DNA due to cytosine deamination. Library amplification was completed with the following parameters: 95 °C for 3 min, then 35 cycles of 95 °C for 20 s, 60 °C for 15 s, 72 °C for 1 min, followed by 72 °C for 7 min. Post-amplification purification utilized a 1.2× AMPure XP ratio. Libraries were generated from a total of 15 samples, one RB, two positive controls and two negative controls.

2.3.3. KAPA Hyper Prep Kit

The KAPA double-stranded DNA library preparations were performed manually at the AFMES-AFDIL using the Roche KAPA Hyper Prep Kit. Unless otherwise noted, library preparation was carried out according to the manufacturer protocol. Again, 5 µL of extract was used for library preparation, and a positive control and negative control were included with each sample set. The positive control was fragmented DNA from a K562 cell line with 1 ng library input. End repair and A-tailing took place in a single step with incubation at 20 °C for 30 min, then 65 °C for 30 min (lid 85 °C), followed by adapter ligation using 15 µM KAPA dual indexed adapters for all libraries at 20 °C for 15 min. Post-ligation clean-up used an increased 2× AMPure XP ratio in order to retain smaller fragments. The full library volume was amplified using KAPA HiFi HotStart Uracil+ ReadyMix and KAPA

Library Amplification Primer mix, according to the manufacturer's recommendations with the following parameters: 95 °C for 3 min, then 35 cycles of 98 °C for 20 s, 60 °C for 15 s, 72 °C for 1 min, followed by 72 °C for 7 min. The same post-amplification AMPure XP purification was utilized as with the SRSLY libraries. Libraries were generated from a total of 15 samples, one RB, two positive controls and two negative controls.

2.3.4. Quantification

To compare the number of DNA molecules converted into library molecules for each of the three library preparation methods, quantitative (q) PCR was performed on the unamplified library products of each method. The qPCR was performed as described in Gansauge et al. [18] at the MPI-EVA with all the libraries on the same plate to remove any possible plate-to-plate variation.

2.4. MtDNA Hybridization Capture

In-solution hybridization capture was used for the enrichment of human mtDNA for the three different types of library preparation methods. Two rounds of capture were performed following the protocol outlined in Fu et al. [19] in 384-well format on a Bravo NGS Workstation B (Agilent, Santa Clara, CA, USA) with adjustments to the number of amplification cycles per library to prevent each from reaching plateau.

2.5. Sequencing and Data Processing

For the comparison of extraction protocols, all resulting single-stranded DNA libraries were pooled for shotgun sequencing. For the comparison of library preparation protocols, each library type was pooled separately (three total pools) for shotgun sequencing and the human mtDNA enriched SRSLY and MPI library sets (two pools). In order to avoid captured libraries with identical indices being sequenced together, the KAPA Hyper Prep human mtDNA enriched libraries were split between nine pools and sequenced with other libraries not included in this study. All sequencing pools were created by combining equal amounts of sample libraries and 1:10 dilutions of controls (RBs and library negative controls). Library positive controls were not sequenced. Sequencing was performed on a MiSeq or NextSeq (Illumina technology) in 2×75 bp paired-end configuration with 8-bp dual-indexed reads. Base calling was completed with bustard (Illumina) and overlapping paired-end reads were merged using leeHom [35]. For shotgun sequencing, reads were then mapped to the human reference genome GRCh37/1000 (Genomes release; ftp://ftp.1000genomes.ebi.ac.uk/vol1/ftp/technical/reference/phase2_reference_assembly_sequence/, accessed on 12 November 2021) and captured library reads were mapped to the revised Cambridge reference sequence [31]. PCR duplicates were then removed using bam-rmdup (https://github.com/mpieva/biohazard-tools, accessed on 15 October 2021).

For the processing of the shotgun results, all sequences less than 35 bp and unmapped sequences were removed. The remaining sequences were then used to calculate the average fragment size, rates of C-to-T substitutions, and number of informative sequences [26] in each sample. The 35 bp cut-off was used to allow comparisons to previous published ancient DNA data.

For the processing of the capture enriched data, the resulting de-duplicated sequences from each library preparation type continued either through the MPI workflow or a CLC Genomic Workbench (QIAGEN, Hilden, Germany) workflow. For the MPI workflow, unmapped sequences, sequences shorter than 30 bp or with a mapping quality less than 25 were removed. The resulting sequences were used to calculate the coverage of the mtDNA genome. For the CLC workflow, the de-duplicated bam files were ingested into the CLC at the AFMES-AFDIL for variant calling, mtDNA haplogroup prediction, and forensic profile reporting using AQME [36], in addition to determining the mtDNA coverage. A minimum read depth of 5 was required for bases to be included in the reported sequence range. Variant detection required a minimum of 4 reads supporting the variant as well as a minimum frequency of 10%. Point heteroplasmy was documented when variants exhibited 10–90% frequency. Length heteroplasmy was reported based on the major molecule; however, this was ignored in concordance assessments due to the impact of differing polymerases on length variants [37]. Additionally, variants consistent with cytosine deamination (C-to-T or G-to-A substitutions) that were low in frequency (<30%) and/or lacking in forward/reverse read balance (<0.30) were excluded. These variant detection parameters minimized the reporting of stochastic error while allowing for the mixture and contamination detection necessary in forensic casework. When processing the SRSLY libraries, contaminant pig DNA was identified as mismapping to the human mtDNA reference genome (rCRS), resulting in spikes of coverage and unexpected variants (Supplementary Figures S1 and S2). The presence of pig sequences in these libraries was confirmed using a pipeline [38] that uses BLAST [39] and MEGAN [40] to assign sequences from sediment samples to different mammalian families (Supplementary Figure S3). To remove these sequences a "pig-out" pipeline was added to both the CLC and MPI workflows as described in Supporting Information Text S1.

3. Results

3.1. Evaluation of Extraction Methods

In order to evaluate the feasibility of integrating ancient DNA methods into a forensic casework workflow, we first evaluated the performance of various extraction protocols with respect to success in recovering DNA fragments. Fifteen non-probative skeletal remains that had been previously tested at the AFMES-AFDIL and were therefore of known quality (Table 1). We selected five different extraction/repair protocols to test: three PCIA-based from the forensic field [32], one from the ancient DNA field ([17], with PB buffer), and one that combined elements of each the forensic and ancient DNA protocols (see Section 2.2). As the bone powder pellet did not go into solution in the initial ancient DNA digestion at 37 °C, a redigestion was performed at 56 °C of the same pellet and each of the fractions was purified. Therefore, six extraction/repair conditions were tested in total (Table 2); however, the two ancient DNA extractions were from the same original powder sample.

DNA extraction performance was assessed using shotgun sequencing data produced from single-stranded libraries constructed following the method outlined in Gansauge et al. [18]. To determine which extraction protocol was most effective, we estimated the number of unique DNA fragments present in each library that mapped to the human DNA reference genome (informative sequences) in each library. For each sample we then determined which extraction protocol resulted in the most recovered informative sequences and took the ratio of the informative sequences from each other extraction protocol to this "best" protocol. This resulted in the relative informative sequences for each sample and extraction combination (see Supporting Information Text S2 for further explanation on how informative sequences and relative informative sequences were calculated). This calculation allowed us to compare the relative informative sequences across extraction types for the different samples (Figure 2A, see Supplementary Data File S1 for which extraction was best per sample). We found that the combined forensic ancient DNA extraction protocol (AFDIL-Dabney) was significantly worse than all other protocols ($n = 15$, Wilcoxon test with correction for multiple testing, p-values: 6.5×10^{-4} to 1.1×10^{-4}). The redigestion at 56 °C with the ancient DNA protocol (aDNA56) recovered significantly more informative fragments than the two forensic extraction protocols that included extra DNA repair steps intended to improve recovery of damaged DNA ($n = 15$, Wilcoxon test with correction for multiple testing, p-values both 2.8×10^{-2}). This loss of recovered DNA is likely, at least in part, due to the addition of extra purification steps. No significant difference in recovered informative sequences was observed between the two ancient DNA protocols and the forensic protocol with no DNA repair (p-values: 6.4×10^{-1} to 1). However, as the two ancient DNA protocols originate from the same bone powder pellet, theoretically if the initial lysis had been performed at 56 °C the DNA recovered in the 37 °C and 56 °C fractions would have been extracted together. If we combine the recovered informative sequences from both of these fractions, the ancient DNA protocol results in significantly more informative sequences than the forensic extraction protocols (n = 15, Wilcoxon test with correction for multiple testing, p-values all <4.8 $\times$ 10^{-4}, Figure 2B). These results indicate that the ancient DNA extraction protocol does improve the recovery of target DNA from historical skeletal remains that are of interest for forensic casework particularly in a MPS workflow.

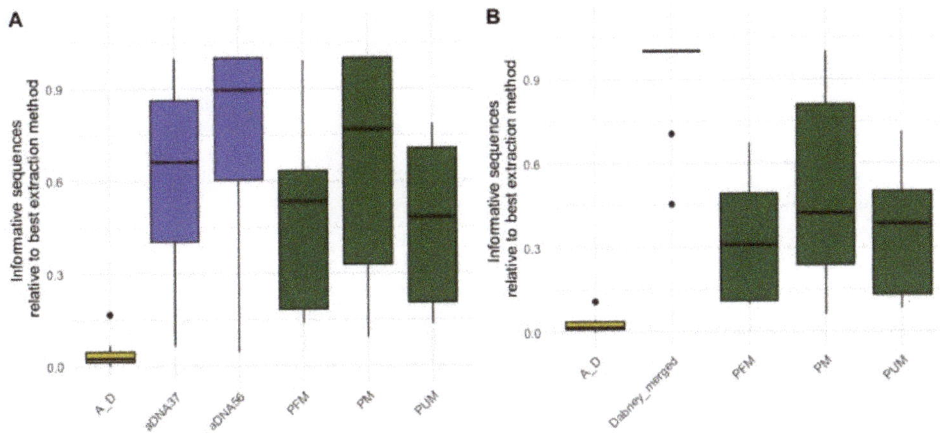

Figure 2. Relative informative sequences recovered per extraction protocol across 15 historical skeletal remains with the ancient DNA extraction fractions (**A**) separate and (**B**) merged. The total informative sequences per library was calculated by multiplying the number of DNA molecules in each library as determined by qPCR by the proportion of sequences longer than 35 bp that mapped to the human reference genome. The relative informative sequences were then calculated by taking the ratio of total informative sequences for each extraction/sample combination to the total number of informative sequences from the best performing extraction protocol per sample. The box plots follow the standard Tukey representation to show the distribution of the relative informative sequences per extraction type (n = 15). The significance of different relative amounts recovered per extraction was evaluated with a Wilcoxon test with a correction for multiple testing. The ancient DNA protocols (aDNA37: 37 °C digestion; aDNA56: 56 °C digestion; Dabney merged: merging of total informative sequences per extraction/sample from aDNA37 and aDNA56) are colored in blue; forensic protocols (PM: PCIA with Min Elute; PUM: PCIA with Min Elute and USER treatment; PFM: PCIA with Min Elute and FFPE treatment) in green; and the combined forensic ancient DNA protocol (A_D: AFDIL digestion with Dabney purification) in yellow.

3.2. Characteristics of Recovered DNA

Single-stranded DNA library preparation coupled with shotgun sequencing allows for the characterization of nuclear DNA recovered from each of these samples. Specifically, we examined the percentage of sequences longer than 35 bp that mapped to the human genome, average fragment size for each sample, and deamination as represented by cytosine to thymine (C-to-T) substitutions. The latter two analyses were performed after removing unmapped reads, PCR duplicates, and sequences shorter than 35 bp or with mapping qualities less than 25. We used the data from the ancient DNA extraction protocol with a 56 °C incubation to investigate each of these factors.

The percent mapped for the samples ranged from 0.13–72.5% (mean 7.88%) and the average fragment size for each of the samples ranged from 44 to 64 bp (mean 49 bp). The observed percent of C-to-T substitutions on the 5′ ends ranged from 8.8% to 30.7% (mean 18.3%) and 8% to 22.3% (mean 13.3%) on the 3′ end. These values are similar to those observed in ancient DNA samples, where the presence of short DNA fragments and deamination are used for the authentication of ancient DNA [41] as well as to disentangle endogenous ancient DNA from modern human contamination [42]. While there have been multiple studies on the impacts of various factors on the DNA degradation patterns from ancient samples [12,22,43] and modern samples [44,45], there is limited data on DNA degradation in the more recent past. Therefore, we compared the average fragment size and deamination patterns of this set of forensic samples to published shotgun data from seven Late Pleistocene modern human specimens (~37 to 46,000 years ago) [46]. We found that the percent of sequences that mapped to the human reference genome (fragment length $\geq$ 35 bp and mapping quality $\geq$ 25) for about half of the historical remains fell within two standard deviations of the mean for the ancient samples (Figure 3A). Additionally, the average sizes of mapped human DNA fragments recovered from all of the historical remains were within the range for the ancient samples (Figure 3B). As the library preparation method used is known to impact the observed 3′ deamination [26], we compared the values on the 5′ end only. In this comparison, many of the historical remains had lower deamination rates than the average ancient sample (Figure 3C). In ancient DNA studies, a cut-off of 10% deamination is often used for the identification of authentic ancient DNA [38,43,47], and the majority of the historical samples exceeded this threshold. When looking at the rate of deamination along the DNA fragments, while the terminal base has the highest rate, elevated rates of deamination continue until the third terminal base for the historical samples (Figure 3D). This trend is known for ancient samples, but this observation indicates that it may be important to consider deamination during the downstream analyses of historical DNA samples, particularly when no DNA repair step is included. In addition, the similarity between the DNA recovered from the historical and ancient samples emphasizes the difficulty of performing identifications for forensic casework when remains may have been formalin treated or are poorly preserved.

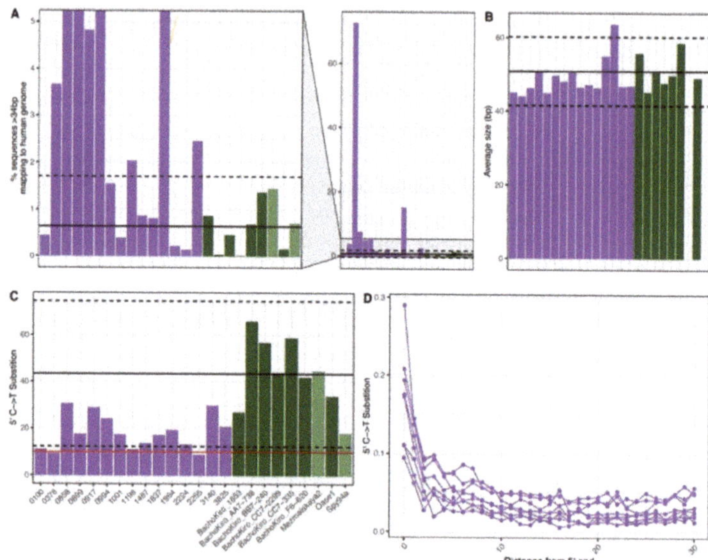

Figure 3. The (**A**) percent mapped (**B**) average fragment size (bp) and (**C,D**) observed 5′ C to T substitution frequencies of DNA recovered from historical and ancient DNA samples. Each bar represents a single sample for fifteen historical samples (purple) and seven Late Pleistocene modern human skeletal samples from ~37,000–46,000 years ago (dark green). In (**A–C**) the x-axis is the same for each and the black line represents the average for the ancient skeletal (dark green) samples and the dashed lines show two standard deviations above and below this average. In (**C**) the red line represents the 10% threshold typically used to determine if a sample contains ancient DNA. In (**D**) each point represents the 5′ C to T substitution frequency at a position from the 5′ end of DNA fragments recovered from a single sample. Note that only historical samples are shown in (**D**).

3.3. Evaluation of Library Preparartion Protocols

The characterization of the DNA recovered from the historical remains confirmed the finding of previous studies that the DNA from these samples is highly degraded [4,15,48]. As the currently validated MPS workflow at AFMES-AFDIL uses a double-stranded library preparation method, it is likely that many of these DNA fragments are lost and not successfully converted into libraries. Therefore, success rates could be improved if a single-stranded library preparation method was used. We tested this hypothesis by taking three 5 µL aliquots from the ancient DNA extracts with a 56 °C incubation and preparing libraries with the KAPA Hyper Prep double-stranded kit (currently being validated for casework by AFMES-AFDIL) [15], the SRSLY single-stranded kit [49], and the single-stranded DNA library preparation method described in [18], which we refer to as the "MPI" method. For the double-stranded KAPA libraries, shotgun sequencing resulted in between 4 and 6997 unique nuclear DNA fragments recovered (two libraries failed during library prep). The two single-stranded DNA libraries resulted in between 23 and 143,388 unique DNA fragments for the SRSLY kit and 908 to 407,183 for the MPI method. It is important to note, however, that none of these libraries were sequenced to exhaustion. As with the extraction method comparison, we determined the relative informative sequences per sample for the three different library preparation methods based on the shotgun data (Figure 4). This confirmed that single-stranded library preparation methods were more effective at recovering informative sequences (n = 15 for the number of samples used for comparisons across the three different library preparation methods, Wilcoxon test with correction for multiple testing, both p-values < 2.0×10^{-5}), although there was no significant difference between the two single-stranded methods (p-value = 0.29).

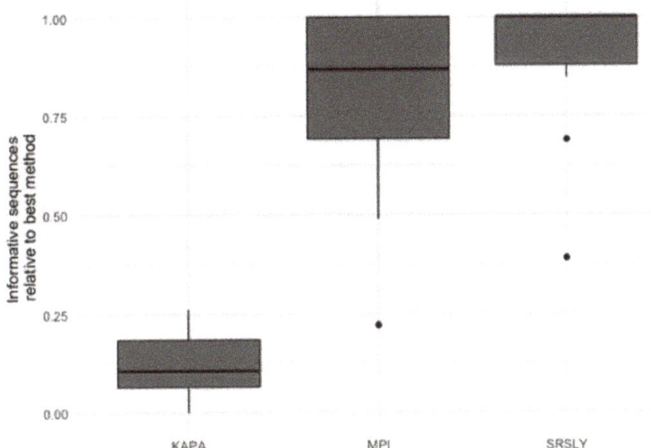

Figure 4. Relative informative nuclear DNA sequences recovered per library preparation protocol across 15 historical skeletal remains. The relative informative sequences per library was calculated as described in Supporting Information Text S2. The box plots follow the standard Tukey representation to show the distribution of the relative informative sequences per extraction type (n = 15). The significance of different relative amounts recovered per library prep type was evaluated with a Wilcoxon test with a correction for multiple testing.

Next, we wanted to evaluate the mtDNA variant calling success rates of the two single-stranded methods for each sample to determine if there was a difference from previous casework attempts. In order to test this, each library was enriched for human mtDNA using hybridization capture. The resulting sequencing data was then processed both at the MPI and using a CLC workflow at the AFMES-AFDIL (see Section 2.5). No significant difference was observed in the percentage of sequences that mapped between the two library preparation methods (Figure 5A, Wilcox test with correction for multiple testing, $n = 15$, $p = 0.57$). However, during the processing of the SRSLY libraries, pig mtDNA was identified as mismapping to the human mtDNA genome (0 to 17 fragments, contributing up to 6.5% of sequences per sample library). Therefore, a "pig-out" alternative workflow was used to remove these sequences via competitive mapping for all the SRSLY libraries (Supporting Information Text S2). The MPI method was found to result in more mtDNA sequences (Figure 5B, p-values adjusted for multiple testing 5.5×10^{-4} for MPI workflow and 7.6×10^{-6} for CLC workflow, $n = 12$ samples compared between library types, Wilcoxon test) with no significant difference in number of unique mtDNA sequences ($n = 40$ sample, library and workflow comparisons, p-value adjusted for multiple testing: 0.24, Wilcoxon test). Importantly, the maximum coverage for the negative controls was 0.3-fold for the CLC workflow, which is lower than typically observed in MPS data using the validated AFMES-AFDIL double-stranded DNA workflow [4], allowing for lowering thresholds below 10-fold for variant detection. For the CLC processing, two standard deviations above mean coverage of the controls was 0.38-fold. Thus the analytical threshold, above which sequence data can be distinguished from background noise, could be set as low as 2-fold ($2\times$) average coverage. The SRSLY library preparation method resulted in 13 samples with an average coverage of at least 10-fold for the mtDNA genome and the MPI library preparation method resulted in 14 samples with at least 10-fold average coverage. While 10-fold was the previous coverage threshold, the low coverages observed in the negative controls supported decreasing this threshold comfortably to 5-fold, well above the 2-fold level of background noise. All samples resulted in at least 5-fold average coverage using either single-stranded library preparation technique (Figure 6, Supplementary Data File S1).

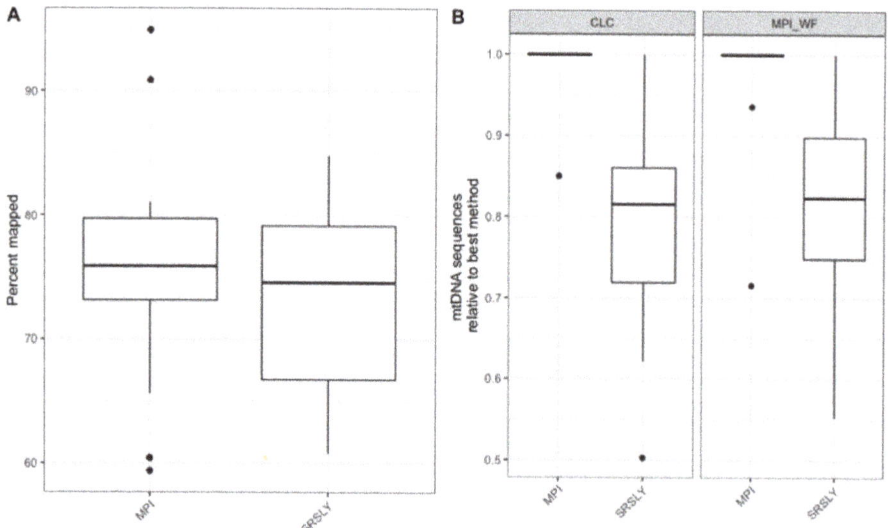

Figure 5. (**A**) The distribution of the percentage of sequences at least 30 bp long that mapped to the human mtDNA reference genome after capture using the MPI workflow. (**B**) The relative number of mapped mtDNA sequences across library preparation methods for both the CLC and MPI workflows. The box plots follow the standard Tukey representation to show the distribution of the relative informative sequences per extraction type ($n = 15$).

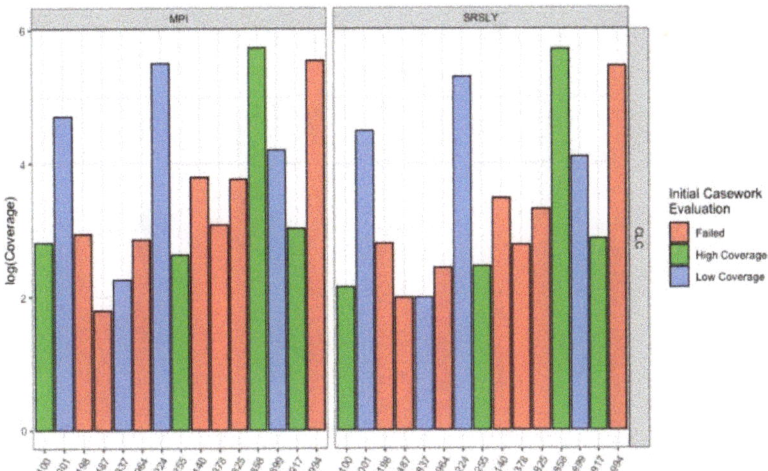

Figure 6. Average coverage of different qualities of samples with MPI and SRSLY library preparations after enrichment for human mtDNA using the CLC workflow. Samples are colored based on the quality as determined from the initial casework evaluation before changing the extraction and library preparation methods (Table 1). The left plots underwent MPI library preparation and the right plots SRSLY library preparation.

For variant calling, only the CLC workflow was used as it applies forensic standards to haplotype reporting that have been previously validated for forensic casework use. When compared with previously generated casework results, the low-coverage and high-coverage sample data were nearly 100% concordant (Tables 3 and S3). It is important to note that the previous casework results were generated from two DNA libraries comprised of roughly 1.0 g of bone powder each; whereas the data in this study utilized DNA libraries comprised of 0.01 g of bone powder. The only discordance was observed in the high coverage sample 2255 at nucleotide position (np) 6755. Heteroplasmy (G6755R) was called in the 473-fold casework data due to a minor guanine (G) variant at 21.1% frequency. However, heteroplasmy was not observed above the set thresholds in either the MPI or the SRSLY data, which both produced a G6755A variant. It is noted that the MPI data exhibited 15-fold coverage at this position, with 13 (87%) of reads exhibiting adenine (A) at this position and two reads (13%) producing a guanine (G) base. The SRSLY data had $11\times$ coverage at np 6755 and produced 100% adenine. This decreased observation of guanine at this position may be due to a combination of lower coverage and cytosine deamination. It is possible that higher coverage, gained through either higher DNA input into library or through combining data produced from multiple libraries and/or sequencing events, would result in improved heteroplasmy detection at this position in either of the single-stranded DNA libraries.

Table 3. Haplotype comparison between previously generated forensic casework data using the methods described in [4] and two single-stranded DNA library preparations (the Max Planck Institute (MPI) [18] and SRSLY [49]) after enrichment for human mtDNA. The AFMES-AFDIL casework minimum coverage threshold was 10-fold and the maximum number of reportable bases was 16,507, as regions of length heteroplasmy are not reported in routine casework. The MPI and SRSLY coverage thresholds were 5-fold. The SRSLY bioinformatics workflow required removal of contaminating *Sus scrofa* mitochondrial DNA (mtDNA) sequences prior to mapping to the rCRS [31].

Sample ID	Casework		MPI			SRSLY (Pig Out)		
	Reported Bases	Predicted Haplogroup	Reported Bases	Predicted Haplogroup	Discordant Sites (Compared to Casework)	Reported Bases	Predicted Haplogroup	Discordant Sites (Compared to Casework)
High Coverage								
2224	16507	H18	16569	H18	0	16568	H18	0
0858	16507	V3c	16568	V3c	0	16569	V3c	0
0994	16507	J1c4b	16569	J1c4b	0	16569	J1c4b	0
2255	16507	J1c3	16268	J1c3/J1c3h/J1c3k	1	16144	J1c3	1
Low Coverage								
0899	16507	H4a1a4b	16565	H4a1a4b	0	16563	H4a1a4b	0
0100	16183	H24a	16181	H24a	0	13585	H24/H24a	0
1001	15765	H1c6	16566	H1c6	0	16567	H1c6	0
3140	16505	U5b1b1-16192	16555	U5b1b1- 16192	0	16515	U5b1b1-16192	0
Failed in Casework								
0378	NA	NA	15951	U5a1a1+16362/U5a1a1d/U5a1a1d1	NA	15681	U5a1a1+16362/U5a1a1d/U5a1a1d1	NA
1837	NA	NA	13504	K1c2	NA	11526	K1c2	NA
1198	NA	NA	16091	H1c3b	NA	15821	H1c3b	NA
1964	NA	NA	16010	L2a1c+16086/L2a1c3b	NA	14871	L2a1c+16086	NA
0917	NA	NA	16386	K1a1b2b	NA	16004	K1a1b2b	NA
3825	NA	NA	16550	H11a	NA	16319	H11a	NA
1487	NA	NA	10715	K1a (and subhaplogroups of K1a)	NA	12009	K1a9	NA

The seven samples that failed to produce reportable mtDNA profiles in routine casework (at a 10-fold coverage threshold) yielded concordant, partial profiles when comparing the 5-fold MPI and SRSLY data. Despite partial ranges, the predicted haplogroups (Table 3) were almost identical between the MPI and SRSLY data for all seven samples. The reason that they are not exactly identical is due to missed/uncalled variants in low coverage regions, in which the minimum 5-fold (5×) coverage threshold was met but the minimum variant count of 4 was not met—either due to cytosine deamination and/or low-level background noise. It is likely that, when merged with sequence data from a second/replicate library, the coverage and variant detection will improve. This merging of data from two independent libraries, as is routinely done in AFMES-AFDIL casework, would likely make these profiles reportable. Notably, only two of the seven failed samples (1837 and 1964) exceeded 5-fold average coverage in routine DNA casework. Thus at a minimum, the MPI and SRSLY methods improved the mtDNA profiling success of the bottom third (*n* = 5) of the poorest quality AFMES-AFDIL samples, from 0% to 100%. In other words, the previous method did not even produce partial mtDNA profiles at a 5-foldcoverage level that could be reported; whereas the ssDNA methods both yielded sufficient coverage for haplogrouping and distinguishing mtDNA profiles.

4. Discussion

The identification of historical remains usually falls within the scope of the forensic science community, particularly with remains from armed military conflicts. The DNA recovered from the samples in this set, which had varied preservation conditions, including formalin treatment, showed similar properties to DNA recovered from remains over 30,000 years old. While it has been previously demonstrated with both artificially degraded DNA and forensic casework samples that ancient DNA extraction methods can increase DNA yields in historical cases [28,30], this study clearly demonstrates the benefits of making this change for the disinterred remains of WWII and Korean War service members. The degraded nature of the DNA recovered from the remains investigated here, possibly facilitated by the powder application and/or formalin-treatment they were subjected to [25,26], made them clear candidates for single-stranded DNA library preparation. For the seven samples that had previously failed to result in data that met the required 10-fold average coverage for casework, six passed this threshold with at least one of the two single-stranded DNA library preparation methods. Importantly, these methods also resulted in cleaner negative controls, which allowed for lowering of thresholds for data reporting, a benefit when working with degraded samples that contain limited amounts of data. In this study, the lowering of the average coverage threshold to 5-fold enabled the reporting of two more samples, which would have failed if we had maintained the previous 10-fold threshold, allowing all samples to be reportable.

Typically, in forensic DNA analysis, analytical thresholds are established based on 2–3 standard deviations above the mean coverage in negative controls [4]. In this study that would place the average coverage threshold at 2-fold. However, we raised this threshold to 5-fold, in order to minimize the reporting of background noise, low-level variants, and contamination. This also raises an important discussion about the detection of contamination. Although both the ancient DNA and forensic fields follow similar clean room practices and maintain negative controls throughout processing, the methods for identification of contamination in sample data differs. Expected elevated rates of deamination in ancient samples allow for the examination of deamination patterns to determine the presence of endogenous DNA and estimate amounts of modern human contamination [41,42], which may result in decisions to restrict analyses to only fragments that have deamination. While the samples in this study showed elevated deamination rates, this is not the case for all forensic samples and cannot be relied upon for confirmation of endogenous DNA content. For this reason, the forensic field has established three pathways for detecting contamination. First, DNA profiles from all staff members and individuals known to have handled the remains are maintained allowing for source identification from any contamination that may arise from the handling of the remains during processing. Profiles among unidentified remains can also be compared this way in case cross-contamination occurs due to commingling of remains. Second, all results from degraded skeletal remains are replicated from a new/second bone powder aliquot that is taken through DNA extraction, downstream processing, and analysis. Finally, each profile is evaluated as being either single-source or a mixture using interpretation parameters established through comprehensive validation studies. For mtDNA, mixed/contaminated DNA samples are known to cause a reduction in variant frequency as well as an excess of heteroplasmy (>3 nucleotide positions across the mitogenome) [4]. Mixed DNA samples are not reportable, and the laboratory work will be repeated in an attempt to determine the source of the mixture. If the bone itself is contaminated, as evidenced by a repeat mixture after a second DNA extraction, the sample results will not be reported. Determining contamination within the bone requires having multi-fold coverage across the mitogenome, which is why we decided to use a threshold of 5-fold. Attempts to lower this threshold further would require the development of other bioinformatic tools for the identification of mixtures from low-coverage data.

Although exogenous human DNA is highly scrutinized, as described above, low-level contaminants from non-human sources can also impact the accuracy of variant calling. We were able to develop a pipeline to remove the identified pig mtDNA contaminant, but currently validated workflows at the AFMES-AFDIL do not include these steps or a way to easily screen for the presence of non-human DNA. There are different taxonomic classifiers and methods used in other fields to identify different species and families in sequence data [39,40,50]. Based on the pig DNA observed in the SRSLY data, it may be worthwhile considering integrating one of these into workflows when working with historical casework. Additionally, the presence of deamination in all samples raises the question of how to ensure this does not impact downstream variant calling. In the presented analysis, variants that appeared to be due to deaminated bases were removed from the profile for concordance purposes. For the typical casework workflow, the impacts of deamination would likely be mitigated by merging the data from multiple extractions and/or libraries. In ancient DNA studies, different methods are used to minimize the impact of deamination on downstream analyses. For example, the terminal three positions of all fragments are often masked or, in extreme cases, only variants that are transversions are used [51,52]. A previous sensitivity study on the impact of DNA degradation on STR and SNP concordance with Verogen's ForenSeq kit also found differences in concordance and heterozygosity balance in comparison to studies with non-degraded DNA [28], indicating that considerations for the analysis of degraded DNA across platforms is of importance. Future studies on the impacts of low-input and degraded DNA for downstream forensics analyses will both help to increase the accuracy when working with more challenging data and open up the possibility of producing accurate, identification informative data from previously inaccessible samples.

In conclusion, we have identified that an altered ancient DNA extraction protocol coupled with single-stranded library preparation increases the amount of recovered mtDNA from disinterred military service member skeletal remains. These findings emphasize the value of exchanging methods between the ancient DNA and forensic fields [29], which are beneficial in both directions as shown from the ancient DNA community integrating bleach treatment to remove contamination from samples [53,54]. The integration of the methods in this study into casework samples with highly degraded DNA has the potential to increase success rates for identifying historical remains.

Supplementary Materials: The following supporting information can be downloaded at https://www.mdpi.com/article/10.3390/genes13010129/s1, Figure S1: The coverage distribution across the mtDNA genome for a SRSLY library negative control before (A) and after (B) CLC pig out workflow. Green portion represents forward reads and red portion represents reverse reads; Figure S2: Sequences mapped to positions 2300–3200 of the human mtDNA reference genome from a SRSLY library (sample 0378) pre- (A) and post- (B) CLC pig out workflow. Horizontal green lines represent individual forward reads and red lines reverse reads. Vertical lines represent differences from the reference (blue = C, yellow = G, red = A, green = T). A maximum of 100-fold in displayed range for (A) and 48-fold for (B); Figure S3: The number of mtDNA fragments assigned to the suidae family for samples that underwent SRSLY library preparation; Figure S4: The (A) informative and (B) relative informative sequences recovered from samples 2018H1198-02A2 across six difference extraction protocols. Table S1: Summary statistics from shotgun sequencing of MPI single-stranded library prepared samples from different types of extracts; Table S2: Summary statistics from shotgun sequenciing and capture of samples from double-stranded and single-stranded libraries; Table S3: Haplotypes reported in routine casework (validated dsDNA workflow), compared with haplotypes observed in MPI and SRSLY DNA libraries.

Author Contributions: Conceptualization, E.I.Z., M.M. and C.M.; data production, E.I.Z., J.T.T., K.S.-A., J.D.-H., K.K.M., A.A.-P., J.R., B.N. and C.M.; formal analysis, E.I.Z., J.T.T. and C.M.; resources, M.M.; writing—original draft preparation, E.I.Z., J.T.T., M.M. and C.M; writing—review and editing, K.S.-A., S.B.-R., G.E.B. and T.P.M. All authors have read and agreed to the published version of the manuscript.

Funding: This research received no external funding and was co-funded by the AFMES and Max Planck Society.

Institutional Review Board Statement: The study was conducted according to the guidelines of the Declaration of Helsinki, and approved by the US Army Medical Research and Materiel Command on September 3, 2014, IRBO Log Number M-10185. No data generated from this project were used for casework.

Data Availability Statement: Data are stored at the AFMES-AFDIL and may be made available to approved laboratories upon written request.

Acknowledgments: We thank Franklin Damann for providing the historical photographs from DPAA; the U.S. Army Quartermaster Museum, Fort Lee, Virginia; COL Alice Briones (AFMES) for administrative support; J. Kelso, J. Visage and L. Skov for help with data processing; and B. Schellbach and A. Weihmann for help with sequencing.

Conflicts of Interest: The authors declare no conflict of interest.

Disclaimer: The opinions or assertions presented hereafter are the private views of the authors and should not be construed as official or as reflecting the views of the Department of Defense, its branches, the Defense Health Agency, the Armed Forces Medical Examiner System, the Defense Personnel Accounting Agency, or the U.S. Government.

References

1. First Criminal Conviction Secured with Next-Gen Forensic DNA Technology. 2019. Available online: https://verogen.com/first-criminal-conviction-with-next-gen-forensic-dna/ (accessed on 2 December 2021).
2. *National DNA Index System (NDIS) Operational Procedures Manual*; Version 10; FBI Laboratory: Quantico, VA, USA, 2021.
3. Greytak, E.M.; Moore, C.; Armentrout, S.L. Genetic genealogy for cold case and active investigations. *Forensic Sci. Int.* **2019**, *299*, 103–113. [CrossRef]
4. Marshall, C.; Andreaggi, K.; Daniels-Higginbotham, J.; Oliver, R.S.; Barritt-Ross, S.; McMahon, T.P. Performance evaluation of a mitogenome capture and Illumina sequencing protocol using non-probative, case-type skeletal samples: Implications for the use of a positive control in a next-generation sequencing procedure. *Forensic Sci. Int. Genet.* **2017**, *31*, 198–206. [CrossRef] [PubMed]
5. Amorim, A.; Fernandes, T.; Taveira, N. Mitochondrial DNA in human identification: A review. *PeerJ* **2019**, *7*, e7314. [CrossRef]
6. Ambers, A.; Bus, M.M.; King, J.L.; Jones, B.; Durst, J.; Bruseth, J.E.; Gill-King, H.; Budowle, B. Forensic genetic investigation of human skeletal remains recovered from the La Belle shipwreck. *Forensic Sci. Int.* **2020**, *306*, 110050. [CrossRef]
7. Cole, P.M. *POW/MIA Issues: The Korean War*; NDRI: Santa Monica, CA, USA, 1994; Volume 1.
8. Keene, J. Bodily matters above and below ground: The treatment of American remains from the Korean war. *Public Hist.* **2010**, *32*, 59–78. [CrossRef] [PubMed]
9. Morris-Suzuki, T. Lavish are the dead: Re-envisioning Japan's Korean war. *Asia Pac. J. Jpn. Focus* **2013**, *11*, 1–8.
10. Coleman, B.L. Recovering the Korean war dead, 1950–1958: Graves registration, forensic anthropology, and wartime memorialization. *J. Mil. Hist.* **2008**, *72*, 179–222. [CrossRef]
11. Gilbert, M.T.P.; Haselkorn, T.; Bunce, M.; Sanchez, J.J.; Lucas, S.B.; Jewell, L.D.; Van Marck, E.; Worobey, M. The isolation of nucleic acids from fixed, paraffin-embedded tissues-which methods are useful when? *PLoS ONE* **2007**, *2*, e537. [CrossRef]
12. Kistler, L.; Ware, R.; Smith, O.; Collins, M.; Allaby, R.G. A new model for ancient DNA decay based on paleogenomic meta-analysis. *Nucleic Acids Res.* **2017**, *45*, 6310–6320. [CrossRef] [PubMed]

13. Holland, T.; Byrd, J.; Sava, V. Joint POW/MIA Accounting Command's Central Identification. *Forensic Anthropol. Lab.* **2008**, *47*, 63–80.

14. Edson, S.; Ross, J.P.; Coble, M.D.; Parsons, T.J.; Barritt, S.M. Naming the dead—Confronting the realities of rapid identification of degraded skeletal remains. *Forensic Sci. Rev.* **2004**, *16*, 63–90. [PubMed]

15. Gorden, E.M.; Greytak, E.M.; Sturk-Andreaggi, K.; Cady, J.; McMahon, T.P.; Armentrout, S.; Marshall, C. Extended kinship analysis of historical remains using SNP capture. *Forensic Sci. Int. Genet.* **2022**, *57*, 102636. [CrossRef]

16. Dabney, J.; Knapp, M.; Glocke, I.; Gansauge, M.-T.; Weihmann, A.; Nickel, B.; Valdiosera, C.; García, N.; Pääbo, S.; Arsuaga, J.-L.; et al. Complete mitochondrial genome sequence of a Middle Pleistocene cave bear reconstructed from ultrashort DNA fragments. *Proc. Natl. Acad. Sci. USA* **2013**, *110*, 15758–15763. [CrossRef]

17. Rohland, N.; Glocke, I.; Aximu-Petri, A.; Meyer, M. Extraction of highly degraded DNA from ancient bones, teeth and sediments for high-throughput sequencing. *Nat. Protoc.* **2018**, *13*, 2447–2461. [CrossRef]

18. Gansauge, M.-T.; Aximu-Petri, A.; Nagel, S.; Meyer, M. Manual and automated preparation of single-stranded DNA libraries for the sequencing of DNA from ancient biological remains and other sources of highly degraded DNA. *Nat. Protoc.* **2020**, *15*, 2279–2300. [CrossRef]

19. Fu, Q.; Meyer, M.; Gao, X.; Stenzel, U.; Burbano, H.A.; Kelso, J.; Pääbo, S. DNA analysis of an early modern human from Tianyuan Cave, China. *Proc. Natl. Acad. Sci. USA* **2013**, *110*, 2223–2227. [CrossRef] [PubMed]

20. Suchan, T.; Kusliy, M.A.; Khan, N.; Chauvey, L.; Tonasso-Calvière, L.; Schiavinato, S.; Southon, J.; Keller, M.; Kitagawa, K.; Krause, J.; et al. Performance and automation of ancient DNA capture with RNA hyRAD probes. *Mol. Ecol. Resour.* **2021**, 1–17. [CrossRef] [PubMed]

21. Vernot, B.; Zavala, E.I.; Gómez-Olivencia, A.; Jacobs, Z.; Slon, V.; Mafessoni, F.; Romagné, F.; Pearson, A.; Petr, M.; Sala, N.; et al. Unearthing Neanderthal population history using nuclear and mitochondrial DNA from cave sediments. *Science* **2021**, *372*, eabf1667. [CrossRef] [PubMed]

22. Zavala, E.I.; Jacobs, Z.; Vernot, B.; Shunkov, M.V.; Kozlikin, M.B.; Derevianko, A.P.; Essel, E.; de Fillipo, C.; Nagel, S.; Richter, J.; et al. Pleistocene sediment DNA reveals hominin and faunal turnovers at Denisova Cave. *Nature* **2021**, *595*, 399–403. [CrossRef]

23. Meyer, M.; Arsuaga, J.L.; de Filippo, C.; Nagel, S.; Aximu-Petri, A.; Nickel, B.; Martinez, I.; Gracia, A.; de Castro, J.M.B.; Carbonell, E.; et al. Nuclear DNA sequences from the middle pleistocene sima de los huesos hominins. *Nature* **2016**, *531*, 504–507. [CrossRef]

24. Meyer, M.; Kircher, M.; Gansauge, M.-T.; Li, H.; Racimo, F.; Mallick, S.; Schraiber, J.G.; Jay, F.; Prüfer, K.; De Filippo, C.; et al. A high-coverage genome sequence from an archaic Denisovan individual. *Science* **2012**, *338*, 222–226. [CrossRef]

25. Stiller, M.; Sucker, A.; Griewank, K.; Aust, D.; Baretton, G.B.; Schadendorf, D.; Horn, S. Single-strand DNA library preparation improves sequencing of formalin-fixed and paraffin-embedded (FFPE) cancer DNA. *Oncotarget* **2016**, *7*, 59115–59128. [CrossRef]

26. Gansauge, M.-T.; Gerber, T.; Glocke, I.; Korlević, P.; Lippik, L.; Nagel, S.; Riehl, L.M.; Schmidt, A.; Meyer, M. Single-stranded DNA library preparation from highly degraded DNA using T4 DNA ligase. *Nucleic Acids Res.* **2017**, *45*, e79.

27. Straube, N.; Lyra, M.L.; Paijmans, J.L.A.; Preick, M.; Basler, N.; Penner, J.; Rödel, M.; Westbury, M.V.; Haddad, C.F.B.; Barlow, A.; et al. Successful application of ancient DNA extraction and library construction protocols to museum wet collection specimens. *Mol. Ecol. Resour.* **2021**, *21*, 2299–2315. [CrossRef]

28. Zavala, E.I.; Rajagopal, S.; Perry, G.H.; Kruzic, I.; Bašić, Ž.; Parsons, T.J.; Holland, M.M. Impact of DNA degradation on massively parallel sequencing-based autosomal STR, iiSNP, and mitochondrial DNA typing systems. *Int. J. Legal. Med.* **2019**, *133*, 1369–1380. [CrossRef]

29. Hofreiter, M.; Sneberger, J.; Pospisek, M.; Vanek, D. Progress in forensic bone DNA analysis: Lessons learned from ancient DNA. *Forensic Sci. Int. Genet.* **2021**, *54*, 102538. [CrossRef]

30. Xavier, C.; Eduardoff, M.; Bertoglio, B.; Amory, C.; Berger, C.; Casas-Vargas, A.; Pallua, J.; Parson, W. Evaluation of DNA Extraction Methods Developed for Forensic and Ancient DNA Applications Using Bone Samples of Different Age. *Genes* **2021**, *12*, 146. [CrossRef] [PubMed]

31. Andrews, R.M.; Kubacka, I.; Chinnery, P.F.; Lightowlers, R.N.; Turnbull, D.M.; Howell, N. Reanalysis and revision of the Cambridge reference sequence for human mitochondrial DNA. *Nat. Genet.* **1999**, *23*, 147. [CrossRef] [PubMed]

32. Edson, S.M. Extraction of DNA from Skeletonized Postcranial Remains: A Discussion of Protocols and Testing Modalities. *J. Forensic Sci.* **2019**, *64*, 1312–1323. [CrossRef] [PubMed]

33. Gorden, E.M.; Sturk-Andreaggi, K.; Marshall, C. Repair of DNA damage caused by cytosine deamination in mitochondrial DNA of forensic case samples. *Forensic Sci. Int. Genet.* **2018**, *34*, 257–264. [CrossRef]

34. *SRSLY NGS Library Prep Kit for Illumina PicoPlus and NanoPlus UDIs and UMIs/UDIs: Unabridged Instruction Manual*; Clarert Biosience, LLC.: Santa Cruz, CA, USA, 2020.

35. Renaud, G.; Stenzel, U.; Kelso, J. leeHom: Adaptor trimming and merging for Illumina sequencing reads. *Nucleic Acids Res.* **2014**, *42*, e141. [CrossRef]

36. Sturk-Andreaggi, K.; Peck, M.A.; Boysen, C.; Dekker, P.; McMahon, T.P.; Marshall, C.K. AQME: A forensic mitochondrial DNA analysis tool for next-generation sequencing data. *Forensic Sci. Int. Genet.* **2017**, *31*, 189–197. [CrossRef]

37. Sturk-Andreaggi, K.; Parson, W.; Allen, M.; Marshall, C. Impact of the sequencing method on the detection and interpretation of mitochondrial DNA length heteroplasmy. *Forensic Sci. Int. Genet.* **2020**, *44*, 102205. [CrossRef] [PubMed]

38. Slon, V.; Hopfe, C.; Weiß, C.L.; Mafessoni, F.; de la Rasilla, M.; Lalueza-Fox, C.; Rosas, A.; Soressi, M.; Knul, M.V.; Miller, R.; et al. Neandertal and Denisovan DNA from Pleistocene sediments. *Science* **2017**, *356*, 605–608. [CrossRef]

39. Altschul, S.F.; Gish, W.; Miller, W.; Myers, E.W.; Lipman, D.J. Basic local alignment search tool. *J. Mol. Biol.* **1990**, *215*, 403–410. [CrossRef]

40. Huson, D.H.; Auch, A.F.; Qi, J.; Schuster, S.C. MEGAN analysis of metagenomic data. *Genome Res.* **2007**, *17*, 377–386. [CrossRef]

41. Briggs, A.W.; Stenzel, U.; Johnson, P.L.F.; Green, R.; Kelso, J.; Prufer, K.; Meyer, M.; Krause, J.; Ronan, M.T.; Lachmann, M.; et al. Patterns of damage in genomic DNA sequences from a neandertal. *Proc. Natl. Acad. Sci. USA* **2007**, *104*, 14616–14621. [CrossRef] [PubMed]

42. Peyregne, S.; Peter, B.M. AuthentiCT: A model of ancient DNA damage to estimate the proportion of present-day DNA contamination. *Genome Biol.* **2020**, *21*, 246. [CrossRef]

43. Sawyer, S.; Krause, J.; Guschanski, K.; Savolainen, V.; Pääbo, S. Temporal patterns of nucleotide misincorporations and DNA fragmentation in ancient DNA. *PLoS ONE* **2012**, *7*, e34131.

44. Rathbun, M.M.; McElhoe, J.A.; Parson, W.; Holland, M.M. Considering DNA damage when interpreting mtDNA heteroplasmy in deep sequencing data. *Forensic Sci. Int. Genet.* **2017**, *26*, 1–11. [CrossRef]

45. Holland, C.A.; McElhoe, J.A.; Gaston-Sanchez, S.; Holland, M.M. Damage patterns observed in mtDNA control region MPS data for a range of template concentrations and when using different amplification approaches. *Int. J. Leg. Med.* **2021**, *135*, 91–106. [CrossRef]

46. Hajdinjak, M.; Mafessoni, F.; Skov, L.; Vernot, B.; Hübner, A.; Fu, Q.; Essel, E.; Nagel, S.; Nickel, B.; Richter, J.; et al. Initial Upper Palaeolithic humans in Europe had recent Neanderthal ancestry. *Nature* **2021**, *592*, 253–257. [CrossRef]

47. Fu, Q.; Posth, C.; Hajdinjak, M.; Petr, M.; Mallick, S.; Fernandes, D.; Furtwängler, A.; Haak, W.; Meyer, M.; Mittnik, A.; et al. The genetic history of Ice Age Europe. *Nature* **2016**, *534*, 200–205. [CrossRef] [PubMed]

48. Marshall, C.; Taylor, R.; Sturk-Andreaggi, K.; Barritt-Ross, S.; Berg, G.E.; McMahon, T.P. Mitochondrial DNA haplogrouping to assist with the identification of unknown service members from the World War II Battle of Tarawa. *Forensic Sci. Int. Genet.* **2020**, *47*, 102291. [CrossRef] [PubMed]

49. Troll, C.J.; Kapp, J.; Rao, V.; Harkins, K.; Cole, C.; Naughton, C.; Morgan, J.M.; Shapiro, B.; Green, R.E. A ligation-based single-stranded library preparation method to analyze cell-free DNA and synthetic oligos. *BMC Genom.* **2019**, *2*, 1023. [CrossRef] [PubMed]

50. Wood, D.E.; Lu, J.; Langmead, B. Improved metagenomic analysis with Kraken 2. *Genome Biol.* **2019**, *20*, 257. [CrossRef]

51. Green, R.E.; Krause, J.; Briggs, A.W.; Maricic, T.; Stenzel, U.; Kircher, M.; Patterson, N.; Li, H.; Zhai, W.; Fritz, M.H.-Y.; et al. A draft sequence of the Neandertal genome. *Science* **2010**, *328*, 710–722. [CrossRef]

52. Meyer, M.; Fu, Q.; Aximu-Petri, A.; Glocke, I.; Nickel, B.; Arsuaga, J.L.; Martinez, I.; Gracia, A.; De Castro, J.M.B.; Carbonell, E.; et al. A mitochondrial genome sequence of a hominin from Sima de los Huesos. *Nature* **2014**, *505*, 403–406. [CrossRef]

53. Hajdinjak, M.; Fu, Q.; Hübner, A.; Petr, M.; Mafessoni, F.; Grote, S.; Skoglund, P.; Narasimham, V.; Rougier, H.; Crevecoeur, I.; et al. Reconstructing the genetic history of late Neanderthals. *Nature* **2018**, *555*, 652–656. [CrossRef]

54. Korlević, P.; Gerber, T.; Gansauge, M.-T.; Hajdinjak, M.; Nagel, S.; Aximu-Petri, A.; Meyer, M. Reducing microbial and human contamination in DNA extractions from ancient bones and teeth. *Biotechniques* **2015**, *59*, 87–93. [CrossRef]

MDPI

St. Alban-Anlage 66

4052 Basel

Switzerland

Tel. +41 61 683 77 34

Fax +41 61 302 89 18

www.mdpi.com

Genes Editorial Office

E-mail: genes@mdpi.com

www.mdpi.com/journal/genes

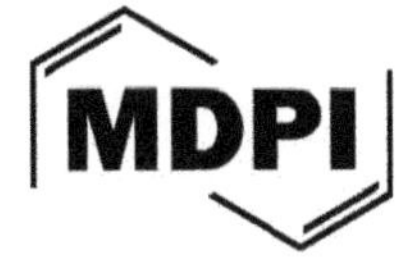